Ourselves, Grow

D1644739

Jean Shapiro is a writer and journalist. For more than twenty years she has been associated with *Good Housekeeping* magazine – for fifteen years as Editor of the family section (for which she wrote articles on education, health, careers, babies and children, disability, the old, the social services, etc.) and now as consultant on a freelance basis. A major part of her job is answering readers' problem letters; this has given her a valuable insight into the experiences and anxieties of 'real' people, and she has been able to make use of this in her several books written since the mid-seventies. *On Your Own: A Practical Guide to Independent Living* (Pandora) and *A Child: Your Choice* (Pandora) are the most recent. A member of an older women's group, she is particularly concerned with the health and welfare of middle-aged and elderly women. Married, with three adult children and five granddaughters, Jean Shapiro has been actively involved in the women's movement for many years.

Books by the Boston Women's Health Book Collective

Our Bodies, Ourselves
Ourselves, and Our Children
Our Jobs, Our Health
The New Our Bodies, Ourselves

Paula Brown Doress and Diana Laskin Siegal and
the Midlife and Older Women Book Project
in co-operation with the Boston Women's Health Book Collective

OURSELVES, GROWING OLDER

Women Ageing with Knowledge and Power

British edition by Jean Shapiro

Fontana/Collins

First published in the United States of America by
Simon and Schuster/Touchstone Books 1987

First published in Great Britain by Fontana Paperbacks 1989
8 Grafton Street, London W1X 3LA

Copyright © Paula Brown Doress and Diana Laskin Siegal 1987

Made and printed in Great Britain by
William Collins Sons & Co. Ltd, Glasgow

Dedication

To my mother, Ethel Brown. Like so many older women, she deserved a much better old age than she got. Despite the ravages of Parkinson's disease, she always enjoyed a good party, and, until her death at age eighty-two, never allowed pain or discomfort or difficult travel accommodations to keep her away from a celebration. It is a great personal sadness that her death came just after Diana and I signed the contract for this book and before our opening meeting/celebration. I regret that she was not able to participate, yet her spirit inspires me daily and has contributed immeasurably to the carrying of this project to its conclusion.

To my father, Abraham Brown. As one of the small but growing minority of caregiving husbands, he cared for my mother with unfailing devotion, risking his own health in doing so. Despite the many difficulties and strains of caregiving, he has never been too burdened to be supportive to his children's and grandchildren's projects. From my dad, I learned that if I keep putting one foot in front of the other I will eventually reach my goal.

To Allen Worters, my new husband, who read early drafts of chapters, made incisive comments, brought flowers at particularly stressful times, was generous when the project overran its advance, and believed me each time I said the book was very nearly done.

PAULA BROWN DORESS

To my parents, Ann and George Laskin, whose outlooks and styles, though very different from each other, combined to inspire me with the desire and the zeal to produce this book. My mother, always the idealist who believes that the world should be a better place for everyone, is the inspiration for the reformer in me. She exemplifies the strength of older women in the way she has continued to grow and rise to new challenges. She gave her full support to this project, including reading chapters, contributing experiences, and providing contacts and clippings. My father started his own business at midlife, demonstrating that one's earlier, seemingly unrelated work may be the necessary preparation for later accomplishment. His sense of humour and his attitude that 'of course' I can do anything I want is the reason I have done what I wanted to do.

To my older, loving, enthusiastic women friends (you know who you are) who kept me going with laughs, parties, meals, movies, and hugs.

To Dick, whose memory will always be with me.

DIANA LASKIN SIEGAL

We both thank Ann and George Laskin, who put up with The Invasion of the Book Project – its staff and its visitors. Ann frequently fed us, George repaired lamps, toaster ovens, and various other items. Together they provided a beautiful garden where we enjoyed our lunch and rested our weary eyes whenever we needed a break from the computer screen.

To our respective children and stepchildren, Naomi Siegal, John Siegal, Hannah Doress, Benjamin Doress, David Worters, and Susan Worters, with our support for the goals and paths they have chosen for their lives, and with our hope that in their older years they will see the results of our efforts.

PBD & DLS

Authors of the American edition listed according to the chapters in that edition:

The Potential of the Second Half of Life, Paula Brown Doress, Diana Laskin Siegal, with Caroline T. Chauncey, Robin H. Cohen, Marilyn Bentov, Lois Harris; *Aging and Well-Being*, Marilyn Bentov, Dori Smith, Diana Laskin Siegal, Paula Brown Doress, with Eve Nichols, Joleen Bachman, Ruth Hubbard, Jane Jewell, Faith Nobuko Barcus; *Massage*, Sylvia Pigors, Marilyn Bentov, Diana Laskin Siegal; *Habits Worth Changing*, Dori Smith, Diana Laskin Siegal, Paula Brown Doress; *Alcohol*, Sandra T. Bierig, Ruth L. Fishel; *Dealing with Pain*, Sylvia Pigors; *Who Needs Cosmetic Surgery? Reassessing Our Looks and Our Lives*, Jane Hyman; *Weighty Issues*, Jane Hyman, Diana Laskin Siegal, Elizabeth Volz, with Esther Rome, Robin H. Cohen, Mary P. Clarke; *Eating Well*, Elizabeth Volz, Diana Laskin Siegal, with Mary P. Clarke, Kathleen I. MacPherson; *Moving for Health*, Elizabeth DuBois, Marilyn Bentov, Diana Laskin Siegal, Dori Smith; *Sexuality in the Second Half of Life*, Aurelie Jones Goodwin, with Lynn Scott, Mary C. Allen, Sarah F. Pearlman, Wendy Sanford; *Birth Control for Women in Midlife*, Paula Brown Doress, Edie Butler, Trudy Cox, with Susan Bell, Judy Norsigian, Suzanne Ollivier; *Childbearing in Midlife*, Paula Brown Doress, Trudy Cox, Edie Butler, with Judy Norsigian, Barbara Katz-Rothman, Phyllis Greenleaf, Jane Pincus; *Menopause: Entering Our Third Age*, Diana Laskin Siegal, with Judy Costlow, Maria Cristina Lopez, Mara Taub (the Santa Fe Health Education Project), Fredi Kronenberg; *Relationships in Middle and Later Life*, Dorothy Frauenhofer, Lynn Scott, Paula Brown Doress, Kristine Rosenthal-Keese; *Mothers-in-law*, Jane Porcino; *Housing Alternatives and Living Arrangements*, Mickey Troub Friedman; *Shelter Poverty and the Housing Shortage*, Caroline T. Chauncey; *Adaptive Environments*, Elaine Ostroff; *Work and Retirement*, Edith Stein, Paula Brown Doress, Mary D. Fillmore, with Tish Sommers; *Money Matters: The Economics of Aging for Women*, Gillie Beram, Caroline T. Chauncey, with Marilyn Rogers, Naomi B. Isler; *Caregiving*, Louise Fradkin, Mirca Liberti; *Finances*, Naomi B. Isler, with Tish Sommers; *Problems in the Medical Care System*, Diana Laskin Siegal, with Norma Meras Swenson, Alice Quinlan; *Nursing Homes*, Susan Lanspery; *Joint and Muscle Pain, Arthritis and Rheumatic Disorders*, Robin H. Cohen, with Jeanne L. Melvin; *TMJ*, Martha Wood, Renée Glass; *Osteoporosis*, Kathleen I. MacPherson; *Dental Health*, Martha C. Wood; *Urinary Incontinence*, Norma Meras Swenson, Diana Laskin Siegal, with Grace Q. Vicary, Mary

D. Fillmore, Neil M. Resnick; *Hysterectomy and Oophorectomy*, Dorothy Krasnoff Reider, with Genevieve Carminati; *Hypertension, Heart Disease, and Stroke*, Ellen Dorsch; *Cancer*, Sharon Bray, Diana Laskin Siegal, with Norma Meras Swenson, Jane Jewell; *Breast Cancer*, Jane Hyman; *Colerectal Cancer*, Edith Lenneberg; *Diabetes*, Dorothea F. Sims; *Gallstones and Gallbladder Disease*, Glorianne Wittes; *Vision, Hearing, and Other Sensory Loss Associated with Aging, Vision Changes*, Ellen Barlow, Diana Laskin Siegal, Faire Edwards, Paula Brown Doress, with Penny Gay, Jane Bailey-Blood Strete; *Hearing Impairment in the Older Years*, Ellen Barlow, Paula Brown Doress, Diana Laskin Siegal, with Judith Chasin, Jessie Buck, Lois Harris; *Memory Lapse and Memory Loss*, Jane Hyman, with Guila Glosser; *Dying and Death*, Mary C. Howell, Mary C. Allen, Paula Brown Doress, with Jane Bailey-Blood Strete; *Changing Society and Ourselves*, Tish Sommers, with Laurie Shields, Fran Leonard.

Chapters rewritten for the British edition by Jean Shapiro:

Housing Alternatives and Living Arrangements; *Work and Retirement* (data from Jane MacKenzie, the Equal Opportunities Commission); *Money Matters: The Economics of Ageing for Women*; *Problems in the Medical Care System*; *Changing Society and Ourselves*. Additional material by Jean Shapiro: *Eating Well*; *Childbearing in Midlife*; *Relationships in Middle and Later Life*; *Caregiving*; *Residential and Nursing Homes*; *Osteoporosis*; *Dental Health*; *Urinary Incontinence*; *Hysterectomy and Oophorectomy*; *Cancer*; *Diabetes*; *Vision, Hearing, and Other Sensory Loss Associated with Ageing (Vision Changes, Hearing Impairment in the Older Years)*.

Contents

Photograph Acknowledgements

p. 11 Randy Dean/VNA of San Francisco's Adult Day Health Center; p. 15 Brenda
Prince/Format Photographers; p. 26 Norma Holt; p. 31 and p. 59 Brenda Prince; p. 66
Marianne Gontarz; p. 76 Mikki Ansin; p. 85 Brenda Prince; p. 90 Norma Holt; p. 105
Marianne Gontarz; p. 111 Brenda Prince; p. 112 Pam White; p. 118 The Dance
Exchange, Dancers of the Third Age/Dennis Deloria; p. 127 Candace Pratt/The Works
Athletic Club; p. 137 Marianne Gontarz; p. 174 Lyn Stirewalt; p. 189 Maggie Murray/
Format; p. 208 Brenda Prince; p. 215 Jerry Howard; p. 227 Brenda Prince; p. 235 John
Cogill; p. 242 Brenda Prince; p. 248 Cathy Cade; p. 250 Nicole Hollander (cartoon);
p. 252 and p. 263 Brenda Prince; p. 266 Marianne Gontarz; p. 268 Maggy Krebs
(cartoon); p. 271 Vicky White/Photo Co-op; p. 281 Marianne Gontarz; p. 287 Andes
Press Agency; p. 294 Camera Press; p. 308 Marianne Gontarz; p. 330 Pam White/
Arthritis and Health Resources; p. 342 Norma Holt; p. 413 Pam White; p. 517 Anne
Chapman Tremearne; p. 519 Ellen Shub; p. 533 Elizabeth Layton; p. 545 Marianne
Gontarz; p. 551 Sarah Putnam; p. 571 Raissa Page/Format.

All medical drawings, Audrey Besterman; lovemaking drawings pp. 152–153,
Roselaine Perkis; diagram p. 346 adapted from an illustration by Nancy Lou Makris in
Herta Spencer, 'Osteoporosis: Goals of Therapy'. *Hospital Practice*, Vol. 17, No. 3,
March 1982, p. 133.

Foreword
(Condensed from the Original Edition)

We are all ageing. The pioneers of the second wave of feminism are advancing into middle age or beyond. In fact, the whole postwar baby-boom generation is moving into midlife, which means that this will be an age group to reckon with in every sense.

Yet the specific concerns of older women are just coming to the fore. There were so many women's issues to be dealt with, and in the 1970s, women of the new wave of feminists were usually quite young. In the area of health, reproductive rights and childbirth issues understandably took precedence. While these remain important to all women because they deal so basically with control of our bodies, there are other concerns which can no longer be ignored.

This book examines the neglected health concerns of middle-aged and older women. The basic principle – that we must know our own bodies and ourselves in order to be free from mistaken notions, the legacy of the patriarchal culture in which we live – continues after reproductive functions have ended. We remain females to the end of our days, and our status as women affects us as long as we live.

Like its predecessor, *Our Bodies, Ourselves*, this book is a collaborative effort. Many women have participated in its writing, and it is based on common experience. It reveals the impact of ageism, compounded with sexism, on all of us. It opens up new ways to free ourselves of both of these, not only in our own minds but also in the society around us. Insights both from the older women's advocacy movement (in the US) and the women's health movement (there and in the UK) are encompassed within it. For older women it is a milestone.

Some of us who have been advocates for older women's issues for a long time are delighted to observe this spread of consciousness. The circle of concern is widening; there are now many approaches, not one; and there is greater organizational and personal interest in the problems of the growing-older female. This book should be a landmark in speeding up that process of consciousness-raising.

Taking control of our lives and of our bodies is the most basic feminist principle there is. This book moves us in that direction, for it breaks down that formidable barrier in our minds – the fear of growing old. It helps us to see that middle and old age are stages of life, as important as any other. Since we can't beat ageing, we had better learn how to join it. That is what this book is about, and I'm very glad to have been part of it.

TISH SOMMERS

Preface to the British Edition

As the co-ordinators of the North American edition of *Ourselves, Growing Older: Women Aging with Knowledge and Power*, it is our pleasure to send greetings to women in the United Kingdom, and to invite them to consider their middle and older years. The ageing revolution has been on our national agenda in the United States for some time; we are just beginning to recognize that the increase in longevity is worldwide. We are pleased that our book will be available to women in the United Kingdom.

Though the second wave of feminism has brought renewed awareness of sexism and a new vision of sisterhood to women in both our countries, it is only recently that the issues and concerns of older women have been raised in the US, within the women's movement itself, within the senior movement, and through new organizations such as the Older Women's League. Since its founding in 1981, OWL has grown to a national advocacy organization of over 25,000 members with local chapters and a national office in Washington, DC. Through working with members of OWL, and in collaboration with the Boston Women's Health Book Collective, our project symbolized a coming together of the older women's movement with the women's health movement.

In our country, there is a growing antagonism to the entitlements of older persons, based on the erroneous belief that elders are better off than formerly, and better off than the younger generations. The purposes of our book are to highlight the differences in ageing by gender, race, and class and to provide information about the neglected health concerns of middle-aged and older women so that we can take control of our bodies and our lives. We encourage women of all generations to work together on issues which affect older women now and in the future.

The US does not have a universal health system though proposals are again under discussion. We applaud the vision of the British people for establishing a system which serves everyone, and want to warn against cutting it and going back to separate systems for the rich and the poor. From US experience we can state that it is very hard to restore programmes once they have been cut.

We congratulate Jean Shapiro for her pioneering effort and splendid work on this adaptation, and for being at seventy-two, a role model of the kind of older woman the two of us in our fifties aspire to be in our seventies. We understand that a few older women, individually and in organizations such as the Older Feminists' Network, have begun to identify the special concerns of older women in the UK. We extend to women in the UK our best wishes for success in mobilizing support for the issues of middle-aged and older women, and hope that this book will be an important resource in building a united women's movement that encompasses the concerns of women of all ages.

PAULA BROWN DORESS & DIANA LASKIN SIEGAL

Notes on the British Edition

When the Boston Women's Health Book Collective completed work on *The New Our Bodies, Ourselves*, several members of the group felt that the 'Women Growing Older' chapter was an important statement of issues which needed further development and elaboration. The present book grew out of that realization. Paula Brown Doress and Diana Laskin Siegal formed the Midlife and Older Women Book Project, which undertook gathering the huge amount of material necessary to present to older women the medical, social and political issues that directly affect all of us in our later years. They had the help of literally hundreds of women, many of whose experiences are incorporated in *Ourselves, Growing Older* and whose words add so much to the impact of the book. They also had the help of the members of the Boston Women's Health Book Collective as consultants.

Of course many of the health concerns of older women are common to women of all ages, and these are addressed in *The New Our Bodies, Ourselves*, a British edition of which, edited by Angela Phillips and Jill Rakusen, is published by Penguin (1989). But there are many other questions, such as the particular difficulties encountered in a society which neglects the housing, employment, financial, and community care needs of older women, and which affect the health of older women. These vital topics are addressed here, and from a British as well as an American perspective.

A work like this encourages confidence and creativity and the acceptance of self-worth at any age. It should help women release the internal brakes we have applied so long, and help us take off in any direction we would like to go. The idea is to enjoy life in later years, to make the most of this most precious season of our lives. This health and living handbook will also increase women's ability to stay well, thereby expanding the growing force of active middle-aged and older women. The way has been shown by the growing influence of the Older

Women's League and other organizations in the US, to make things easier for the next generation coming along. Women in the UK can learn a great deal from the experience of their American sisters. For older women *can* change the circumstances of ageing for all women, and men as well.

Such efforts expand the concept of sisterhood across generations, with women in midlife providing a crucial bridge. Together we can build a new road to ageing, and at the same time that road will be building us. Young women have as great a stake in our efforts as older women do, for their turn is coming.

When we finally bridge the generation gap, women will be a magnificent force for positive change in society. For we are the compassion experts – we've been socialized in that direction. Humanizing the social fabric is our special domain. We're the nurturers and informal healers, even though professionals of both sexes have medicalized the process, leaving only the unpaid part to us.

At present we're caught within the confines of a health care system which is not only distorted in its priorities but is increasingly under attack by the very government that should be safeguarding its future. Privatization and chronic under-funding threaten the whole basis of the National Health Service and, as always, it is women, the poor and defenceless who are suffering. But given a long view, and our involvement, that, too, can be changed. Knowledge is the first step. The second is taking more control over whatever aspects of our own health that we can. From dependence on 'experts' we must move towards greater interdependence, which means taking more responsibilities for our own bodies, as well as for the policies which affect us.

We do believe that women will take the lead in remodelling the health care system of the future, and those of us in midlife or older will play an important part in the defence of all that is good in the National Health Service, and its eventual transformation. Why? Not only because we are the compassion experts – but also because we have the least to lose and the most to gain by that defence and transformation. Women of all ages, by changing their own health habits and affecting others around them, by speaking up and then becoming involved with all aspects of the health service will, we predict, have far greater influence than we can now imagine in redesigning the whole system. But first we must start with ourselves. Then we should move on to try to understand the influences that are at work, the interests that bolster the drive for 'economy' and the power of those forces that put profit before people. Then we will be able to create a health service worthy of the name.

This book was edited at a time when almost daily changes in the government's response to crises in the social services, the NHS and education were being published. The vast majority of these changes have been perceived by consumers and professionals alike as attacks on the freedom and welfare of the ordinary citizen. Because of the ever-changing scene, it has not been possible to incorporate here everything that has occurred since mid-1989 – such important documents as the government's response to the Griffiths Report on Community Care, for instance, arrived too late for us to summarize it in the following pages. For up-to-date information, readers are asked to refer to the relevant statutory services and our address lists at the end of the book.

In editing this book I have attempted to follow as far as possible not only the content but the format of the original. Obviously some chapters have had to be totally rewritten in order to meet British conditions; others have needed only minor modifications of the American text. Footnotes have been largely retained (see end of each chapter for numbered notes); thus most of the references are to material published in the US, although the bulk of the journals and research reports mentioned are available in academic libraries here. To counterbalance this American orientation, after each chapter there is a list of British books and publications for the general reader, most of which are easily obtained in bookshops and public libraries.

The New Our Bodies, Ourselves presents the claims of 'alternative' health practitioners in some detail. In this book, reference is made to alternative medicine wherever this option seems appropriate. Readers who want to study what 'non-medical' medicine has to offer are referred to *The Handbook of Complementary Medicine*, edited by Stephen Fulder (Oxford), which presents a detailed picture, written by the practitioners themselves, of what each alternative therapy does for a patient. It also includes a comprehensive directory of about 250 organizations.

Some of these groups are included in the directory of women's, health, and other organizations to be found at the end of this book. Many of these are referred to by title in the text, and so can be easily identified. Others have titles incorporating their purpose or special interest – for example, the name of an illness or disability, the age-group they represent and so on – and are listed alphabetically accordingly. A reader finding difficulty in identifying a particular group should look under 'Association of . . .'; 'National Association of . . .'; 'British Association of . . .'; 'Society of . . .'; 'Standing Conference on . . .', etc. Addresses and telephone numbers were correct as this book went to press. If an organization has moved in the meantime, a forwarding address or telephone number will normally have been arranged.

JEAN SHAPIRO

Acknowledgements

I am very grateful to the British women whose ideas and experiences are quoted along with those of the Americans who contributed to the original edition.

Many thanks, too, to the following for their valuable information and advice:

Age Concern; Toni Bellfield (Family Planning Association); The Commission for Racial Equality; Zelda Curtis and the Older Women's Project, Pensioners' Link; The Fawcett Library; The Health Education Authority; Jan McHarry and Friends of the Earth; Jane MacKenzie and the Equal Opportunities Commission; Kathy Meade; Rose Shapiro; Shelter; The Women's Health and Reproductive Rights Information Centre.

My personal thanks to my family, and particularly to Monte, whose practical help, encouragement (and tolerance of the paperwork that invaded our living space for several months) made editing this book so much pleasanter. My North London older women's group's positive reactions to what I was doing kept up my morale – I thank them. My gratitude, too, to JoAnne Robertson, for being such an approachable and compatible editor, and Rebecca Armstrong for so conscientiously checking through the 'Books and Publications'.

JS

The Potential of the Second Half of Life

This book grows out of our conviction that the decades after forty can be rich and fulfilling, a time when we as women can come into our own. One in eight British people is now over sixty-five. Older women are survivors, living an average of six years longer than men, enjoying longer life spans than we might as young women have expected to or planned for. Life expectancy for women is just under seventy-eight years; those already over sixty-five can expect to live well into their eighties. We can and do use our added years in ways that please us – learning new skills, travelling, and living out long-delayed dreams. Yet, as survivors, women are also likely to face more of the challenges of ageing: chronic health conditions; inadequate income; caregiving responsibilities; lack of care when we need it;* and perhaps most devastating of all, the deaths of family members and friends. In this book, we have tried to give equal attention to both the promise and the challenge of the later years.

Why a Book About Both Middle-aged and Older Women?

The economic problems of older women grow out of women's early experience of sex discrimination in the workplace and the prejudicial belief that women do not need to earn enough money to support themselves. The two poorest groups in the UK today are women raising children alone and women over sixty-five living alone. Whether we have been poor all our lives or have experienced downward mobility in our middle or later years, many of us find that we do not have adequate financial resources for the second half of our lives. A feminist analysis is an important tool to help us become aware of the ways that we women are programmed from our earliest years toward financial and emotional dependency. At midlife, we can begin to make changes in order to avoid the isolation, poverty, and ill health that mar the later years of so many older women.

*We cannot rely on family ties for care. By the age at which most women need care the majority of those who had married are widowed; many others have never married; and 25 per cent of women over seventy have no living children.

In the role of traditional caregivers, women at midlife are in closer contact than any other group, except for the ageing themselves, with the problems that arise when public policy fails to meet needs such as old people's housing, long-term care, and in-home care. When such needs go unmet by public services, it is middle-aged women who are expected to give their unpaid labour to provide the services required. Frequently, our personal aspirations and careers suffer when we do so. Also, our future security suffers if we fail to earn pension credits in those crucial middle years. Policies that require women to care for the elderly for free at home are short-sighted. Such policies sow the seeds for another generation of impoverished older women. We must demand the resources for respite care, long-term care, and housing and support services that will provide alternatives to the limited choices of unsupported independent living versus a nursing home.

Many of us become so habituated to caring for others and helping others achieve that we lose sight of our own goals or never get around to formulating any. In the second half of life, many of us have an opportunity to pay attention to ourselves and our own needs and aspirations, perhaps for the first time. The added years we gain with increased longevity can be ours to grow spiritually and intellectually. Midlife is often spoken of by women in metaphors of birth and rebirth, a time to nurture our own talents, casting off the external criteria by which we may have devalued ourselves and blossoming in new ways.

If we think of our future years as providing an opportunity to develop our creativity, our passions, and our activism, we can look forward to our older years with confidence and enthusiasm.

Ageing and Ageism

Whole Woman of the ^ Year

Have you ever known a woman named 'November'?
Neither have I.
Now 'May' and 'June' and 'April' have their namesakes –
Ever ask why?

We rarely picture woman as autumnal;
Female is spring.
Please, someone, name a newborn girl 'October'
And hear her sing

Of harvest cut and growth complete and fruit mature,
Not just of birth.
Oh, let a woman age as seasons do;
Love each time's worth!

MIRIAM CORCORAN

Ageism – the belief that a person's worth and abilities are determined solely by chronological age – is the enemy that threatens the creative, growing future we envision for ourselves. Research shows that intellectual capacity remains stable throughout life – the ability to learn new things continues unabated and, when actively exercised, enhances our well-being.[1] Yet ageism declares us obsolete at a socially defined deadline. At age sixty we find ourselves defined as 'Senior Citizens' or OAPs, forced to retire whether we like it or not.

In a youth-oriented society, both middle-aged and older women struggle with ageism. Because of the double standard, women are labelled 'old' at an earlier age than men are.[2] The sexist beliefs that relegate women to child rearing and domestic work exclusively seem to mark us as obsolete when children leave home and our childbearing potential is at an end. Such archaic beliefs are irrelevant to most contemporary women, yet we continue to suffer the discrimination which is their legacy, especially when we enter or re-enter the work force or change jobs in our middle years.

We live in a society that values the quick fix and the slick package. As one woman put it, 'I'm a lot more interesting than I was at twenty-five or thirty-five, but it's a lot harder to get anyone to pay attention.' We can fight such attitudes by actively reaching out and valuing one another. At a social or community gathering, if you seek out one of the oldest women and get acquainted with her, you will be amply rewarded.

I went to a women's get-together where most of the women ranged from the mid-thirties to the mid-fifties. I was curious about one much older woman who turned out to be a sculptor in her seventies. She invited me to visit her at her studio. I drove down with a photographer friend, bringing a picnic lunch, and enjoyed a delightful afternoon viewing her recent work, each of us sharing her experiences as a woman trying to do creative work at different times in the life cycle. [a forty-four-year-old woman]

At a wedding where I did not know many people I noticed an older woman in her seventies who seemed to have a visual disability. No one was speaking with her, so I struck up a conversation. I found out she was a founding member of a self-help organization for people with low vision and did counselling on the telephone from her home for others with low vision. It was fun to meet and talk with such a gutsy lady. [a forty-eight-year-old woman]

Unity and Difference Among Women

When you read the experiences of the women quoted in this book, do not automatically picture a white, middle-class, heterosexual, able-bodied woman. We reached out to and heard from a great variety of women – white women, black and Asian women, middle-aged and old women, heterosexual and lesbian and bisexual women, able-bodied women and women with disabilities. Because the book is primarily about ageing, we identified the speaker by age alone unless another characteristic was significant to her story and not apparent in what she said.

SEXUAL PREFERENCE

At least 10 per cent of women, perhaps more, are lesbian. It is sad that homophobia, the irrational fear and hatred of homosexuality and bisexuality, is still so prevalent that many lesbian women are reluctant to acknowledge openly their preference. Many women who have found a way to survive and thrive in a woman-centred community still hide this important part of themselves from their heterosexual friends and colleagues.

In gathering personal experiences for this book, we found that the lesbians (mostly middle-aged) who are part of an organization or network with other lesbians welcomed an opportunity to discuss the satisfactions of living a woman-centred way of life. We were less successful in reaching the oldest and most isolated lesbians who grew up and lived in even more repressive circumstances. Their fear of exposure and learned discomfort with openness has rendered them understandably reluctant to share their experiences and even keeps them isolated from all but a few of their lesbian sisters. This is a loss to all of us who could learn from their life experiences as women surviving on their own.

We must unite as women to fight against the ageism, sexism, racism, homophobia, and discrimination against persons with disabilities that blight all our lives, especially in our later years. Our unity will be more powerful and effective if we can honour our differences and work toward inclusiveness of all groups. Each of us, whether heterosexual, lesbian, or bisexual, can examine our own attitudes and practices. We may be able in our own social circles to build a climate of inclusiveness and openness that will make every woman feel accepted and affirmed for who she is.

AGEING AND DISABILITY

It is a mistake to equate disability with a particular age. Some women have lived with severe limitations from birth or an early age, while others become disabled later in life as a result of an accident or disease. Even the longest-lived women may remain free of limiting disabilities, but a number of women must learn to manage a disability in the middle and later years. If that happens to us, we may have to learn about adapting our living space, demanding access to buildings, and a whole host of other situations we may never have had to deal with before. In that situation, there is much we can learn from other women with disabilities and from the disabled people's movement. Yet groups representing older people rarely communicated with those representing the disabled, at least until an American conference on ageing and disability in 1986.[3] We hope this communication will be the beginning of a dialogue about ageing and disability.

In the past, when it was more common for people to die at earlier ages, many people feared that premature death would close off the chance of accomplishing their life's goals. But today, many people fear pain, illness, and dependency more than death – a fear of 'dying socially' before biological death occurs – or they fear 'living too long'.[4] Much of the fear of ageing and the ageism that results is our own fear of disability. If we can work for a society in which disability does not mean social death, we can make it a better society in which to grow old.

Health and Ageing

Experts on ageing have described a phenomenon they have tagged with the unlikely name of 'youth creep'. As life expectancy lengthens, people stay youthful longer. Thus, those over seventy-five used to be called 'old-old', but now this term refers to those over eighty-five, as the group from seventy-five to eighty-four stays healthier and lives more independently than before. Some use the term old-old to refer only to those who are ill or disabled, while those who are in good health and independent even in their eighties and nineties are counted as young-old.

Most of the health and medical problems we face in our later years are chronic rather than acute, and require innovative approaches to people's needs for personal support, caregiving, and housing. However, the National Health Service tends to be geared to medical intervention for acute medical problems, and is frequently at a loss in responding to the chronic conditions more common in our later years. Ageing is part of the life span and should not be turned into a medical event. We can help ourselves and one another in maintaining our good health, and in other situations in which we have been taught to turn to professionals for answers.

Women and Policy for the Elderly

Women make up the majority of the over-sixty-five population, and outnumber men in the over-eighty population by two to one. Therefore, the needs of older women should be central to public policy for the elderly. More women than men have to claim income support and other benefits to bring their standard of living up to the 'poverty line'. Women outlive men an average of six years, so nearly all once-married women experience widowhood for some part of their later years. Eighty-five per cent of surviving spouses are women.[5] Once widowed, we are much less likely than men to remarry. Men over age sixty-five are seven times more likely to begin a new marriage – and they usually marry younger women.[6] Although most older men are married, most older women are not. And older women living alone are more likely to be poor than those living with a partner or others. Women from 'ethnic minorities' in the UK can expect to earn less than the average 74.8 per cent of men's wages, and Pakistani and Bengali women's employment rate is exceptionally low, so that their incomes in later years are even lower than those of the general population. It is important to bear these facts in mind when we're told that pensioners today are more affluent than ever before. Most single older women must have strong community ties and substantial family support just to maintain an adequate standard of living.

The growth in numbers of older women gives us greater political clout. We have a lot to contribute to society and to ourselves. We know what the world felt like before the nuclear bomb made apocalypse a grim possibility. We won the vote, worked to feed families in the Depression, ran factories when men went off to war, raised children who in adulthood brought fresh winds of change to our society, and learned to confront racism and sexism. Now we are learning to confront ageism.

The supports we build for ourselves through organizing, community building, networking, and political activity can help change negative stereotypes of age, of women, of the powerless – and those we have of ourselves. Our friendships with women can be lifelong relationships as important as family, often outlasting family ties. Being open to meeting new people and building on old and new friendships are important ways to counter the isolation that can occur as we sustain losses in our later years.

National and local organizations, pensioners' associations and network groupings such as the Older Feminists' Network and the Older Lesbian Network are beginning to make the voices of older women heard. We have a long way to go before we can compare our level of organization with that of the American Older Women's League and the Gray Panthers – but in a variety of local actions such as those undertaken by groups of older women co-ordinated by London's Pensioners' Link we are beginning to learn to use our experience and sense our power for change.

NOTES

[1] K. Warner Schaie and Sherry Willis, 'Can Decline in Adult Intellectual Functioning Be Reversed?' *Developmental Psychology*, Vol. 22, No. 2, 1986, pp. 223–32.

[2] Susan Sontag, 'The Double Standard of Aging'. *Saturday Review*, Vol. 95, No. 39, 23 September 1972.

[3] Irving Kenneth Zola, 'Policies and Programs Concerning Age and Disability: Towards a Unified Agenda'. In Sean Sullivan and Marion Ein Lewin, eds., *The Economics and Ethics of Long-Term Care and Disability*. Washington, DC: American Enterprise Institute, 1988, pp. 90–130.

[4] Matilda White Riley and John W. Riley, Jr, 'Longevity and Social Structure: The Added Years'. *Daedalus: Journal of the American Academy of Arts and Sciences*, Winter 1986, pp. 51–75.

[5] Coalition of Women on the Budget, 'Inequality of Sacrifice: The Impact of the Reagan Budget on Women', March 1984. Distributed by National Women's Law Center, 1616 P St, N.W., Washington, DC 20036.

[6] *Older Women: The Economics of Aging*, Women's Studies Program and Policy Center at George Washington University, 1980.

BOOKS AND PUBLICATIONS

The Women's Health and Reproductive Rights Information Centre publishes a variety of broadsheets and leaflets on women's health. Broadsheets discuss aspects of women's health from a feminist, social and political viewpoint. The leaflets describe a problem or situation and give practical solutions.

Subjects include information on a range of topics, including general health, disability, food, poverty and unemployment, and a useful rundown on Well Woman Services nationwide. Menopause, hysterectomy, contraception and cancer are among other subjects covered – the leaflets on cancer being produced in Bengali, Gujerati, Hindi, Punjabi and Urdu as well as English.

For a list of publications, with prices, and an order form, send a stamped addressed envelope to WHRRIC, 52 Featherstone Street, London EC1Y 8RT.

1
Ageing and Well-being

At My Age

Last summer our vegetable garden yielded small
bounty: round pink tennis ball tomatoes ripening
among the marigolds in an inferno of sun, captives
of ninety degree days, of unwavering heat, fitful
squalls of rain that released, not a drenching cool,
but drops of water that glanced off tight shiny skins
the way globules hiss from a sizzling fry pan.

One day I looked into the patch and there was one
tomato seamed and split, a deeper fruitier juicier
red inside, but with a frayed and largely open look.

I wanted to cup it into my hands and not lose a drop.

DORIS PANOFF

A Plan for Ageing Well

Many of us want to live long lives, but fear the infirmities or disabilities that
may come with advancing age. In this chapter we will emphasize that ageing
well is more than the absence of disease. It is a harmony of mind, body, and
spirit. Each of us can take an active role in our well-being as we age – a holistic
approach that involves sharing with others, reducing stress, and participating
in community life.

*I have so many things I want to do, and I have to be well to do them. I don't want to
live to be eighty or ninety unless I am well enough to be active. I don't want quantity
of life without quality.* [a fifty-seven-year-old woman]

*Whether I am healthy because I can be busy and happy or whether I am busy and
happy because I am healthy is a question. I can do many things that I never had time*

to do before. Among my activities, I play the recorder in two groups, make ceramics, take part in a book group, go to concerts, plays and lectures, garden with the help of a young man, and volunteer at a pensioners' club. For the good of my somewhat achy leg, I swim three or four times a week, take a yoga class, and sometimes cycle. Life gets somewhat hectic but there's nothing I want to stop because I really enjoy the things I do very much. [a seventy-four-year-old woman]

At any age, we may have disease or disability to contend with, but we can still be as healthy and active as possible.

I am multiply disabled – legally blind, with chronic pain from head and neck injuries. Instead of drugs (I was using narcotics), much of my pain can be relieved by physiotherapy. Every day, in addition to aerobics, I do forty-five minutes or so of muscle stretching and isometrics, push-ups, sit-ups, etc. I am taught by my physiotherapist that these changes I am making in my life-style must be permanent, daily, lifelong. [a forty-one-year-old woman]

The self-care necessary to be well begins with self-value. *Deciding* on wellness reflects and fosters that self-value. We can prolong our healthy, active years by paying attention to good nutrition, activity and movement, solitude and rest, good relationships, and our links to the communities in which we live and work.

I'd been depressed and anxious and using sleeping pills for a number of years. With the help of a friend who was a therapist, I became aware of a lot of anger I'd been holding toward my mother and father – and toward my husband. I started adopting some new habits – like taking care of myself physically. I was in bad shape – I started jogging and I took yoga to learn to relax. Feeling better physically bolstered my self-esteem and gave me the courage to confront my husband about the inequities in our relationship and to push for changes. [a woman in her fifties]

Studies show that older people who give themselves a better health rating than their doctor does frequently prove, in time, the greater accuracy of their own intuitive feelings about the state of their health.[1]

The best way I know to stay healthy and alive is to stay away from pills and keep active. [a ninety-year-old woman]

To keep involved and growing, we must recognize and fight ageism in all of its manifestations. We can deal with ageism more effectively if we have energy and strength.

Ageing is Not Old Age

There is a difference between 'ageing' and 'getting old'. 'Ageing' encompasses all the biological changes that occur over a lifetime – for example, increase and decrease in height, onset and cessation of menstruation, and shaping of the young-adult and middle-aged body. Changes in thymic hormones are sometimes used as a sign of the ageing process because the thymus gland, a pyramid-shaped gland beneath the breastbone involved in regulation of the immune system, begins to shrink slowly after the age of two.[2] The pace of biological ageing differs among individuals. In all people, some organs age faster than others. The impact of genetic and environmental factors on biological ageing is just beginning to be understood.

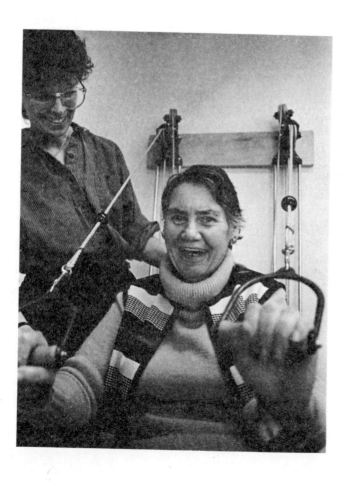

'Getting old', on the other hand, is a social concept, and our feelings about it may only be slightly related to the biological processes of 'ageing'.

It is not surprising that women have such feelings about being identified as ageing; our culture has a strong prejudice against older women. Traditional cultures often hold their elders in high regard, seeing them as storehouses of wisdom to be transmitted to the next generation; older women, especially, are often seen as healers. The Pueblo Indians, for example, believe their elders' rituals help the sun to rise each morning. Imagine how it would feel to believe oneself so vital to life itself!

For as long as I can remember, I've cherished an image of my future self as a 'wise old woman'. I can see myself now – my silver hair provides softness around my face. I live in a cottage by a stream, and my fireplace walls are decorated with well-used iron skillets and copper pots. I'm preparing to receive young guests who come regularly to visit me. I find my fulfilment in teaching them the wisdom gained over my lifetime. This image has sustained me through many dark hours in which I feared I would never make a contribution to life. [a forty-three-year-old woman]

It is especially important to distinguish physiological ageing from the capacity for intellectual growth and social participation. Even very ill or frail old people can continue to learn and to be socially involved. If ageing well is our goal, it is important to view health as the World Health Organization defined it in 1946: 'A state of complete physical, mental, and social well-being, not just the absence of disease or infirmity.'[3] Continued engagement and productivity is the best way of delaying the onset of frailty in the older years. Robert Butler argues that 'health and productivity are interacting conditions: the unproductive human is at higher risk of illness and economic dependency and the sick person is limited in productivity and is, therefore, at higher risk of dependency.'[4]

Scientists have learned a great deal about senescence, the biological changes that occur in different cells and tissues over time, but they still have fundamental questions about how and why these changes come about. Some think that ageing is controlled by a genetically programmed 'biological clock', but others think that ageing results from cumulative damage to certain systems in the body. It may be many years before we know which theory or combination of theories explains biological ageing.

Research is currently exploring factors that seem associated with longevity, in the hope of finding a formula for extending human life expectancy or minimizing conditions associated with ageing. We must be careful to differentiate between test results in the laboratory and what happens in our own bodies. For example, rats and mice placed on a diet containing 30 to 50 per cent fewer calories than the normal diet for caged laboratory rodents but containing essential vitamins and minerals live longer than control animals.[5] But studies of the relationship between longevity and weight in humans have produced conflicting results.[6]

Commercial manufacturers sometimes take advantage of highly publicized laboratory results to promote products that have no proven value. Superoxide dismutase (SOD) is found in animals with long life spans. Advertisements may tout SOD as an anti-ageing drug, but in fact, SOD is broken down during digestion and cannot be reassembled in the body.[7] Thus, such diet supplements have no effect on human longevity and are a waste of money.

Laboratory studies of the effects of vitamin and mineral supplements on the ageing process also must be evaluated carefully. The possible anti-cancer action of vitamins A and C and the anti-ageing actions of the mineral selenium deserve further investigation, but the evidence available does not support the contention that these supplements either prevent cancer or extend life.[8]

It is unlikely that researchers will find a single intervention to stop ageing. Indeed, any promise of extraordinary benefit probably indicates something of which the buyer should beware. In the future, scientific advances in many areas may delay specific ageing processes, such as the decline in immune function, but, until then, we should be cautious about claims for the life-extending or rejuvenating properties of any anti-ageing agents or regimes.[9]

The term 'life expectancy' refers to the average number of years of life expected for an individual in a given population. 'Life span' is the maximum number of years of life possible for a species. Researchers involved in efforts to increase understanding of the ageing process have found ways to increase both the life expectancies and the life spans of experimental animals.[10]

The average life expectancy in developed countries has increased steadily during the past two hundred years as a result of improvements in housing, nutrition, health care, and sanitation. In England and Wales, the average life expectancy at birth is 77.8 years for a girl; for a boy it is 71.8 years (1983–5 figures). More people are living to an old age than in past centuries, but the human life span has remained fixed at about 115 years for all of recorded history.

Although the prospect that the life span might be increased is exciting, we believe that the present focus of ageing research should be to improve the quality of life for all members of society. One of the ways to do this is by perfecting techniques for the prevention and treatment of disease (including illnesses previously thought to be unavoidable signs of ageing) and by changing the view that old age involves declining function.

Women and Research

The major problem with most clinical studies on ageing is that until recently very few of them have involved women. For example, the Baltimore Longitudinal Study of Ageing, which began in 1958, did not admit women volunteers until 1978. This omission was due to the traditional tendency to view males as the norm for the species. Processes that occur only in women have generally attracted less interest than male-related processes. In addition, studies focusing on one gender are less expensive, recruitment of subjects is easier, and data analysis is less complex.

Researchers have now begun to recognize that comparisons of women and men can contribute significantly to knowledge about age-related diseases and the ageing process in general. For example, premenopausal women are less prone to cardiovascular disease than men. A better understanding of the reasons for this difference and of the changes that occur after menopause could lead to new preventive and therapeutic measures for both women and men. Similarly, studies comparing bone loss in men and women could lead to new ways to maintain our muscles, bones, and tendons over time and to prevent fractures from osteoporosis.

Health statistics indicate that life expectancy at birth is greater for women than for men in most parts of the world, but that the length of time varies significantly depending on the country. For example, both women and men live longer in Sweden than they do in the United States, but the longevity gap between the genders is much smaller in Sweden. Research designed to help us understand the reasons for these differences could help improve the quality of life for all people.

Changing Health Habits

Science is developing information about the ageing process which strongly suggests that our health choices – positive or negative – greatly affect how we age. Growing old well – maintaining, even improving, physical and emotional health – is something over which today's women in midlife and beyond have more control than ever before.

There are no magic wands or potions for good health, no fountains of youth, no products that cure all ills, no vitamins that prevent all ailments. A wellness programme requires effort, planning, and persistence, but it is an investment that pays unbelievably high interest. When we feel good we are more likely to exercise, eat well, and take care of ourselves, all of which in turn are likely to make us feel better. Thus we create a 'virtuous cycle'.

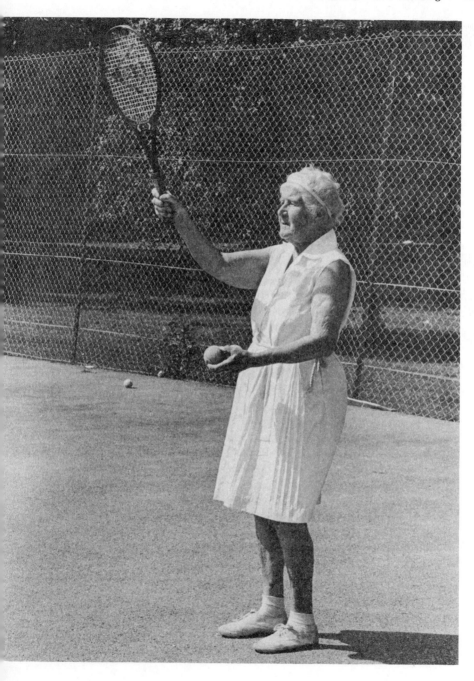

Habits are like the 'backbones' of our lives – the firm structures upon which we can rely. It helps not to have to think about every step we take – to have comfortable routines in our lives. But as we grow older, some habits may no longer serve us well. The morning mad rush routine that helped us get ourselves and a whole family off to school and work may no longer be necessary. We may be happier and calmer with fifteen minutes of quiet meditation before starting our day. Illness may require us to change from a vigorous exercise programme to a more gentle one. Or we may be inspired by new information or changes in our lives to pay better attention to ourselves, to pursue renewed health and vitality by dramatically altering our pattern of health habits.

It is not true that as we grow older, we become less flexible, less able to change. Change and renewal are possible at any age.

As I've got older, my idea of time has changed. I used to be rather proud of myself for keeping up with younger people. But recently I've realized that I don't have to rock-climb or undertake half-marathons. The fact that stopping these activities means that I'm slowing down doesn't worry me. I just know that I'm lucky to have been able to keep so very fit for so long, although I'm still only fifty-five, and long walks at weekends are enough to keep me well and active without competing with younger people.

A 'clean slate' approach may be your style of change, and can be very helpful when you're ready.

I got in the habit, over a number of years, of 'needing' a variety of legal drugs: tea, six to eight cups a day, to keep my spirits up; alcohol before bedtime to calm me down; a couple of aspirin to make sure I didn't wake up with a headache; then in the morning I really needed that tea to get going. Eventually, I was exhausted all the time and prone to illnesses. My doctor suggested that all these bad habits supported each other, and she was right. I was able to stop after some good introspection about getting my real needs met. I went on a one-week 'cleansing fast'* of fruit juices and spring water. I rested, walked and watched clouds. Two months later, I had dropped all my unhealthy habits and I began to know what my own energy feels like – and I like it! It feels great to depend on myself, not on all those stimulants and depressants. [a forty-two-year-old woman]

A gradual approach may be more successful for many of us. You may want to

---

*Some holistic health practitioners believe that fasting – going without food and taking only water and juices for a very brief time – is helpful in making the transition to a natural diet. Get guidance from a health practitioner, especially if you are older or have physical problems.

begin with a single change. Identify the roots of the problem. Ask yourself these questions: When did I first establish the habit? What need did it serve then? Does it now? Can other habits provide more satisfaction? Become aware of your *real* needs – for example, when you reach for a cigarette or coffee, you may be looking for a relaxing break or sociability. Fulfil them directly and in healthier ways.

Make changes in small, manageable steps. Many habits interact, so changing one may help you change others that are harder to break. For example, if you are trying to stop smoking, drink milk, fruit or vegetable juice, or herbal tea instead of coffee to break the coffee-and-cigarette association.

No matter which approach to change you choose, take on a habit when you feel strong and have no other major issues pressing on you. But watch out for procrastination. When you feel overwhelmed, phone a friend, change environments if possible, or change your activity. Get support from others to help you change. Form a partnership with a friend to support each other's new habits.

I spent a holiday at a lake with an old friend swimming, canoeing, and eating the macrobiotic style of food combinations and preparation which she has studied. I knew I didn't want to change my meals so drastically but enjoyed sampling her cooking. I also realized I felt better with more activity. A year later I am still following the changes I made. I am walking more, eating more whole grains and less fat in my meals than before. [a fifty-four-year-old woman]

For those who can afford it – and most of us can't – a week or more at a health farm can help to re-educate us and change our life-styles. However, it *is* possible, though not so easy, to 'do-it-yourself' through reading books such as this and those listed at the end of the section. If you can do this with a friend or a group, you'll be able to support each other.[11]

ENJOYING LIFE WITH LESS ENERGY

BY PAULA BROWN DORESS, LOIS HARRIS, JANE HYMAN, AND DORI SMITH. SPECIAL THANKS TO LUCY MITCHELL, BETH ROSENBAUM, AND ELSIE REETHOF.

Finding ourselves with physical limitations can bring frustration, sadness, and a strong sense of loss. We miss the things we are no longer able to do.

If you have anything wrong with you it makes all the difference in the world. Six years ago I was trying out lots of new things and the world was more or less my oyster. I had fun with music, I had fun with painting, and I was having fun with poetry. Anything seemed possible to me. Then I got rheumatoid arthritis, and I got it badly. I had three major operations in five months, and two new shoulders and one new knee. And at age seventy-three, three major operations take a lot of getting over. I still have the disease and feel lousy a great deal of the time. I don't quite feel that the world is my oyster anymore. [a seventy-nine-year-old woman]

We resent health problems when they are painful, make us feel weak and tired, and restrict our movements and our lives. We get angry with our bodies because we want to do everything the way we used to and we can't.

When joints ache, I calculate each step. I don't automatically get up and get a drink of water, or to put something away . . . I wait and take these steps in conjunction with some other necessary steps. I don't do things on the spur of the moment anymore. . . . Will our eyesight grow worse? Will we become increasingly hard of hearing? Will the arthritis be harder to control? and so on. . . . It makes no sense to let our thoughts wander in this direction, but inevitably they do. [a woman in her late eighties][1]

Usually, the first change we make is to reorganize our environment as much as possible to accommodate our conditions. Basically, this means keeping all regularly used objects in the same place and within easy reach, and finding new ways to accomplish daily chores.

I always put my glasses and keys on a very attractive plate that I keep in the centre of my apartment so I'm not always hunting for them. This is a way I conserve my energy. [an eighty-two-year-old woman]

Learn about ways you can adapt your environment to make the most of your abilities and reduce the impact of physical changes (see pp. 362 and 524). The disability rights movement is redefining the term 'disability' as an improper fit between a person and an environment rather than a fault of the person.[2] In other words, if you can no longer get out of a chair by yourself, you get a chair that helps you get up.

Your local Social Services department can supply various aids for people with disabilities; the British Red Cross lends out some appliances; and the Disabled Living Foundation (see Organizations) has a permanent exhibition of aids to easier living which you, your helper or physiotherapist can visit by appointment.

Support from others becomes a necessity. We may need the help of friends and family as everyday activities we took for granted – cooking a meal, doing the laundry, shopping – become difficult. We also need moral support. We want others to believe in us, that we can do it, that we can fight weaknesses. We need to believe it too.

The mind is terribly important. If I really believed I was ninety, I would think I couldn't do anything. But I'm still interested in many things and can make people happy. [a woman who maintains a high level of involvement living in a residential home]

For most women, energy eventually becomes an issue, whether they have health problems or not. If, through most of our sixties and seventies, we have been 'the marvellous old woman' whose vitality everyone admired, we may feel we are letting people down as well as letting go of a valued image of ourselves.

I have reached a stage in my life that I had not given much thought to. Somehow I had thought that I would continue as active as I had been in the past. This is not so. I am now eighty-one and I think something is happening to me that may happen at an earlier or a later age for many women. It's a new stage – one that can be looked upon as negative, or it can be looked at simply as a continuation of the life span. [a woman in her eighties]

The first step in self-help is what many women with illnesses and disabilities had to learn earlier in life – to stop blaming themselves for limited energy and to plan realistically for it. If you have been very active in your job or voluntary work it may be necessary to reassess your activities and cut out those that tax your strength too much or are no longer personally rewarding.

After I retired, I was often asked to serve on committees. After a while, I learned to refuse to be a token old person on a committee and accepted only those appointments which seemed to value *what I uniquely had to offer. I do not feel that I can continue attending as many meetings as I have in the past. There are other aspects in my life now to which I need to give more time and attention.* [an eighty-two-year-old woman]

Look at your assumptions about what you *have* to do, and see how much isn't essential. You will feel better if you can pare down obligations while keeping up the pleasurable part of your commitments.

Everything I do takes so much longer – just getting dressed – I have to choose how to spend my time. I choose not to cook anymore because my back won't take it; all our family celebrations are now in my children's homes. My grandchildren have to accept that when they visit me they won't get chicken soup and potato pancakes anymore. [a seventy-nine-year-old woman]

When I think about packing and moving I feel overwhelmed. I can't do at seventy-eight what I could do at seventy-two. For the first time I am considering letting my son help me or paying the movers to do the packing.

Think of energy-conserving ways in which you can handle your needs.

The supermarket is about fifteen or twenty minutes away. I wouldn't think of going out to shop without my trolley. I am experimenting with taking along a small folding chair and a book, so I'll sit down and rest when I get tired and also have a chance to read something. [an eighty-one-year-old woman]

Regular physical activity and exercise help improve energy and increase stamina and endurance, but don't assume that you have to continue your leisure activities at the same pace, or give them up entirely. Try walking, gardening, swimming, and exercising at a slower pace, or for shorter periods of time. Women often find they enjoy these activities more when they ignore any feelings of haste or need for achievement.

Thinking, meditating, watching, and listening are as worthwhile as more strenuous activities. In our younger years, we were often too busy and rushed for reflection. Now that we cannot rush, we can turn to these quieter pursuits if we wish.

Life Review

Reflecting on the past is a natural process that helps us gain perspective on our lives and count our contributions and our blessings. We can also look at our mistakes and disappointments, but it is vital to do this in a positive framework, letting go of guilt or sense of loss. We can arrive at a conviction of the utter rightness of our lives.[3]

I've had a wonderful life. Tell me, what could I have changed? There's nothing I could have made any different. Everything was the way it had to be. [a ninety-eight-year-old woman]

This is the time of life to write about your life's journeys, share experiences with others, and think about integrating past, present, and future. Your children or other loved ones will appreciate the legacy of your autobiography. Writing it – or tape-recording it – can motivate you to reflect on your life, and on the events you've witnessed or taken part in. Be sure to include rich details to bring the picture to life – what you wore, what the furniture looked like, the sounds and smells. This can be a way of maintaining links between generations, so much needed in our life today.

One custom worth adapting for the twentieth century is the 'ethical will'. In medieval times, parents wrote extensive letters to their children and grandchildren advising them on the morals and values which had given meaning to their own lives.[4] You may wish to look back on your life, and write about the most important thing about you that you'd like your friends and family to remember after you're gone. What about you has made a difference in the world?[5] What are you most satisfied and proud of?

You can also relive the high points of your life. Think back to a peak experience – a time when you were in love, or viewing a beautiful sunset, or had a creative insight. Relive that experience. Then ask yourself, what are the essential qualities of that experience? How can you give that to yourself in your life *now*?[6]

There are many ways to reflect on your experiences. One is called the 'Stepping-stones' process.[7] In it, you review your life and identify specific events that stand out as signposts. Reflect and write about each one, using these words: 'It was a time when

' . . .' If you read what you've written out loud in a group of friends or write letters to family members, you may find added significance.

Some local women's groups or pensioners' clubs compile personal and local histories contributed by their members. There may be an Adult Education Centre in your area which runs classes in local history and welcomes accounts of the past from older students. Age Exchange (see Organizations) is a 'Reminiscence Centre' which works with groups of all ages collating personal histories and helping set up displays and museum exhibits. If there is no local group, why not get together with friends and start your own?

[1] Janet Neuman, 'Old Age: It's Not Funny'. *Perspective on Aging*, November/December 1982, published by the National Council on Ageing.

[2] Irving Kenneth Zola, 'Policies and Programs Concerning Age and Disability: Towards a Unified Agenda'. In Sean Sullivan and Marion Ein Lewin, eds., *The Economics and Ethics of Long-Term Care and Disability*. Washington, DC: American Enterprise Institute, 1988, pp. 90–130.

[3] Based on Erik Erikson's theory of adult development, in Erik H. Erikson, 'Eight Ages of Man'. *Childhood in Society*, New York: W. W. Norton & Co., 1963, pp. 268–9.

[4] 'Ethical Wills: Twelfth and Fourteenth Centuries', pp. 311–16 in Jacob R. Marcus, ed., *The Jew in the Medieval World*, New York: Atheneum, 1974.

[5] Adapted from Janette Rainwater, *You're in Charge: A Guide To Becoming Your Own Therapist*. Marina del Rey, Cal. DeVorss & Co., 1985, p. 203.

[6] Ibid., p. 44.

[7] Ira Progoff, *At a Journal Workshop*. New York: Dialogue House Library, 1975, pp. 119–30.

Disarming Stress

Old Age Must Be Like This

Alone and sick at three in the morning
She relives each mistake
wonders if there's enough money in the bank
But it's her life that's overdue
She's made too many plans
Who did she think she was
in those hectic days of health –
magic legs moving from sink to stove
from barn to the woodpile
– and the telephone lifting itself so easily
off the hook

the throat making all those intricate movements
in order to speak
Now simple tasks
laundry
dinner
fetching the mail –
can't be done
Dishes pile up in the sink
wood stays in the barn
She turns the electric blanket higher
wonders who will feed her birds –

MARILYN ZUCKERMAN

How we manage the stress in our lives is an important component of whatever disease-prevention and health-promotion regime we undertake. In a dangerous situation, our bodies go 'on alert', ready to take immediate action – to fight the threat, or to run away. This is called the 'stress response' and is normal and evolutionarily significant in humans as in other animals. However, in modern society the threats we experience are not often direct physical dangers, but are more generalized and ongoing, such as the pressure of a job, or the lack of one, sex and age discrimination, losses of relationships, and global dangers such as the threat of nuclear war. Sometimes, stress occurs when we feel emotionally threatened – such as when we perceive a neutral event or situation as threatening, or exaggerate a danger in our minds. There is a profound connection between thinking, feeling, behaviour, and what happens inside our bodies.

Stress can become a problem when it is continuous or ongoing, because the body does not return to its normal, non-aroused state. Chronic triggering of the fight-or-flight response has been shown to lead to many health problems, including hypertension,[12] elevated sugar levels, an overworked endocrine system, and possible brain-cell loss.[13] By adopting new habits to reduce stress and reverse its harmful effects, we can prevent the damage that can result from continual or chronic exposure.

Signs of Stress

How can you tell that you are under stress? Our bodies usually send us warning signals, but we may ignore them or cover them up with pills or minimize their importance. Sometimes we are not even aware that we are under stress.

The first time I realized that feelings affect my health was during a routine physical exam. I was worrying, just a little, about a decision I'd made. But my blood pressure was up – so much higher than usual that I knew I was anxious, terribly so, more than I wanted to believe. [a fifty-six-year-old woman]

Signs of stress that we all experience include muscle tightening, clenching, shallow breathing, headaches, and digestive disturbances. We may feel driven to compulsive behaviour such as excessive eating, drinking, smoking, or talking. We may turn to alcohol, drugs, caffeine, or tranquillizers. Depression, difficulty in sleeping, sleeping too much, lack of concentration, or irritability – even getting a fair number of irritable responses from other people – are all signs that we are not handling stress effectively.

Special Stresses of Middle-aged and Older Women

As middle-aged and older women, we face special stresses caused by sexism and ageism. We women face sexism throughout our lives. But we face ageism earlier than men do, sometimes even before forty, because of the double standard of ageing. This compounding of ageism and sexism brings with it added stresses. Each experience of prejudice – each rebuff, dismissal, act of condescension – is new and painful. Poverty deepens all other stresses and contributes to a feeling of despair. Each chips away at our self-esteem. Growing older in a society that has few respected roles for older people can bring a multiplicity of stressful experiences.

Caregiving is a role that frequently falls to women in the midlife and older years and can be extremely exhausting, isolating, and stressful. Bereavement, one of life's most painful experiences, occurs most often in the second half of life. Sometimes we face a series of losses in quick succession.

It seems like everything happened at once. I had to put my mother in a nursing home, where she suddenly died. I didn't have time to grieve, because I had to work for weeks to settle her affairs. About then, my seventeen-year-old daughter was preparing to leave home. I now had the freedom to move where I wanted to but I had a hard time leaving my home. What could I let go of? Every little thing had meaning for me. I had to go slow in packing – I kept injuring myself and I kept getting rashes. I'm still grieving, months later. Healing from my mother's death will take a long time. [a forty-nine-year-old woman]

In the scale below, adapted from the research of psychologists T. H. Holmes and R. H. Rahe, a series of life events were rated by 394 persons according to the amount of 'social readjustment' they required. Among the life events ranked most stressful are those that are frequently faced by middle-aged and older women.

Life Events Rated for Stressfulness[14]	Stress Rating*
Death of a spouse	100
Divorce	73
Death of a close family member	63
Personal injury or illness	53
Marriage	50
Retirement	45
Change in financial status	38
Death of a close friend	37
Children leaving home	29
Beginning or finishing school	26
Christmas	12

As older women, our lifelong socialization as nurturers can contribute to our feeling stressed. When we allow ourselves to be too generous to others with our time and energy, we risk overextending ourselves with too many commitments, some of which are neither vital nor beneficial. Thus we may damage our own well-being.

We are taught from early childhood to control our aggressiveness and suppress our anger. In fact, most of us don't even admit having aggressive feelings. Behind the mask of 'being nice' often lurk anger, lack of self-esteem, and frustration. When we repeatedly suppress our negative feelings out of fear or concern for others, we turn our accumulated anger and frustration against ourselves, and the chronic stress can damage our health.

I learnt a meditation technique, but it didn't help. I couldn't suppress my anger at the way life – and people – had treated me. I knew I needed to 'get it all out' and in the end I found I could when I went to a martial arts course and was encouraged to shout and kick an imaginary opponent. Before long I could cut down on the various pills I'd been taking, and today I don't have any medicines and I feel much better mentally and physically [a fifty-one-year-old woman]

Learning to use our anger in appropriate and constructive ways helps us preserve ourselves, prevent stress, and make needed changes. Organizing to change society's laws and attitudes as well as making use of community

---

*Participants were asked to rate each life event on a scale of 0 to 100, where marriage was rated 50.

resources can help us counteract the stress that comes from feeling powerless and anxious.

Most of the time we react automatically to stressors with feelings, words, thoughts, behaviours, and attitudes that we learned a long time ago – things which worsen the stress. An important part of coping with stress is learning to become less automatic in our responses.

It's been suggested that the way to cope is to stop fussing about small problems – and all problems are little ones, really: if you can't fight them, and you can't escape them, then try to use stress-management techniques so they won't bother you so much.[15] Some people find that sharpening their conscious awareness of stress and how it affects them helps them interrupt harmful patterns and adopt more constructive ways of coping. You can learn about your patterns through keeping a diary, talking with your friends, or seeing a psychotherapist. You can achieve a sense of *real* control by understanding what makes you tense, knowing what you can and cannot do to change or avoid those things, and knowing you can discharge the tension in various short-term and long-term ways.

- Paying attention to yourself, your desires, aspirations, and needs is a first step toward identifying who or what might be causing stress.
- Elicit the help of people around you. Develop, cherish, and nurture friendships. Take care to maintain multiple friendships and roles. These can be a buffer when one relationship or role is in conflict. In times of stress, friendships are especially important.
- When the cause of our stress is too big and powerful to tackle alone, you can join together with friends, co-workers, neighbours, and others to work for change in movements and organizations.
- Laughter actually has stress-reducing effects on the body. Read funny stories and watch comedies on TV.[16]
- Catch yourself when you notice you are dwelling on negative thoughts without working toward problem-solving. Concentrate on your strengths and accomplishments.
- In many situations, you can clearly express your dissatisfaction and work out a mutually satisfactory solution. For example, people respond better to 'I' statements than to 'you' statements. Don't say '*You* are giving me a headache with that radio.' Instead say, '*I* can't think when the radio is so loud.'[17] The idea is to express clearly your own discomfort and to avoid blaming anyone for it. Thus you enlist co-operation in solving a problem. Blaming passes your stress on to others – and it may bounce back.
- Scientists have proved what pet lovers already know – pets can be very beneficial to human health. Pets give and receive affection and touch.

- Eating well, especially foods that are high in vitamin B complex and vitamin C, can help you manage stress better. Cut down on beverages containing caffeine (coffee, chocolate, tea, and carbonated soft drinks) because too much caffeine can cause nervousness, irritability, and problems with digestion and sleep. If you are having trouble falling asleep or in sleeping soundly, you might consider that the caffeine in the tea you drink in the evening and before bed may be affecting you. Switching for a week or two to a tea with no caffeine, warm milk, or even plain hot water will give you a chance to test the effect of the tea.

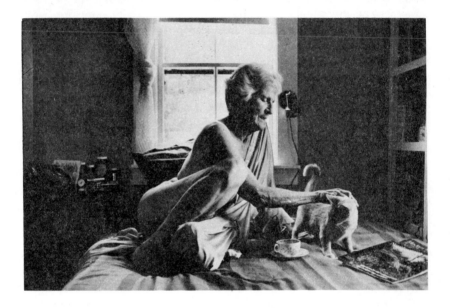

- Getting enough sleep is very important. Many people report needing less sleep as they age, so if this is true for you, allow time for rest and quiet instead. Don't try to solve problems at night or when you are tired.
- Have fun. Develop hobbies that you enjoy. Gardening, photography, amateur theatre, and pottery all provide many hours of pleasure. Take advantage of adult-education classes in which you can learn and meet people at the same time.

I draw and paint. It gives me a sense of accomplishment. When you are all alone and living on a fixed income like I am, you have to find things to keep you occupied without spending a lot of money. I go to public auctions, local fairs, museums, or I window shop. I also like to keep my mind stimulated and do crossword puzzles and read novels, mysteries, and history. I watch games on TV. I do sitting-in-the-chair exercises while watching TV. [a sixty-three-year-old woman]

- Exercise helps reduce the effects of stress by bringing blood to the muscles and brain, and by stimulating production of chemicals called endorphins and encephalins that give you a sense of well-being. Any expressive body movement can help make creative use of the pain of anger, fear, grief, or depression. Try dancing to a favourite record and using rhythm and strong movement to say what you feel. Any prolonged regular movement will loosen you up, such as a fast walk, a long swim, skipping, or simply stretching hard while doing rhythmic breathing.

The Relaxation Response

The Relaxation Response[18] is a simple meditation technique that synthesizes Eastern teachings with Western knowledge. The basic components are:

- A quiet environment and uninterrupted time.
- A sound, word, or short phrase of your own choosing repeated silently. The word 'one' is suggested – or a word from a prayer or meditation that is consistent with your culture or belief system.[19]
- A receptive attitude (the most important element). Clear your mind and visualize nothing. Keep your palms up as if you were open to whatever would happen.

Follow these simple steps:

1. Sit or kneel quietly in a comfortable position.
2. Close your eyes.
3. Deeply relax all your muscles, beginning with your feet and progressing up to your face. Keep them relaxed.
4. Breathe through the nose. Become aware of your breathing. As you breathe out, silently say the word or phrase you have selected. Breathe slowly and naturally.
5. Continue for ten to twenty minutes. When you finish, sit quietly for several minutes with your eyes closed and then for a few more with them open. (It is better to open your eyes when you feel the need to check the time than to use an alarm.)
6. Do not worry about whether you are successful in achieving a deep level of relaxation. *Permit relaxation to occur at its own pace.* If distracting thoughts occur, acknowledge them and let them go. Return to repeating your word or phrase.

Practise the technique once or twice daily, but not within two hours after any meal.[20] Once you are comfortable with it, you can utilize the technique in a waiting room or even a train, or almost any place you wish. You will feel quiet inside, mentally clear, alert, and in charge.

A second relaxation method is Progressive Relaxation.[21]

1. Lie comfortably on your back in a quiet place. Allow yourself to relax.
2. Begin by taking a few deep breaths and then relaxing into your natural breathing rhythm.
3. Tense and release groups of muscles, one group at a time, beginning with your toes. Tense the muscles; hold for a count of five and then release. Do this same thing to each group of muscles until you reach the top of your head.
4. Notice what the tension feels like as you contract each muscle group. Focus on the experience of *letting go* of this tension as you progressively relax parts of your body. You might imagine the *letting go* as a warm sun that's melting your icy body, or as water flowing around whatever part of your body you're relaxing. Allow the tension to float out of your muscles as you let them go as limp as you can. You are gradually relaxing yourself into a state that is almost bodiless until you feel that you are floating in space.

Many Local Education Authorities organize yoga or relaxation classes, and Yoga for Health Foundation (see Organizations) can give you the address of a local teacher for individual or group learning. They also market a relaxation course on cassette tape, and large record shops have relaxation tapes for sale.

Music and Imagery

Music and imagery can help you reach either a relaxed or an energized state, and can even help heal stress-related illnesses.[22] Try various kinds of music to see what states of awareness or mental pictures they encourage.

One older woman finds listening to Beethoven's Pastorale Symphony helps her imagine herself in a peaceful, lovely mountain-side scene; another enjoys Dixieland jazz to get her going for the day.

Self-Hypnosis or Self-Talk

After you master deep breathing and relaxation, you can learn to achieve a meditative state using self-hypnosis, sometimes called autogenesis. With self-hypnosis you can suggest relaxation (or other desired states such as alertness or joy) to your unconscious mind, which then causes your body to respond appropriately. You can practise it in any environment – at your desk, waiting in a queue, or trying to fall asleep at night. To practise, sit or lie down. Loosen clothing (ties, belts); become comfortable. Allow gentle concentration. Let your day's experiences pass through and out of you. Concentrate on a sensation and suggest it to yourself. Repeat it three times and take it to each part of your body as you say it; for example, if you say, 'I am at peace,' imagine an area of tension and fill it with peace; peace may be a colour, sensation, image or something that conveys deep peace to you.

To relieve a migraine, try decreasing blood flow in the head by saying to yourself, 'Blood is flowing away from my head and down through my body.' Concentrate on making that happen. Imagine a cool breeze going through your head; imagine the vessels dilating, expanding, and letting the blood flow rapidly.

I could not sleep because of all the noise outside. I decided that there was nothing I could do except not make it worse. If I couldn't sleep, I would rest. I just told myself things that would relax me. 'I will be better tomorrow. This rest is worth more than sleep.' I relaxed each part of my body, thinking, 'I am sinking into a profound state of rest that is even deeper than sleep.' I told myself that if the noise stopped I might doze off for only a few minutes before being awakened again but in those few moments I would have several hours of rest and would feel refreshed. The next day I felt fine and taught one of the best lessons I have ever given. [a fifty-five-year-old woman]

Prayer and Meditation

As we grow older, many of us find the spiritual aspects of our lives becoming more important. As our consciousness of our own mortality increases, we ask ourselves the meaning of our lives and of our places in the world. This can be especially true for women with physical limitations. As energy wanes and our movements are restricted, the pleasures of the mind and the spirit grow stronger. Some women continue an earlier bent for religion, philosophy, science, or literature, finding that their lives' experiences make study richer and more meaningful than ever before; some develop new interests.

Meditation and prayer can help you find spiritual strength and achieve a state of physical and emotional calm. Whether you choose meditation or prayer or a combination of the two will depend on your beliefs.

Some women find that, as they grow older, their religious beliefs and practices change. Some leave established religious groups, others renew their faith or find a new spiritual community. A growing literature on spirituality and its relation to well-being, healing,[23] and feminism[24] is available in libraries and bookshops.

Sharing Touch – Massage

As we get older, some of us fear that if we are not in a sexual relationship we may never be touched or held. We touch to express non-sexual tenderness and affection, to acknowledge each other's presence non-verbally, to comfort, to support, and to soothe. The misconception that touching always involves sex and is only appropriate in a sexual context causes real deprivation. People need to touch and be touched throughout their lives.

Some of us worry about touching or hugging others, especially other women, and so deny ourselves pleasure, comfort, and closeness. Some of us come from families where touching is limited to ritual holiday kisses. Intergenerational or homophobic taboos may make it hard to exchange hugs with friends or family members. But if we are able to free ourselves of these constrictions, we open ourselves to a whole array of rich experience.

Those who are disabled or very ill continue to need touching. Family members, friends, and staff members must recognize that patients in hospitals and residents in nursing homes need friendly touching every day. The wish for emotional intimacy and physical touching of another caring person is inseparable from other needs. Providing massage, allowing and encouraging patients to touch one another, and affectionate hugs and non-sexual touching on the part of staff members should all be part of the life of nursing-home residents. Staff members must be sensitive to individual and cultural differences in residents' acceptance of touch.

Since we never outgrow the need for warm physical touch, we may experience 'skin hunger'[25] if we rarely touch or are touched. One way to meet this need is through giving and receiving massage.

Massage has had a bad reputation because of the tendency to equate pleasurable touching with genital sexual arousal and the association of massage parlours with prostitution. Yet most massage is not sexual. Massage has a respected history in both East and West as a form of physical therapy. Massage offers many physical benefits, such as lowering blood pressure and stimulating circulation. In addition to its physical benefits, massage is one of the most pleasurable ways to relax. It is energizing yet relaxing to both the giver and the receiver.

Connecting with each other through caring touch is deeply satisfying and fun. We can form 'touch partnerships' with one or more friends and exchange massages regularly.

I enjoy sensuality. I gathered a group of women with whom I could do massage. Our group members would call each other up and exchange massages – twenty minutes

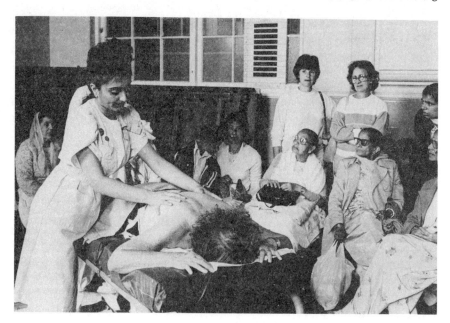

each. We took lessons and learned techniques. We became fast friends. [a sixty-five-year-old woman]

Giving and receiving warmth and caring is healthy and imparts a sense of being connected with your own body. The message given by caring massage is, 'I care about you just as you are.'

Massage makes me feel re-created; it's so pleasant. When I look in the mirror, I'm lean and gaunt-looking, but I don't feel like that when I'm being massaged. [a seventy-seven-year-old woman]

It is also possible to use similar techniques to massage yourself, communicating your caring for your own body.

Keep conversation to a minimum during the massage. Silence deepens the experience, allowing both giver and receiver to pay more attention to what's happening. It is important for the person receiving massage to give feedback on what feels good and what doesn't. Often the clearest feedback comes without words in a sigh of relaxation or in a slight contraction against pressure that's too hard or too sudden.

Before starting a massage, be sure to ask about injured areas to be avoided.

Do not massage a blood clot, or areas that are swollen, inflamed, or tender.

If you or the person you are massaging feels shy, start with foot and hand rubs, or head, neck, and face. A rapping motion with sides of hand, cupped palms, or loosely closed fists feels great on the arms, legs, back, and shoulders – try it on yourself first, then with each other. Finger-tapping feels good on the head and face. Kneading, squeezing, and rolling or rocking can be done over loose clothing. In order to glide smoothly over skin, use a lubricant such as light vegetable oil with or without perfume, or a bar of cocoa butter. Do not use mineral oil or products that contain it, such as baby oil. Hand lotions and creams are too quickly absorbed and do not provide enough lubrication, but cream may work well for facial massage.

The person receiving the massage will be most relaxed if she lies on a firm, comfortable surface, but you can also work on her as she sits. The person giving the massage should always work in a comfortable position. Deepen your own breathing as you remind the person you are massaging to deepen hers. When finishing a particular area, use long, light brushing strokes with fingertips. To finish the massage session, place your hands gently on the head or feet for a long moment, visualizing the person as healed and whole. Your public library should provide books on the various techniques, but the best way to learn is to share massages with a friend or attend a massage therapy course yourself.

Technique is less important than transmitting a sense of caring through your hands. Remember that you are touching a person, not just skin. As you touch, allow yourself to be fully attentive and aware of the uniqueness of the person you are massaging. The experience of giving massage is as heartwarming as receiving it.

I always enjoy massage, whether from friends or from massage therapists. I tend to hold all my tensions in my back and so suffer from stiffness and pain. Exercise and relaxation techniques, including massage, help. When I visited my daughter, who is a massage therapist, she gave me a Trigger Point [deep muscle work] treatment that kept me pain-free for several months. I found someone where I live who is helping me on a regular basis so the pain won't start again. [a fifty-four-year-old woman]

You may, as you are being massaged, feel an opening awareness of emotion, as massage is more than just physical manipulation. It is your decision whether the person giving the massage is the person with whom to discuss the feelings that come up during a massage. Alternatively, you may want to think through these issues yourself, write in a diary, talk with a friend, or discuss them with a psychotherapist.

Dealing with Depression

Research has shown that 25 per cent of the British population suffer from diagnosed or undiagnosed depression – and twice as many women as men (see Memory Loss chapter). Why the discrepancy?

Throughout this book we've noted the many ways in which women are disadvantaged – personally, socially and economically. Most of us older women have spent years looking after children, partially or totally dependent on a male partner. Sometimes it's a true partnership, real sharing of responsibilities in which 'who earns and who cares' are irrelevances; but for very many women caring for a family can feel like living in a trap. Deprived of adult contact for many hours of the day, meeting the unrelenting demands of the children and their father, denied any possibility of leading their lives in the way they would really choose, they become withdrawn and unconfident. When the trap-door finally opens, some are no longer capable of escape.

While there's some evidence to show that some people's brain chemistry may make them more vulnerable to depression, it's the isolation and powerlessness of women that must explain why so many feel so low and hopeless about themselves that they can be described as 'clinically depressed'. We may imagine that with a radical change in the way society treats women this situation may change, too. But in addition to working for such a change, what must concern us here and now is what we can do as individuals to overcome our feelings of worthlessness.

The first, and often the best resource is the friendship and support of other women. It isn't easy when we live on an isolated housing estate or a high-rise block to approach total strangers – especially when our children are older and there's no longer the opportunity for school-gate chat that made us friends in the past. But many lasting friendships are formed when women get together on common issues – problems with the housing department or landlord, hospital closures, transport cuts and so on. Activity of this kind, and the feelings of unity and purposefulness that it brings, are excellent antidepressants.

Women's groups, whether they're branches of national organizations such as the Women's Institutes or the National Women's Register, or feminist consciousness-raising groups formed by friendship networks or through advertisements in *Spare Rib* magazine, can be very supportive. Many women have been saved from severe depression by talking through their problems in a safe and confidential setting. Contact the Older Feminists' Network (see Organizations) for information about London meetings and any local groups.

When we're so depressed that taking any kind of social initiative can seem too daunting, we may need to seek professional help. For most of us, that means first seeing our GP. The medical model is similar for 'mental' as for physical problems. The GP may diagnose and treat (probably with anti-depressant drugs, rarely with some form of psychotherapy); or refer the 'patient' to a consultant psychiatrist. He – usually a male – will treat her in accordance not only with his diagnosis, but along the lines of his particular preference. This could be with antidepressants; by some form of psychotherapy; by group therapy; or by referring her on to a clinical psychologist for treatment, perhaps along 'behaviourist' lines or by psychotherapy or a combination of both approaches. (For a detailed discussion of these and alternative treatments see the chapter on mental illness in the British edition of *The New Our Bodies, Ourselves*.)

It's very difficult for most women, dependent as we are on the National Health Service, to make an informed choice about the kind of treatment we may meet if we are labelled 'depressed'. If we have good rapport with our GP we can ask her about her experience with different consultants; whether these are so unfavourable that she feels more confident about prescribing treatment herself; whether the consultants are so biased and opinionated that they may treat us as deviant if we are lesbians, or in a racist way if we are black; or whether she can suggest a counsellor or local group which could be helpful. The fact is that many GPs have little confidence in the psychiatric services available in their area, and, as we so often experience when we're referred to a consultant for *any* problem, there's no guarantee that we'll see that consultant at all; or if we see him once, that we'll ever see him again.

The result may be that however much we've tried to inform ourselves about the kind of treatment we're likely to get, we could find ourselves in the hands of a psychiatrist, psychologist or psychotherapist with whose approach we are uncomfortable or whose treatment seems to be useless or actually harmful. If this happens, we must overcome our tendency to accept whatever the 'expert' hands out, and withdraw. That is our right. It is only if we are 'sectioned' (see p. 297) that we can be compulsorily detained in a hospital.

The care of our friends and relatives for us can be vital in preventing the development of a severe depression or supporting us through one at home; but it is also important if we do find ourselves in a psychiatric ward. A regular visitor should make her presence known to staff. She should ask about progress and question treatment, and be ready with support if the patient believes it may be in her best interest to discharge herself. If hospital staff know that there's someone outside who is monitoring the situation, neglect or even ill-treatment are far less likely to occur.

MIND (see Organizations) has an excellent information and advice service, and has recently set up a policy group on women and mental health. They can also put you in touch with a Black and Ethnic Minority Mental Health Development Team in North London, as well as local MIND groups.

For those able to consider alternative forms of therapy, the Women's Therapy Centre in London offers individual and group help, and may be able to put women in touch with sympathetic therapists elsewhere, including Centres in Birmingham, Bristol, Edinburgh, Leeds, Nottingham and Oxford. A feminist therapy centre in South London is the Pellin Centre (see Organizations). Fees at these centres are much lower than private therapists! Depressives Anonymous is a national association which runs some local self-help groups and a penfriend service.

I Have Held Hands with Fear

I have held hands
with fear;
We have gone steady
together.

Sorrow has been
my mate;
We have been bed-
companions.

The days of my night
have been long.
They have stretched
to eternity.

Yet have I outlived
them.
And so shall you.

MITZI KORNETZ

BOOKS AND PUBLICATIONS

Dorothy Rowe, *Depression: the Way Out of Your Prison*. London: Routledge & Kegan Paul, 1983.

Women in Mind, *Finding Our Own Solutions – Women's Experience of Mental Health Care*. London: MIND, 1986.

Sheila Ernst and Lucy Goodison, *In Our Own Hands – a Book of Self-Help Therapy*. London: Women's Press, 1981.

Kathy Nairne and Gerrilyn Smith, *Dealing with Depression*. London: Women's Press, 1984. See also the extensive list at the end of the mental health chapter in *The New Our Bodies, Ourselves*.

Getting in Touch with Others – Friends and Support Groups

We have the power to enrich our lives and those of others through our personal relationships. Research has shown that those who maintain strong bonds with family, friends, or neighbours actually have lower death and illness rates. When we feel isolated, it takes courage and initiative on our part to reach out to make new friends. A ten-year study of seven thousand people across America found that the mortality rate among people with poor social bonds was 2.5 times higher than among people with a good support system of friends and relatives.[26]

One thing that our society lacks, from my point of view, is that people don't have groups of friends. You have one individual friend. And if something happens to him or her, you have no one to talk to. And you wind up at the psychiatrist. . . . I have friends who let me talk things out. Through the talking, I realize what I must do. [a woman age eighty][27]

When we were younger, local women often gathered to talk over coffee, discussing child rearing, sharing homemaking tips, and enjoying the pleasure of conversation. At work, people band together to help each other survive the pressures of the job. Now that we are older, these natural groups may have fallen away. And as society becomes more mobile and fragmented, with family members often far away, there's a vital social gap to be filled. Friends become our family of choice on whom we depend.[28]

Though many groups meet for specific purposes, simple friendship can be a sufficient reason for gathering. One group of women of all ages, fearing a future alone, call themselves 'Just Friends'. They meet not only for the enjoyment of being in a group of women of all ages, but also to help each other.

Self-Help Groups

Specific shared issues can be a good catalyst for bringing people together. You, perhaps with a friend, may wish to form a self-help group of women who share a common problem, such as a troubled relationship with an adult child, arthritis, allergies, or urinary incontinence. You can also join a group such as Cruse (see Organizations), or a hospice group that supports you after the death of a loved one.

Self-help groups often have practical results. A good example is the effect an older women's group had in helping older people stay in their homes. The group organized a pool of younger volunteer and paid workers who helped with housekeeping, repairs, transport, companionship, and a variety of other personal services.[29]

Self-help groups are different from old-style authoritarian groups, and it takes some adjusting and patience to get one working well. Here are some pointers:

A self-help group sets its own goals. Begin by discussing, in democratic fashion, what the group members' needs are. It is assumed that each member is an expert on her own problems, needs, and goals. Avoid letting one member take over; encourage those members with professional expertise to participate as equals, without reference to credentials.

Leaderless self-help groups ensure that each woman's needs, goals, and experiences are equally respected. The results are well worth the time and trouble. Another approach is to rotate leadership among group members, or to appoint one member as a facilitator to keep the group focused. Whoever leads the group has the same needs as the other members and must be given time to air her concerns while another member fills in as leader. In such groups, we learn new skills of openness and flexibility, and develop our natural leadership and communication abilities.

I was a member of a support group that had started off with a leader. When we became independent, I sometimes felt frustrated, so I thought, 'What would Ann [the former leader] say if she were here?' and then I would try it. Now we all share the responsibility of keeping the group moving. [a woman in her fifties]

In my women's group we divide up the tasks of leadership and take turns doing them. At each meeting one woman keeps track of the time allowed for each person to speak. Another woman is responsible for keeping the discussion on track, so that as each woman speaks she is free to concentrate solely on what she is saying. [a forty-seven-year-old woman]

Groups in the UK that are run along these lines include the Older Feminists' Network and the Older Lesbian Network (see Organizations).

NOTES

[1]Asenath La Rue et al., 'Health in Old Age: How Do Physicians' Ratings and Self-ratings Compare?' *Journal of Gerontology*, Vol. 34, No. 5, 1979, pp. 687–91.

[2]Marc E. Weksler, 'Genetic and Immunologic Determinants of Aging'. In *Proceedings of the Second Conference on the Epidemiology of Aging*. Bethesda, Md.: US Department of Health and Human Services, National Institutes of Health, 1980, pp. 15–22.

[3]Robert N. Butler, 'Health Productivity and Aging: An Overview'. In Robert N. Butler and Herbert P. Gleason, eds., *Productive Aging: Enhancing Vitality in Later Life.* New York: Springer, 1985, p. 8.

[4]Ibid., p. 12.

[5]Mary Anne Kurz, 'Theories of Aging and Popular Claims of Extending Life'. *News and Features from NIH*, Vol. 85, No. 4, 1985, pp. 8–10.

[6]Edward L. Schneider and John D. Reed, Jr, 'Life Extension'. *New England Journal of Medicine*, Vol. 312, No. 18, 2 May 1985, pp. 1159–68.

[7]Kurz, op. cit.

[8]Schneider and Reed, op. cit., p. 1161.

[9]Ibid., p. 1165.

[10]Gene Bylinsky, 'Science Is on the Trail of the Fountain of Youth'. *Fortune*, July 1974, p. 134.

[11]K. Warner Schaie and Sherry Willis, 'Can Decline in Adult Intellectual Functioning Be Reversed?' *Developmental Psychology*, Vol. 22, No. 2, 1986, pp. 223–32.

[12]B. Folkow and E. H. Rubinstein, 'Cardiovascular Effects of Acute and Chronic Stimulations of the Hypothalamic Defense Area in the Rat'. *Acta Physiologica Scandinavica*, Vol. 68, 1966, pp. 48–57. Quoted in Herbert Benson, *The Relaxation Response.* New York: Avon Books, 1976, p. 70.

[13]R. M. Sapolsy et al., 'Hippocampal Neuronal Loss During Aging: Role of Glucocorticoids'. Paper given at Conference on Aging and the Dementias, Montefiore Centennial Series, Rockefeller University, New York, 24 October 1984.

[14]Excerpted from T. H. Holmes and R. H. Rahe, 'The Social Readjustment Rating Scale'. *Journal of Psychosomatic Research*, Vol. 11, 1967, p. 213.

[15]Robert Eliot, a Nebraska cardiologist, quoted in Claudia Wallis, 'Stress: Can We Cope?' *Time*, 6 June 1983, p. 48.

[16]Norman Cousins, *Anatomy of an Illness.* New York: W. W. Norton & Co., 1979.

[17]Thomas Gordon, *Parent Effectiveness Training.* New York: P. H. Wyden, 1970.

[18]Herbert Benson, *The Relaxation Response.* New York: Avon Books, 1976.

[19]Herbert Benson, *Beyond the Relaxation Response.* New York: Times Books, 1984. How to harness the power of faith and personal belief in the healing process.

[20]Benson, *The Relaxation Response*, p. 163.

[21]Steve Kravette, *Complete Relaxation.* Rockport, Mass.: Para Research, 1979, pp. 21–37.

[22]Carolyn Latteier, 'Music as Medicine'. *Medical Self Care*, Issue No. 31, November–December 1985, pp. 48–52.

[23]Benson, *Beyond the Relaxation Response*, op. cit.

[24]*Ms.*, December 1985, special issue on women and spirituality.

[25]Flora Davis, 'Skin Hunger – An American Disease'. *Woman's Day*, 27 September 1978, p. 156.

[26]Lisa Berkman and S. Leonard Syme, cited in Judy Foreman, 'Friends: As Vital as Family'. *The Boston Globe*, 3 February 1982.

[27]Grace Chu, in Jane Seskin, ed., *More Than Mere Survival: Conversations with Women Over 65.* New York: Newsweek, 1980, p. 223.

[28]Karen Lindsey, *Friends as Family.* Boston: Beacon Press, 1982.

[29]Mike Samuels and Nancy Samuels, *Seeing with the Mind's Eye.* New York: Random House, 1975, pp. 56–64.

BOOKS AND PUBLICATIONS

The Boston Women's Health Book Collective, *The New Our Bodies, Ourselves*. London: Penguin, 1989.

Norman Cousins, *Anatomy of an Illness as Perceived by the Patient: Reflections on Healing and Regeneration*. London: Bantam, 1987.

Gordon Inkeles, *The New Massage: Total Body Conditioning for People Who Exercise*. London: George Allen & Unwin, 1981.

Clare Maxwell-Hudson, *The Complete Book of Massage*. London: Dorling Kindersley, 1988.

Dr Tony Smith (ed.), *The British Medical Association Family Doctor Home Adviser*. London: Dorling Kindersley, 1986.

Jean Shapiro, *On Your Own: A Practical Guide to Independent Living*. London: Pandora Press, 1985.

Aleda Erskine, *The Time of Your Life: Handbook for Retirement*. London: Help the Aged, September 1984.

Susan Hemmings (ed.), *A Wealth of Experience: Lives of Older Women*. London: Pandora Press, 1985.

Barbara Macdonald and Cynthia Rich, *Look Me in the Eye: Old Women, Ageing and Ageism*. London: The Women's Press, 1984.

Janet Ford and Ruth Sinclair, *Sixty Years On: Women Talk About Old Age*. London: The Women's Press, 1987.

Health Education Authority, *Your Right to Health*. Booklet in English and twelve non-English languages giving information on health and social security provision.

2
Habits Worth Changing

We live in a substance-abusing society. We are surrounded by billboards, store displays, and ads in all the media touting alcohol, over-the-counter drugs, cigarettes, soft drinks, coffee – all promoting a glamorous and happy life. The message is, 'Reach for a [whatever it is] and all your problems will be solved.' Physicians are also bombarded by drug-company salespeople and medical-journal ads offering drugs for every symptom. But these substances – tobacco, caffeine, alcohol, and drugs – when turned into habits are so common and damaging that they warrant special attention. They also interact with each other in ways that increase their danger.

Smoking

Cigarette smoking is the chief avoidable cause of death in our society, and the most important health issue of our time.[1] Smoking is on the rise for women. Since World War II, women have been smoking in large numbers and now our smoking-related disease patterns are beginning to resemble men's. In fact, our favourable advantage in life span over men (77 years to men's 71 years, as of 1983) may change for the worse as a result.[2] Lung cancer is now the number one cancer killer of women, exceeding both breast cancer and colorectal cancer.[3]

The dangers of 'passive smoking' – smoke inhaled from other people's cigarettes – are also very high. 'Secondhand smoke' contains thousands of chemical compounds, including some deadly ones. It contains fifty times more ammonia, five times more carbon monoxide, and *twice as much tar* as the smoker inhales.[4] Awareness of the rights of non-smokers has been heightened in recent years by the efforts of activist groups such as ASH (Action on Smoking and Health, see Organizations). Local groups such as GASP (Group Against Smoking Pollution) in Massachusetts and other American states support efforts to create no-smoking areas in public places and the workplace and to ban both the sale of cigarettes in hospitals and the distribution of cigarettes to minors.

The risks of smoking increase with age and with the number of years you've smoked. These risks include osteoporosis, glaucoma, a full range of cardio-vascular and respiratory diseases, and many more kinds of cancer than the obvious lung cancer. Smoking accounts for about 30 per cent of all cancer deaths.[5] There is an increased danger of cardiovascular disease among users of oral contraceptives who smoke, and an increased risk of cancer of the mouth, pharynx, larynx, and oesophagus among people who both drink and smoke. Smoking also increases wrinkles.

Nicotine is by no means the only dangerous ingredient in cigarettes. We must also count carbon monoxide (in an amount eight times greater than the amount industry is allowed to release into the air), tars, and even the heat itself. Chemical additives and modern tobacco-curing processes apparently add to cigarette smoking's deadly results.

The good news is that smoking is avoidable. The highest mortality rates are among current smokers, and stopping *at any age* causes the mortality rate to drop. In the case of coronary heart disease, stopping causes a 50 per cent drop in death rate within twelve months, and after a decade or more of not smoking the mortality rate from coronary heart disease approaches that of non-smokers.[6]

HOW TO CELEBRATE A TWENTY-FIFTH SMOKELESS ANNIVERSARY BY BETH ROSENBAUM

It is now twenty-five years since I smoked my last cigarette. In 1960 I inhaled the last nicotine into my then fifty-four-year-old lungs. For thirty-four years a cigarette had been my constant companion, my picker-upper, my relaxer, and my security blanket. 'Put me in a padded cell,' I told my family, 'if you want me to stop smoking.'

In the Roaring Twenties the cigarette was the flapper's logo of sophistication. 'Cigarette me, big boy,' said Joan Crawford, and we all bought carved ivory holders. 'Be non-chalant, light a Murad,' said the elegant smokers on the American billboards.

Now the Department of Health, doctors, and health organizations warn, cajole, raise consciousness, modify behaviour, hypnotize, segregate, and abuse smokers – with questionable success.

But in my twenty-fifth Smokeless Anniversary year, I offer my method free to all nicotine addicts. No coupons to clip. No salesperson will call. No obligations.

First: Build up a strong guilt feeling. Guilt can be very productive if used constructively. How can one feel guilty about smoking? Many ways. You don't want to give your children and grandchildren unhealthy habits, do you? More children of smoking parents become smokers than the lucky offspring of non-smoking parents. No children? Think of all the money you could give to your favourite charity; at today's cigarette prices, several hundred pounds a year. Besides, don't you feel uneasy about all the air you're polluting? Your loved ones are breathing it, not to mention innocent strangers. So, pick the guilt that suits your situation and dwell on it.

Second: Choose a day with a spiritual, mystical, or sentimental association for you. I chose Yom Kippur – the Jewish Day of Atonement – after reading in the service: 'This day ... I have set before you life and death, blessing and curse; therefore choose life, that you and your descendants may live' (Deuteronomy 30:19). Good advice, I decided, from an authorized source. Or choose your birthday, surely a symbolic day. You came into this world with clean, rosy-pink lungs. Do you really want to go out with dirty black lungs? Don't choose New Year's Eve. Decades of bad jokes about New Year's resolutions have conditioned us to break the ones we make.

Third: Think upbeat. Make a little ceremony around smoking that last cigarette. Tell yourself, out loud: 'This is the last time in my life I'll smoke. I am not giving anything up. I'm starting something new.' You, yourself, built the habit of smoking. You can build a new habit. After you eat anything, even a snack, use a toothpick vigorously. Keep that toothpick in your mouth or put it in an ashtray. You'll find your own substitute habit. Sweets and coffee won't help. They tend to make you want to eat and smoke . . . a never-ending cycle. Concentrate on something – like a crossword. Occupy your mind and hands. It works.

Fourth: Enjoy it. It's a great ego-booster. Feel superior to all those lily-livered, black-lunged weaklings who think their very lives depend on a tiny, dangerous, expensive paper tube stuffed with straw.

Fifth: Declare a victory. A poet and soldier described World War I as 'damned dirty, damned dull, and damned dangerous'. *You* have just won a war, also dirty, dull, and dangerous. Congratulations. You deserve a medal to pin on your healthier chest.

Take heart in knowing that a high percentage of those who try to stop succeed, even if it takes several attempts. The 'frontal attack' on the smoking habit – going 'cold turkey' – may work. But there's a risk: if you don't succeed, the habit may grow stronger, and you may feel less powerful in relation to it. If you make a slip – take one cigarette – you may feel like a failure and go into a full-scale relapse. The motto of Alcoholics Anonymous, 'One day at a time', can be helpful to anyone trying to quit. Many quit on their own, assisted by self-help literature. For others, self-help groups and cessation programmes (the cost of which may be covered by the NHS if prescribed by a doctor) are essential.

Smokers reach for cigarettes to relieve boredom, to fill time, to do something when feeling tense or anxious. One reaction to tension is to hold your breath or to take little, shallow breaths. If you smoke, inhaling a cigarette may be your only way to take a full, deep breath. Try taking three deep breaths when you crave a cigarette. You may actually crave oxygen.

Smoking a cigarette may be the only socially accepted way of taking a break at your workplace. You may have to fight for acceptance of a more healthful break, like going for a short walk, or just to the door or window for air, or getting up to stretch.

Some women are working to create a smoke-free environment where they are employed. Sadly, when some women approach their trade union to try to get workplace smoking banned, or confined to certain areas, they meet a brick wall. One woman, who tried for months to get her employers to agree to set up a no-smoking area, succeeded only when the office was reorganized for other reasons, but she did get a 'You are now entering a non-smoking zone' notice put up on the door to the office where she and other smoke-haters worked. Attempts are being made to enforce a smoking ban in certain areas of the civil service – especially in the Department of Health.

Smoking is a hard habit to break, and for various reasons women have a harder time quitting than men. Stopping smoking often requires that we confront these obstacles:

- Tobacco manufacturers spend millions on special advertising efforts to expand their markets among women. The financial clout of the tobacco industry inhibits the flow of anti-smoking information while assuring that the pro-smoking messages remain in the media – a serious infringement of freedom of the press.[7] Earlier advertising attempted to link smoking with sexiness. Now the ads play on a caricature of feminism that links smoking to women's struggles for equality and feeling 'tough' and 'cool'. The only way smoking helps you to 'come a long way, baby' is by catching up to men's lung-cancer rates.

- Nicotine is a physiological addictor. When you smoke, you reward yourself for smoking, and when you try to quit, it feels like you are punishing yourself. You can reverse this by developing a reward system for every cigarette you do *not* smoke. One suggestion is to set aside the money you spend on cigarettes for a present for yourself. By *not smoking* you can spend the money on something you will enjoy longer than a cigarette.

Smoking is higher among groups stressed by job pressures and unemployment – especially women. Figures released by the government in 1988 show that smoking among young women and teenage girls is increasing, at a time when fewer men and boys are hooked. This has serious implications for the future – it's well known that pregnant women who smoke tend to have low birth weight babies, and their children can be badly affected by passive smoking.

- Women learn to suppress anger, and some of us tend to reach for a cigarette when feeling angry.

It took me eight years to stop smoking completely. The last cigarettes I gave up were the ones I 'cadged' at work when I didn't feel free to say what I really thought. My close co-workers would ask me after the meeting, 'What didn't you like?' [a fifty-four-year-old woman]

- Many women use cigarette smoking to reduce calorie intake, picking up a cigarette instead of a dessert. We fear gaining weight if we quit. Cigarette manufacturers play on such fears through advertising.

When you give up smoking, food will taste and smell better without cigarettes, but weight gain is not inevitable. Instead, try non-caloric or low-calorie substitutes like gum or carrot sticks rather than resorting to high-calorie foods to sate your reawakened appetite. Try chewy, satisfying whole grains like brown rice to restore the B vitamins lost in smoking. Drink extra fruit and vegetable juices to speed elimination of nicotine from your system. Increase your walks or other exercise. Try swimming; nobody smokes in a swimming pool.

When you stop smoking, you can expect to feel pretty bad for a few days, and tense for a few more. Being prepared for this experience is half the battle. Try to arrange to stop on a day when you don't expect to meet problems and difficulties at work or at home, get support from family and friends. Contact ASH for helpful literature; talk to your doctor.

Before long you'll feel more energetic, enjoy your food more, get rid of 'smoker's cough'. The long-term rewards are incalculable in terms of better health and the feeling of being in control.

Caffeine

Tea and coffee are the 'drugs of choice' for millions of people. We use coffee as fuel for our industry and business, making typists type faster and executives work longer hours. Caffeine and related compounds are found in coffee, colas, tea, and chocolate.

What caffeine in fact achieves is partial responsibility for a wide range of disorders: panic attacks,[8] chronic nervousness and irritability; digestive difficulties, including heartburn, indigestion, and ulcers; fibrocystic breast lumps; migraine headaches; and low blood sugar. It can lead to increased risk of pancreatic and bladder cancers,[9] and, as a heart stimulant, is linked to blood-pressure abnormalities and myocardial infarction. In a 1973 study of 440 patients with acute myocardial infarction, the disease was seen 60 per cent to 120 per cent more frequently in coffee drinkers.[10]

'Decaffeinated' coffee is only half decaffeinated. It still contains about 3 per cent caffeine compared with ordinary coffee's 6 per cent, as well as other substances such as tars, acids, and oils that may be part of the coffee/disease picture. If you drink several cups of decaf, you are still getting a lot of caffeine. The safest way to remove caffeine from coffee is the water-processed method. Some health-food shops may sell water-processed decaf. Chemically processed decaf has been specifically implicated in pancreatic cancer.[11]

The coffee mornings which developed among local women to inject a little sociability in a day filled with chores and isolation, is often just an excuse to sit down together. You can still have the sociability without the dangers of caffeine.

What can you do if you want to switch? Cut down gradually. When you feel like having a cup of coffee, find other ways to increase circulation and oxygen to the brain, such as aerobic exercise. Drinking milk, vegetable juices, unsweetened fruit juices, herbal beverages, and grain-based coffee substitutes (iced or hot) may add a new flavour dimension to your life. Don't forget your need for water. Evaluate your priorities, and see if you are pushing yourself harder than necessary using coffee as a whip.

Alcohol

During their middle and later years, women undergo significant life changes and cultural pressures. Trying to cope with these changes and pressures is very difficult, and a drink or a tranquillizer may seem like an easy way to cope. Women can often trace changes in their drinking habits to upsetting events in their lives.[12] But drinking opens a door to a nightmare of alcohol abuse and possible addiction.

If we are having trouble sleeping, we may be tempted to have a drink before bed to encourage sleep. To add to this danger, doctors may prescribe drugs that can eventually control us physically, mentally, and spiritually, and can interact dangerously with alcohol.[13]

If we have already spent several decades using alcohol as an accompaniment to life, it is difficult to imagine that it can suddenly take over completely. Yet it can do just that!

When I was living alone with no car, I felt really alone. I had a morbid fear: suppose I lost my mind or something? I'd open a can of beer and make a gin and tonic, and have a sip of one and then a sip of the other. It was so warm and soothing. But it was dangerous. [an eighty-eight-year-old woman]

Are we overstating the case, being alarmist? After all, most people drink. It is a customary part of our social life. Sometimes there is social pressure to drink. We are more apt to drink, or to drink more than we usually do, in a group, for the sake of sociability. It is important to remember that we have the right to abstain.

When I was going through the menopause I found that any alcohol triggered severe hot flushes and so asked for mineral water or juice. I was amazed at the pressure from people (not from my close friends) who were unrelenting in trying to get me to drink alcohol. I finally started to lie and told them I was taking medication that could not be taken with alcohol. Then they were sympathetic and stopped pressuring – until the next time. [a fifty-five-year-old woman]

Relatively little is known about the effects of alcohol on women of any age because most research on alcohol and drug abuse is still being done with men as subjects. We do know that women's average body weights are lower than men's, so the same quantity of alcohol hits us harder. Even at the same weight, alcohol enters our bloodstreams faster because of our higher proportion of body fat, which doesn't absorb alcohol. Twenty-five per cent of women who become alcoholics do so between the ages of forty and fifty-five,[14] and anywhere from 1 to 5 per cent succumb to the disease after age sixty.[15] The 'safe' level of alcohol consumption for women is 14 measures a week – in other words, two standard glasses of wine per day.

My family and friends knew there was something wrong with me, but they just couldn't put a finger on it. The changes had been too subtle. They could see that I was drinking a little too much, now and again. What they did not know, because I went to great pains to hide it from them, was that the times I drank had become more and more frequent, and the times between shorter. [a woman in her fifties]

Many women fall prey to problem drinking without realizing it is happening. If alcohol becomes a problem for you, will you realize it? Will you know how to handle it? Will you want to do so? We owe it to ourselves to be aware of certain telltale signs of problem drinking in ourselves or in others close to us.

No one starts life with the goal of becoming an alcoholic. The onset of alcohol abuse is usually very slow and insidious.

My tolerance to alcohol grew so that I had to drink more to achieve the same effect. My daily activities began to be planned around my drinking time, and more and more often, drinking became my main activity. My dependence on the alcohol was growing as my addiction took hold. I could manage to rationalize anything if it meant defending my right to drink. At that point, of course, my 'right' was a synonym for my physical and emotional need. [a fifty-one-year-old woman]

While it is not possible to predict exactly who will or will not become an alcoholic, the following questions can provide some early clues. Are you, for example:

- Drinking faster or more frequently? Are you gulping your drinks or trying to maintain the feeling drinking gives you, while looking for more opportunities to drink and feel okay about it?
- Changing your daily pattern of drinking? Has a nightcap been expanded to include a before-dinner drink?
- Changing companions? Are you breaking dates with old friends and trying to find new ones who drink as you do?
- Having trouble maintaining your activity level at work or at home? Do lunches include an alcoholic beverage when tea or coffee used to be enough? Is it increasingly difficult to return to work afterwards? Have you lost interest in activities that used to make you happy but did not include drinking?
- Becoming unable to resist when you want to drink, even at times you would normally consider inappropriate? Are you planning ahead to ensure your supply? Finding reasons to justify drinking? Can you rationalize almost anything if it means you can drink when you want to do so?
- Denying that anything has changed? Are you lying to yourself and others about the frequency of your drinking and your need to continue it? Are your friends and family members making excuses for you? Is your relationship with them changing for the worse?
- Experiencing blackouts? Are you beginning to have times when you cannot remember things you did while drinking?

'The quality of life returns as we learn a day at a time how not to drink.' As these words were spoken at an AA meeting recently, there flashed before me the scene of a Christmas morning in my living room – and the faces of my husband and son – as I stood shakily before them following what I hope is my last drunken blackout, seven years ago. [a seventy-two-year-old woman]

- Having more accidents? Are you falling more, or getting burns or cuts without being able to explain how?

Until I almost fall down, or become ill, or wake up the next day with a massive hangover, I don't truly recognize how drunk I am. [a fifty-year-old woman]

Facing Problem Drinking

Drinking is considered to be inappropriate behaviour for women, especially for older women. Women who drink to excess are judged harshly, their value as people and women challenged. Those of us who grew up during the times when women were more restricted socially may feel this prejudice more keenly, but few of us are free of it entirely.

I rang AA at least three times over my last five years of heavy drinking. Each time I called with a different story, a different lie! Once I said I was phoning because my son drank too much. I don't remember the other lies. I even disguised my voice because I felt so ashamed. [a forty-nine-year-old woman]

As well as robbing women who drink too much of their self-esteem and security, this attitude keeps many from getting help. Most women are reluctant to seek treatment, even privately, because of the stigma attached. Seventy per cent of women who drink to excess hide their drinking for as long as possible, some better than others.[16] Women who live by themselves or with partners who are absent frequently can do so more easily. Women in higher income brackets may also be able to hide problems more easily because expense is less of an issue and because they rarely come to the attention of social workers or the criminal justice system.

However, no one is exempt from addiction. Although it often seems as if no one wants to admit it, the woman alcoholic or problem drinker can be anyone – a next-door neighbour, a fellow-worker, or a close relative. She can be a lesbian, a member of an ethnic minority, a strict churchgoer, a professional, an eighty-five-year-old great-grandmother, or you.

Alcohol and the Lesbian

Most women over thirty-five did not know the freedom growing up that our younger sisters have today. The experiences of older lesbians involved the painful conflict of fear of being found out versus a deep need to socialize. The situation was made more complex by the fact that social life in past years centred around bars.

Too many older lesbians still feel isolated, guilty, ashamed, and have low self-esteem because of society's homophobia. Alcohol, first used as a temporary relief from those pressures, grew to be a constant need for almost one third of all lesbians in America.[17]

I so deeply suppressed my homosexual feelings that I was no longer aware that they existed. Married at twenty-three, I lived the role of a traditional mum and wife. I had always felt different from my friends, and I thought that something must really be wrong with me. Having a drink before supper was a nightly event for my husband and me. Gradually, however, this one drink became two or three for me. I really looked forward to those drinks because they were the only times that I felt able to relax. Gradually, over the years, I lost control of my drinking and became an alcoholic.

Fortunately, at forty-two, I found AA and began my road to recovery. In the process, my old feelings began to resurface and I could no longer deny that I was both emotionally and sexually attracted to other women. While these feelings frightened me, I could no longer suppress them. Instead I began actively to seek out other women like me. While I had been afraid that going to bars would be my only way to find them, I discovered that the AA actually listed several gay meetings.

I was very nervous about going, in case someone I knew might see me, but when a woman in the group stood up to introduce herself with the words 'My name is Kathy and I am an alcoholic and a lesbian' tears of relief streamed down my face. [a forty-nine-year-old woman]

There are a few groups for older lesbians to be found in London and other large cities, and in most, smoking and alcohol are restricted.

Social Effects of Alcohol Abuse

A long list of social troubles can be the outcome of problem drinking and alcoholism. Choosing to take a mood- or mind-altering substance instead of dealing with issues that come up in daily life also causes problems. We can lose friends and lovers, see our marriages break up, lose jobs, run up debts by spending money to ensure our supply rather than paying our bills, be picked up for drunk driving, and so on.

As I began to drink more, I began to be late for work. At first it was just once in a while, and then more frequently. Finally I started missing days completely. When I was at work, the quality of my work was becoming more uneven. At first my friends covered up for me, but eventually they were less and less willing to do so. Finally my boss began to notice. I was warned a number of times, and people bent over backward to help me, but I was unable to see what was happening to me. When I lost that job I rationalized that it hadn't been much of a job anyway, and I would be happier without it. [a fifty-one-year-old woman]

Health Hazards of Alcohol Abuse

Heavy alcoholism over a period of years adversely affects every organ and system of the body. Some of these damaging effects can be reversed, but many cannot.[18] When we drink, we might like to think that any long-term effects will happen only to others, but they can happen to us. The possibilities include:

- Memory loss caused by brain atrophy
- Digestive problems, including inflammation of the pancreas, gastritis, fatty liver, hepatitis, and cirrhosis. Heavy drinking can impair the absorption of vitamin B_1 (thiamine), which can contribute to both brain damage and many problems of the intestinal system.
- High blood pressure and cardiac arrhythmia (irregular heartbeat), coronary artery disease and alcohol cardiomyopathy (heart muscle damage)
- Nerve and muscle disorders resulting in weakness, the gradual wasting of muscles, and even paralysis
- An increased susceptibility to infection. Alcohol suppresses the production of white blood cells and impairs their ability to get to the site of an infection quickly.
- An increase in the effect of carcinogens (cancer-causing substances) such as tobacco. Alcoholics with cancer have a poorer chance of survival and a greater chance of developing another primary tumour than do non-alcoholics with the same cancer.
- Malnutrition. Alcoholics often neglect their nutrition, leading to anaemia and increased tendency to bleed.

It cannot be overstated that, in addition to the above, there can be severe, sometimes fatal, effects as a result of combining alcohol with other drugs, even those drugs which are necessary for various health problems.

My friend Margo had a serious thyroid problem which was controllable with medication. She was also one of those unfortunate people who suffered from long- and short-term memory loss related to alcohol use. Over the years of heavy drinking her thyroid condition worsened because she would forget to take her medication, increasing the burden on her overworked heart. Ultimately her heart did give out and Margo died when she was just fifty-two years old. The death certificate stated that she died of heart failure, but it was her alcoholism which was the real cause.

Getting Help

If you cannot stop drinking when you want to; if, on any given occasion, you find you are taking drugs more than you want to; or if you know deep inside that drinking or drugs are affecting any part of your life in a negative way, help is as close as your telephone. Even if you are only beginning to wonder if you have a problem, it is never too early to seek help, nor is it ever too late.

Finally, after twenty years of drinking, I went to my GP to whom I confessed out loud for the first time that I couldn't stop drinking. In his ignorance of the disease of alcoholism, he said, 'There, there, dear. You are just a little neurotic. A few pills and you should be all right in a few months.' In my own ignorance and desperation, I actually believed this man. He started me on Librium and then when that didn't work, Valium. Two and a half years later he had tried thirty-one different drugs on me, including Ativan because I shook so much from the combination of all these drugs. I now know that Ativan is particularly dangerous when used in combination with alcohol. When he gave it to me, this doctor knew that I had not stopped drinking. I had always told the truth about that.

At last I told this doctor that I felt I was getting nowhere, and that I planned to go to AA. Though he had been unable to help me, he did not encourage me to go. He believed that AA is only for people who are down and out and he told me that I would never find a group in which I could be comfortable. Instead, I found hope and love and warmth from my first AA meeting. I have been sober for several years now, and my life has changed dramatically for the better. [a forty-nine-year-old woman]

You no longer have to be alone, feel guilty, or hide. Help and support are available in every neighbourhood. Your anonymity will be protected.

You must first get sober and stay sober. You may need a detoxification regime* to get sober, and AA to keep sober. Once you are sober, you may want to work on your problems. If you choose to work with a therapist, it is important to find someone who has a clear understanding of AA and can help you to use both systems effectively.[19] Many therapists will urge an alcoholic to go to AA if she is not already doing so. DAWN (see Organizations) is a campaigning group which can give information about help in the London area.

Helping Someone We Care About

When someone we care about has a drinking or drug problem, it is not easy to find the best way to help. Helping a friend or family member acknowledge that

---

*In Britain it will probably be necessary to get a referral to a special addiction unit in a psychiatric hospital or to 'go private' at considerable cost. Your GP can advise, but for both NHS and private referrals you must 'come clean' with her as a first step.

she or he has a problem can be one way to make a difference.

My best friend became an alcoholic and was progressively getting worse. She came from a teetotal family, and I knew how the conflict between her upbringing and her secretive drinking was tearing her apart, in addition to the physical destruction of alcoholism. I assumed she would deny any accusation with vigour, and was very fearful that she might be so angry she would end our friendship, an outcome I would find intolerable. After three years, I knew that I could no longer call myself a friend if I continued to ignore what she was doing. I arranged a day's outing and confronted her. She was so relieved! Nobody in her family had acknowledged what she was doing and she had concealed it from her doctor. As always, with confrontation, my only regret was that it took me so long to be able to do it. [a fifty-seven-year-old woman]

When we are closely involved with alcoholics – whether our spouses, lovers, parents, or children – we tend to become caught up in the illness as well. We spend prolonged periods of time trying to change our loved ones and convince them that they are destroying themselves by continuing to drink. We find ourselves fighting a losing battle to maintain some semblance of normality, unable to believe that the presence of alcoholism in our lives is permanent. The sooner we get help for ourselves or for our teenaged children from Al-Anon, the sooner we will learn how to live our own lives, how to put the responsibility on the alcoholic for her or his own behaviour, and not shoulder the blame ourselves.

We women are such good nurturers that we are usually loyal to our relationships even when we suffer as a result. Alcoholism is one disease in which the effort to smooth over and solve problems all by ourselves is misplaced. We can become what has been called a co-alcoholic or para-alcoholic, exhibiting the same denial, guilt, and blame as the alcoholic. The responsibility for alcoholism should rest squarely on the alcoholic – where it belongs. Even after many years of unhappy marriages and other close relationships with alcoholics, women have been able, through AA and other organizations, to reconstruct their own lives.

Over-the-Counter and Prescription Drugs

Although people over sixty-five make up 11 per cent of the US population, they use about 25 per cent of all dispensed drugs,[20] and figures for the UK are similar – and growing. In Britain, women are prescribed twice as many psychotropic (mood-changing) drugs as men – most of them tranquillizers –

while some doctors prescribe other drugs to women for conditions that in men don't get treated with medicines. In fact, men use more over-the-counter (OTC) drugs than women. In the United States in 1986 consumers spent an estimated $21.3 billion on 1.51 million prescription drugs.[21] Latest figure (1986) for NHS prescriptions in England and Wales was £323 million (not including hospital dispensaries).

Many of these drugs may be needed, even life-saving, but many are not. Often old prescriptions are not re-evaluated for continued need and for interactions with new prescriptions and with OTC preparations. 'Polypharmacy' is the term used to describe taking too many, or excessive amounts of, drugs at a time. It is common among older women who may be seeing several physicians for different conditions.

Drug companies, in business for profit, have offered new products to the market while sometimes failing to report adverse and life-threatening reactions to drugs.[22] The US Food and Drug Administration and its British equivalent, the Committee on the Safety of Medicines, continue to permit drugs on the market that later prove harmful and have to be withdrawn. Do not agree to use a drug which has been on the market for less than four years unless you are willing to be part of an experiment.[23]

Harmful effects from drug interactions are too numerous to list here, so always inform your doctor of everything you are using (prescriptions, OTC, and vitamin supplements) and always double-check with your pharmacist. OTC drugs and vitamins, herbs, and supplements from health-food stores can be just as potent and dangerous as prescription drugs. Do not take leftover or other people's medicines.

Most drug dosages should be adjusted to the size and the age of the person taking the drug. Women at any age may require lower drug dosages than men because of women's lower body weight and mass. We become even more sensitive to drugs over time because, as we age, drugs are metabolized more slowly, the kidneys and the liver excrete them more slowly, and so they remain in the body longer. Also, as we age, some muscle mass turns to fat, so many drugs that can be stored in fat tissue, such as tranquillizers, stay in the body a longer time, increasing the likelihood of addiction even from low, infrequent doses. Drug companies have only recently started testing the effects of drugs on older people and still do not distinguish the more severe effects of drugs on people over the age of seventy from the effects on the whole group over fifty. Drugs may be harmful or may be taken in too high doses if individual adjustments and frequent re-evaluations are not made. One study of older persons admitted to an American state mental hospital found that 15 per cent were actually suffering from drug toxicities rather than from dementia or other mental illness.[24] There are similar findings in the rest of the older population.

Over half the adult women in the United States have used tranquillizers, sedatives, and amphetamines (stimulants often used in 'diet pills'). These drugs are legally available in Britain, too, and are the most commonly abused classes of drugs among older women. The practice of some doctors freely to write prescriptions for these types of controlled drugs has declined in Britain in recent years, following media publicity highlighting their terrible addictive properties and the publication to doctors of guidelines pointing out the dangers of repeat prescriptions. In theory, tranquillizers should now be prescribed for limited periods only, but we still hear from women who have been taking them for years and are finding it difficult to convince their doctors that they need help in weaning themselves off the drugs. Information is available from SCODA, TRANX and Release for groups and individuals (see Organizations).

Tranquillizers can't cure anything by themselves. Their use is an attempt to treat medically what is really a social problem – the stress and isolation many women (especially older ones) experience. For information about groups offering support, contact the Council for Involuntary Tranquillizer Addiction and the National Tranquillizer Advice Centre (see Organizations).

We don't know the long-term effects of illegal 'recreational' drugs. We do know, though, that marijuana can damage the respiratory system and that cocaine is addictive and can cause sudden death through its action on the heart. The continued use of such substances will add to the health problems of future generations of older women who started using such drugs when they were young.

It's also important to be aware of the possible dangers of combining prescription or recreational drugs with alcohol. Doctors don't always warn their patients about this, and there have been deaths or serious accidents caused by people topping up pills with alcohol.

It is essential that medical schools include more courses on alcohol and drug abuse and related illnesses. Pharmacists should write warnings on bottles and caution their customers. Despite the fact that these addictions are national problems with enormous impact on the public, only a few medical schools teach their students anything at all about them. Doctors often assume we do not feel satisfied with our visit unless we come away with a prescription. One study, however, showed that 72 per cent of the patients surveyed preferred a non-drug remedy when it and a drug were both offered and fully explained.[25] We might benefit more from explanations, answers to our questions, support, and sound practical advice than from drugs. Unfortunately, training of doctors in these approaches is even weaker than their training in pharmacology.

It is important to know what the drugs we take can do for us and to us. Antihistamines, for instance, frequently cause drowsiness. Some other cold medicines contain drugs to clear stuffy noses (vasoconstrictors), which may make you feel jumpy, and caffeine to keep you active when you probably should be resting in bed. Most liquid cold preparations and mouthwashes contain alcohol; many preparations and vitamins contain sugar. Be fore-warned: the advertising for many products never mentions that the drugs they contain could cause dependency or undesirable interactions with other drugs.

When considering any medication, consult your doctor or practice nurse and your chemist. Bring a list of all the prescription and non-prescription preparations you are using. Report any allergies or reactions to medication you suffered in the past. Seek the answers to the following questions:[26]

1. What are both the brand name and the scientific (generic) name of the medication, and what is it supposed to do?
2. How do I store it and take it, and for how long? What should I do if I miss a dose?
3. What foods, drinks, other medicines, and activities should I avoid while taking this medicine? What do I especially need?
4. What other effects might I have while taking this drug, and what should I do if they occur?
5. Is there any written information available about this medicine?

Find out as much as you can so you can take the medication in the most beneficial way. Do not, for example, crush a coated tablet, for the coating has been put on to protect you or to improve the drug's absorption.

Two common problems for which too many women habitually use harmful drugs are insomnia and constipation. Both are better dealt with by non-pharmaceutical methods.

Dealing with Insomnia

Some changes in sleep patterns may occur as we get older but at any age we need adequate, deep sleep for good health. Do not assume you have a problem just because you get less sleep than you used to. Judge by how you feel, not just by the number of hours you sleep. Some women have problems falling asleep; others may readily fall asleep, but wake up after only a few hours and have trouble going back to sleep. There are many things we can do to sleep better.

Worries and depression can cause sleeplessness. Many women will focus on the sleeplessness rather than on the causes of the worries and depression. If you seek and find the right kind of help for the underlying cause of the problem, you may be able to sleep better. Labelling the problems as insomnia will not solve either the problems or the insomnia, and may make it worse by starting a cycle in which you go to bed each night worrying about whether your 'insomnia' will keep you awake.

Many activities can interfere with sleep. Among them are eating late at night (especially sugar); having unsuspected caffeine in soft drinks, cocoa and chocolate, and tea; taking vitamin B or C before bed; not getting enough protein in your diet. Tryptophan is an amino acid which induces drowsiness. Since many tryptophan-rich foods are high in protein (milk, turkey, fish, meat), many people who avoid these foods may have trouble sleeping and may be helped by taking tryptophan (available at health-food shops and some chemists). This should be used only before bedtime and in small amounts.

Drugs are a common cause of sleep problems. Caffeine is not the only one. The complete list of prescription and OTC drugs that interfere with sleep is too long to include here. Just a few are: nicotine in cigarettes; pain relievers and cold remedies that contain caffeine or antihistamines; appetite suppressants; decongestants; drugs for asthma, high blood pressure, heart rhythm, and thyroid problems; and many others. Antihistamines (contained in cold remedies and OTC sleeping pills) and alcohol cause drowsiness initially but interfere with later sleep and can cause early awakening. The insomnia caused by certain conditions such as an overactive thyroid will be relieved when treated appropriately – not by sleeping pills.

Medications formulated to help you sleep, including sleeping pills, tranquillizers, and anti-anxiety drugs, can cause sleeplessness after their use is discontinued. They can also be addictive. Sleeping pills may make older people less alert, aggravate memory loss, and have other adverse effects, all which may be confused with dementia. Their use increases the likelihood of falls, and resultant broken hips or other broken bones. Chloral hydrate, still sometimes prescribed, interferes with rapid eye movement sleep (REM, the time when we dream), which is vital for mental health. While you might choose to use sleeping pills for a few nights in some special situation, you should be especially cautious as you get older. Smaller than usual doses will probably suffice.

Sleeping pills slow down respiratory function in some people and are particularly dangerous for people with sleep apnea (the sudden cessation of breathing during sleep) or heavy snoring. Sleep apnea may occur from a few times to several hundred times a night with or without heavy snoring. If your bed-partner or roommate tells you that your breathing seems to stop during sleep, you should seek medical advice, because this behaviour often signals a more serious problem.

To deal with sleeplessness:

- Try to go to sleep and get up at regular hours in whatever pattern suits you best. You may want to avoid daytime naps in order to sleep more hours at night, or you may feel better sleeping fewer hours at night and taking a daytime nap.

- Exercise during the day, not just before bed.
- Soak in a hot bath before bed, unless you have diabetes.
- Don't go to bed hungry but avoid eating a huge meal before bed. Being too full may disturb sleep. Try milk before bed, warm if you like. The tryptophan in milk will help you sleep.
- Try relaxation techniques. If something is on your mind, make a note to deal with the problem the next day and then try to forget it.
- Make your surroundings as comfortable as possible, including the bed, temperature and humidity, sound and light.
- Develop the association between bed and sleep. Follow the same rituals every night before going to bed. Do not read or write in bed. If you can't sleep, get out of bed and go back later.
- Keep a diary of your sleep patterns to help you identify problems and the success of changes you try.

I have a tape of the sound of ocean waves on a cassette by my bed. If I wake up in the middle of the night, I reach over and turn on the tape. It seems to crowd out distracting thoughts and lulls me back to sleep. [a fifty-five-year-old woman]

Dealing with Constipation

Laxatives are another commonly overused medication. Many of us were taught that we were supposed to have a bowel movement each and every day. In fact, though two thirds of the women in a survey claimed one bowel movement per day, the normal variation was between three times a day and twice a week.[27] Consider yourself constipated only if your customary pattern changes or if you have hard, difficult-to-pass stools.

Changes in diet can alleviate constipation. White flour products with or without sugar are the most common culprit. Add more natural fibre by eating plenty of vegetables, fruit, and whole grains as well as breads and cereals that contain bran. Drink eight to ten glasses of fluid each day, more on very hot days or if you are sweating heavily from work or exercise. Fresh fruit and fruit juices, especially prune juice, can have a laxative effect. Additional fluids are necessary if you add bran to your diet in order to prevent the stool from becoming too bulky and hard. Large amounts of caffeine usually cause diarrhoea but in some women may cause constipation. Withdrawing from coffee may also cause constipation temporarily.

Activity is needed to keep the bowels active. A little exercise each day, especially walking, does wonders. Exercise also alleviates stress, anxiety, and depression, which can all cause constipation. Strengthening weak abdominal and pelvic muscles can help elimination. It is particularly important to keep the stool soft if you have a weakening in the wall of the rectum (a rectocele) in which the faeces can collect.

Many women become constipated because they are too busy to take time in the toilet. They may 'hold it' too long, just as they hold urine too long, losing awareness of their need to 'go' (see Urinary Incontinence chapter). Go to the toilet at regular times but do not strain. Holding the breath while pushing can raise blood pressure. If you can't move your bowels, relax and try later.

Common medications and vitamins can affect bowel movements. You will have to make the decision for yourself. For example, magnesium-aluminium antacids are the most effective for people who suffer from wind and other problems that might be relieved by an antacid. However, milk of magnesia can cause diarrhoea, so the aluminium is added to counteract it.[28] Aluminium antacids interfere with the absorption of calcium. Iron supplements often cause constipation. Taking vitamin C increases the absorption of the iron and also helps alleviate the constipation. Many other drugs, especially painkillers, slow down the bowels.

One of the most common causes of chronic constipation is the use of laxatives. The body can become habituated to the laxatives and lose the ability to function normally without them. Laxatives also interfere with the body's absorption of vitamins, minerals, and many medications. If you are used to laxatives, try tapering off gradually while improving your eating habits and exercising regularly.

While you are tapering off, use the type of laxative most suitable for your problems. Read the labels so you will know what you are taking. Bulk laxatives (such as psyllium seed) add bulk to the stool. Lubricants (such as docusate sodium) encourage water to enter the stool, thereby increasing its bulk and softness. Salt laxatives (such as milk of magnesia) also hold water, making the stool softer and bulkier, but are not recommended for those on low-salt diets. Irritant drugs (such as castor oil or senna) stimulate the intestinal nerves, thus increasing bowel activity. Glycerin suppositories stimulate the bowel muscle and lubricate the stool already in the rectum. Mineral oil helps lubricate stools higher in the intestines but prevents absorption of many needed nutrients. If it is necessary to use mineral oil, take it at 6 a.m. and take a supplement of fat-soluble vitamins at 6 p.m.

Dealing with Pain

Many people overuse and misuse pain medication. They may become addicted to pain medication and continue its use long after the pain has stopped. Others suffer needlessly from pain because they fear reliance on medication, or addiction. Our instinct to pull away from something painful – such as a hot cooker – has great survival value. Pain can be a signal to protect ourselves or a warning for us to pay attention. Ignoring pain can put us in great danger, and even cause death. People vary in how they interpret and tolerate pain signals, and there are as yet few ways to measure how much pain people feel. Understanding our bodies will help us know when to seek help.

We have to cope not only with pain, but with what the pain means to us – usually our fear of what we think might be causing the pain, or fear that the pain will not end. Sometimes we ignore pain that could easily be helped because we fear a more serious cause. Stress and pain have a close relationship. It's easy to understand that being in pain stresses us. But stress can also cause or intensify pain. When pain does not have a clear-cut cause or, worse, is interpreted as signalling a dangerous illness, it can feel more intense. Factors such as tension or tightening up, anxiety, depression, and fatigue can modulate the pain threshold.

There are many pains for which no specific cause can be found, or for which there is no single effective cure. That does not mean that our pain is imaginary or should be dismissed. Unfortunately, many doctors believe that much of women's pain is imaginary or a device for getting attention. All pain is real. We should not be told that we must just learn to live with pain; we should be given specific suggestions on how to do it.

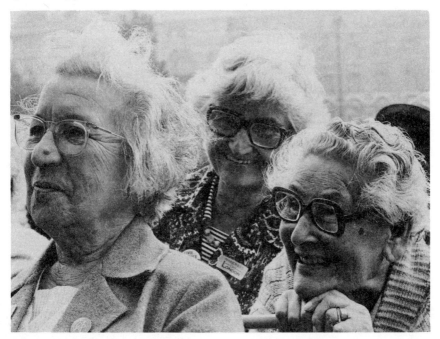

Traditional healing methods, many from Eastern medicine and philosophy, approach pain as if it were blocked energy. The practitioner of such methods should be our partner in exploring the possible connections between our present pain and our entire life-style – day-to-day habits of eating, exercise, emotional patterns, social relationships, occupation, creative and spiritual connections – as well as possible disease. We can learn to use deep breathing and relaxation exercises to control and manage pain. Some of us have used the techniques learned in childbirth classes throughout our lives. Techniques such as relaxation, meditation, massage, yoga, and acupuncture are helpful for managing pain. Although these techniques seem to work particularly well with chronic pain (pain lasting more than six months), they can also help us with acute pain. In a situation of acute, even life-threatening, pain that requires immediate emergency medical care, such as a heart attack, techniques learned from relaxation, meditation, and self-hypnosis can help us avoid panic and cope with pain.

Western medicine tends to see pain as an enemy, to be destroyed as soon as possible. The focus is on the specific body parts that hurt: what is the cause, what is the cure? The doctor is the expert and has the primary responsibility for finding the cure. But Western medicine is beginning to combine Eastern mind-body concepts with modern technology to develop techniques – such as biofeedback – which can be useful in pain control. Other new methods include TENS and PCA. TENS (transcutaneous electrical nerve stimulation) sends measured pulses of electric current to the pain sites through electrodes attached to the skin, providing significant but temporary relief for up to 70 per cent of the users. Some researchers think TENS causes the body to release natural opiates called endorphins; others think it interferes with the transmission of pain signals. Patient-controlled analgesia (PCA) is an innovation that provides individualized pain control. This technique utilizes a device that permits intravenous self-administration of narcotic drugs within limits of dose and frequency established with the doctor.[29]

Pain clinics, which now exist in some cities, focus on the whole person and may use both Western and traditional techniques appropriate to the individual. As one client in a pain-relief clinic said, 'It's a relief to be treated as a person, instead of as a hip problem.' This approach, which should be used by all health care providers, invites us to be more active on our own behalf, befriending those parts of us that have hurt for so long that we may have given up on them – our stiff knees, miserable back, perpetual headaches.

I've changed my attitude toward pain. I don't think of my foot that's hurting as a separate, bad part of me – something to be angry at. I now try to take a more caregiving approach, to see what kind of special attention it wants. I massage my feet and calves every night. The trouble with having the doctor be the only one who can treat you is that, if he can't do it, then you're a goner. It's good I've found some things I can do for myself to help myself feel better. [a thirty-five-year-old woman]

Once we adopt a body-befriending approach to pain management, we can create many self-help techniques. There are many things that alleviate pain, such as exhaling or panting rather than holding the breath while we do physical work, thinking about something else more pleasant while the dentist drills, stopping negative self-talk, soothing painful areas with light strokes. Many others are well known: taking a hot bath or a cold shower, taking a walk, distracting ourselves by doing some favourite thing. It's difficult to feel depressed when we are singing or to feel anxious while we are taking slow, deep breaths.

There are many painkilling drugs, including aspirin, paracetamol, Brufen, codeine, and morphine. All pain-relieving drugs have undesirable and potentially harmful effects. They may cloud our consciousness at the very time when we might wish to get as much out of life as possible.

On the other hand, many of us are so fearful of pain medication that we deprive ourselves of comfort and help when we could most use it. Pain is very tiring; pain can use up the energy we need for caring for ourselves and managing the condition causing the pain. Often a moderate and careful use of pain medication can help us have the strength we need for dealing with the cause. Using the non-drug pain-relief methods already described can reduce our need for medication. Smaller, more frequent doses of pain medication may keep us comfortable and result in use of less medication than if we wait until the pain becomes so severe that we need massive doses to feel relief. Avoid drugs or combinations of pain-relieving drugs that make you sleepy without reducing pain.[30]

When faced with severe pain, we should be able to choose the extent of pain relief that suits us. Each woman has her own level of pain tolerance. When death is imminent, we need not fear addiction. Especially at that time we should be able to remain in control and be able to choose among all options.

NOTES

[1] US Office of the Assistant Secretary for Health and Surgeon General, *The Health Consequences of Smoking: The Changing Cigarette. A Report of the Surgeon General*. Rockville, Md.: US Department of Health and Human Services, Public Health Service, 1981.

[2] G. H. Miller and D. R. Gerstein, 'The Life Expectancy of Nonsmoking Men and Women'. *Public Health Reports*, Vol. 98, 1983, pp. 343–9. Quoted in Jonathan E. Fielding, 'Smoking: Health Effects and Control'. *The New England Journal of Medicine*, Vol. 313, No. 8, 22 August 1985, p. 491.

[3]American Cancer Society, *1985 Cancer Facts and Figures*, p. 9.

[4]Massachusetts Department of Public Health/ Massachusetts Hospital Association brochure, 'Are You Really a Non-Smoker?'

[5]American Cancer Society, op. cit., p. 17.

[6]Miller and Gerstein, op. cit.

[7]Susan Okie, 'The Press and Cigarette Ads: Smoke Gets in Their Eyes'. *Healthlink*, March 1986, pp. 54–5.

[8]Paul Raeburn, 'Caffeine Tied to Panic Attacks in Over 2 Million People'. Associated Press, printed in *The Boston Globe*, 19 October 1986, p. 23.

[9]Frances Sheridan Goulart, *The Caffeine Book: A User's and Abuser's Guide*. New York: Dodd, Mead & Co., 1984. Thorough coverage of health effects of caffeine-containing foods and beverages.

[10]Hershel Jick et al., 'Coffee and Myocardial Infarction: A Report from the Boston Collaborative Drug Surveillance Project'. *The New England Journal of Medicine*, Vol. 289, No. 2, 12 July 1973, pp. 63–7.

[11]Goulart, op. cit.

[12]Jean Kinney and Gwen Leaton, *Loosening the Grip*. St Louis, Mo.: C. V. Mosby Co., 1978, p. 223.

[13]Barbara Gordon, *I'm Dancing as Fast as I Can*. New York: Harper & Row, 1979, pp. 304–5.

[14]*Report on the White House Mini-Conference on Older Women*, Alcoholism and Drug Abuse Section, 1980, p. 36.

[15]Jacob A. Brody, 'Aging and Alcohol Abuse', in *Nature and Extent of Alcohol Problems Among the Elderly*. Presented at the White House Conference on Aging, Washington, DC, 1981, p. 305.

[16]Jonica D. Homiller, *Women and Alcohol: A Guide for State and Local Decision Makers*.

Washington, DC: The Council of State Authorities, Alcohol and Drug Problems Association of North America, 1977, p. 15.

[17]Nancy Taylor, *Alcohol Abuse Prevention Among Women: A Community Approach*. Presented at the National Council on Alcoholism, Washington, DC, 1982, p. 1.

[18]C. Samuel Mullin, *Medical Consequences of Chronic Alcohol Abuse*. Boston: Massachusetts Department of Public Health, Division of Alcoholism, 1983.

[19]Alvin Rosen, 'Psychotherapy and Alcoholics Anonymous. Can They Be Coordinated?' *Bulletin of the Menninger Clinic*, Vol. 45, No. 3, 1981, pp. 229–46.

[20]Annabel Hecht, 'Medicine and the Elderly'. *FDA Consumer*, September 1983, p. 20.

[21]Estimate obtained by Carlos Ortiz of CVS from Prescription Drug Services of Phoenix, Ariz.

[22]'Prescription Drug Pushers' and 'Five Dangerous Drugs'. *Health Letter*, Vol. 3, July– August 1986, pp. 1, 12.

[23]'Another Dangerous Drug'. *Health Letter*, Vol. 2, No. 1, March–April 1986, p. 1.

[24]Report of the Public Health Service Task Force on Women's Health Issues'. *Public Health Reports*, Vol. 100, No. 1, January– February 1985, p. 96.

[25]Gail Povar et al., 'Patients' Therapeutic Preferences in an Ambulatory Care Setting'. *American Journal of Public Health*, Vol. 74, No. 12, December 1984, pp. 1395–7.

[26]Adapted from the National Council on Patient Information and Education.

[27]Marie Feltin, *A Woman's Guide to Good Health After 50*. An AARP Book. Glenview, Ill.: Scott, Foresman & Co., 1987, p. 174.

[28]'Gas, Heartburn and Antacids'. *Living Healthy*, Vol. 3, No. 3, August 1980, pp. 1–12.

[29]National Institutes of Health, 'The Integrated Approach to the Management of

Pain'. *Consensus Development Conference Statement*, Vol. 6, No. 3, 19–21 May 1986.

[30]Kathleen M. Foley, 'The Treatment of Cancer Pain'. *The New England Journal of Medicine*, Vol. 313, No. 2, 11 July 1985, pp. 84–95.

BOOKS AND PUBLICATIONS

Bobbie Jacobson, *Beating the Ladykillers: Women and Smoking*. London: Pluto Press, 1986. How to stop smoking.

J. and J. Chick, *Drinking Problems*. Edinburgh: Churchill Livingstone, 1984.

Brigid McGonville, *Women under the Influence*. London: Virago Press, 1983 (out of print but probably available from libraries).

Celia Haddon, *Women and Tranquillizers*. London: Sheldon Press, 1984.

National Extension College, *That's the Limit*. Booklet on alcoholism, free from local health education units.

Health Education Authority, *A Smoker's Guide to Giving Up*.

Health Education Authority, *Breathing Other People's Smoke*.

Janette Pleshette, *Overcoming Addictions*. Wellingborough: Thorsons, 1989.

3
Our Looks and Our Lives

Herstory – in a Plate

Her face reminds me of my
  grandmother's antique plate –
    cracked with fine-lined patterns
    of living.
I can see either the beauty or the imperfection –
  Usually I see the beauty,
    except when she irritates me, or my
      fears of my own mortality block my vision.
We are both – mortal and perfect –
  beautiful and imperfect –
    a crazed pattern of sanity
    in a cracked world –
  a throwback to another time,
    and a vision yet
    to be.

MOLLY SMITH STRONG

As we get older, we have to come to terms with our changing appearance and others' reactions to it. We get wrinkles, our hair turns grey, and our body weight changes and is redistributed. Chronic diseases or disabling conditions can also affect the way we see our bodies. Such challenges require fresh sources of strength and a reassessment of our interests, abilities, and needs.

Looking Older – What It Means to Us

Those of us who grew up knowing and loving our grandparents or other older people probably remember loving their wrinkled faces. In the years before we learned to think of the signs of ageing as 'unattractive', a wrinkled face was often the most loving and the most beloved face we knew. However, as adults we live in an environment in which standards of beauty are important, narrow, and restricted to the young.

I have no passion to look eighteen forever, but I still have vanity. I rather hate looking at that network of wrinkles that looks like a traffic jam – but there it is! What can you do about it? [a sixty-nine-year-old woman]

Looking older can be hard on us, since as women we are brought up to please others rather than ourselves, and to value ourselves by how pleasing we are to others. This makes us especially vulnerable to the idea that through makeup, hair dyes, face-lifts, diets, and clothes we can – and must – live up to a certain ideal of beauty. Many of us were very hard on ourselves in our younger years, not beginning to accept or like our faces or bodies until we were in our late thirties or early forties. We may have hardly overcome early prejudices against ourselves – hips too large, nose too small – when we are faced with another: ageism.

When I was thirty-eight I looked at my naked body in the mirror, and for the first time in my life thought, 'Wow, nice!' And then I started ageing. [a fifty-two-year-old woman]

The quest for physical perfection may be taken more seriously by women in the United States than by women in other countries. America is a young and powerful country and it admires the young and powerful. The message in Britain, too, is that we only count if we are white, slender, attractive, able-bodied – and young. For some women, especially in midlife, this narrow standard of acceptability leads to a period of grieving over the loss of 'peak' years. Barbara MacDonald (age sixty-nine), co-author of a book on ageism, reflects on her own ageing:

Sometimes lately . . . I see my arm with the skin hanging loosely from my forearm and cannot believe that it is really my own. It seems disconnected from me; it is someone else's. It is the arm of an old woman. It is the arm of such old women as I myself have seen, sitting on benches in the sun with their hands folded in their laps; old women I have turned away from. I wonder now how and when these arms I see came to be my own – arms I cannot turn away from.[1]

Middle-aged men are a possible exception to the generally narrow standard of looks. According to one study, they are considered even more attractive than young men. This same study showed that middle-aged women are considered less attractive than young women, and that old men and women are both considered less attractive than the young or middle-aged. Some researchers think that middle-aged men gain in attractiveness because others see them as being at the peak of success in their social roles. Conversely, middle-aged women, seen primarily as mothers, are considered to be past their social usefulness because they are no longer bearers of children.[2] If looks are associated with usefulness and power, it may be that the looks of old age are considered unattractive because the elderly are seen as useless and powerless. As middle-aged and older women become more powerful, others may see them as more attractive. We may see ourselves as more attractive as well.

Sometimes I think of the alternatives to looking older, and I wonder what it would be like to have my face frozen the way it was in my thirties, and I think – that would be ridiculous! That's not me, that doesn't reflect the years I've lived and all the things I've experienced. I don't want to deny my experiences and I feel that if I dislike my ageing looks I'm denying all the wonderful parts of my life. I don't want to do that. [a forty-eight-year-old woman]

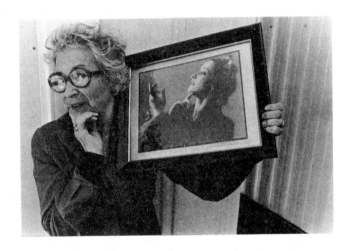

Women's responses to looking older vary greatly. Women who grew up in warmly affectionate families where they were hugged, kissed, and cuddled, for example, tend to accept their bodies as they are. There are indications that women whose families provided opportunities for physical activity or who were athletes at school and college feel more positive about their looks than women without such experiences.[3] In general, warm, close family relationships and physical activity foster self-confidence and high self-esteem. When self-esteem is high, body image is often positive. Considering the importance of athletics and self-esteem, it is no surprise that studies show that men (always encouraged to participate in sports) *over*rate their body image, thinking that others have a higher opinion of their looks than they actually do, while women *under*rate their body image, thinking others have a lower opinion of their looks than they do.[4]

If you were considered unusually attractive as a younger woman, looking older may be more difficult for you than for a woman who never set great store by her looks. A woman who is constantly praised for being pretty may come to believe that her worth as a person depends on her looks. A woman who never considered herself pretty, however, has already dealt with that issue and gone beyond it.

Women who are concerned about looking older seem to experience this concern during midlife up to their middle or late sixties. In fact, many women in midlife like *getting* older; they feel freer and more confident. What they don't like is *looking* older.[5]

I'm forty-three now and this whole past year I've felt a sense of getting older which I never did before. When I look in the mirror, I don't like what I see, so I don't look at myself. When I go somewhere I try to forget about what I look like, and that isn't the way it used to be. I used to think, 'Today I look good!'

In later years, this concern tends to disappear. It seems that the anticipation of looking older is more distressing than the actual experience. Perhaps with the years we learn to place greater value on our inner qualities. Also our own or our partner's health and energy become more important, and losses or other concerns can become paramount.[6]

Body changes as a result of health problems can also cause a temporary or permanent difference in the way we see ourselves. Skin diseases, scaly dryness or chapping of the skin, a stoop due to osteoporosis, and swelling of the joints as a result of arthritis are all visible changes.

I am trying to recognize that my hands are indeed a part of me, and a part of me that I love. Because I do a great deal with my hands, of course, and they are very capable despite the fact that they have arthritic swelling. And I realize that I have indeed been taken in by what a woman's hands should look like, and mostly they're supposed to look pretty useless. My hands don't look useless at all. In fact they look as though they've been used a great deal. [a sixty-four-year-old woman]

Appliances such as a hearing aid, pacemaker, stick, or walking frame can change our body image, especially when we first begin to wear or use them. They often seem much larger and more conspicuous to us than to anyone else. The effects of drugs, scars or a limp from operations or accidents, and amputated limbs or organs can profoundly influence our body image. Integrat-

ing such changes into our self-image is an important factor in feeling whole
again despite the loss.

*In a bathing suit I'm not so hot because there is a huge gouge where one hip was taken
out, and the incision got infected. That is hard for small children to have to look at so
I wear very matronly bathing suits. So my image of myself as a sexy-looking woman
went, and I decided to be quaint – a quaint old lady.* [a sixty-nine-year-old
woman]

As we grow older we may become slightly shorter due to the gradual drying
of the discs of the spine or compression fractures caused by osteoporosis.
Otherwise, most of the visible changes associated with age occur in the skin,
hair, and underlying muscles and fatty tissue.

Since the skin is susceptible to influences from inside and outside the body,
it is hard to distinguish between 'normal' signs of ageing and those caused by
environmental damage, such as overexposure to sunlight. Skin changes which
normally occur with time can be accelerated by exposure to the elements,
especially radiation from the sun. Black and olive-skinned women experience a
slower rate of change with age, partly because of the larger amounts of melanin
(pigment) in their skin. Some women find as they age that they sunburn more
easily. All women can protect themselves against skin damage and skin cancer
by avoiding tanning and sunburning.*

Skin cells grow more slowly with age, and the outer layer of skin is not shed
and replaced at the same rate as in younger years. Changes in a protein called
collagen make the skin stiffer and less pliable, and some sebaceous glands
which provide oil for the hair and skin become less active. With age, cells lose
some of their ability to retain water, causing dryness. Some women relieve
dryness and itching by patting themselves dry after washing, and applying
cream or oil while the skin is still moist. It can also help to bathe less often and
to use only a mild or creamy soap or no soap at all on trouble areas.

As the skin loses tone and elasticity it sags and wrinkles, especially in areas
where there is frequent movement, such as the face, neck, and joints. Sagging
is also caused by the pull of gravity over the years. The underlying muscles and
fatty tissue undergo similar changes. Small blood vessels become more fragile
due to thinning of the vessel walls, and can cause frequent black-and-blue
marks. 'Age spots' (also called 'liver spots') may appear. They would be more
appropriately called sun spots, since they are caused by exposure to sunlight
over the years. Hair becomes thinner as hair follicles decrease their activity,
and greyer as cells stop producing a colour-determining pigment. These

---

*See page 103 on need for obtaining vitamin D from sunlight.

gradual changes are a part of the cycle of life, and everyone who lives long enough will experience some of them.

How Weight Influences the Way We See Ourselves

As we grow older, many of us tend to gain weight. Since our metabolism slows down, our bodies need fewer calories, yet we often consume the same amount of food as in our younger years (see Weighty Issues chapter). Many of us get less exercise or have disabling conditions that keep us sedentary. Weight gain in our older years can be particularly hard to accept because we are also trying to come to terms with other changes in our bodies.

I went to Weight Watchers and lost eight pounds. But I gained them right back. Then last summer I fractured my shoulder. I was at home a lot. It was a terribly hot summer. The only exercise I got was a little walk every day. That walk always included a stop for an ice cream. Now I look in the mirror and I say: 'You are fat!' and I don't like it. [a seventy-three-year-old woman]

Studies have shown that the value placed on thinness in advertising has a strong impact on us. Many women live in constant fear of gaining another pound. We tend to see ourselves as overweight even when we are within what is generally considered a desirable weight range. Women want to be even thinner than men want them to be.[7] The influence of advertising is also evident in the growing incidence of eating disorders such as anorexia and bulimia in middle-aged women.[8]

It isn't easy to fight the effects of advertising single-handedly. Through body-image workshops, reading, or exercise, we can make our image of ourselves more positive. It is worth trying to accept our size rather than using our energy disliking our bodies and going on unnecessary diets.

When I swim or walk regularly I feel stronger and more energetic and my body is more flexible. My weight stays the same but people say to me, 'You've lost weight!' as if only pounds mattered. [a fifty-three-year-old woman]

Some women think that if they learn to accept and love their bodies they will just eat everything and gain more weight. Only punishment through diet can work, they believe. But, in fact, many women have found that if you punish your body you cannot lead it to a positive, healthy state. 'You have to love your body *before* you can change it – if indeed you wish to change it once you love it.'[9]

Belly dancing is an example of an exercise only weighty women can do well.

The movements make you feel sensuous, not heavy. Belly dancers love their bellies, have fun 'throwing their weight around', and benefit from the exercise.

The 'Beauty' Business

As they grow older, many women attempt to mask or alter their physical appearance. Even the poorest women spend money on cosmetics.* Some of us wear makeup, or more of it, and dye our hair. According to one survey, most women who colour their hair do so to cover the grey. This is most common among women in their forties and fifties. Forty-five per cent of American women dye their hair.[10]

It is hard to resist the temptation to alter our appearance, since in every store we see bottles, tubes, and jars containing cosmetics advertised to make us more attractive and younger-looking. The cosmetics industry makes millions of pounds by reinforcing the message that we need not, dare not, look older. As the population ages, advertisements abound for products which are said to prevent or hide wrinkles.

Advertisements for skin care preparations and advice columns in the women's magazines spell out an impossible prescription: clear, fresh, firm, and youthful [skin] . . . in short, a skin that shows no sign of physical maturity, hard work, aggravation, exhaustion, hormonal changes, the effects of pregnancy, or the normal wear and tear of daily living.[11]

Cosmetics manufacturers are not required to obtain Committee on Safety of Medicines approval before putting their products on the market. Responsible manufacturers test their products for safety before marketing. Still, many cosmetics contain dangerous substances. One hundred cosmetic ingredients are suspected chemical hazards, according to the American National Institute of Occupational Safety and Health.[12] Many of these hazardous substances can be absorbed through the skin, including the scalp. Be wary of cosmetics that list hormones in the ingredients. They usually contain oestrogen, which can affect the body's hormonal balance. Reported effects of hormonal cosmetics include vaginal bleeding in women over sixty-five.[13] Lipstick enters the body through the throat along with food and drink. Many lipsticks and other cosmetics contain colour additives that cause cancer in laboratory animals.

---

*There are signs that more and more men, new victims of the youth culture, are becoming intensely concerned about looks and ageing. More men buy cosmetics and undergo plastic surgery and hair transplants than ever before. Shari Miller, 'A New Image', US *Vogue*, January 1985, p. 243.

These colours include reds and orange (azo dyes) with 'E' numbers which must be shown on processed foods' labels, and some of which may provoke hypersensitive reactions.[14] Petroleum-based hair dyes, mostly in dark shades, cause cancer in laboratory animals. If you do colour your hair, a hair crayon, available from a beauty-supply store, can help you use less hair dye by extending the time between hair-dyeing applications.

For a small but growing number of women, the need to look young or thin may be so strong that they choose to undergo surgical procedures such as face or eyelid lifts, or surgery that slenderizes the abdomen, thighs, or buttocks, or de-wrinkles hands.* Women seem to be choosing such operations earlier, between forty and fifty – even in their thirties. Some women hope that plastic surgery will lead to a major life change, but surgery is no guarantee that a woman will get or keep a partner or a job, nor is it a cure for low self-esteem.

Plastic surgery increased 61 per cent between 1981 and 1984, making it one of the fastest-growing medical specialties in the US.[15]

The risks of plastic surgery include scarring, severing of a facial nerve, infection, haemorrhage, and blockage of a blood vessel in the lung or brain. The latter three risks can cause severe impairment and, in rare cases, even death.[16] Other complications include blindness caused by bleeding behind the eyes. High blood pressure can cause excessive bleeding during surgery. Women who take large amounts of aspirin should stop five to seven days prior to surgery, since the drug interferes with clotting. A recent study showed that 10 per cent of people who had face-lifts experienced skin slough, the death of skin from inadequate blood supply, after surgery. The majority of those who experienced skin slough smoked more than one pack of cigarettes a day.

In Britain, plastic or cosmetic surgery can be done under the NHS in cases where there is severe disfigurement or conditions which are causing mental distress to the patient. However, it is still possible to get cosmetic surgery in private clinics advertised in the press, and it is *essential* not only to get a referral to a reputable surgeon through your GP, but to make sure that the surgeon is a member of the British Association of Aesthetic Plastic Surgeons. 'Cowboy' plastic surgeons have irretrievably damaged many women undergoing face-lifts, breast augmentation, and the like.

Yet at a time of life when our risks of medical complications are going up, why expose ourselves to the additional hazards of unnecessary surgery and anaesthesia?

---

*Wrinkles, sags, and fat deposits are called 'deformities' in medical literature on cosmetic surgery.

The Social Impact of Looking Older

Relationships with Men

Many women fear that looking older means losing the power to attract men. This can mean losing the excitement of sexual attraction and the warmth of physical intimacy. For many women, men have played the role of the great critics of their lives. Men's opinions of our outward appearances, their acceptance or rejection of us based on our looks, have strongly influenced the way we see ourselves.

Last year when a much younger man I was very attracted to told me what he really wanted was friendship, I felt shattered. I assumed that he rejected me sexually because of my age, and that started a whole train of bad feelings about myself – about growing older and not having anybody love me anymore – especially men. That blow has been repaired by the love and attention of another man, which is wonderful. Yet it bothers me that I seem to be so reliant on the opinions of men, as though I didn't have it within me just to care about myself. It's amazing – since I met this other man I feel much, much better about myself. It's as though I look in the mirror and see a different person – as though my whole outward appearance changes in my own eyes, to be built up or torn down by someone else. [a forty-five-year-old woman]

Unattached women seeking a sexual partner are often more concerned with signs of age than those who feel secure in a marriage or relationship.[17] Midlife divorce can heighten a woman's sense of competition, throwing her back into the 'dating game'.

Women who feel sexually dissatisfied in long-standing marriages or relationships may be frustrated because they believe that their age makes it impossible to have new sexual experiences.

I have tried to talk about sexuality with my husband but it's been a long time, a long marriage, and it's very hard to change things. Then when I read The Hite Report *I suddenly found myself validated. I hadn't known that I had any sexual rights and that the desires that I had were normal desires of a so-called normal woman. It made me feel a lot better, but also it made me feel that I'd been cheated. I was fifty or so and I felt that I could not retrieve some of these things or start over again because I was not sexually attractive enough anymore. I thought that these are privileges of the young. You have to have a smooth body, no wrinkles – be 'juicy', as I call it. This voice kept telling me, 'You're too old for that; who would want you?' And I was angry, at being 'too old'.* [a sixty-one-year-old woman]

Some women who are in generally unsatisfactory marriages or relationships may stay in the relationship, afraid that they are too old to find another partner.[18]

With the years we may feel that our partners turn away from us, and this can cause or reinforce negative feelings about our looks. It helps to realize that low self-esteem can cause us to perceive rejection when none was intended.[19] Finding a new relationship or a new source of self-esteem can help us overcome negative feelings.

It's nice to be appreciated. I can tell by the way he looks at me that he loves my face and my body, as old as it is. [a sixty-eight-year-old woman, remarried five years]

Now, I feel I have to press ahead in the world out of some inner sense of myself rather than with the help of my looks. And that's exciting because it makes me more adventurous. I'm working on my Ph.D. and preparing for a life of teaching and scholarly writing. As a younger woman I wouldn't have had the courage to embark on such a challenging career. [a forty-three-year-old woman]

I'm no longer the completely lonely person I was before because I have established an inner strength. I find new patience and compassion with others. I had always thought that the emptiness in me could only be filled by someone else. I'm finally discovering that I can be a complete and happy person through my own inner resources. [a sixty-eight-year-old woman]

Some women have found their relationships unsatisfactory and burdensome, and are not concerned about looking young for men.

Now that I'm fifty-two – who needs an old man around! And he'll be retired pretty soon and sitting around all day. It's different when a woman retires because she has friends and can get around with other women. But when a man retires you've still got to cook for him and wash. He doesn't have any friends – he just sits there, in the way.

Relationships with Women

Some lesbian women may be less concerned with weight gain and ageing than heterosexual women. Loving another woman can change the way a woman sees her body.

When I came out as a lesbian at thirty-seven, my body image changed. My lover's body was like mine, with breasts and curves, yet different. Our love was based on mutual respect and caring, bodies came second. I remember looking in the mirror a couple of years after we met and noting that my body seemed to have changed. My breasts hung lower, were less prominent. But mostly it was the feeling inside me that had changed. My breasts were part of a whole, not something to be leered at or mauled. I found myself looking at my breasts and body with pleasure. I liked what I saw. I claimed my body. [a forty-two-year-old woman]

Although I do have difficulty with ageing, I believe that it is easier as a lesbian. I am less self-conscious about cosmetic perfection, about weight gain and wrinkles – and feel that I have more sexual/romantic opportunities than a straight woman of my age. I cannot say that I love getting older. However, I am more comfortable with myself than I have ever been before. And peaceful. I feel confident, for the most part, attractive and assured. My life is rich, full, adventurous and really quite wonderful. [a fifty-year-old woman]

But many lesbian women feel a strong pressure to look young and see themselves at a disadvantage in finding partners.

I cannot say that I am unselfconscious or not preoccupied at times with ageing. Most of my self-esteem as a young woman was based on my looks and it has been a shock and an adjustment to have wrinkles and look older, especially when I feel so young inside. I am self-conscious about approaching younger women, worry about being inappropriate and question what younger women see in me in terms of my looks. My lovers have all been much younger than me, which is a concern. I worry that I will not remain attractive to them and what their reactions will be to my ageing and possibly declining health. [a fifty-year-old woman]

Work

For many of us, our main concerns about looking older centre on our power to earn money and to be valued as workers. As we look for jobs, or want to change from an unsatisfactory job, we become aware that looking older can mean being unemployable.

I do freelance work in a young business. All the people I deal with are my age or younger, and each time I have a new project interview I go thinking, 'Do I look young enough, do I look young?' I'm afraid people will stop employing me, because you don't appoint fifty-year-old women to do this kind of stuff. I'm scared about what it means for me professionally. [a thirty-nine-year-old woman]

Sometimes we can counteract employers' or colleagues' ageist attitudes with the help of our own strong self-esteem and/or the support of other older workers.

At first it seemed strange to me that everyone in the department is about thirty-five years younger than I am. But then I thought, if they have trouble dealing with a colleague old enough to be their mother, that's their problem! [a sixty-nine-year-old woman]

If you use your beauty to get a job, a man, then you are always indebted to it. You're always chasing it, looking in the mirror to see if it is still there. Once you stop that and realize you can use your head, your whole person, nobody can take that from you! You are powerful if you realize you have a brain and can use it. Society says: 'You are no longer valuable because you aren't gorgeous.' We say we are valuable, because we think and do. [a sixty-five-year-old woman]

Some women find that being older brings more respect and power on the job. Looking older increases our credibility and authority. Being older brings better judgment and wisdom. We can speak more freely and be listened to. These advantages depend on the kind of work we do, and seem to be greater in the professional world.[20]

As a therapist my age really is an advantage. I have a much larger store of experiences and understanding of what makes people tick and of what kinds of things happen to people, just because I've lived so much longer. [a seventy-nine-year-old woman]

Being older has helped me in my profession. I have much more authority. With my students I don't have to prove that I know something; they take that for granted. Certainly it would be much more difficult at twenty-five to be the authority I am. It would be impossible! Whatever my fears may be, whatever my private problems, what my students see is a woman of power. [a fifty-six-year-old woman]

Age and Identity

We live in a culture that rejects us for our looks just when we have the most to offer. Some women feel betrayed by such a society. Some of us, however, feel sorry for those who cannot see through our wrinkles and grey hair to our talents and abilities.

When I was younger I was considered more attractive than I am now. I no longer feel as though people look at me and say 'Oh, wow, what an attractive woman', which they did when I was younger. And I feel sorry for them because I am really a much more interesting person now than I was then. But that's their problem. [a sixty-five-year-old woman]

Our culture's view of how older women should look and behave is constricting to them and detrimental to society as a whole. Many women refuse to be confined by set images of what they should look like, be, and do. They dress and move according to their tastes and their personalities. They are as emotionally and physically involved with life as their wishes and their health allow. They see ageing as a new experience for which they are setting the pace.

Getting old can be wonderful if you're not imposed on by other people's rules about how you should be when you're old. I consciously break as many as I can because then I'm breaking through oppression. [a sixty-five-year-old woman]

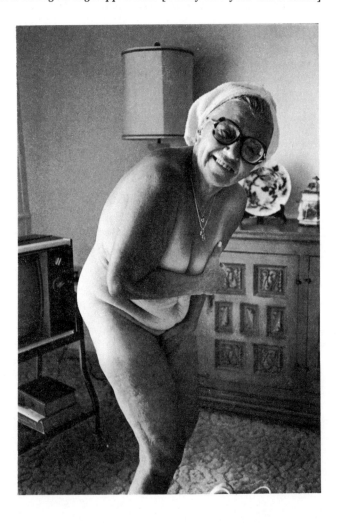

Life's less confusing for me now, things are falling into place. In a way I feel happier than I did at thirty – I like myself much better. And I think that's a key point – to like oneself, to be your own best friend. [a fifty-seven-year-old woman]

We can choose whether or not to use the technology – cosmetics, plastic surgery – offered us to look younger. And, in fact, many women find that instead of wanting to look different they see an inner and outer beauty in themselves and other older women that they didn't see before. Some of us find that we like signs of ageing and that they make a face more interesting than the smoothness of youth. We respond to other, lasting qualities of appearance, such as bone structure, or an alert, lively expression.

I know a lot of handsome older women. They have character! They're people! They've lived! One friend my age has the most animated, humorous, charming face. She would really beguile anybody! [a seventy-nine-year-old woman]

Self-confidence brings us a freedom many of us never felt in our younger years; we no longer feel obliged to be youthfully 'feminine' sex objects. We feel free to be ourselves, to be honest and outspoken, and are relieved and relaxed with this freedom.

You can make conscious efforts to change your own and others' ideas of beauty. Older women can learn, from the impact of the phrase 'Black is beautiful', how to raise self-esteem. One way to do so is to tell your older friends how good they look, how alive and interesting. Tell them how fine and handsome are the visible signs of years, experiences, and character. This is an important way women can help each other deal with our culture's negative attitude toward age.

NOTES

[1] Barbara MacDonald and Cynthia Rich, *Look Me in the Eye*. San Francisco: Spinsters, Ink., 1983, p. 14.

[2] Gwendolyn T. Sorell and Carol A. Nowak, 'The Role of Physical Attractiveness as a Contributor to Individual Development', in Richard M. Lerner and Nancy A. Busch Rossnagel, eds., *Individuals as Producers of Their Own Development: A Life-Span Perspective*. New York: Academic Press, 1981, pp. 389–446.

[3] Jan Benowitz Eigner, 'Interaction and Building of Body Concept and Self Concept Over the Lifespan: A Study of 20 Women Age 40 to 60'. Unpublished dissertation, St Louis University, 1984.

[4] Daniel Goleman, 'Dislike of Own Body Found Common Among Women'. *The New York Times*, 19 March 1985, pp. C1, C5.

[5] Diane White, 'An Age-Old Problem'. *The Boston Globe*, 26 October 1983.

[6] Carol A. Nowak, 'Does Youthfulness Equal

Attractiveness?' in Lillian E. Troll, Joan Israel and Kenneth Israel, eds., *Looking Ahead: A Woman's Guide to the Problems and Joys of Growing Older*. New York: Prentice-Hall, 1977.

[7]Jennifer Robinson, 'Body Image in Women over Forty'. *The Melpomene Report*, Melpomene Institute for Women's Health Research, 316 University Ave., St Paul, MN 55103, October 1983, pp. 12–14.

[8]While eating disorders are epidemic among adolescent women, their incidence, although small, is growing alarmingly among middle-aged women.

[9]Marcia Germaine Hutchinson, author of *Transforming Body Image*, quoted in 'Body Hatred'. *McCall's*, April 1985, p. 136.

[10]Clairol, 1983, as cited in Robin Marantz Henig, *How a Woman Ages*. New York: Ballantine Books, 1985, p. 61.

[11]Susan Brownmiller, *Femininity*. New York: Fawcett, 1985.

[12]Jane E. Brody, 'Personal Health'. *The New York Times*, 19 September 1984.

[13]*The Medical Letter on Drugs and Therapeutics*, 21 June 1985.

[14]*Health Facts*, Center for Medical Consumers, Inc., New York, October 1985.

[15]Report of the American Society of Plastic and Reconstructive Surgeons, cited in *Newsweek*, 24 May 1985.

[16]Robin Marantz Henig and the editors of *Esquire, How a Woman Ages – Growing Older: What to Expect and What You Can Do About It*. New York: Ballantine Books, 1985, p. 28.

[17]Cleo S. Berkun, 'Changing Appearance for Women in the Middle Years of Life', in Elizabeth W. Markson, ed., *Older Women*. Lexington, Mass.: D. C. Heath/Lexington Books, 1983, p. 24.

[18]Berkun, op. cit., p. 28.

[19]Troll, Israel and Israel, op. cit., p. 51.

[20]Berkun, op. cit., p. 24.

BOOKS AND PUBLICATIONS

Frigga Hang (ed.), *Female Sexualization – A Collective Work of Memory*. London: Verso/NLB, 1987.

Wendy Chapkis, *Beauty Secrets: Women and the Politics of Appearance*. London: The Women's Press, 1988.

Jo Campling (ed.), *Images of Ourselves: Women with Disabilities Talking*. London: Routledge & Kegan Paul, 1981.

4
Weighty Issues

In this country we are preoccupied with weight. Every women's magazine has articles on diets and 'fitness'. In the general mania for thinness, many of us think we are overweight when we really are not.

Many women avoid healthy foods they think are fattening and skip meals in an effort to lose weight. 'Fat phobia' – the fear of being fat – can interfere with proper nutrition. We can feel well and strong without being exploited by the multimillion-pound weight-loss and fitness industries. Our money is better spent on healthy foods and activities that are fun, sociable, and cause no injury.

Another Look at Dieting and Weight

Each of us has a unique size, shape, and body chemistry strongly determined by heredity.[1] How much we weigh is a function of energy input (food), energy used (activity), our own body's rate of using energy (metabolism), and other factors that are not well understood. The amount of energy we use to perform tasks, including sedentary activities such as office work and reading,[2] can vary from woman to woman. Studies show that fat women generally do not eat more nor are they less physically active than thin women.[3] The difference is in the fat woman's naturally larger build and in her rate of metabolism.

Because of the constant pressure to be thin, many women try sporadically or constantly to lose weight by reducing the calories they consume. This is so common that to most of us the term 'diet', which in its original meaning simply refers to what we eat, has come to mean a plan to lose weight. Dieting to lose weight can become a way of life. Most dieters never learn healthy food habits. When you go on a low-calorie diet, your body reacts as if it were being starved and tries to preserve as much energy as possible by decreasing its rate of metabolism. Your rate of metabolism may slow down more with each diet and remain slower once you return to your usual eating habits. Ironically, this means that after each diet, unless you drastically increase your exercise, you may gain weight more easily than before, since your body adds more fat to protect itself in case you deprive it of food again. This partially explains why 90 to 99 per cent of dieters regain their weight within five years, or even regain more than they lost.[4] It also explains why some researchers say that repeated low-calorie dieting may be a major cause of weight gain.[5]

Women are frequently encouraged to lose weight not only because 'thin is in' but because medical authorities believe that being 'overweight' puts us at risk for a variety of diseases and even death. But studies done on weight and health contradict each other, and many are faulty. Some studies find a relationship between high weight and early death, and others do not. Many studies do not take into account other known health risks such as cigarette smoking, repeated dieting, or hereditary factors, and most studies do not include women. One study which included women (but did not ask if they repeatedly dieted) did find an increase in death rates among women who for many years were 55 per cent to 65 per cent over the average weight charts.[6] But this means that, depending on your height and build, you would have to be about 65 to 110 pounds 'overweight' for many years to be adversely affected.

One of the problems in interpreting weight studies is knowing what the term 'overweight' means. We tend to read weight charts with the assumption that 'overweight' is bad no matter how old we are, what kind of body tissue we have, and where it is located on the body. But weight can mean many things. Poundage by itself is not a measure of fat; skin-fold measurements and water-immersion tests are better indicators. The weight we add as a result of exercise and body conditioning is not a hazard to our health. Increasing our weight by increasing our muscle mass will strengthen our bones and help prevent osteoporosis.

In addition, recent research shows that when studying the association between weight and disease, not only fat mass but the distribution of fat has to be considered. Fat tissue that was once considered an inert mass on the body is apparently involved in a number of metabolic functions that vary in different parts of the body. Women ages forty to fifty-nine with fat distribution predominantly on their waists and upper bodies have significantly more hypertension (high blood pressure), diabetes, and gallbladder disease than women with fat predominantly on their lower bodies. Relatively more fat from the waist up (as compared to hips) is associated with higher rates of these diseases even among women with comparable total body fat. Arthritis is associated with fat on the hips in some women. In the case of arthritis, factors such as added weight on the joints or the effects of fat tissue on posture and motion appear to be more important than the metabolic activity of the fat tissue.[7] Thin women who jog may be stressing their joints just as much as fat women who walk.

Moreover, our bodies' needs change with age. Some research shows that the ratio of weight to height associated with long life rises with age. Therefore, healthy people should not be concerned if they gain some weight as they move from early adult years to late middle age. The weights in the often-quoted Metropolitan Life Insurance Height and Weight Chart were increased in 1983 but are still too restrictive for women in their fifties and sixties. There are advantages for women in being a little heavier than previously thought – gaining a pound a year is apparently healthy.[8]

As we grow older, some lean muscle tissue is replaced with fatty tissue. Even if we stay the same weight, we will have more fat proportionately at eighty than we did at forty. Since it takes less energy to maintain fat tissue than to maintain muscle tissue, we would have to cut our calories* by 10 to 15 per cent from age twenty to age sixty just to maintain the same weight.[9] But if we cut our intake, we may not get adequate nutrition.

Emphasis on 'ideal' weight dictated by weight charts masks the damage caused by the constant pressure on women to be thin. Fat women suffer more from discrimination against fat than from any weight-related health problems. Many dieters experience emotional disturbances due to the effects of starvation on the body. Studies show that weight-related emotional disturbances are related to overeating, disparagement of body image, and the complications of dieting. Eating at night, insomnia, and skipping morning meals are associated with stressful life circumstances and often related to depression,[10] perhaps made worse by fruitless dieting attempts. A group for heavier women is the Fat Women's Support Group (see Organizations).

The following 'diets' have dangers in addition to the general hazards mentioned above.

- The use of 'diet pills'. Just because a drug is prescribed by a doctor doesn't mean that it is either effective or safe. Many prescription 'diet pills' contain amphetamine, a stimulant that speeds up the body's processes and can cause insomnia and diarrhoea. It is addictive, toxic, and can even cause violent behaviour and death. Also, don't assume that, because something is sold over the counter (OTC) without a prescription, it is harmless. Most OTC diet pills contain phenylpropanolamine (PPA), which is chemically similar to amphetamine. PPA raises blood pressure and alters brain function, but is not a proven aid to weight loss. It is also used as a nasal decongestant and is found in many cold remedies. Many diet pills and cold remedies also contain caffeine, which heightens the effect of PPA. Even recommended doses can cause confusion and hallucinations; high doses can cause heart damage, seizures, strokes, and even death. **A person can easily overdose by combining diet pills and cold remedies**.
- High-protein/low-carbohydrate, and sometimes high-fat diets. These raise

*A calorie is simply a way of estimating the energy available in a particular food.

triglycerides (fats) in the blood, promote dangerously high levels of ketones in the blood, increase calcium loss, and trigger carbohydrate 'binges'. Very low carbohydrate intake can cause fainting spells and depression.

- Grapefruit, banana, egg, or other limited-food diets. No single food is a 'magic' way to reduce weight. No enzymes in them melt away or otherwise remove fat from our bodies. High-egg diets are also high in cholesterol. These diets lack the nutrients you can obtain only by eating a variety of foods.

- Powdered-protein or high-protein liquid diets. These products (also called protein-sparing) are supposed to protect the lean body mass. They have many adverse effects, such as causing irregular heartbeats and even sudden death.[11] They should be used only under the close supervision of a research physician skilled in weight loss.

- Special supplement combinations, such as vinegar, lecithin, kelp, and vitamin B_6. These substances by themselves do not cause weight loss. Rather, weight loss is achieved through the limited-calorie diet which is supposed to accompany the supplements.

- Cellulose-based 'slimming aids' which reduce appetite by inducing a feeling of fullness may prevent you eating an adequate amount of necessary food for health; and they do nothing to re-educate you into eating a healthy balanced diet when you stop slimming.

An increase in two severe eating problems which primarily affect women, anorexia nervosa and bulimia, reflects the general tendency in society to promote thinness at all costs. Anorexia is a form of severe and initially deliberate self-starvation; bulimia is an eating pattern of bingeing and then purging, usually by vomiting or laxative usage. Anorexia is more common among young women, but it is increasing among older women. Bulimia seems to be found among all age-groups. Anorexia and bulimia can result from severe psychological distress as well as cause it. Both create many physical problems, including loss of tooth enamel (from regurgitated stomach acid), loss of ability to absorb food properly, loss of the gag reflex, and imbalances in the body's fluids severe enough to cause death. Even some bestseller diets encourage these methods as ways to lose weight.[12]

Therapists who treat people with eating problems agree with the feminist critics who first pointed out that anorexia and bulimia affect women more than men because of women's lack of power in society and because of the constant messages that women should be thin.

I felt out of control in my life. This was the one place where I could exert control – over my eating – and I did. Ultimately, however, I didn't have control of it – it had control of me. I could not stop when I wanted to. [a forty-five-year-old woman]

Being Thin

With all the emphasis on thinness, we may be so proud of ourselves if our weight is low that we do not realize when we are malnourished. Thin people are more susceptible to certain diseases, including lung diseases, fatal infections, ulcers, and anaemia.[13] Studies show that older people who are 'significantly underweight' die sooner than those who are not.[14] But the term 'underweight' is just as controversial as the term 'overweight'. (Underweight is usually defined as 10 to 15 per cent below the Metropolitan Life Insurance weight-for-height charts.) Many weight studies do not take into account smoking and pre-existing diseases that might have caused both the thinness and the early death.

Being thin is just as natural for some women as being heavy is for others. However, as older women, we frequently lose weight simply because we fail to eat enough. This may be a consequence of depression or loneliness, lack of interest in preparing or eating food, physical conditions that make preparing food or chewing difficult, not being able to afford enough to eat, and changes in the ability to taste food as we age. Certain drugs and certain illnesses, such as Type I diabetes, overactive thyroid, and cancer, can also cause weight loss. If you lose weight and are not sure why, or if you have no appetite, you should see your doctor or health visitor to make sure there is not an underlying problem.

Feeling Well: Achieving a Healthy Food/Activity Balance

The entire concept of an 'ideal' weight for any woman or group of women should be abandoned.[15] Instead, we should focus on getting plenty of good food and exercise. We need to create new patterns for dealing with food and activity if old patterns are not serving us well. Here are some suggestions.

- *Listen to your own body's feelings of hunger and fullness.* Years of dieting and bingeing can cause us to lose awareness of our body's signals. Eat when you are hungry and stop when you are full.
- *Learn good nutrition.* Basically, this means cutting down on high-fat foods and replacing them with whole grains, vegetables, fruits, and legumes. If you ate four chocolate bars a day you would get 1600 calories but you wouldn't be feeding your body what it needs.
- *Exercise.* Begin slowly. Don't do more than feels comfortable, or you won't keep it up. Statistics from many studies show that if you use 300 to 350 calories a day in exercise (2100 to 2500 per week), you will feel happier, more energetic, and stronger. Some people take two or more years to work up to that level. In 20 minutes you consume about 90 calories in light

housework, 100 calories in brisk walking, and 240 calories in swimming. In one study, weighty women who simply added a half-hour walk to their daily routines without changing their calorie intake lost twenty pounds in a year.[16]

Months of pain and inactivity had seriously limited my ability to move. I love to swim, but at first I could only walk the length of the pool, though the support of the water made it easier. When I felt well enough to swim one length, I had to rest until my heart stopped pounding. It took twenty months, with setbacks from illnesses which meant I had to work up slowly again, for me to be able to do thirty lengths in one hour. Now with swimming, some walking, and stair-climbing, I've reached my goal of 2000 calories of exercise a week. [a sixty-one-year-old woman]

- *If your caloric intake is too low, try to eat more.* This is usually best accomplished by eating small, frequent snacks that are high in nutrition and calories, such as ice cream, puddings, milk shakes, cheese, nuts, nut butters, and whole-grain scones, cakes and biscuits. Choose the vegetables and fruits that have the most calories. Drink Complan or similar products *in addition to* your regular foods. Flavour your food with herbs and spices. Arrange to eat with others when you do not feel like eating.
- *Keep records.* Keep daily records of exercise, and of what and how much you eat (written within fifteen minutes of eating). If you discover you are gaining or losing more weight than you wish, a review of accurately kept records can be enlightening. One woman thought she should cut calories by giving up bread. Keeping a record showed her that eating bread helped her avoid overeating. Consider the records over a period of a week rather than for each day.
- *Set goals for success.* Unrealistic food and exercise goals set you up to fail. Sometimes the only achievable goal seems small (one day a week I'll carry a piece of fruit to work instead of buns), but the fact that you *do* achieve it helps you take the next step.
- *Control your environment.* Make your meals as attractive, tasty, and fun as possible. Try moving your TV into the bedroom and take your planned snack with you to enjoy during late-night watching. Don't skip parties and celebrations because you want to avoid food. Enjoy yourself and choose nutritious food – or bring your own.
- *Enjoy what you choose to do or to eat.* For example, when choosing among several kinds of biscuits, remember that an oatmeal-raisin biscuit gives you more nutrients than a chocolate biscuit. A glass of skim milk and a potato have approximately the same number of calories as the same size glass of Coke and ten to fifteen potato crisps. But the first two provide protein,

calcium, vitamins A and D, and other nutrients while the latter provide calories and little else. If you decide on the chocolate biscuit or the potato crisps, enjoy them. When you decide to treat yourself to a favourite food, whatever it may be, this is an informed choice, not a 'failure'.

Last night at a restaurant I chose fried prawns and chips because I wanted them. I didn't fool myself by ordering steamed fish and a baked potato which I really didn't want and then pretending I wasn't adding extra butter. I felt satisfied and know I won't binge the way I used to when I felt deprived. [a fifty-eight-year-old woman]

I have developed such a sweet tooth in my old age. I just can't resist sweets when I have them in the house. My neighbour told me about a wonderful substitute: frozen banana slices. You freeze the banana peeled and wrapped in foil, then slice as many slices as you want with a sharp knife and rewrap the rest. It's amazing how much a banana tastes like a sweet when it is frozen. [a seventy-five-year-old woman]

I keep my favourite nutritious snacks in the refrigerator – low-fat coleslaw, cold boiled potatoes, and steamed broccoli – to counter the conditioned siren-call to high-

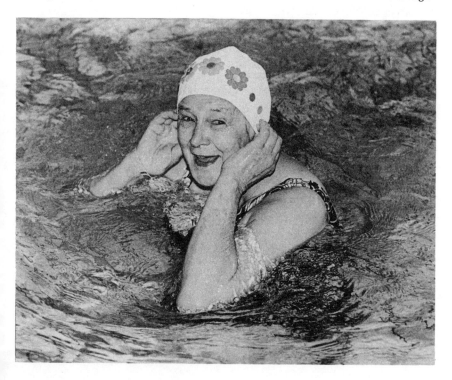

fat foods that fills TV, magazines, and newspapers. Sometimes I feel the whole world is out to get my money, and to hell with my health. [a sixty-one-year-old woman]

NOTES

[1]Albert J. Stunkard et al., 'An Adoption Study of Human Obesity'. *The New England Journal of Medicine*, Vol. 314, No. 4, 23 January 1986, pp. 193–8. Though the title mentions only obesity, the study showed that the relationship between biological parents and adoptees was not confined to the obesity weight group but was present across the whole range of fatness – from very thin to very fat. The conclusion was that family environment alone has no apparent effect. Obesity is usually defined as at least 20 per cent over the 'ideal weight' according to life insurance weight tables.

[2]Susan C. Wooley, O. W. Wooley and Susan R. Dyrenforth, 'Theoretical, Practical, and Social Issues in Behavioral Treatments of Obesity'. *Journal of Applied Behavior Analysis*, Vol. 1, Spring 1979, p. 8.

[3]Susan C. Wooley and O. W. Wooley, 'Obesity and Women – I. A Closer Look at the Facts'. *Women's Studies International Quarterly*, Vol. 2, 1979, pp. 69–79.

[4]W. Bennett and J. Gurin, 'Do Diets Really Work?' *Science*, Vol. 82, March 1983, p. 43.

[5]Wooley and Wooley, op. cit.

[6]Artemis Simopoulos and T. Van Itallie, 'Body Weight, Health, and Longevity'. *Annals of Internal Medicine*, Vol. 100, No. 2, February 1984, pp. 285–95.

[7]Arthur J. Hartz, David C. Rupley and Alfred A. Rimm, 'The Association of Girth Measurements with Disease in 32, 856 Women'. *American Journal of Epidemiology*, Vol. 119, No. 1, 1984, pp. 71–80.

[8]Reubin Andres, 'Impact of Age on Weight Goals'. *Health Implications of Obesity*, Program and Abstracts, National Institutes of Health Consensus Development Conference, 11–23 February 1985, pp. 77–80. More complete information is available in Reubin Andres et al., eds., *Principles of Geriatric Medicine*. New York: McGraw-Hill, 1985, pp. 311–18.

[9]Daphne A. Roe, *Geriatric Nutrition*. Englewood Cliffs, NJ: Prentice-Hall, 1983, p. 64.

[10]Albert Stunkard and Thomas A. Wadden, 'The Adverse Psychological Effects of Obesity'. *Health Implications of Obesity*, NIH Consensus Development Conference, 11–13 February 1985, pp. 59–62.

[11]Rafael A. Lantigua et al., 'Cardiac Arrhythmias Associated with a Liquid Protein Diet for the Treatment of Obesity'. *The New England Journal of Medicine*, Vol. 303, No. 13, 25 September 1980, pp. 735–8.

[12]O. Wayne Wooley and Susan Wooley, 'The Beverly Hills Eating Disorders: The Mass Marketing of Anorexia Nervosa'. *International Journal of Eating Disorders*, Vol. 1, No. 3, 1982, pp. 57–69.

[13]Paul Ensberger, 'Fat and Thin Not Black and White'. *Radiance*, Vol. III, Spring 1986, pp. 21–2.

[14]Simopoulos and Van Itallie, op. cit.

[15]T. R. Knapp, 'A Methodological Critique of the "Ideal Weight" Concept'. *Journal of the American Medical Association*, Vol. 250, 1983, pp. 505–10.

[16]G. Gwinup, 'Effects of Exercise Alone on the Weight of Obese Women'. *Archives of International Medicine*, Vol. 135, 1975, pp. 676–80.

BOOKS AND PUBLICATIONS

University of Bradford, School of Science and Society, 'Diet and Cardiovascular Disease' for *British Agriculture, Implications of the Committee on Medical Aspects Reports on: A Commentary.* Wheelock & Fallows, March 1985.

Geoffrey Cannon and Hetty Einzig, *Dieting Makes You Fat.* London: Sphere, 1984.

Kim Chernin, *Womansize: The Tyranny of Slenderness.* London: The Women's Press, 1983.

Hilde Bruch, *Eating Disorders – Obesity,*

Anorexia Nervosa and the Person Within. London: Routledge & Kegan Paul, 1973.

Susie Orbach, *Fat is a Feminist Issue*, Part 2. London: Arrow, 1984.

Susie Orbach, *Hunger Strike.* London: Faber & Faber, 1986.

Janet Polivy and C. Peter Herman, *Breaking the Diet Habit: The Natural Weight Alternative.* London: Basic Books, 1984.

Julia Buckroyd, *Eating Your Heart Out.* London: Macdonald Optima, 1989.

5
Eating Well

Food is important to us on many levels. What we eat is connected to our health, our feelings about ourselves, our social and family ties, our ethnic backgrounds, and our roles as women.

When I was sick with the flu as a little girl, my mother used to make me chicken soup. To this day I never smell chicken soup but what I remember how much better it made me feel then. Even now when I'm feeling bad, I'll want some soup like my mother made for me. This canned stuff is not a good substitute. [a sixty-eight-year-old woman]

Many of us are experienced in meal planning and preparing food. We may have spent many hours trying out new recipes or preparing our family's favourites over and over again. Often, being responsible for one to three meals a day, seven days a week, however, can dampen our enthusiasm for cooking. Many of us are more familiar with taking care of others than with taking care of ourselves. It may be hard to prepare a nice meal for ourselves when we feel lonely. Or we may enjoy the freedom from fixed schedules and complicated meals but fail to pay attention to our nutritional needs.

Since my husband died and my youngest daughter left home, I find it hard to prepare real meals for myself. If I haven't planned ahead, I'll stand at the refrigerator and eat whatever is handy – pickles, ice cream, cold sausages, whatever. [a fifty-five-year-old woman]

I gained ten pounds after my husband died. I like sweets, but he had so many restrictions on what he could eat when he was ill, and I just ate what I prepared for him. When it was over, I felt a certain release and indulged myself in eating all those 'forbidden' goodies.
Now I plan more what I am going to eat. I cook ahead and freeze small portions in packets that can be dropped into boiling water when I am ready to use them. I bake a large cake, freeze half and keep half in the refrigerator, so it will be there when I want it, but I won't be tempted to eat it all at once. [a woman in her eighties]

Mass advertising promotes high-profit processed foods and soft drinks, promising fun and eternal youth but delivering only empty calories. Health-food stores and the still rare food co-ops are good sources of foods not easily found in supermarkets, but in a growing number of communities, supermarket managers are responding to increased consumer sophistication about nutrition by stocking whole-grain breads and biscuits, tofu,* and a wider variety of fruits and vegetables. Shops now also contain a variety of ethnic and new foods which can improve our food selections and broaden our pleasures. A good tip for supermarket shopping is to begin by going around the edges of the shop where the unprocessed food is – dairy, meat, fish, and produce. Use the centre aisles mainly to restock staples and paper products.

Eating in healthier ways usually means deciding to change and then doing it slowly. One way to start is to learn more about what a healthy diet is. Healthy unprocessed foods can be flavourful and interesting. One woman who suffered from gastritis and constipation reports:

I decided to put into practice some of the nutritional advice which I'd been reading. I stopped eating white sugar in any form. No more processed food, including white bread, white rice and pasta; in came more fresh vegetables and grains. That was five years ago and today all the ailments I mentioned earlier are completely gone. No more of that headachy feeling from constipation. I count my blessings for being freed from this condition from which I suffered so long. [a fifty-seven-year-old woman]

Making Eating Sociable and Easy

The company of others can seem particularly important at mealtime. Try to make eating a happy sociable event. Plan to share a meal or two a week with friends. Consider going out to lunch – food is sometimes cheaper then and it may be easier to arrange time with friends at midday. For people over sixty, in some areas, there are special pensioners' lunch centres. Though some women avoid these because they mistakenly perceive them as only for the economically needy or because they don't want to be associated with 'old people', those who do go enjoy it a lot and frequently become 'regulars'.

I live alone but I am rarely by myself, due to a steady stream of family, friends, and international visitors, and many activities. I enjoy eating at the lunch club. This is

---

*Tofu is a bland, custardlike food from East Asia. Made from soybeans, it is high in protein and calcium, low in calories and carbohydrates, and has no cholesterol. Tofu is available in Asian food markets and health-food stores, and increasingly in supermarkets.

how I solve my problem of thinking of a meal as a true communion. I urge others to try it. [an eighty-seven-year-old woman]

Not all of us are able to travel or live in a group setting, but we can certainly

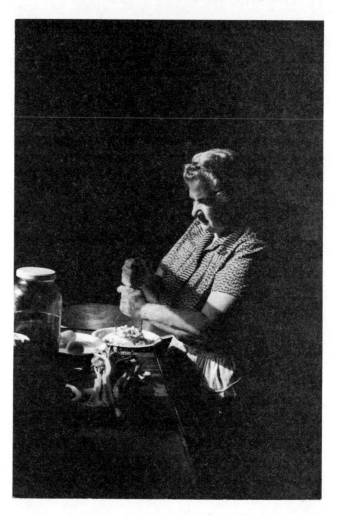

make our home a place where people want to be – and then ask them over! Potlucks are popular, economical, and fun.

For the housebound there's a Meals-on-Wheels service, provided either by the local authority or a voluntary organization. Welcome as this is, it's important to try to supplement these meals with some fresh fruit or uncooked vegetables, as the meals provided are usually rather short on both.

You can eat well more easily if you simplify the storing and cooking of food. For example, if you have freezer space, cook food ahead of time, divide it into meal-size packages, and freeze it. You don't have to make a complicated meal to have nutritious foods. Fresh or frozen vegetables can be cooked in five to ten minutes in a steamer (for about £2 you can buy one that fits any saucepan). Small pieces of chicken, fish, or meat can be quickly prepared. Low-fat dairy products such as skim milk, cottage cheese, and yogurt can make convenient, nutritious snacks. In addition to cooking grains such as brown rice, whole grains can be eaten in cereals (shredded wheat, oatmeal, muesli, wheat germ, bran cereal) or by eating whole-grain bread, biscuits, and pasta.

Other circumstances can affect how we eat. For instance, living too far from a shop or having too many stairs to climb can limit the amount of food you can get into the house. You may have too little storage space, or refrigerators or cookers that don't function properly. Poorly fitting dentures can be an impediment to good nutrition. Sometimes help can be found in the form of a friend or neighbour to shop or eat with, or through the social services and Home Helps scheme.

Eating Well for Less Money

For many of us, the kind and amount of food we eat are influenced by the cost. Most families spend an average of 15 to 20 per cent of their income on food. Poor older women may have to spend 30 per cent or more of their income on food.[1] For these women, the choice may come down to paying the rent or buying food.

Some suggestions that may help those on a limited budget are:

- Buy only as much as you can use or store. Split cheaper 'economy size' packages with a friend.
- Buy foods that are 'nutrient dense' – in other words, unprocessed foods that give you the most nutrition for your money. For instance, eggs, low-fat cottage cheese, dried beans, whole chickens, protein-enriched spaghetti products, peanut butter, oatmeal, low-fat milk, whole-grain cereal, inexpensive fish, and hamburger.
- Avoid highly processed foods when possible. They seem economical but aren't. For instance, a cup of canned beef-noodle soup or a frozen dinner are in about the same price range as the foods mentioned above. Their percentage of protein, however, is far less.
- Fresh vegetables and fruits are cheapest in season. Frozen vegetables are

often less expensive than fresh and have approximately the same nutritional value. Avoid frozen vegetables packed in sauces because they cost more and contain more salt and fat. Canned vegetables can be quite inexpensive although there is some nutritional loss. For instance, four ounces of canned green beans contain one third the amount of vitamin C of fresh or frozen beans.

- Meals at a meal centre are inexpensive. You can also save cooking time and meet new friends.
- Make sure that you are claiming any benefit to which you are entitled (see Money Matters chapter).

Food in Institutions

People in nursing homes and hospitals often don't have much choice about what they eat. Institutional food is often high in refined carbohydrates and fats and low in fresh fruits and vegetables. This can be a very difficult situation to deal with. If you, a friend, or relative is in this situation and find the food lacking in nutrition or taste, one solution is to bring in or have brought in small amounts of food from the outside. Another is to put pressure on the institution to provide better food. Discussing this with your doctor or dietitian can often be useful. If that doesn't improve the situation, talk with other residents informally and then bring it up in the residents' council, if you have one.

What is a Good Food Plan?

No single dietary plan is right for everyone. We all have different nutritional needs as well as different physical and economic limitations. Advertisements, books, magazines, and television all present conflicting information.

I still don't know what I should eat or how much. I try to keep up with nutrition through magazines and newspapers, but I am never sure I'm getting what I need. [a fifty-five-year-old woman]

The purpose of this chapter is to help us evaluate what we read and hear so that we can eat healthier food.

Little solid research has been done in the area of nutrition for older women. The US Department of Agriculture's (USDA) Human Research Center for Aging is currently studying the nutrition of healthy older people. After this research is done, we may have more answers about diet and ageing, but we will still have questions about the different dietary needs of older women and men.

Nutrients – carbohydrates, fats, proteins, vitamins, water, and minerals –

work together in our bodies to provide heat and energy, regulate bodily processes, and provide material for repair and growth. Each nutrient has its own functions, so the food we eat must contain all of the nutrients for our bodies to function really well.

Recent legislation in the United Kingdom lays down rules about the labelling of packaged foods with information about the proportion of fats, sugars, etc. they contain. But it is up to the customer to work out whether these meet the nutritional requirements of the individual. Our Department of Health Recommended Daily Allowances (RDAs) vary from those of some other countries, and most authorities would now say that, in any case, they may represent the *minimum* amount of certain vitamins and minerals needed to prevent actual deficiencies. Some food manufacturers are beginning to provide fuller information than the bare requirements demanded by the legislation, and with Britain's increasing tie-up with the European Community this may become universal. Additives (colourings, flavour-enhancers, etc.) have 'E' numbers which now appear on packages (but not on unpackaged foods) and if these mystify you – as well they may – the books listed on page 106 are enlightening.

In neither the US nor the UK does labelling include all the essential nutrients.[2] More useful are the findings of the Committee on the Medical Aspects of Food Policy (the COMA report), which you could ask for in your public library, as well as some of the books on our list (pp. 105–6).

The US Senate Select Committee on Nutrition and Human Needs concluded that Americans, especially the poor, are not well nourished, and in Britain the position is similar, with older people in particular being at risk. Even among middle-class Americans, the committee found that 40 to 50 per cent suffer from at least one nutritional deficiency.[3] The committee also found that although the country has far more than its share of agricultural resources, nutrition has suffered as a result of the extent to which processed food has become an ever-increasing part of American diets.

Our food supply has changed from reliance on whole, unrefined foods such as fresh fruits, vegetables, meats, dairy products, and whole grains to highly processed, 'fortified', preserved, synthetically manufactured 'convenience' foods. The latter take up at least half the space in any supermarket. Our use of fats and oils increased by about 50 per cent from 1910 to 1980. Our use of sugar and other sweeteners has also increased, largely because of the use of hidden sugars in processed foods and beverages.[4]

The following suggestions are adapted from the goals set by the Senate committee and from the *Dietary Guidelines for Americans* published jointly by the US Department of Agriculture and the US Department of Health and Human Services. The suggested guidelines in Britain are similar.

- **Increase consumption of complex carbohydrates.** This category includes fruits and vegetables; nuts; legumes such as split peas, lentils, chick peas, lima beans, and navy and other beans; whole grains such as brown rice, bulgur, and buckwheat; and whole-grain products such as whole-wheat bread, whole-grain biscuits, bran cereals, non-instant oatmeal and oat bran, and shredded wheat.
- **Reduce consumption of refined sugars.** This category includes processed foods that list sugars as first, second, or third ingredients. Sugars may have a variety of names, such as corn syrup or corn sweetener, sucrose, dextrose, maltose, lactose, fructose, or levulose. 'Natural' sugars such as honey, barley malt, maple syrup, apple concentrate, and molasses are only slightly better for you and should be eaten only in small quantities.
- **Reduce overall fat consumption.** Foods to cut down on include fatty meat, processed meats (cold meats, sausages), deep-fried foods, butter, margarine, mayonnaise, high-fat cheeses, pastries, crisps, and other 'snack' foods. Good substitutes for some of these foods are lower-fat animal products such as fish, poultry without the skin, low-fat dairy products, and vegetable proteins such as grains and beans. Unbuttered popcorn is an excellent snack.
- **Change the ratio of saturated to unsaturated fats, reducing the use of saturated fats.** Saturated fats are generally solid at room temperature and include animal fats, hydrogenated (hardened) vegetable fats, and coconut and palm oils. Unsaturated fats are liquid at room temperature and include vegetable or nut oils such as canola, safflower, sunflower, soy, corn, linseed, and walnut oils. Saturated fats raise cholesterol levels while unsaturated fats lower them. Mono-unsaturated fats, like peanut or olive oil, are liquid at room temperature but solidify easily with refrigeration. Mono-unsaturates have no effect on or may lower cholesterol levels and can be used in cooking, as they remain stable at high temperatures. The fats in fish (including shell-fish, the cholesterol levels of which were previously overestimated) contain omega-3 fatty acids, which actually lower cholesterol and triglyceride levels in the blood (see the chapters on arthritis, hypertension and heart disease).
- **Reduce sodium consumption.** Eat only small quantities of salt-cured foods, most condiments, salty snack foods, soy sauce, foods containing monosodium glutamate (MSG), most canned vegetables and soups, and any processed food in which salt or sodium is high on the list of ingredients. Keep track of your use of salt in cooking and at the table. Be aware that some water softeners work by adding salts. Avoid over-the-counter medicines high in sodium, including many antacids. However, some sodium is essential for our well-being and cutting intake too low for our needs can result in weakness.

CARBOHYDRATES

Carbohydrates should provide 50 per cent or more of our energy needs and supply the glucose necessary for brain function. Adequate carbohydrate intake keeps the body from using protein as an energy source, so that protein can be conserved for body-building functions.

Carbohydrates are usually divided into two categories – simple and complex. Simple carbohydrates are sugars such as table sugar, honey, and the sugar in fruits (glucose and fructose). Complex carbohydrates are starches such as grains, starchy vegetables, fruits, and beans. All sugars and starches are converted by digestion into a simple sugar called glucose, which is released into the bloodstream. However, the glucose from starches is digested and absorbed more slowly than that from sugar, avoiding the rapid rise and fall of blood sugar that can come from eating too many simple sugars at one time. Whole foods with complex carbohydrates such as grains also furnish essential nutrients and fibre, while simple carbohydrates such as sugar and refined flour tend to be 'empty calorie' foods – they supply too many calories for the nutrients they provide. White flour loses most of the twenty-three of its vitamins and minerals in the refining process and is then labelled 'enriched' when only four are replaced.

Choosing Our Food

What should we eat on a daily basis for the nutrition we need? Nutritionists traditionally dealt with this question by dividing food into four groups: (1) fruits and vegetables; (2) dairy products; (3) breads and cereals; and (4) meats and other protein foods. Since these groups don't take into account such things as levels of saturated fat or different ethnic eating habits, we have changed the groups somewhat to make the recommendations a little more flexible. However, if you ate all of the minimums, for every group, you would be eating too little; if you ate all of the maximums, you would be eating too much in total calories.

- **Vegetables** 2 to 5 servings (one serving is half a cup cooked). Includes all fresh, frozen, or canned vegetables. Generally, the deeper the colour of the vegetable, the more nutritious it is in vitamin A, so tip the balance in favour of dark green leafy and yellow/orange vegetables. Also include starchy vegetables such as sweetcorn, peas, and potatoes.
- **Fruit** 1 to 4 servings (one serving is one average-size fruit, or approximately half a cup). Includes all unsweetened fruit – fresh, frozen, canned, dried, or

juiced. Whole, raw fruit is generally the most nutritious. Include a vitamin C fruit or vegetable source daily.

- **Dairy products** 1 to 3 servings (one serving is approximately one cup of liquid like milk or yogurt, or 1 to 1½ ounces of cheese). Includes milk, yogurt, all cheeses, or ice cream made with real cream. Be sure to include low-fat dairy products such as skim milk, low-fat yogurt, and low-fat cottage cheese.
- **Whole grains, including bread and cereal** 3 to 6 servings (one serving is half a cup of grain or cereal, or one slice of bread). Includes all whole grains – rice, barley, millet, cracked wheat, corn; whole-grain breads and cereals – oatmeal, bran, shredded wheat; whole-grain biscuits, pasta, and tortillas. If you are not used to whole grains, start gradually to substitute them for white-flour products and eat only as much as your digestive system can comfortably handle. For example, you can cook a combination of brown and white rice, gradually shifting toward more of the whole grain.
- **Protein** 2 to 3 servings (one serving is approximately 3 ounces of cooked lean meat, chicken, or fish, 5 ounces of tofu, 2 large eggs, 1 cup cooked beans, or combinations such as ⅓ cup beans with ⅔ cup rice). Many women over age seventy do not eat enough protein.

Protein is the second most plentiful substance in the body. It is important for the growth, development, and repair of all body tissues. Proteins are composed of units called amino acids. The body requires approximately twenty-two amino acids to make human protein. All but nine of these can be produced by the body. These nine are called 'essential amino acids' and must come from the food we eat. Animal proteins from foods such as meat, poultry, fish, dairy products, and eggs contain all of the amino acids in adequate amounts and are therefore called 'complete proteins'. Many vegetables, grains, beans, nuts, seeds, and other complex carbohydrates contain proteins but are 'incomplete' by themselves and have to be combined to have sufficient amounts of all of the amino acids. Combined vegetable proteins have the advantage of being lower in fat, higher in fibre and minerals, and generally lower in cost than complete proteins.

Many traditional food combinations yield complete protein – such combinations as grains and beans, beans and nuts or seeds, grains and nuts or seeds, and any vegetable protein with any animal protein such as potatoes with dairy products. For more information on combining foods to make complete protein, see one of the vegetarian cookbooks listed on page 106.

- **Essential fatty acids** approximately 1 to 2 tablespoons per day in salad dressing or cooking. This is not really a food group, but we do need small amounts of oil and fat in our diet for good health. Fats are part of the basic structure of every cell. Furnishing more than twice the number of calories per gram as carbohydrates and proteins, they provide the most concentrated form of energy in the diet. Fats act as carriers for fat-soluble vitamins (A, D, E, and K) and provide insulation and protection for our organs and the skeleton. Oils high in essential fatty acids (in descending order) are fish oils, linseed, walnut, soy, safflower, sunflower, and corn oils. If you eat a diet which is high in fatty fish, whole grains, seeds, and nuts, you may not have to add extra oil.

- **Water**, although it is not a nutrient, is the most important element for life and is frequently overlooked. Our bodies are made mostly of water, which is vital to maintain life and health. Water is essential for proper functioning of both the kidneys and the bowels, and is an important vehicle for disposing of poisonous substances. It is the basic transport system of the body, moving all nutrients, hormones, blood cells, waste products, and oxygen through the body.

  As we age, our mechanisms for controlling fluid balance become less efficient. Most of us need six to eight cups of water daily, and more in some circumstances. Water can also be obtained from soups, juices, beverages, fruits, and vegetables. Coffee and other beverages containing caffeine actually push fluids and minerals out of the system and should be taken in small amounts only.

- **Fibre**, although not a nutrient, is nonetheless a necessary component of a well-balanced diet. Fibre serves primarily as a vehicle for holding water, binding both toxic and essential nutrients, and providing the soft bulk that absorbs body waste. Because of these properties, fibre helps our intestines work more smoothly. This is particularly important as we grow older and our intestines lose some of their elasticity and mobility, increasing the tendency toward constipation. Adequate fibre intake may also help prevent such conditions and diseases as diverticulosis, gallbladder disease, colitis, colon cancer, and high cholesterol.[5]

  Different forms of fibre have different functions; for instance, oat bran lowers cholesterol, whereas wheat bran does not. Pectins from foods such as apples and beans prevent diarrhoea and help excrete cholesterol. Cellulose and other fibres from whole grains help prevent constipation and colon cancer. It is therefore important to eat a variety of fibrous foods, including whole grains, beans, fruits, vegetables, nuts, and seeds. Beware of fibre-enriched white breads. Some contain harsh products. Fibre has its negative side as well. High fibre intake can cause wind and bloating. More seriously, wheat bran can interfere significantly with calcium, iron, and zinc absorption.[6] So far, there are no established recommendations for fibre intake for older women. A prudent course is to have enough fibre (and adequate fluid) to make our bowel movements soft and easily passed.

- **Vitamins** are organic compounds found in living things. Their function is to act as catalysts for chemical reaction. Some chemical processes require the presence of several vitamins simultaneously. Vitamins themselves do not furnish energy, as they have no calories, but they are necessary for metabolism.

    Vitamins are soluble in either fat or water. The fat-soluble vitamins – A, D, E, and K – require fat in order for the body to absorb them from the intestinal tract. They are also easily stored in the body and can become toxic at high doses. This is particularly true for vitamins A and D. Water-soluble vitamins are the B complexes and vitamin C. Because they are water-soluble, unneeded amounts can be disposed of easily in the urine. And because they are not stored easily in the body, we need to be more careful to get them daily. They are generally not toxic except at very high levels.

- **Minerals** are inorganic compounds that originate in soil, rocks, and water. Approximately seventeen minerals are necessary for human nutrition; several others are thought to have at least a minor role in body processes.

    Like vitamins, minerals act as catalysts for many chemical reactions in the body. These include regulation of muscle contractions, transmission of messages through the nervous system, and aiding the digestion and metabolism of foods. Certain minerals also constantly adjust our internal water balance and regulate the flow of substances in and out of cells. They control the acid balance in our blood and tissues. The essential 'macrominerals', those present in relatively high amounts in the body, are sodium, potassium, calcium, magnesium, and phosphorus. The essential 'trace minerals', those present in only very small amounts, are iron, copper, zinc, manganese, chromium, selenium, vanadium and molybdenum.

Should We Take Nutrient Supplements?

Unfortunately, there is no simple way to know how well nourished you are. One technique, hair analysis, is useful in discovering toxic levels of minerals such as lead, arsenic, and mercury. It does not, however, give accurate information about the nutritional condition of various tissues of the body. It can even give false readings about nutritional status if, for example, certain shampoos are used before testing. Whereas zinc in hair can be low if a diet is deficient, it can also be normal if hair is slow-growing because of semi-starvation.[7]

There are some conditions under which you may want to consider taking a supplement: when you don't have control over the food you eat (for instance, in a nursing home); when you are on a medication which can interfere with

FOR WHAT IT'S WORTH

We may do our best to follow all the rules of sensible, healthy eating and still be consuming harmful substances. Britain lags behind other countries – the United States and most European nations – in failing to control the use of doubtful additives in many pre-prepared foods; allowing harmful pesticides, banned or controlled elsewhere, to contaminate fruit and vegetables; and using the public as guinea-pigs for secret experiments in increasing milk production by injecting hormones into cows and then mixing the milk with 'ordinary' milk from other sources. The pharmaceutical and agrochemical industries themselves provide almost all the 'experts' who sit on the various committees charged with the job of advising the government on the safety or otherwise of a large number of possibly doubtful additives and other substances – and *their reports are never published.** What can we do? We should try to

buy organically-produced food and/or encourage shops and supermarkets to sell them. And we can

- become familiar with the 'E' numbers now marked on packaged foods and reject those that may be harmful even though legal in the UK. (Two books listed at the end of this chapter will help.);
- thoroughly wash all green vegetables before eating or cooking;
- wash, or if practicable, peel all fruit before eating;
- join and campaign with consumer groups, environmental organizations and political parties concerned with environmental questions;
- encourage women's organizations and pensioners' associations to take up these issues.

For a fuller discussion on the impact of pollution, agrochemicals and additives on the development of cancer, see Cancer chapter.

absorption of nutrients; if you indulge in cigarettes, alcohol, or caffeine; if you haven't yet changed to healthy food habits.

Remember that supplements are supposed to do just that – supplement your diet. You cannot use them to replace food or to make up for a nutritionally unsound diet. A good vitamin-mineral supplement is low in the fat-soluble vitamins A and D (A – 15,000 IUs or less, D – 400 IUs or less), contains a complete B complex (B_1, B_2, B_6, B_{12}, biotin, folate, niacin, pantothenic acid, choline, inositol, and PABA), vitamin C, vitamin E, and minerals such as magnesium, iron, selenium, chromium, manganese, and zinc. If you feel you need more than a general supplement or are confused about what to take, you can consult a nutritionist or dietitian, through your GP.

*Information from Channel 4 programme, *4 What It's Worth*, 20 September 1988.

Special Needs for Women Over Forty

The specific nutritional needs of older women have not been determined. The nutritional levels of the healthiest of the elderly – those who are largely free of disease and are mobile – are remarkably similar to those of younger people. Unfortunately, what is clear is that as many as 50 per cent of women over the age of sixty-five are malnourished because they consume too few calories, proteins, and essential vitamins and minerals for good health.[8] Specifically, many do not get enough thiamine (B_1), riboflavin (B_2), vitamins B_6, B_{12}, C, D, K, folic acid, magnesium, zinc, and iron, as well as calcium.[9] *Adequate daily calcium intake is vital throughout our life span.* In the US, the RDA remains at 800 mg per day for adults, while in the UK it is only 500 mg. The following chart, compiled from several sources, lists recommendations higher than 800 mg per day.

Calcium Needs of Women

Age	Milligrams per Day
9–19	1200
If pregnant	1500–2000
If breastfeeding	2200
20–50 (premenopausal)	1000
Postmenopausal or for early natural or surgical menopause	1500

A thousand milligrams of calcium can be obtained in one day by eating all of the following: two half-cup servings of cooked green vegetables, one ounce of cheese, and two cups of skim milk. Adding a sesame-seed bun, a serving of sardines or yogurt, and increasing the two green vegetables to one-cup servings will increase the calcium to 1500 mg for the day.

All dairy products are rich in calcium. Skim or fat-free milk is commonly recommended,[10] but one recent book states that small amounts of fat improve calcium absorption because the absorption of calcium and fat is interrelated.[11] Whole milk contains only about 3 per cent fat. You can drink one or even three glasses of whole milk daily and still keep your cholesterol level low. You can add additional low-fat powdered milk to pancakes, soups, custards, puddings, and casseroles.

You can still obtain calcium if you are lactose intolerant. Try consuming small amounts of dairy products and note how you feel. Most people can tolerate half a glass of whole milk with each meal and can eat yogurt, cheese, and buttermilk without discomfort.[12] Tablets containing the enzyme required to digest milk and lactose-free milk are now available in some health-food shops.

Good Calcium Sources

Food	Portion Size	Mg of Calcium
Whole milk	8 fl. oz.	290
Low-fat (2%) or skim milk	8 fl. oz.	300
Buttermilk	8 fl. oz.	285
Non-fat dry milk	1 oz. powder	377
Cheddar cheese	1 oz.	205
Cottage cheese	2 oz.	77
Parmesan cheese	1 oz.	320
Yogurt, plain low-fat	3 oz.	290
'Real' ice cream	$\frac{1}{2}$ cup	90
Greens, cooked	1 cup	150–350
Parsley	$3\frac{1}{2}$ oz.	203
Spinach, cooked	4 oz.	150
Broccoli, cooked	4 oz.	130
Sardines (with bones)	$\frac{1}{4}$ lb.	300
Salmon (canned with bones mashed in)	$\frac{1}{4}$ lb.	225
Oysters (fresh)	$\frac{1}{4}$ lb.	210
Shrimp	3 oz.	147
Brazil nuts	2 oz.	140
Almonds	2 oz.	80
Tofu made with calcium sulphate	4 oz.	145
Corn tortilla	6 in. diameter	60
Kelp	$\frac{1}{2}$ oz.	150

Some magazines now carry ads for calcium supplements, playing on our fears of bone fractures. Because of these ads, some women may now be adding *too much* calcium to their diets. This may interfere with the absorption of iron and other nutrients, and may cause imbalances in calcium metabolism. Adding a calcium supplement to bring the total daily intake from food and the supplement up to 800 mg on days when we can only eat less than 800 mg of calcium is certainly safe, but high-dose supplementation should probably be reserved for women with established osteoporosis or a high risk of osteoporosis. If you have a history of kidney stones, check with your doctor about calcium levels that are safe for you. For most women, however, a maximum calcium intake from *food and supplements* of 2000 mg a day is considered safe. Make sure to divide your intake throughout the day and save the final for bedtime, as the body tends to lose calcium during sleep. Calcium before bed may prevent leg cramps during the night. A glass of milk before bed also contains tryptophan (which will help you sleep), protein, and vitamins.

There is no agreement that calcium supplements are desirable for public health. The labels on some calcium supplements now list the percentage of elemental calcium in the supplement based on the assumption that 1000 mg per day is the recommended amount. If the label lists 200 mg of elemental calcium, then that is the actual amount in the supplement.

HOW MUCH CALCIUM IS IN THE SUPPLEMENTS?

- Calcium carbonate   40%
- Tricalcium phosphate   39%
- Calcium chloride   36%
- Calcium phosphate   23%
- Calcium lactate   13%
- Calcium gluconate   9%
- Bone meal*   31%
- Dolomite*   22%

To find the actual amount of calcium contained in each tablet, multiply the percentage of calcium contained in that particular form by the number of milligrams of the entire tablet. For instance, a 500 mg calcium carbonate tablet actually contains only 200 mg of elemental calcium (500 mg of calcium carbonate × .40 = 200 mg of calcium).

The question is not only how much calcium you are eating, but how your body is using it. It is doubtful that the calcium in these supplements is absorbed as well as the calcium in food. Calcium carbonate is not water-soluble and is not absorbed well, especially as we get older. Water-soluble calcium in calcium citrate, gluconate, aspartate, and lactate is more readily absorbed. Do not use calcium lactate if you have lactose intolerance. Many women, nevertheless, prefer to use calcium carbonate, which can be purchased at pharmacies in an inexpensive powdered form. Calcium carbonate is also found in some antacid tablets, which may also contain sugar. Be careful not to use an antacid containing aluminium as it can cause calcium to leave the bones. In addition, all calcium supplements are harder on the stomach than the calcium in food. For some women, calcium carbonate causes constipation, wind, or 'acid rebound' with heartburn. If you have an insufficient amount of hydrochloric acid in your stomach, which is common in older people, these products may make digestion difficult and can interfere with the absorption of other nutrients.

*Taken in small amounts as an occasional supplement to a healthy diet, the traces of toxic minerals reported in these sources of calcium are not harmful.

Vitamin D and magnesium are two important nutrients necessary for calcium absorption and utilization. Because vitamin D is formed on the skin in the presence of light, vitamin D deficiency can occur when we are not often exposed to sunlight. Although only one half-hour of sunlight daily on 20 to 30 per cent of the skin is needed, getting enough sunlight can be a problem for women who are housebound or institutionalized, or who spend the winter months in cold climates.[13] Vitamin D is not found in many foods. Cod-liver oil and other fish oils contain the highest amounts. You may be vitamin D deficient if you have reduced your consumption of egg yolks, butter, liver, and vitamin-D-fortified dairy products in order to reduce saturated fats and avoid lactose.[14] If you need to supplement your diet with vitamin D, 400 IUs per day is a reasonable amount. Magnesium is plentiful in green leafy vegetables, whole grains, nuts, seeds, and fruits. If you take a dietary supplement with calcium, it is a good idea to increase magnesium intake to half the level of your calcium intake.

DRUG EFFECTS ON NUTRIENT ABSORPTION

Drug	Effect	Drug	Effect
Over the Counter		Phenytoin	decreases
Aspirin	iron loss	(Epanutin)	vitamins D, K,
Antacids	phosphate loss, thiamine deficiency		and folic acid
		Phenobarbital	decreases vitamin D
Laxatives	decrease in potassium, calcium, magnesium, zinc, vitamins A, D, and E	Indomethacin (Indocid, Imbrilon) and other anti-inflammatory drugs	iron loss
Prescription		Chlorpromazine hydrochloride	decrease in riboflavin
Antibiotics	can decrease riboflavin, vitamin C, and calcium absorption and destroy the bacteria in the intestinal tract that produce vitamin K	(Largactil) and Thioridazine (Melleril)	
		Tricyclic antidepressants	weight gain or loss
		And many others. Check with your pharmacist.	

Chronic diseases as well as changes in cardiac, respiratory, liver, and kidney functions can affect our nutritional needs. In addition, many medications interfere with the absorption or utilization of nutrients. Eating well will help us stay healthy and resistant to disease.

FACTORS THAT DECREASE CALCIUM ABSORPTION

- Foods containing oxalic acid in combination with calcium interfere with calcium absorption. These are spinach, rhubarb, Swiss chard, sorrel, parsley, beet greens, and unhulled sesame seeds. None of these foods should be used as a main source of calcium, but can and should be added to a diet that is varied.
- Foods containing phytates (a substance found in the outer layers of grain seed, such as wheat bran) may also make calcium unavailable for absorption. Sprouted-grain breads contain no phytates, but unprocessed bran does. Phytates may be broken down more in breads baked with yeast than in unleavened breads and crackers. If your general calcium intake is varied, however, you do not need to worry about phytates.
- The absorption of calcium and that of fat are interrelated. Small amounts of fat improve calcium absorption; too much fat is unhealthy.
- High stress levels decrease absorption.
- Calcium absorption tends to decrease with age in both women and men.
- Caffeine and alcohol act as diuretics and can cause loss of calcium in the urine. Alcohol also directly interferes with calcium absorption.
- Drugs that impede calcium absorption include tetracycline, laxatives, corticosteroids, E panutin, diuretics, heparin, caffeine, antacids containing aluminium, and nicotine.
- There is a direct relationship between high salt intake and loss of calcium in the urine.
- While some phosphorus is needed, too much interferes with calcium absorption. Avoid excess red meat, cola drinks, and processed foods that have phosphorus additives.

NOTES

[1]Agriculture Research Service, *Family Economics Review*. Washington, DC: US Department of Agriculture, No. 1, 1983, p. 31.

[2]Jeffrey Bland, *Nutraerobics*. San Francisco: Harper & Row, 1983, p. 54.

[3]Rudolph Ballantine, *Diet and Nutrition*. Honesdale, Pa.: Himalayan International Institute, 1978, p. 10.

[4]Bland, op. cit., p. 59.

[5]C. W. Suitor and M. F. Crowley, *Nutrition: Principles and Applications in Health Promotion*, 2nd ed. Philadelphia: J. B. Lippincott Co., 1984, p. 152.

[6]Ballantine, op. cit.

[7]K. M. Hambidge, 'Hair Analysis: Worthless for Vitamins, Limited for Minerals'. *American Journal of Clinical Nutrition*, Vol. 36, November 1982, pp. 943–9.

[8]Erik Eckholm, 'Malnutrition in the Elderly: Widespread Health Threat'. *The New York Times*, 13 August 1985.

[9]Jeffrey B. Blumberg, 'Nutrient Requirements for the Healthy Elderly'. *Contemporary Nutrition*, Vol. 11, No. 6, 1986; Janet R. Mahalko et al., 'Nutritional Adequacy in the Elderly'. *The American Journal of Clinical Nutrition*, Vol. 42, September 1985, pp. 542–53; and Institute of Food Technologists' Expert Panel on Food Safety and Nutrition, 'Nutrition and the Elderly'. *Food Technology*, Vol. 40, No. 9, September 1986, pp. 81–8.

[10]Jane Fonda, *Women Coming of Age*. New York: Simon & Schuster, 1984, p. 195.

[11]Betty Kamen and Si Kamen, *Osteoporosis: What It Is, How to Prevent It, How to Stop It*. New York: Pinnacle Books, 1984.

[12]Jeanne Goldberg and Jean Mayer, 'Milk Isn't Natural for Everybody'. *The Boston Globe*, 2 May 1984.

[13]M. L. Freedman and Judith C. Ahronheim, 'Nutritional Needs of the Elderly: Debate and Recommendations'. *Geriatrics*, Vol. 40, No. 8, August 1985, pp. 45–62.

[14]Daphne A. Roe, *Geriatric Nutrition*. Englewood Cliffs, NJ: Prentice-Hall, 1983, p. 127.

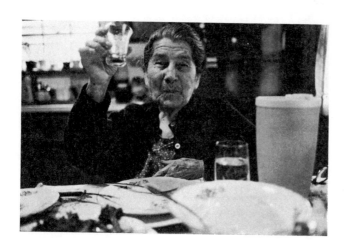

BOOKS AND PUBLICATIONS

Health Education Council, *Food For Thought*. Free from local health education units.

Joint Advisory Committee on Nutritional Education, *Eating for a Healthier Heart*. London: HMSO.

London Food Commission, *Report of the Food*

and Black and Ethnic Minorities Conference, 1986.

NACNE Report 1983. (A report on British diet and recommendations for healthy eating.) Free from local health education units.

Christopher Robbins, *Eating for Health.* London: Granada, 1985.

Leonard Mervyn, *The Dictionary of Vitamins: A Complete Guide to Vitamins and Vitamin Therapy.* Wellingborough: Thorsons, 1984.

Pamela Westland, *High Fibre Cook Book: Recipes for Good Health.* London: M. Dunitz: Macdonald Optima, 1982.

James Erlichman, *Gluttons for Punishment.* London: Penguin, 1986 (out of print but probably available from libraries).

Maurice Hanssen, *The New E for Additives.* Wellingborough: Thorsons, 1987.

Felicity Lawrence (ed.), *Additives: A Survival Guide.* London: Century, 1986.

Janet Pleshette, *Health on Your Plate.* London: Hamlyn, 1983. Foods must be combined in order that a complete diet of amino acids can be obtained from them, and hence the protein necessary for our diet. Vegetarians should be particularly aware of the amino acid content of foods, since non-vegetarians obtain most of their protein from meat. This book offers an excellent discussion on this subject.

Eating Well on A Budget. Mitcham: Age Concern. Recipes for pensioners from the BBC *Food and Drink* programme.

Health Education Council, *Guide to Healthy Eating.* Free leaflet from local health education units – based on COMA and NACNE reports.

Stephanie Lashford, *The Residue Report: The Action Plan for Safer Food.* Wellingborough: Thorsons, 1988. Includes a comprehensive bibliography on pesticide, hormone, etc. pollution.

6
Moving for Health

Many women walk, lift, bend, and stretch daily in their work. Increasingly, however, we are becoming more sedentary. Our desk jobs offer us little relief for the strain and inactivity imposed on our bodies. The washing machine and the car have replaced arm and leg power. Decreased energy, illness, age-related problems, and partial immobilization also make it easy to slip into sedentary habits.

There is strong evidence that appropriate levels of physical activity not only safeguard health, but improve it at any age, even if you have disabilities. In an experimental exercise programme at the University of Southern California, sixty- and seventy-year-old women and men became as fit and energetic as people twenty to thirty years younger. The older people in that programme who improved the most had been in the poorest shape![1]

I was having back pain, so I started to swim at the local baths. When I began, I was forty-six. I thought twenty-five lengths a day was terrific for my age. Now I'm fifty-four and I swim almost a mile (seventy-two lengths). My resting heart rate is fifty-three. That's the rate for a young male athlete.

After stopping exercises for one year for personal reasons, I got stiff, sluggish, flabby, and had aches and pains. I felt old and tired all the time. My spirit was low, too. When I started a regular regime again three times a week, I improved after three months. I felt alive again, got my stamina and good spirits back. [a seventy-five-year-old woman]

People who are active and who exercise tend to suffer less from headaches, chronic back pain, stiffness, painful joints, irregularity, and insomnia. Women often report renewed sexual energy and enjoyment, and the alleviation of hot flushes. Inactivity causes depression, poor circulation, weak muscles, stiff joints, shortness of breath, loss of bone mass, and 'that tired feeling'.[2] It's hard to get started if you're tired all the time.

But where to begin? We have to overcome society's prejudice against women being physically active, especially in their later years.

My son told me that he's embarrassed to have a mother who dances at seventy-five. He thinks I ought to be just sitting knitting.

When we exercise as hard as our bodies allow us to, we're actually being kind to ourselves. Joints develop or regain flexibility, muscles become strong, blood pressure lowers, bone density improves, our cardiovascular system becomes more efficient, and food digests better. We have more, rather than less, energy for everyday living. Feelings of alertness, well-being, and energy from exercise provide us, in turn, with reasons to stay active.[3]

I run several miles a week and I try to work out on a Nautilus machine twice a week. If I'm feeling depressed or tired, just having a half-hour run really helps. I know that if I'm feeling a bit depressed, I have a way out, running, and it really does help. It increases my energy level. [a forty-three-year-old woman]

Age is not the crucial factor in determining and improving fitness. More important are our general state of health and, to some extent, inherited characteristics. Patterns of activity adopted today will affect the strength and agility of our bodies tomorrow and in the years to come. Regardless of what we did in the past, today is the time to start living healthier, more active lives.

Getting Started

Shedding

My skin scares me. It feels tight.
I envy the snake who sheds his. Mine
binds me in limited space.
I circle, move more slowly, less,
a running-down top.

taking three deep breaths I
soar make
spirals that sweep
add more space
am alive

LOIS HARRIS

Unless you've been consistently exercising, start your new activities slowly and gradually. For example, find ways to increase the amount of time you spend walking each day. Try parking a block or two away from your destination or getting off the bus a few stops from where you're going, and walking the rest of the way. Add a few stairs whenever possible. Find reasons to walk instead of using your car.

No matter where you are, you can begin moving by stretching your fingers and toes, rotating your ankles, wrists, and shoulders, stretching out your arms and legs, and breathing deeply.

My idea of a woman in motion is me: I walk instead of riding; I climb stairs instead of using the escalator or lifts. I do these in addition to normal lifting, bending, carrying, stretching. [a seventy-two-year-old woman]

There are hundreds of daily opportunities to move – look for them! Try tightening abdominal and pelvic muscles while waiting for a bus, or swinging arms and legs while watching TV.

While daily activities keep us moving, they are usually not sufficient to promote and maintain the degree of fitness that promotes radiant health. Unless we do them correctly, many movements such as vacuuming, making beds, lifting, and even standing actually put added strain on the body, especially the lower back. To counteract inactivity or movements that potentially tire or strain our bodies, we need a complete exercise programme which includes stretching, strengthening, corrective posture, and cardiovascular conditioning. Among the activities that help achieve these are folk dancing, ballroom dancing, ballet, belly dancing, walking, running, biking, camping, boating, yoga, Tai Chi, jogging, hiking, weight training, swimming, skating, skiing, tennis, bowling, golf, squash, volleyball, and – you name it!

Some activities promote contact with other people. You can cultivate new friendships while you get fit at community centres, parks, adult education centres, YW and YMCAs, community schools, and colleges. Folk dancing and square dancing traditionally attract people of all ages. Clubs exist for people of all ages who like swimming, walking, bowling, golfing, or cycling.

If you can't find the activity or kinds of people you enjoy, you can always start something yourself. Many older women are seeking adventurous outdoor activities such as hiking and backpacking, fell walking, and adventure training.

When I was working I was a member of a climbing club attached to my workplace. I retired at sixty-five, and this coincided with the onset of some arthritic pain. A physiotherapist suggested that I needed to keep moving, but that I shouldn't overtax myself. Now I still enjoy visiting my old haunts, but I look up at the mountains instead of down at the valleys – and it's all just as beautiful on a two-mile walk as on a whole day's climb. [a seventy-one-year-old woman]

Your movement programme should be varied and should be compatible with your preferences and physical limitations.

When my mother was in her seventies and wheelchair-bound with Parkinson's disease, she was very excited and proud of learning to play 'basketball' – aiming the ball at a wastebasket in the centre of a circle of fellow-players in wheelchairs. My mother emigrated here from a very traditional community, where girls' sports were virtually nonexistent, so she was learning to play for the first time. [a forty-eight-year-old woman]

I am blessed with quite good health. I have arthritis, which I ignore.* I have a bike and ride whenever I can, but every morning I take a standing-still ride on an exercise bike in my bedroom. I also have a series of exercises which I do each morning to get my bones moving. I live very close to the centre of the city, and can walk practically anywhere I want to go. [a seventy-five-year-old woman]

Finding time for exercise despite all the demands of jobs and a busy home life can be difficult but empowering.

A good plan of exercise will allow for improvement in the four areas that comprise total fitness: flexibility, cardiovascular endurance, muscular strength, and body composition (ratio of body fat to lean body mass). We can set realistic and achievable goals for ourselves.

KEEPING OUR JOINTS SUPPLE

Flexibility is the ability of a joint to move freely about its axis. Chronic joint stiffness can lock us into painful fixed positions and keep us immobile and unable to do what we want to do. Gentle activity warms the gel that surrounds joints and that acts as a fluid lubricant. It's a good idea to exercise in the morning to liquefy the gel and lubricate the joints. Always warm up with about five minutes of walking, light jogging on the spot, stationary biking, or any activity that gently accelerates heart rate, breathing, and circulation. Try gentle swinging motions of arms and legs, circling of the wrists and ankles, and shoulder shrugs.

When I wake up I take a warm shower, run up and down the stairs a few times, ride a stationary bike while my cereal is cooking, and then am 'warmed up' enough to do my stretches before I eat. [a fifty-year-old woman]

Once the body is warmed up, do stretches by holding each one for ten to twenty seconds, letting gravity gently increase the stretch. Breathing should be

---

*In fact, she is not ignoring her arthritis but is helping it with exercise (see Joint and Muscle Pain, Arthritis and Rheumatic Disorders chapter).

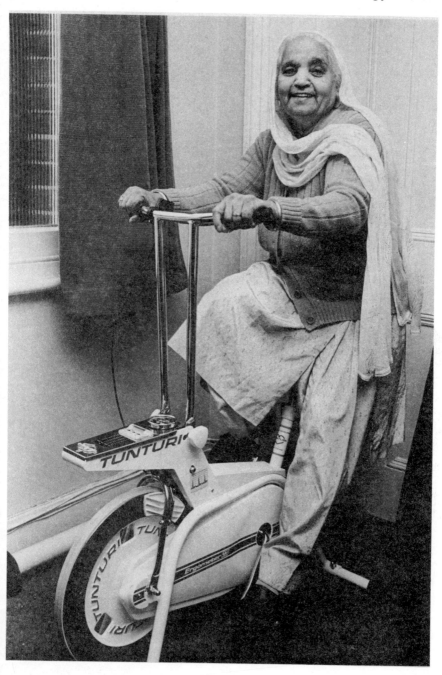

continuous and normal. This is called static stretching, which helps increase the space between joints and keeps the spine flexible. Do not do the bouncing, pulsing kind of stretches (called ballistic stretching), which can tear connective tissue, and do not stretch 'cold' muscles without sufficient warmup.

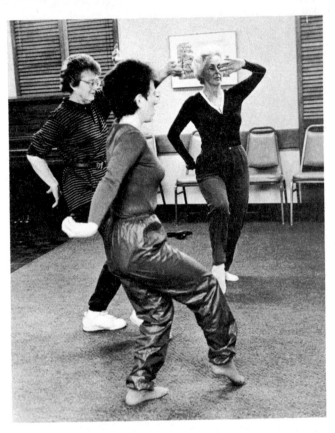

Be *especially gentle* when doing the following: (1) bending or rotating the head (it is best to go forward and side to side – not back); (2) dropping the head and body over the legs from a standing position (don't lock your knees when doing this); (3) extending the legs (lift, don't kick); (4) standing knee bends (always keep the knees over the toes and do not bend lower than 90 degrees); (5) arching the lower back (always be cautious: don't do 'donkey kicks' on your hands and knees, bringing the knee to the chest and then lifting the leg straight back, and don't do 'fire hydrants' on hands and knees, lifting the leg like a dog peeing); (6) don't do forced two-person stretches or bouncing stretches.

PUTTING YOUR HEART INTO IT: AEROBIC EXERCISE

The lungs, heart, and blood vessels, working together to carry oxygen to every cell in the body by means of the blood, comprise the cardiovascular system.

Aerobic (meaning 'in the presence of oxygen') exercise is any physical activity which uses the major muscle groups of the body in a rhythmic manner and which is performed at an intensity that raises the heart rate to between 60 and 85 per cent of its maximum capacity for twelve or more minutes. At this rate, the heart and lungs can keep up with the body's demand for oxygen and a conditioning effect takes place.

The benefits of such conditioning are a lowered pulse rate both at rest and during exercise, due to a larger and stronger heart muscle which allows more blood to be pumped with each beat, decreased blood pressure because of more elastic and stronger blood vessels, and more efficient removal of carbon dioxide – the end or waste product of breathing. Such conditioning can lengthen life.

Anaerobic exercise is any activity done so vigorously that the heart and lungs cannot keep up with the body's demand for oxygen and cannot carry away the chemical byproducts of exercise. Anaerobic exercise cannot be done continuously for long periods of time. Examples are sprinting and weight lifting.

Naturally, a beginner must get into aerobic exercise gradually. Start with three to five minutes of stationary biking, walking, or simple dance steps. Take your pulse count for ten seconds at rest, and then several minutes into your exercise routine. A pulse count is your only way of monitoring aerobic progress. In time, the aerobic portion of your exercise routine can last thirty minutes or longer, three times a week – or more. The safe way is to warm up, stretch, do your aerobic workout, then to cool down with slow walking or another gentle movement.

I have a series of yoga-type stretches I have done every morning for years that stretch every part of my body. They take ten minutes to do. Then I go out for a brisk thirty-minute walk. When I come in from my walk I am ready for my breakfast and feel energetic enough to face the day's work. [a sixty-year-old woman]

A second advantage to aerobic activity is that it causes excess fat to burn more efficiently than by any other means. A well-designed aerobic-exercise programme combined with proper eating may actually *increase weight* by increasing muscle and bone mass, but will *decrease fat*.

THE STRENGTH FACTOR

In order to perform many of our daily activities and to be able to bear the weight involved in many forms of aerobic exercise, our bodies must be strong.

HOW TO DETERMINE YOUR HEART RATE

1. Resting Heart Rate: Take your pulse for sixty seconds. Most people will get a 60, 70, 80, or 90. Take your pulse several times during the day to determine your average.
2. Maximum Heart Rate: Subtract your age from 220. This is the fastest your heart can beat. DO NOT EXERCISE AT THIS RATE!!!
3. Training Heart Rate, or Target Zone: Subtract your resting heart rate from your maximum heart rate; multiply by .60 and by .85; add to each your resting heart rate; the result is your training heart rate, or target zone, per minute. To find the rate for ten seconds, divide by six.

Example: A fifty-five-year-old woman has a resting heart rate of 85 beats per minute. To calculate the target zone (or range of heartbeats per minute within which she should carry on an aerobic activity):

$220-55$ (age)$=165$ (Maximum Heart Rate)
$165-85$ (Resting Heart Rate)$=80$

$80\times.60+85=133$ beats per minute
$80\times.85+85=153$ beats per minute
$133\div6=22.2$ (22 beats per 10 seconds)
$153\div6=25.5$ (26 beats per 10 seconds)

When this woman exercises, she should maintain a heart rate of 133 to 153 beats per minute (22 to 26 beats per 10 seconds).

Those on beta-blockers, blood-pressure medications, or other medications that may affect heart rate should check with their doctor about computing their maximum heart rate and about the percentage they should use in calculating their target zone.

Once you have calculated your target zone, take ten-second pulse checks at regular intervals (every five or ten minutes) during aerobic activity. Keep moving as you count, as heart rate drops rapidly when exercise is stopped. All you have to remember are the two ten-second figures – don't go below or above those numbers. It's also best to work near the lower or middle end of your target zone. The beneficial results are the same, and you are running no risk of injury if you are in normal health.

That's where muscles enter the picture. When a gradually increasing demand is placed upon muscles, they respond, given sufficient rest between exercise sessions (at least forty-eight hours), by becoming larger and stronger. Also, as muscles contract during exercise, they act beneficially on the bones, causing calcium to be properly deposited within them to make them denser and stronger.[4] This reduces chances of brittle, easily breakable bones – the condition known as osteoporosis.

Conventionally, girls and women have not been encouraged to be strong. Fortunately, that picture is changing.

I train people of all ages on Nautilus and on free weights. At least 50 per cent are women and they love the results. They stand taller and are stronger and have more endurance and muscle strength for walking, dancing, aerobics, skiing, and swimming. I'm a living example. My posture is great and I have a resting heart rate of 51. So – it can be done! (And I am fifty-one years old!)

Initially, and perhaps predictably, weights were considered a man's domain. After all, men were the more muscled of the species. Though men tend to develop greater muscle mass than women do, this does not mean that women cannot or should not develop their muscular potential to the fullest. Society has stereotyped women as soft, round, weak, and submissive. We can and must break that image. Our very health and survival depend on it.

Making gains in the development of muscular strength need not be difficult. Each day find ways to use your leg, arm, chest, back, and buttock muscles to lift, carry, support or move weight. When lifting, always bend your knees, use your leg not your back muscles, and keep objects close to your body. You can add weights to your home exercise programme by holding objects such as small cans of food or by purchasing a set of light hand and ankle weights with instructions. Some women make weights from mattress ticking filled with sand.

If you have experienced bone fractures because of osteoporosis, check with your doctor before working out with weights. Other exercises to strengthen the muscles and bones should be done first.[5]

POSTURE: STANDING TALL

Posture? We'd all like it to be good; but, aside from appearance, does it matter that much? Yes, it does, because posture profoundly affects physical and mental health.

Simply sitting for hours at a job, even slightly bent over, can induce high states of anxiety. The reason is that in this position the lungs are constricted, oxygen intake is reduced, and thus the amount of glucose (fuel for brain cells) that reaches the brain cells is greatly diminished. Sitting bent over can contribute to round shoulders, which can reduce breathing capacity, elevate blood pressure, and contribute to the formation of a dowager's hump.

Poor posture can affect digestion and elimination, contribute to hernias, haemorrhoids, intestinal diverticuli,[6] and bladder-control problems. With prolonged poor posture, some muscles shorten while others lengthen and weaken. A ripple effect takes place: one disturbed set of muscles, especially around a joint, affects others, and they, in turn, affect still others. Gradually, posture becomes increasingly faulty and injurious.[7]

Good posture permits free movement and offers the best starting point for any physical work or exercise. Since posture affects us all the time, it is advisable to pay attention to body alignment and body co-ordination while walking, standing, sitting, stooping, lifting, or doing more complicated movements. You can begin to change poor postural habits by strengthening abdominal, back, and chest muscles.

As one whose posture was poor all of my life, I speak from experience. No amount of urging me to 'stand up straight' on my mother's part or my own efforts to do so ever improved my posture one iota. At fifty-plus years of age I stand taller and prouder than ever before in my life. I owe it all to weight training. We have to be aware of what is holding the body upright. It's not bone. It's not fat. It's not water or blood. It's muscle – the active tensing of moving muscle tissue pulling upwards against the downward pull of gravity.

Designing Our Own Fitness Programme

The major muscles of the body that we need to strengthen are the abdominal muscles, the chest and back muscles, and the muscles of the legs and arms. Without fancy equipment and expensive clubs, we can use the most effective method of strengthening muscles – moving against the force of gravity. Walking, swimming, cycling, and dancing strengthen our muscles and improve the cardiovascular system. At any age, these are the most all-round beneficial, easily accessible, and least expensive kinds of activity.

In planning your activities, consider safety factors. Dress comfortably, wear proper shoes and a bicycle helmet when biking outdoors. Campaign with others for bike paths, safe streets, snow removal, and swimming lessons for the disabled and other adults in your community.

WALKING

Vigorous walking helps accelerate blood flow: the veins in the legs get squeezed with every step, sending the blood back to the heart. Brisk walking, including a few hills, can be an effective aerobic exercise. Keep your target zone in mind and calculate your pace. You might begin with $\frac{1}{4}$- to $\frac{1}{2}$-mile walks or even shorter ones daily. When that distance becomes easy, increase it gradually. When you can walk a mile without tiring, try walking that same distance a little faster. Then add a little more distance. Then more speed, etc. Walking provides the same benefits as jogging without the extra stress on joints.

SWIMMING

Swimming sets off a reflex action that enlarges the heart, causing it to pump more blood than it does in land sports, and also increases flexibility. Swimming does increase bone density, especially in the upper body, which is not strengthened by walking.

In swimming, as in other aerobic activities, when you hit your stride, your mind is free to wander, plan, solve problems, imagine.

I've learned to keep my pencil and a pad of paper in my locker so I can write down all the solutions that come pouring into my head after I've done about a third of my laps in the pool. [a fifty-four-year-old woman]

BICYCLING

Cycling is an excellent exercise for the cardiovascular system. There are adult three-wheeled bicycles that are easier to balance than two-wheelers. Stationary bicycles are also convenient for those who never learned to ride and for exercising while watching television, reading, or listening to music.

DANCING

Dancing is perhaps second only to walking as the most beneficial form of exercise. Besides developing flexibility and strength, it gives a natural 'high' and a feeling of well-being. Moving to a beat or to music is one of the oldest activities on earth.

As I dance, I affirm the beauty of my rounded belly that bore two babies who are now adults, of my heavy hips that carried them, the beauty of my breasts that nursed them, of my skin that is hard from years of heat and cold. As I dance, I affirm the strength of these legs that have laboured up fifty-six years of steps. I insist that my asthmatic lungs still work for my pleasure, and my curved back still supports my desire. As I dance, I reach out to other women and say, 'Look, we are beautiful; no one need tell us so; we know it; and we love each other.'

Furthermore, you can dance alone in the privacy of your own home to a record or the radio, as well as socially at gatherings, clubs, dance groups, and parties.

I learned how important it was for me to do some kind of movement as I got older. I developed an exercise and yoga programme for the elderly people at a senior citizens' club. Our movement leader was an enthusiastic fifty-nine-year-old dance therapist. At first, people were reluctant to get up from the lunch tables. But a seventy-eight-

year-old Chinese woman got up, smiling and dancing, and gradually others joined her. (She told us later that old people in China are very active. She was feeling depressed about being old here before she discovered us.)

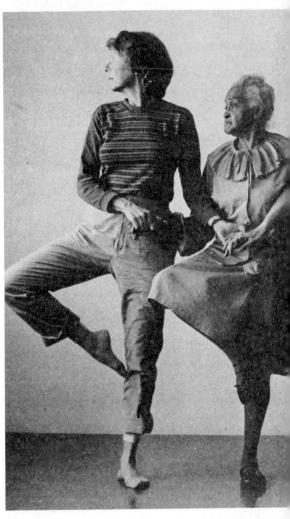

People came regularly for about three months. We saw women begin to unbend locked elbows and to twist heads and torsos that had stiffened into one piece. Once after a two-hour session, they didn't want to leave. So we did circle dances with tambourines, castanets, drums, ribbons, and scarves for another half an hour. While we were dancing, one woman, in her late eighties, turned to me and said: 'My

husband would never believe this if he saw me.' Another, who always carried a stick, left and forgot it. The therapist joked: 'And the lame shall walk.' But she had tears in her eyes. So did I. [a fifty-four-year-old woman]

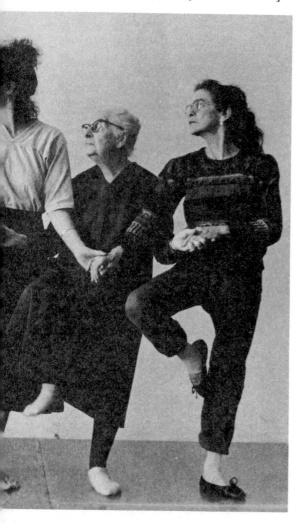

HATHA YOGA

Hatha Yoga is one of the best exercises for attaining total body flexibility. Its fringe benefits can include inner peace, relaxation, help with insomnia, decreased blood pressure, and relief from anxiety and stress.

Hatha Yoga has a great calming effect. It's good for stress reduction and flexibility. I was immobilized at age fifty-two by an arthritis attack. My yoga exercises helped me return to being as flexible as anyone.

Yoga is particularly useful as we age because its stretches keep joints flexible. Yoga positions help strengthen abdominal muscles and foster good posture – both areas that are vital to the health of older women.

TAI CHI

Tai Chi is a beautiful exercise and 'martial art' developed in ancient China. In modern China, it is considered especially appropriate for the old. Tai Chi is a continuous sequence of forms that includes gently moving all the joints and paying attention to the effect of breathing on the ebb and flow of energy. Tai Chi is becoming increasingly popular and available in this country because it has such positive effects on physical and emotional fitness.

In some countries, inner or spiritual growth through exercise is considered to be a major aspect of an ageing person's daily life. The disciplines from the East, such as yoga and Tai Chi, not only develop flexibility and strength, but also inner awareness and concentration.

I learned once, in a dance class, that it's important to talk to your body. It's like mothering a child. Instead of getting upset or angry because it isn't behaving the way you'd wish, you praise your body for small achievements, comfort it when it hurts, promise it pleasure, and encourage it to push just a little harder. In this way, I've learned that my body and I, though we feel separate, are different parts of the same being. [a fifty-four-year-old woman]

METHODS TO CHANGE HOW WE MOVE

Several movement/awareness approaches, such as the Feldenkrais method and the Alexander technique, use movement for improving both physical and emotional health. These methods are especially useful for learning how to move easily without pain despite disabilities and physical restrictions.

Some forms of psychotherapy also use the body to diagnose and treat emotional problems. The two best known, bioenergetics and psychomotor therapy, attempt to break through chronic muscle tensions developed early in life in response to emotionally disturbing situations. These methods can also improve co-ordination.

HOW MUCH OF A GOOD THING?

The average woman should start slowly and work up to three to five hours a week in a combination of flexibility, cardiovascular, and muscle-strengthening exercises to create and maintain fitness. Let your body be your guide. It helps to keep a diary for several months after starting a movement plan to clarify needs, expectations, and feelings about the programme you've started.

When Movement is Limited

There are times when we can't be active – during illness, or when recuperating from an illness or an operation. Some of us suffer from disabilities that greatly restrict movement. If you have a disability, you can still benefit from exercise. Even if you are bed- or wheelchair-bound, you can improve lung capacity, muscle strength, and flexibility with consistent daily exercise tailored for you. Few conditions require total rest or immobility. Ask your physiotherapist to guide you in designing a medically sound movement programme.

It's difficult and discouraging to exercise when we're feeling weak or in pain. But there is no question about the importance of exercise in rehabilitation. A moderate and regular exercise programme helps many problems.

A massive stroke impaired my ability to function independently. The effects seriously damaged my physical and emotional stability. Learning to swim was one of my most effective coping techniques. Two swimming sessions (forty-five minutes each) weekly increased my strength and endurance. The encouragement from the therapist and members of the group for even a small accomplishment was a tremendous morale booster. We adopted the motto 'Press on regardless'. The formation of new friendships was essential in helping to develop emotional security. [a thirty-eight-year-old woman]

Close to 100 per cent in a survey of women with arthritis mentioned that regular exercise decreased their pain.[8]

If you are confined to a chair or bed, exercise can help maintain strength and flexibility of joints and muscles, good digestion and bowel movements, good blood circulation, and a better mental outlook. It can prevent bedsores, and it makes things easier for the caregiver as well. Community nurses and nursing home personnel should be trained to provide exercises for persons in beds or chairs.

Here is a list of things you can do at your own pace. Try them for a few days and experience the relaxation and the gentle glow of energy that simple movement can give you. Do the exercises with energy and concentration to enhance their effectiveness. Start slowly and do more each day. *Many of these exercises are the same ones that women in more fit condition will find useful also.*

1. Breathe deeply.
2. Contract and relax any muscle group you can control. While breathing regularly, tighten the muscles for several seconds, and then slowly release. Be aware of the relaxation that follows.
3. Pelvic floor exercises and 'tummy blops' (see pp. 124–6).
4. Exercise your face muscles by making 'funny faces'. Move your lower jaw from side to side and forward and back. Open eyes wide, then squeeze shut. Wiggle your ears if you can.
5. Stretch and limber the neck slowly, carefully. In bed your neck is protected from bending too far backward. Rotate the head in wide circles, in both directions. Alternately look slowly to the ceiling, stretching the front of the neck, then look slowly down, being aware of a stretch in the back of the neck ('Yes'). Then turn the head from side to side ('No').
6. Placing hands on shoulders or by your sides, rotate shoulders in both directions.
7. Stretching arms out to your sides, twist them in both directions. Make small circles with your hands and then with your arms. Then open and close fists. Alternately stretch each arm upward from the shoulder as if picking apples.
8. Circle wrists as far as they can go. Quickly open and close fists several times, stretching fingers. Circle your ankles in both directions. Flex feet backward and forward, then clench toes and release.
9. Tie a rope to the foot of your bed (or have someone do this for you) and slowly pull yourself to sitting position, then lower again.
10. 'Walk' against the footboard of the bed.
11. If you can, pull your knee to your chest; then the other knee; then both.
12. If you can stand, hold on to the back of a chair while rotating your legs, one at a time, from the hip. Rotate in both directions. Then extend your leg forward and slowly swing your lower leg backward and forward.

Avoiding Injury

The best way to avoid injury is to get a medical checkup before you start an exercise programme. The examination should make you aware of potential problem areas and possible limiting factors, and help you to set realistic goals. Particularly if you decide to undertake demanding movement programmes like tennis, badminton, use of Nautilus or other weight-lifting equipment, or if you have physical disabilities, it's best to get a medical evaluation to prevent injury, to get the maximum benefit from what you do, and to set realistic goals. Your doctor may refer you for a stress test, which monitors your heart while you are performing an ever-increasing work load on a treadmill, to discover and make you aware of any hidden heart disease. It isn't infallible, however, especially for women, and may be too stressful (p. 436).

In the long run, only you can choose how much caution (or precaution) to use before starting your exercise plan. Most important, always pay close attention to how you feel.

Normal Reactions to Exercise:
Increased depth and rate of breathing
Increased heart rate
Feeling/hearing your heart beat
Mild to moderate perspiration
Mild muscle aches and tenderness at first

Abnormal Reactions to Exercise – STOP IMMEDIATELY:
Severe shortness of breath
Wheezing, coughing, difficulty in breathing
Chest pain, pressure, or tightness
Lightheadedness, dizziness, confusion, word slurring, fainting
Cramps, severe pain, severe muscle ache
Nausea
Severe, prolonged fatigue or exhaustion after exercising

If these symptoms recur with further exercise, check with your doctor. You might need special guidance.

Some General Precautions

1. Lubricate *all* joints with gentle bending and swinging (shoulders, elbows, wrists, knees, ankles), contraction and release (fingers, toes, arches, spine), and stretches.
2. Don't hold your breath; co-ordinate full breathing with each movement.
3. Drink fluids before and after exercising. It is common as we age not to feel thirsty, even when dehydrated.
4. When ill, do only mild stretches, joint lubrication, and deep breathing. Gentle movement that doesn't cause you to tire will allow your body to use its energy for rehabilitation. This is a good time to practise deep breathing and meditation.
5. No two bodies are alike. Achieve what is possible for yourself; do not compare yourself to others.

6. Wear any comfortable clothing that breathes (natural fibres like cotton are best), that doesn't bind in the crotch, around the shoulders, or at the waist. There's no need to spend money on expensive sportswear unless you want to. *Never* wear rubberized or plastic sweat suits. They can cause high internal temperatures (hyperthermia), dehydration, and even death. Supportive shoes with arches are necessary to soften impact on your organs and spine. If you decide to jog, buy running shoes; if you do aerobic dancing, buy aerobic shoes. They are not the same. Running shoes have more support in the heel and aerobic shoes have more support under the ball of the foot.

Exercises for All Women

Two problems that are special issues for women are very much affected by exercise. These are:

- Bladder control to prevent loss of urine, particularly when we cough, sneeze, or laugh. The strength of the muscles in the pelvic floor, abdomen, and back is very important.
- Loss of bone density due to inactivity, resulting in osteoporosis and bone fractures.

Exercises to Develop Your Own 'Girdle'

These exercises are often called 'Kegel' exercises after Dr Arnold Kegel, who first began his pioneering research in the 1940s in the US, in response to women's complaints of leaking urine.[10] He later demonstrated how strengthening the pubococcygeal muscle (also called the levator ani muscle) not only improves bladder control, but also contributes to increased sexual satisfaction and more comfortable childbirth. In Britain these exercises are called 'pelvic floor' exercises in reference to the muscles supporting the internal organs, not because they must be done lying on the floor.

When you exercise the pubococcygeal muscle you will become aware of your vagina. A surprising number of adult women have to be taught how to locate this muscle and how to exercise it; they have been living for years with a kind of inertness or numbness in this region. Others, even at an advanced age, still do not know that there are three separate openings in the pelvis of the female body. One woman in her seventies wanted to use tampons in her vagina to absorb urine leakage.

When women use cloth and elastic girdles, they are trying to compensate for the loss of control over abdominal muscles. Keeping these muscles in shape not only improves the contours of the body, but also contributes to the support of the internal organs and the back.

A good way to locate the muscles that support the bladder and uterus is to spread your legs apart and start and stop the flow of urine. Other methods are to tighten around one or two fingers inserted into the vagina or around a man's erect penis during intercourse. Your ability to do these indicates how strong your muscles are.

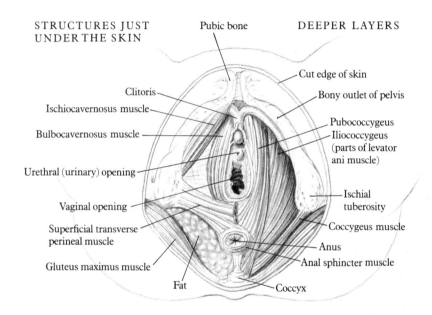

STRUCTURES JUST UNDER THE SKIN

Pubic bone

DEEPER LAYERS

Cut edge of skin

Clitoris

Ischiocavernosus muscle

Bulbocavernosus muscle

Urethral (urinary) opening

Vaginal opening

Superficial transverse perineal muscle

Gluteus maximus muscle

Fat

Bony outlet of pelvis

Pubococcygeus
Iliococcygeus
(parts of levator ani muscle)

Ischial tuberosity

Coccygeus muscle

Anus

Anal sphincter muscle

Coccyx

Start these exercises by lying down, as there will be less pressure on the pelvic floor from the weight of the pelvic organs. If you cannot feel the muscle working in this position, raise your buttocks on a pillow and use gravity to assist. As you progress and the pelvic floor strengthens, do your exercises while sitting or standing rather than lying down.

As you should with all exercises, breathe naturally when doing them. You may combine these exercises, but in order not to strain or overwork your pelvic floor, do no more than fifty contractions a day.[11]

Exercise 1: Contract or draw up the pelvic floor, hold for three seconds, and relax. Repeat five times. Repeat the series occasionally during the day, building up to ten groups of five contractions. If the muscle feels sore, reduce the number of contractions or stop for a day or two until this temporary soreness disappears, and then increase gradually.

Exercise 2: Think of your bladder and uterus as a lift which you are trying to raise to a higher floor, and visualize pulling them up into the abdominal cavity toward your stomach. When you reach the top, go down floor by floor again, gradually relaxing the muscles in stages. When you reach the basement, let go of all the tension and think release. Then come back up again to the ground floor, so the pelvic floor is slightly tense and able to hold the organs firmly in place.

Exercise 3: Raise the entire pelvic area, as though sucking water into the vagina. Relax and repeat five times. This series of five contractions may be repeated four to six times a day, building up to twenty to thirty contractions a day.

The following exercises will strengthen the upper and lower abdominal muscles. In order to do them effectively and protect your back, tighten your abdominal muscles before you start rather than doing them with your abdomen sticking out.

For the upper abdominals, do modified bent-knee sit-ups. Lying on your back with knees bent and feet flat on a bed or the floor, lift the head and shoulders while reaching forward with the hands to touch the knees, then lie back again, keeping eyes looking up and shoulders off the bed or floor. Reach for your left knee with your right hand as you twist your waist slightly, then do the same with the right knee and left hand. As you become stronger, you can do these sit-ups with your hands behind your head (do not pull up on your head – use hands only to support your head on the way down), reaching your elbows toward your knees. Do not do sit-ups with straight legs.

For the lower abdominals, lie on your back with legs extended straight up overhead. You may find this easier to do with your buttocks against a wall. 'Walk' your feet in the air in place or toward your head. 'Bicycling' with legs as high as possible also strengthens the lower abdominals.[12] Also while standing, tighten your abdominal muscles with tummy 'blops'. On an empty stomach only, inhale fully, exhale fully, then tighten and release stomach muscles three or four times. Then inhale, and repeat the cycle several times. Another way is to lie on your side with your knees drawn up. Contract your belly muscles so that you pull your knees and head closer together.

Exercising for Strong Bones

Remember that when we are physically active, the body uses calcium efficiently for bone growth and maintenance. When we are inactive, calcium is not absorbed well into the bones but is 'dumped' and excreted in the urine. The depletion of bone cells (osteoporosis) can lead to a dowager's hump and to bone fractures. Many doctors now treat osteoporosis with special exercises.[13]

For older women, fast walking is the best exercise to increase bone density in the lower body. If you have no spinal or skeletal problems, jogging may be all right, but it is more stressful on the joints. Exercise the upper body as well so calcium will be deposited in all the bones. Weight training, which develops muscle, is especially beneficial because it also increases the strength of the connective tissues, tendons, and ligaments. Exercise also improves balance and co-ordination so we are less likely to fall or, if we do fall, more likely to fall safely.

'Going Formal': Choosing an Exercise Class

If you want to undertake a conditioning programme that requires special facilities or instructions, take time to find the best place. Any fitness centre should provide safety, well-trained instructors, and personal attention. It should be reasonably priced, easily accessible, and suited to your personal needs. In considering whether you can afford instruction, keep in mind the

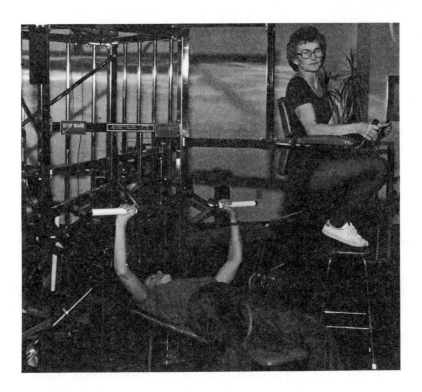

intangibles that aren't price-tagged: better health can give you time otherwise spent in illness; you will feel better about yourself and life.

What should you look for in a fitness centre or exercise class?[14] First, find the place that has the activities you want. Next, check further about each: Are their hours convenient? Can you get there easily? If you have special needs, will they be met there? Are the costs reasonable?

Then, arrange a tour of centres that meet your criteria, and ask questions. What credentials do the staff have?

In recent years there has been a boom in the 'fitness industry' in the UK, and it has been possible for totally untrained people to set themselves up as exercise class leaders or fitness experts. Ask around and find out from friends whether they've been satisfied with any centre they've attended. Fitness teachers should hold a certificate in physical education or be members of a recognized teachers' organization.

In some areas you will find a special Over Sixties keep-fit class at an adult education centre, and there you can be sure that the class leader is properly trained. Fees are much lower than those for commercial fitness centres, too.

When you do visit a privately-run fitness centre, try to go at the busiest time of day, or at a time you will want to use the centre. Ask some of the clients how they like the centre, and what some of the problems are. Look to see whether equipment is in good condition and whether showers and other wet areas are clean. Beware of places that push 'lifetime contracts'. A life membership lasts only as long as the life of the centre unless another operator takes over and honours the existing contracts. Buy the shortest-term package to try out before committing a lot of money. Does the centre take a medical history? Do they take blood pressure and pulse rate before, during, and after exercise? Can you get personal guidance in the use of equipment? Some centres have special rates for club usage during the midday hours, when it is least busy. If those hours are convenient for you, this may be an ideal arrangement, as it benefits both you and the club.

Don't make a decision on your first visit. Beware of high-pressure salespeople who offer you bargains if you 'make a decision today', or who refuse to allow you to take the contract home to review before signing. The right choice can make a big difference in whether you use the centre regularly, consistently, and safely.

Finally, guard against giving up instead of accepting limits and going on.

I used to like to go mountain climbing. When I couldn't do that, I went hill climbing. Now I walk on more level ground. You don't have to give up your dream. You just shape it differently. [an eighty-two-year-old woman]

NOTES

[1]Herbert A. deVries with Diane Hales, *Fitness After Fifty*. New York: Charles Scribner's Sons, 1974, pp. 9–11.

[2]James Blumenthal and R. Sanders Williams, Duke University Center for the Study of Aging. *Center Reports*, Vol. 6, No. 3, December 1982, p. 4.

[3]Robert S. Brown et al., 'The Prescription of Exercise for Depression'. *The Physician and Sports Medicine*, Vol. 6, No. 12, December 1978, pp. 52–8.

[4]A. Chamay and P. T. Schantz, 'Mechanical Influences in Bone Remodeling: Experimental Research on Wolff's Law'. *Journal of Biochemistry*, Vol. 5, 1972, pp. 173–80; and E. L. Smith, Jr et al., 'Bone Involution Decrease in Exercising Middle-Aged Women'. *California Tissue International*, Vol. 36, Supplement 1, 1984, pp. 129–38.

[5]Joseph Lane, 'Post Menopausal Osteoporosis: The Orthopedic Approach'. *The Female Patient*, Vol. 6, November 1981, p. 54.

[6]Gerda Hinrichsen, *Body Shop: Scandinavian Exercises for Relaxation*. New York: Taplinger Publishing Co., Inc., 1976, p. 46.

[7]Joseph T. Freeman, 'Posture of the Aging and Aged Body', in *Health Aspects of Aging*. American Medical Association Committee on Aging, Chicago, 1965, pp. 49–55.

[8]*Hot Flash*, Vol. 3, No. 2, Winter 1984, p. 1.

[9]Stephanie Fallreek and Mollie Mettler, *A Healthy Old Age: A Source Book for Health Promotion with Older Adults*. Wallingford Wellness Project, Seattle, Wash.: University of Washington School of Social Work, 1979; and Henry C. Barry, 'Exercise Prescriptions for the Elderly'. *American Family Physician*, Vol. 34, No. 3, September 1986, pp. 155–62.

[10]Arnold Kegel, 'The Physiologic Treatment of Poor Tone and Function of the Genital Muscles and of Urinary Stress Incontinence'. *Western Journal of Surgery, Obstetrics, and Gynecology*, Vol. 57, 1949, pp. 527–35.

[11]With thanks to the Adelaide Women's Community Health Centre, North Adelaide, Australia, for their instructions, 'Exercising and Strengthening the Pelvic Floor, Kegel Exercises'; and Sheila Kitzinger, *Woman's Experience of Sex*. New York: Penguin Books, 1985, pp. 48–50.

[12]Personal communication from Maggie Lettvin.

[13]Lane, op. cit., p. 54.

[14]Adapted from Gretchen M. Von Mering, *The Fitness Directory: A Guide to Exercise, Nutrition, and Recreation Programs and Services in the Greater Boston Area*. Boston: The Medical Foundation, Inc., 1983, pp. 5–15.

BOOKS AND PUBLICATIONS

Sports Council, *Exercise. Why Bother?* Fitness for all age groups.

Which? 'Report on the effects of various forms of exercise'. London: Consumers' Association, February 1984.

Take Care of Yourself: Health Handbook for Older People. London: Help the Aged/Buckingham: Winslow Press, January 1988. Includes a section on exercise.

Eira M. Davies, *Let's Get Moving: Group Activation of Elderly People*. Mitcham: Age Concern, February 1975. Handbook for group facilities.

Sports Council, *50+ All to Play For*. Free leaflets on a variety of leisure and sporting facilities, from regional Sports Council Offices.

Audrey Cloet and Chris Underhill, *Gardening is for Everyone*. London: Human Horizons/Souvenir Press, 1982.

Russell Gibbs, *Exercise for the Over-50s*. London: Jill Norman, 1981.

7
Sexuality in the Second Half of Life

*Letter to My Children**

If we
could start again
You, newbegotten, I
A clean stick peeled
of twenty paper layers of years
I'd tell you only what you know,
Teach one commandment,
'Mind the senses and the soul
Will take care of itself
Being five times blessed.'

ANNE WILKINSON

We affirm ourselves as we experience pleasure through our senses. Now that we are older, if we attend to the wisdom of our minds and bodies, we can enhance our sexual pleasure. The pleasures of the body, and specifically sexual pleasures, provide us with release, shared intimacy, communion with our inner selves and with our partners, and a chance to express ourselves physically. We can give ourselves pleasure through masturbation, whether or not we are in a sexual relationship with another person. Sex allows us intimate connection with someone we love, or adventure with a new partner. Our senses provide us with pleasure and our thoughts and feelings give meaning to our experience.

Almost all of us who are middle-aged or older grew up in an environment where attitudes toward sexuality were more rigid than they are today. We may have learned that we should not talk about sex and that women do not or should not enjoy sex as much as men, or that men should always initiate sex. Because of this early training, we may still feel embarrassed or ashamed over sexual issues. Paradoxically, we may believe that because of the 'sexual revolution' we

*From *Collected Poems of Anne Wilkinson*, A. Smith, ed., Macmillan Co. of Canada Ltd, 1968, p. 94.

shouldn't be uncomfortable, or that we ought to have more sex than we do. A double standard of sexual behaviour still exists, particularly among middle-aged and older people. This chapter is intended to affirm and support our sexuality and to help all of us enjoy our sexuality more fully.

Two misconceptions occur when women are stereotyped by ageist thinking. Older women are considered neither sexually attractive nor sexually active. Those men who are available often choose younger women or women who look young as partners. Things are changing slowly in this respect. According to a recent article in *Time*, 'The average age of desirability in American women seems to have risen by a dozen years or more.'[1] Yet we are still expected to project a youthfully glamorous image. These stereotypes make it hard for us to fully accept our sexuality. Believing the stereotypes leads to fear and denial of ageing, and takes a toll on our self-esteem when we see the signs of ageing in ourselves and in those we love.

As we age, some physical changes occur which may affect our sexual activity. But there is no physical reason based on age alone why we cannot continue to enjoy sex for as long as we live. Despite social pressures, many of us are accepting and enjoying our sexuality more freely than ever. One way we can help ourselves in this respect is to break through the barrier of silence and talk with each other about sexuality. Although it may be hard to talk openly with other women about sex if you have never done so, it is such a positive experience that it is worth the effort. By listening to older women in our families or in women's groups, we can recognize negative messages about sex which we received as children, and then re-evaluate our attitudes. Talking to family members about sex can be especially difficult; yet it is often liberating.

Women's groups in which we talk about sexual experiences and feelings have developed since the late sixties as an outgrowth of the women's movement. There are women's groups and a few women's centres in the UK, and the Older Feminists' Network with contacts in London and some other cities. It is common to hear women exclaim, 'I never knew anyone else felt the way I do!' One long-married woman, age fifty, who had complained of lack of sexual interest, returned to a women's group to say, 'After our discussion last week I went home and talked with my husband and we had an absolute orgy!'

Myths and Realities about Women, Sex, and Ageing

Sexism, ageism, homophobia, and Victorianism all interact to create a pervasive mythology about sex and the older person. These myths do the most damage when we ourselves accept and act on them, and in so doing give up pleasures that are an important and valuable part of our humanity. Consider the following:

Myth 1: Older people are no longer interested in sex and sexuality and no longer engage in sexual activity. Sex is for the young.

This myth has its roots in several notions that link sex and youthfulness. Since society equates attractiveness with youth, it follows that, according to the myth, when you are no longer young, you are no longer desirable.

This myth also connects sexuality with romantic love. In the media, in stories, songs, and the general folklore of our culture, romantic love is the exclusive province of young heterosexual women and men.[2]

The reality is that if you are interested in sex and want to act on that interest, you are just like many other people your age. A recent study of people sixty to ninety-one years old revealed that 91 per cent enjoyed sex for a variety of reasons: it reduces tension, makes women feel more feminine, helps people sleep, and provides a physical outlet for emotion. The people studied engaged in sexual relations an average of 1.4 times a week – about what they averaged when they were in their forties.[3] Both the Kinsey research and Masters and Johnson found that women and men continue their accustomed sexual patterns throughout their later years. If you led an active sexual life when you were younger, you can look forward to continuing to do so. If you found sex a burden, you may decide to cease sexual activity as you grow older. Masters and Johnson's research confirmed what many women have discovered for themselves: that there is no time limit on women's sexual capacity. Although our responses may slow down, we can continue to enjoy sex and orgasm throughout our lives.[4]

It is often especially difficult for adult daughters and sons to accept us as sexual beings – they continue to see us as asexual, as they did during childhood.

Myth 2: Changes in hormone levels which occur during and after menopause create a 'deficiency disease' that causes women to find sex uncomfortable and unpleasant.

Menopause has been the subject of many fallacious myths, several created and perpetuated by doctors, psychiatrists, and drug companies. The notion that menopause produces a deficiency disease[5] has, among other things, fostered widespread use of hormonal supplements. In fact, menopause is a normal life transition, not a disease. Women continue to feel sexual and enjoy sex until very late in life.

Myth 3: Women who are beyond childbearing years lose their desire and their desirability.

Sexuality and sex appeal are not the same as fertility. For many older women and men sex is actually *better* in the later years. Many women experience a reawakening of sexual interest when pregnancy is no longer a worry. Couples often have more time to relate to each other sexually after children are grown up. A divorce or other life change which has nothing to do with fertility may also contribute to a reawakening of sexual interest.

Myth 4: In order to have a full and complete sex life, a woman must have a male partner.

Although the majority of women do have relationships with men, we can be sexual in a variety of ways – with a man or a woman or by pleasuring ourselves alone. The choice is ours to make.

Myth 5: The only truly satisfying and acceptable sex is through intercourse, culminating in mutual orgasm. All other sexual activity is 'foreplay' and doesn't count.

While sex is sometimes defined in terms of intercourse, it is not true that intercourse is the only satisfying form of lovemaking. As we age, our experience of intercourse changes. Older women and men need more time for sexual stimulation before they are ready for intercourse. Once we learn that gratifying sexual experience without penetration is a possible choice, we can feel free to explore the variety of other caresses that can provide pleasure.

Older people report in several studies that oral sex is a favourite activity.[6] Cuddling, caressing, and manual stimulation are also satisfying. Lovemaking may continue to be satisfying whether one, both, or neither party has an orgasm.

Sex and Ageing: Some Women's Experiences

People have this idea that sex is somehow naughty for older people. They picture serene and wise grandparents. Older people are not supposed to be feeling and passionate. But at fifty I thought, 'Hey, I'm old enough to do as I damn well please.'

There is a current of sexuality in everyday life. I find him a very attractive man and he finds me a desirable woman and we tell each other that without words all the time. There's a kind of flow. [a fifty-eight-year-old woman whose husband is seventy-five]

After I came out as a lesbian I danced more than I had in the previous thirty-five years. People ask if I feel foolish – not at all! It's good for the young to know you can keep right on doing, and not pay attention to the wrinkles. [a woman in her eighties]

When searching for a new partner, I often felt discouraged about looking older and worried that I would no longer be appealing to men. Once I was in a relationship, the years I've lived became a plus; I felt proud of my experience and skill as a lover, something I did not have as a younger woman. [a forty-eight-year-old divorced woman]

I've worked at learning to let go of rational thinking during sex. I say I'm going to experience the moment. Here is a wonderful experience I'm going to have, a dedicated time and place. I'm going to live it fully. I soak up the feelings, immerse myself in the sensation and pleasure. The more I do it, the better it gets, like turning a golden key. It is very beautiful to me. [a single woman in her late fifties]

At seventy-three, being sexual feels right, comfortable, and just plain satisfying, but it wasn't always like this. Growing up with Victorian spinster aunts, the family disgrace of a flapper cousin who 'had to get married', and baffling warnings to always be careful on infrequent dates left me with feelings of being ugly and unwanted. Where I am today is one stage in a constant process of growing. I learned to love and be loved, helped by friends and lovers. I bore a child at age thirty-eight and raised him, developing my own changing value system.

When I was growing up women worried about being thought bossy or wilful when we were outspoken or assertive. Now my husband has become more nurturing and accepting of my assertiveness. Our relationship is more balanced. [a woman in her sixties]

We could be equals. We could be friends. I didn't need anything from him and I was free to be me. We were like two kids playing in a sandbox. Oh Lord. A chance to play! [a divorced woman in her fifties]

Now I can just enjoy it. I don't have to be such a good citizen. When I was younger I worried so much for my partner that I never got much real pleasure for myself. [a woman in her fifties]

I have earned the right to express what I like and expect to get it. I want pleasure, joy, fun, and passion during sex for the rest of my life. My contribution to a partner is to give her the same. [a woman in her fifties]

I feel more accepting than I used to – if I don't have an orgasm, if he doesn't have an orgasm, if we stop in the middle, or if we just go to bed and hold each other – it's much more all right than it was when I was younger. [a fifty-five-year-old divorced woman]

Last year I spent several months without sex. I masturbated occasionally, but I even stopped that after a while. I simply didn't miss it; it didn't seem terribly important. I was working pretty hard. Now I'm enjoying it again, but I could do without it. I don't find myself with that rush about sex any more – that feeling of getting hit in the stomach – none of that passion. I still have orgasm, but I seem to have lost my passion, lust. In a way, that's restful. [a fifty-five-year-old woman]

I used to enjoy masturbation and orgasm. But now I don't have any desire for that or a sexual relationship. [an eighty-year-old woman]

Sex was fine but it was only a part of our marriage and I was happily married for thirty years. Since my husband died I've never looked at another man. I masturbate occasionally, but it's not important to me. Knowing another person – that is what matters. I get as much pleasure from my work as I might get from sex. [a sixty-year-old woman]

I miss the intimacy, the love letters, but I'm back solidly celibate. I never could masturbate. It's not the orgasm I crave, but the intimacy – the candles, the flowers, the feeling of another body. [a seventy-two-year-old woman commenting on the ending, several years ago, of a relationship with a woman]

Pleasuring Ourselves*

Masturbation is one way of giving ourselves pleasure. Most of us enjoy a variety of sensual pleasures and view pleasure as a good thing, yet many of us were taught to believe that giving ourselves *sexual* pleasure is bad. Whether we masturbate or not is our choice. Pleasuring ourselves through masturbation can be a satisfying alternative to sex with a partner. If you have lost a partner with whom you enjoyed good lovemaking, you may not be ready to start over with someone new.

After my divorce masturbation was an important part of my life that made it very nice to go to bed. It's still a special occasion. [a seventy-eight-year-old woman]

If you do have a partner, masturbation can be a good way to learn about your own sexual responses – what fantasies you enjoy, what kinds of touch arouse you and please you – without having to worry about your partner's needs and opinions. Then, if and when you choose, you can tell or show your partner

---

*The expression 'pleasuring ourselves' as an alternative for the word 'masturbation' was suggested to us by Eleanor Hamilton, a seventy-five-year-old pioneer in sex education who has written a great deal about cultural biases against pleasure and sex. Hamilton objects to the word 'masturbation', which is derived from the Latin meaning 'to pollute with the hand'.

what you've learned. Some of us incorporate masturbation into our lovemaking with a partner as a way to enhance pleasure and to reduce pressure on both partners to 'satisfy' the other.

If you have never masturbated but would like to try, it may take some time to adjust to the idea and to find the way that gives you the most pleasure. The Books and Publications note on page 161 lists some excellent books that offer specific suggestions. Deliberately setting the mood in much the same way you would with a partner – candles, incense, and music – can enhance the experience. A soothing bath or a glass of wine may help you relax and focus on yourself for an interlude of personal sexual pleasure. You may enjoy the feelings of arousal whether or not you have an orgasm.

Those of us for whom masturbation is not an acceptable choice can still enjoy sensuality – luxuriating in a bubble bath, feeling the sun on our skin, exchanging a massage with a friend. These body experiences can enrich our lives and help us feel alive and vital.

FANTASIES

Sexual fantasy can help arouse, maintain, and increase sexual excitement. It is particularly helpful to women who lose their concentration during sex. A fantasy can be a story or stories, or a series of erotic images. Sometimes partners share their fantasies.

We have a wide variety of scenes. I am the rampaging female who leaps into bed in a comical way. Or when I'm very tired he says, 'You rest, I'll do all the work.' Or we play who gets to be the baby – or other psychological conditions – we play with them and we don't feel threatened. [a woman in her late fifties]

We may feel disloyal to a partner if we fantasize while lovemaking or worry that something we imagine is bad or 'sick'. Yet creating erotic images is just a way of allowing ourselves to experiment without risk. It may take a while to accept our fantasies and understand that we can enjoy them without having to act on them.

Sexuality and Relationships

During the second half of life, we face major physical and emotional changes affecting our sexuality. Many long-time partners feel increasingly more comfortable over time as they learn how to give sexual pleasure to each other.

In a long-term relationship, lovemaking provides a way to express our deepest feelings of tenderness and mutual caring. Lovemaking can also provide comfort during times of loss and change.

We were feeling so troubled and unhappy we just went to bed and made love to give each other some solace for this terrible sadness. [an eighty-two-year-old woman]

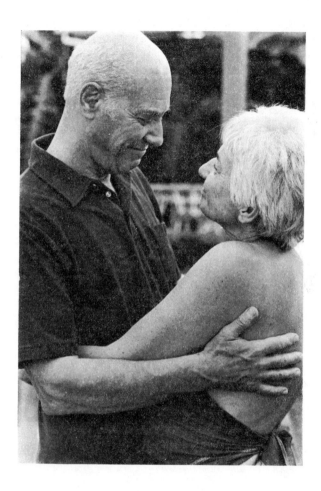

A loving partner who understands and accepts us and is willing to compromise is an important element in a satisfying sexual relationship.

We have a generalized sexual relationship. We're very sexy with each other in a continuous way. It doesn't show a lot . . . just through little things like touching fingers in the movies. [a fifty-eight-year-old woman]

There are several factors that can diminish interest in sexual activity between long-term partners. Recent research shows that the sexual activity of married women seventy or older is directly influenced by physical disability, illness, or loss of their male partners.[7] In many instances, when a male partner loses his interest in sex, his self-confidence, or his ability to have an erection, all sexual activity ends. Sometimes when both partners retire they feel they are spending too much time together; each person feels emotionally crowded. Women in long-term lesbian relationships often share the same activities and friends; they may be even more likely to find themselves struggling with this problem. For all couples, having some separate interests, activities, and friends can help keep each partner and their mutual relationship vital and interesting.

Sometimes sadness, unresolved anger, or disappointment with a partner can block sexual feeling. Allowing your feelings to surface, acknowledging them, and discussing them with your partner may renew sexual desire.

A number of studies suggest that in marriage, satisfaction increases after child rearing is finished and children leave home.[8]

We didn't have choice of time when the kids were young. Now we have time during the day. We seldom make love at nighttime. Now we can choose. It might be 10 a.m., or 2 p.m. – whenever we're feeling turned on. [a sixty-five-year-old woman]

Because of the double standard of ageing, some women as they grow older worry about losing their partner to a younger woman.

My husband is going through some kind of change – he's on a strict diet and runs several miles a day. I have to admit to myself he looks fifty. Me, I look my age. He's got this young woman at work – says she's like a daughter and he's helping her – she keeps calling for this and that. Joe wants me to invite her to dinner but I'm not fooled by this daughter business. I think he's trying to hold on to youth. I keep suggesting things we can do together. We joined a theatre group and sometimes we go out dancing with another couple. [a sixty-five-year-old woman, married forty years]

Because women on average have a longer life expectancy than men, most of us will experience the loss of a partner through death. If your relationship has ended with your partner's death, you may not feel sexual for some time while you mourn the loss.

After he died I was celibate for a long while and then went through a long stretch of mourning and masturbation, always with a tremendous sense of grief. [a seventy-eight-year-old woman speaking of a time when she was in her fifties]

After a time of grieving most of us redefine ourselves as survivors with continuing needs for love, affection, and sexual expression. Then we may be ready to consider a new sexual partner.

When partners separate, some of us – particularly those who didn't initiate the breakup – may also lose interest for a while in expressing ourselves sexually as we grieve over the end of the relationship. Our self-esteem may be low and it may take us a while to regain sexual confidence. Or we may be ready to resume sexual activity right away. We may be surprised or even embarrassed by unexpected feelings of sexual desire.

Whereas married people sometimes take sex for granted, single people face continuing decisions about their sexuality, including the choice of being sexual with one person or with more than one.

I have been single for ten years and had many lovers. I like sex a lot; I went through what I call my sport fucking phase. I didn't have to love him – if I felt like having sex I had sex. Now I have two lovers. Sex is very nice with both these men. In fact it's better than it's been for a long time. [a fifty-five-year-old woman]

Many women want more emotional intimacy than can be found in a casual sexual encounter. Some of us have difficulty finding male partners who care about intimacy as much as we do.

It's hard to get emotional closeness and great sex to come together in one relationship. I had an affair and enjoyed it but we didn't have a commitment as I did with my husband. It's true what the books say: sexuality goes on all your life. But you can't split sexuality from emotion. To me sexuality means intimacy. [a seventy-year-old woman]

If we are dating again for the first time in many years, we may feel awkward and unsure of what to expect. How far will my date expect me to go? Can I get by with a goodnight kiss? Often, both men and women would be happy to have a friendly, non-sexual relationship, but feel pressured by certain expectations.

After I got divorced at forty-eight, I expected to have a man courting me like my husband did when I was a teenager. I was very naive, so I had some surprises. I went out with a man and then he asked me to go up to his apartment to listen to music. So I said, 'We just came from listening to music!' I was naive, but I wasn't stupid! I wanted someone to hold my hand and say nice things, not to jump into bed with someone I didn't really know. [a fifty-nine-year-old woman]

Now I enjoy flirtations; when I don't worry about whether we'll have sex, it's totally fun. [a forty-eight-year-old divorced woman]

After about two years of brief and unsatisfactory relationships, I met a wonderful, warm, caring man, with a surprisingly developed feminist consciousness. How delightful to find that in bed he was exciting, passionate, and playful. [a forty-four-year-old divorced woman]

The man shortage, a hot topic among women of every age, can become critical in the second half of life. Today one out of every five middle-aged American women is single,[9] whether out of choice, widowhood, or divorce. Among older women, the majority are unmarried; in fact, older women are twice as likely to be unmarried as older men.[10] Men over sixty-five are seven times more likely to remarry than women over sixty-five, and when they do, they usually marry younger women.[11]

Whenever I have been between relationships I have prided myself on being independent and not needing a man in my life. But now that I have no man in my life – now that I am not even casually dating, now that I have cut my ties with my long-distance lover – I realize that what I miss most is the physical contact. I am not even necessarily talking about sex, although that is very important to me. I miss the cuddling and holding and touching with affection. [a woman in her fifties]

Being single I miss that flow in marriage – when I was married if we didn't make love one day there was always tomorrow. [a divorced woman in her fifties]

What the hell. I'm really nicer than I used to be and now no one's looking. [a divorced woman in her sixties]

I wasn't only mourning my husband, I was mourning that there might never be someone else. [a seventy-eight-year-old widow]

Women who have lost a partner find many different solutions to the problem. Some marry again. Others choose a less formal although not necessarily less committed relationship, dating one male or female partner exclusively but maintaining separate living quarters, or living with a partner without marrying. Some women who are having trouble finding suitable sexual partners are learning to initiate both social and sexual interactions more often. Some of us, even some who never dreamed we would choose an unconventional life-style, are considering or trying out new kinds of relationships.

I keep wondering – is this the end of lovers? I can't really believe that. Yet in my experience few men my age are interesting and vital. Younger men? Sure, why not. But not too much younger or the experience gap becomes too much. I meet lots of interesting women and I am enlarging my circle of women friends. If I really connected with someone would I consider a lesbian relationship? Maybe. In the meantime, I am accepting myself in a new and differ∂nt way. I am learning to treat and to nurture myself by doing the things I want to do and not doing what I don't want in a more honest way than ever before. [a woman in her fifties]

I feel such intense body hunger – for touching and stroking and for good old-fashioned sex. Sometimes I get together with an old friend. Neither of us wants it to be more than what it is now – good old friends with sex sometimes. [a forty-nine-year-old divorced woman]

I met a man fourteen years younger. We can laugh and talk and it feels so relaxed. He is very uninhibited sexually. We spend our time laughing and doing fun things. I relate so much better to younger men; they are less rigid about sex roles than older men. I like their values. [a forty-eight-year-old divorced woman]

I know a woman who is fifty-two who has a forty-year-old lover. She told me I have a hang-up about age, but I'm fifty-three, I'm afraid of getting hurt. Still, there's something to what she said: 'If you're alive and beautiful inside, with all the experience and patience older women have, no twenty-two- or thirty-year-old can really compete. A fascinating older woman can be irresistible for certain types of younger men.' I'm thinking about this and loosening up.

Sexuality between two women can be deeply satisfying. Some middle-aged or older women are, for the first time, considering or having sexual relationships with women.

I had an orgasm during a non-sexual massage which another woman was giving me. I thought, 'What difference does it make what gender the hands are?' [a woman in her fifties]

My first sexual experience with a woman was at age forty. I found myself very suddenly and very intensely turned on to a good friend who was gay. No sexual involvement was possible since she was in a long-term relationship with another woman, but the feeling was clearly there. That summer I began to seek out women as sexual partners while on holiday. I was absolutely captivated by the sensations of holding and physically loving another woman. The combination of delicacy and strength was thrilling. And the softness . . . that double twofold softness of two women together. [a fifty-year-old woman]

I spent years trying to make it in the heterosexual world because my sexual identity was 'wrong'. When I finally allowed myself to love another woman fully, it was like coming home – home at last. [a woman in her sixties]

I grew up loving women – the way they walk, smell, feel; wanting to touch them, cherish them, love them passionately and overtly, but it was not until years later that I actually fell in love with a woman. I found it extremely liberating and also a wonderful way to develop deep friendships and associations in one's old age. I am part of a group of women who are developing mutual interests and commitments. [a seventy-eight-year-old woman]

Although it is sometimes suggested that heterosexual women would be more sexually active if they would consider women as partners, a recent survey of one hundred lesbians aged sixty to eighty-six found that 53 per cent had had no sexual contact in the past year. One-third of the 53 per cent consider themselves celibate, but three-quarters of that number are not celibate by choice.[12] It may be that the issue is not the gender of our partners, but our own socialization, which conditions us to wait for someone else to initiate a sexual relationship.[13] Another study of twenty-five lesbians over sixty found none had casual sex after sixty, but most had sex an average of three times a month, which is comparable to or more frequent than lesbian couples of all ages.[14] It is difficult to know how to interpret findings such as these because research on older lesbians is very limited.

Early in my life I knew that I never wanted to have children and I never wanted to marry. I had crushes on older girls and some girl friends, but I also had boy friends. At forty-five for the first time in my life I suddenly wanted to get married. My menopausal crisis! My lover was willing but then I realized that while it was a good relationship for a weekend in another city, I couldn't imagine being married to him. I decided marriage was not right for me and then I was celibate for twenty years. When I was sixty-five I fell in love with a woman who was twenty-three years younger than I was. Making love with a woman was not that much different from experiences I had had with men. But this was the most complete relationship of my life. It was romantic, passionate, sharing, intellectual. It was everything I had read about but never experienced – such fullness and balance. When the relationship ended I decided to go back to celibacy, the way I had lived happily for twenty years, but it was the hardest thing I ever did. Maybe I'm into twenty-year cycles and can look forward to another love when I'm eighty-five. That would be nice. [a seventy-two-year-old woman]

Many middle-aged and older women are celibate. Some lack the opportunity to meet partners, others prefer to be celibate rather than change a lifetime pattern of being involved in one special relationship.

Whether you are celibate out of necessity or by choice, you can still lead a happy and satisfying life, enjoying affection, the company of friends, and sensual pleasures.

Sex and Ageing: Physiological and Emotional Changes

As we age, we experience changes in our bodies that affect our sexuality. It's important to distinguish between the effects of the ageing process itself, temporary hormonal changes we undergo during and after menopause, and the effects of illness, disability, and relationship difficulties. We don't need to resign ourselves to sexual problems as a natural, irreversible part of ageing. As women, we have learned to come to terms with changes in our bodies; we can understand and accommodate ourselves to the changes of ageing just as we did during menstruation and pregnancy. If you connect your sexual identity with the ability to have children, after menopause you may experience a sense of loss and a *temporary* drop in sexual desire. Some women report a need to mourn the ending of fertility, although such feelings are usually short-lived.

I know I wouldn't ever want to get pregnant again. Yet I'm aware that we derived great satisfaction from the thought that we could get pregnant if we wanted to. Sometimes we fantasize that we are making a baby, but it's not the same. [a fifty-one-year-old woman]

Many women in their fifties experience a reawakening of sexual interest once they no longer need to prevent pregnancy and once the pressures of child rearing are past.[15]

It's wonderfully freeing. I always hated the mess and the interruption of birth control. I was always anxious about getting pregnant and that put a damper on sex. [a forty-nine-year-old woman]

At times, hot flushes during menopause can interfere with sexual enjoyment.

My lover and I have had to be very creative to find suitable positions for lovemaking which take into account that one of us is bound to have a hot flush in the middle of it all. We discovered that lying next to each other, toes to head, gives us a good vantage point for genital play (toes are good for sucking too) without overwhelming each other with our wacky temperature controls. We'll be damned if such a thing can slow down our sexual pleasuring. [a lesbian in her fifties]

Orgasm

For many women, clitoral stimulation leads to orgasm. Yet until the mid-1960s, medical texts and marriage manuals followed Freud's famous dictum that the 'mature' woman had orgasms only when her vagina, not her clitoris, was stimulated. Then sex researchers found that much of the sexual pleasure women experience occurs because of direct or indirect stimulation of the clitoris.[16] This information electrified the newly developing women's movement and contributed to a revolution in women's understanding of ourselves as sexually autonomous beings rather than sexual objects.[17] More recent research indicates that orgasm may occur as the result of clitoral stimulation, vaginal[18] and uterine stimulation, or a combination of both.

For many women, continuous clitoral stimulation is what most surely brings orgasm. Some women enjoy orgasms brought on by penetration of the vagina which they describe as feeling 'deep' or 'uterine', and may find clitoral stimulation distracting if continued during vaginal penetration. In addition, increasing attention is being given to those women who report a loss of sexual feeling after hysterectomy;[19] they may miss the jiggling of the pelvic muscles and cervix which they had formerly felt during deep penetration. These new understandings lend further support to the idea that women's sexuality is complex and multifaceted. The main thing to remember is that you are the expert about yourself, and you can adjust your sexual pleasures to meet your changing needs.

Women who have uterine contractions during orgasm sometimes find that after the menopause these are less intense, more spasmodic and irregular, and fewer in number. A few older women experience painful contractions, somewhat like menstrual cramps, during orgasm. This is more likely to occur if orgasm is infrequent. If this happens to you, try not to get into a cycle of worrying about it, because this condition is similar to the discomfort we experience when any seldom-used muscle is exercised and is less likely to continue if you have orgasms more frequently. If you have sex with a partner infrequently, or if the anxiety about the contractions interferes with your orgasm with a partner, you can help yourself by masturbating to orgasm until you feel more relaxed and the contractions go away or become less painful.

SLOWER AROUSAL TIME

As a result of ageing, both women and men become aroused more slowly.

You know you are middle-aged when a 'quickie' takes forty-five minutes. [a fifty-one-year-old woman]

It's true that I need more time to be turned on, but everything balances out because I enjoy sex more once I do get aroused. [a forty-nine-year-old woman]

I've never been quick to have an orgasm and now it takes longer and I can't always count on it. I choose to make love because I want to be touched and stroked. [a fifty-five-year-old woman]

The slowing of sexual responses is similar to other ways in which our bodies slow down physically. If we believe social attitudes that 'virility' or 'sexual allure' means instant arousal, we may become alarmed as our bodies respond more slowly. This may lead to further anxiety and affect our confidence in ourselves. However, slower arousal time has its compensations.

When Jay used to lose his erection I would think that I had failed as a woman because I couldn't keep him aroused. But now I see that it can mean more time to play around and a chance to start over again so that lovemaking lasts longer. [a forty-nine-year-old woman]

VAGINAL CHANGES

As we age, the lips of the vagina, or the labia, become less firm, and less fatty tissue covers the mons, or pubic bone. This reduction in fatty tissue may decrease the pleasurable sense of fullness that was formerly part of your sexual response. The length of the vaginal canal may seem shorter, since the tissues are less elastic. The stretching of these delicate tissues may hurt on penetration or deep thrusting. In addition, thinner vaginal walls offer less protection to the bladder and urethra during intercourse and may result in bladder irritation or infection. Drinking a glass of water before sex and urinating after sex, as well as washing your genitals before and after sex, may help this condition. A hot bath feels good and helps relieve irritation after lovemaking.

The lower oestrogen levels that accompany middle age may cause dryness or itching of the vagina, making intercourse less comfortable or even painful. You may need more stimulation before you are lubricated enough for penetration. Dryness can also make it uncomfortable to have the vulva or clitoris caressed. Changing your lovemaking to allow more time to get aroused and expanding your repertoire to include more caresses – especially oral sex, which provides its own lubrication – before or instead of penetration may be all that is necessary.

A lot of hand play is wonderful because it does start the juices flowing. [a woman in her seventies]

I've always loved sex and I could make love for hours. Now, even though I'm excited, my vagina doesn't have enough juice. It's so frustrating – I want to, but it hurts. We have found that after penetration if he just waits and doesn't move for a while it stops hurting and then it's fine. [a fifty-one-year-old woman]

We can incorporate lubricants into our lovemaking now even if we never used them earlier in our lives. Try an over-the-counter product such as a non-contraceptive lubricating jelly. Knowing that you are already lubricated may help you to relax and let your feelings of arousal build until your natural lubrication takes over. Artificial lubricants should not be expected to replace natural lubrication, since without some of her own lubrication a woman is neither physically nor psychologically ready for intercourse.[20]

If a woman feels pressured by her partner for rapid penetration, she may experience even less lubrication. Susanne Morgan notes that 'lubrication is more than wetness: it is the first indication of arousal'.[21]

Some authorities suggest using only water-based lubricants because oil-based lubricants don't flush out of the system as readily, and in older women may cause vaginal infection.[22]

After my hysterectomy I started to experience discomfort with intercourse; my vagina was becoming very dry. There was no longer any pleasure in the activity; sex became something to avoid. Early on I started to use a personal lubricant with unsatisfactory results. Being a resourceful person, I dug deep into my past experience and remembered that the introduction of the spermicidal jelly with an applicator (which I used to use with my diaphragm) always produced the side advantage of easier intercourse. So I dug out my old plastic plunger-type applicator and filled it with the lubricant as in days gone by. The result was tremendous! My husband and I instantly noticed the improvement. The problem of getting the lubricant where I needed it the most was resolved. [a woman in her late thirties]

Some doctors prescribe oestrogen for a dry vagina. This is a powerful drug which should not be taken without first considering all of its potential effects. (See chapter on Menopause and p. 359.) An alternative to taking oestrogen orally is the use of low-dose oestrogen cream. It is important to note that oestrogen is absorbed even more quickly when used vaginally than when taken orally. Because oestrogen cream bypasses the liver, the risk of liver and gallbladder problems is reduced. However, the risk of cancer of the uterine lining (endometrium) and the risk of other effects of oestrogen are still present. If nothing else helps and you feel you must try oestrogen cream, use as little as possible for as short a time period as is necessary to get the desired results. Apply the cream to the area which is most sore, usually the entrance to the vagina. A week of such treatment will usually relieve soreness. British researchers found that only one-eighth of the dosage usually recommended by American doctors is enough to plump up vaginal tissues.[23] The cream comes with an applicator and you will have to estimate a one-eighth dose as the 4-gram applicator isn't marked. If you can't use oestrogen, androgen cream (which is made of 1 to 2 per cent testosterone in a water-soluble cream) is another way to treat vaginal soreness and is used in the same fashion as oestrogen cream (see p. 403 for the risks of using testosterone). These powerful substances are medications. They should never be used as lubricants at the time of lovemaking.

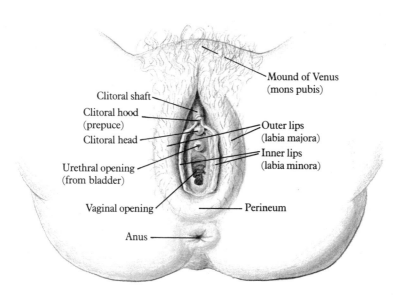

CLITORAL CHANGES

The clitoris is always highly sensitive and grows even more so as we age. The hood of skin that covers the clitoris may pull back, so that the clitoris is fully exposed. If your clitoris becomes hypersensitive, you may not be able to tolerate having it directly touched or rubbed without lots of lubrication. Touching the mons, the clitoral hood, and the labia will stimulate the clitoris indirectly and provide pleasure.

MEN ALSO CHANGE

Men as well as women undergo changes in their sexuality as they age. Lower testosterone levels are sometimes a factor in loss of sexual interest for some men. Their sexual responses may slow down, and they may need a longer time of non-demanding genital stimulation before they attain a full erection. Once lost, the erection may take longer to regain.

A woman can help her partner to gain a full erection by putting pressure on the base of his penis, and massaging it away from his abdomen. This will press against the major blood vessels and hold the blood in the penis, creating an erection. It is important not to pull it up toward the abdomen, since this will drain the blood from the penis and diminish the erection. Another technique which some men like is to stuff a partially erect penis into the vagina and then the woman tightens her vaginal muscles rhythmically as a form of stimulation for both partners.[24]

Middle-aged and older men also experience changes in orgasm. They often don't need to ejaculate at the end of each sexual experience and may opt for orgasm every two or three episodes rather than every time they make love. Older men also need a longer time to renew their sexual energy after an orgasm before they can have another erection. But by delaying ejaculation and not pushing for orgasm after each lovemaking session, an older man can often rapidly become erect again. This means that both partners can enjoy frequent lovemaking and have orgasms when it feels right.[25]

My lover's divorce had left him feeling sexually rejected and vulnerable. When our relationship grew intimate, I made it clear that I didn't regard sex as a competition, but as a way for two people to express warmth and caring. My friend's 'problem', delayed ejaculation, allowed us to prolong our lovemaking until both of us were ecstatically exhausted. Instead of the conventional problem of 'would I come?' I worried at first when he didn't come, but he assured me that he didn't need to come every time. Sometimes we would resume our lovemaking in the morning and then he would have his orgasm, while I would sometimes have another. As we grow to love each other more, our delight in giving each other pleasure deepens. [a forty-seven-year-old woman]

Now there is longer playing around . . . and without fussing about whether or not it's going to be intercourse. We can bring each other to orgasm at any time. It's no longer goal oriented, so it's wonderful. [a woman in her late seventies]

Impotence is the inability to maintain an erection long enough to have intercourse. It is usually temporary. Sudden onset of impotence is usually the result of some unusual stress. Once the stress is removed, potency often returns.

I was getting angry because he seemed to be giving up sex. I was being solicitous – doing oral sex because I wanted it to work the first time after his operation. Then oh! It worked just like it used to! [a sixty-eight-year-old woman]

We enjoy each other. As far as sex is concerned, he is sensible. He understands he can't do what he used to do. Some men can't admit this and blame the woman, but not him. [a sixty-eight-year-old woman in a second marriage of thirty years]

He can't maintain an erection, so we mutually masturbate and it's very satisfying. [a sixty-five-year-old woman]

Although there is a sharp upward turn in male impotence after age fifty, a high percentage of men who become impotent after years of normal sexual activity can be helped by sex therapy. Worries about career and money or illness, fatigue, heavy meals, and too much to drink can all contribute to impotence. 'This sensitivity to mental fatigue is the biggest difference between the aging population and younger men,' say Masters and Johnson. 'There is no way to overemphasize the importance that the "fear of failure" plays in aging males' withdrawal from sexual performance.'[26]

My husband was anxious about prostate trouble. He had been very ill and had a history of impotence. I want to say to him, 'Relax, it's going to be okay,' but I don't want to touch on the subject because I'm afraid he'll consider it a demand. He seems to be getting back his feelings of sexiness, but it's a slow process. When it's been so long [since we had sex] that I'm taking it personally or feel far away from him, I initiate it by doing something romantic. I dress up and do a dance, or I arrange a sexy situation of some sort – and it works. But he prefers to get it going himself because he's never sure if he's going to have an erection. [a sixty-five-year-old woman]

Recent evidence has shown that up to 50 per cent of male impotence (more than was suspected) may be caused by physical problems such as arteriosclerosis.[27] There are other, rarer conditions which may require investigation, and it is always a good idea for a man to overcome his natural reluctance and consult his doctor, who may refer him to a specialist. But when a partner has sexual problems or slows down sexually, whether because of physiological or psychological problems, we may interpret it as rejection, or fear that it has something to do with our diminished 'attractiveness'.

Social stereotypes that men are 'supposed' to have stronger sex drives than women and that women are 'supposed' to be passive but alluring recipients of sex only aggravate the situation.

My husband became impotent. One of the grimmest things was the sense of helplessness and guilt. I wondered what I could do differently but was not able to speak about it openly because it was a big, bad, sad problem. We went months without sex and every time I would realize this I became enraged that he didn't want it. I thought maybe I should take the initiative, but he saw that as aggressive and as a demand, and he wouldn't even play around. I found that painful – we couldn't be physically intimate in any way without his seeing it as a threat. When we became preoccupied with his erections, I didn't have orgasm any more. I was left hanging in the air. [a woman in her fifties]

SEXUAL AIDS

Many older women are enjoying sex aids which are available through mail-order catalogues or 'sex shops'. Although some people may find such toys objectionable, others delight in playing with them. Generally, women find vibrators more effective stimulation than men do, and prefer electric vibrators that are not shaped like a phallus. These provide intense stimulation to the nerve endings around the vulva and clitoris.

I'd never be without one again! Sometimes I just want to be soothed and the sound and continuing vibration does that. Other times if I want to get really excited I know I can if I use my vibrator. For me it's a sure-fire way to have an orgasm. [a forty-nine-year-old woman]

The weak vibration of some small, battery-powered vibrators often advertised in sex magazines does not provide sufficient stimulation to bring about orgasm, but women who enjoy deep penetration may prefer them.

Many women report that they like a sensation of fullness inside the vagina, and use dildoes for this purpose. You can order dildoes from sex magazines or you can make your own from candles or vegetables (either raw or partially cooked). It is important never to use glass objects or anything which might hurt you or break. Always wash anything which has been in the anus before inserting it in the vagina.

Some couples like to look at erotic films, magazines, or books, or to listen to sexy music or relaxing tapes or records of environmental sounds such as surf, forest sounds, or falling water. 'White noise' such as the hum from a fan or air conditioner can block distracting noises and allow you to concentrate on your intimate environment.

Accommodations in Lovemaking

Illness may bring about a temporary loss of sexual interest or ability to engage in sexual activity. Most illnesses do not mean the end of sexual activity but may require different ways of giving and receiving pleasure. With problems such as arthritis or back pain, fear of causing pain or being hurt can affect spontaneity. If a partner holds back in lovemaking or rarely initiates sex, her or his concern about illness may be misinterpreted as rejection. In fact, good sex can actually help relieve pain. It is distracting, and sexual stimulation releases neurotransmitters in the brain which block pain and produce pleasure.[28]

People sometimes fear returning to sexual activity after an illness or surgery. Through masturbation, you can rediscover your sexual self in private communication with your own body, trying out degrees of arousal that feel safe and comfortable. Once you feel reassured that your body is still capable of responding with pleasure, you may be ready to ask your partner to join you. Satisfying intimacy can hasten the healing process. Many women find they are more comfortable with a gradual resumption of lovemaking – touching, hand-holding, and caressing at first as a way to express closeness until they feel ready to resume full sexual relations.

If one person is unavailable sexually because of illness, it is always possible to lie together and hold each other and let feelings flow in a warm and close embrace. The most important thing to remember is that if you are open to trying new ways of making love you *will* be able to continue having sex. Even when you can't enjoy penetration or intercourse, you can still give and receive pleasure using a variety of techniques.

My husband had a series of operations last year – a penile implant – and he's still unable to enjoy sex. That doesn't matter so much to me. We still make love and hold and kiss. [a sixty-five-year-old woman, married forty years]

The following ideas may help when one of the partners is having physical problems.

Sex researchers encourage exercising sexual organs through pelvic floor exercises, masturbation, or lovemaking to help maintain muscle tone and lubrication. If you have not been sexual in a while, you may feel tight or dry at first, but you can overcome this with pelvic floor exercises (see p. 124) followed by gentle and slow resumption of sexual activity.

Let your partner know what feels good and what hurts during sex. You may want to do this by talking or by guiding your partner's hand away from tender areas, or toward places that feel especially good. Tell your partner what your present sensations feel like. Once you feel secure about being understood, you

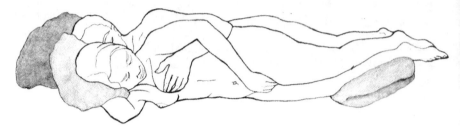

The 'spoon position', where both partners lie on their sides and one has her back to the other, is excellent for cuddling and for lovemaking with or without inter-course. You can stimulate your own clitoris and breasts in this position or ask your partner to do so.

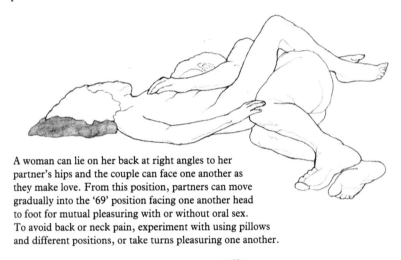

A woman can lie on her back at right angles to her partner's hips and the couple can face one another as they make love. From this position, partners can move gradually into the '69' position facing one another head to foot for mutual pleasuring with or without oral sex. To avoid back or neck pain, experiment with using pillows and different positions, or take turns pleasuring one another.

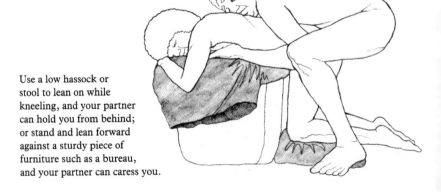

Use a low hassock or stool to lean on while kneeling, and your partner can hold you from behind; or stand and lean forward against a sturdy piece of furniture such as a bureau, and your partner can caress you.

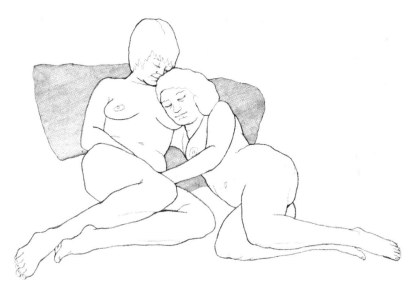

Having one partner on top of the other may be too stressful if either partner is
having physical problems. Partners can caress one another or have intercourse in
a sitting or reclining position. It can be comfortable to sit in an armless chair where
one person sits in the chair and the second person sits on her partner's lap. Make sure
the chair is sturdy. Sit so that both partners' feet touch the ground; this way
neither person bears too much weight.

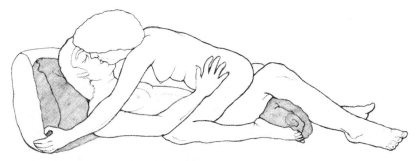

Change positions to allow for fatigue. The person who is ill or tired can lie on her
or his back while the other partner kneels above. Several pillows can be used to
advantage to support a back or be placed under the knees.

will be better able to relax and surrender to sexual pleasure without fear of pain.

Before making love, agree on a clear signal which you both know is a sign to stop if something hurts you. If a favourite position has become uncomfortable because of temporary or permanent aches and pains, experiment to find a position that feels better.

Ask for what you want in a positive way. Offering an alternative sexual activity which you enjoy is easier on your partner's ego. Some women find it easier to discuss sexual issues during non-sexual times together. Look for a private time when you won't be interrupted.

Communication is important between partners regardless of gender. We cannot assume that a woman partner will know what we want and enjoy – women have to make the effort to be clear and explicit with each other. It's easy to hide our own embarrassment or reluctance to ask for what we want behind the assumption that 'She must know, for, after all, she is a woman like me.' It's important to understand that every woman is different.

Choose a time of day when you are both feeling comfortable. Making love in the morning when you are rested can help if you tire easily. Men are more likely to have an erection in the morning. Time lovemaking to coincide with maximum effectiveness of pain medications. Turn up the thermostat; a warm room helps you feel supple.

Creating a relaxed sexy mood with your partner can be a way to increase intimacy and release sexual energy. Changing the time and place for sex may keep it from seeming routine. The setting can make a big difference in whether you feel a surge of desire – an attractive, tidy bedroom free of reminders of illnesses can be an asset. Simply moving all the pill bottles into the bathroom may lift our spirits and put us in the mood for lovemaking.[29]

Mild exercise, yoga, massage, breathing and relaxation exercises, meditation, and prayer all reduce stress, counteract stiff muscles, and can be good preludes to making love. Taking a bath or shower together, listening to music, sharing a relaxing meal or quiet talk can help you and your partner feel close and connected.

Getting Help

Usually sexual difficulties can be resolved by talking things through in a spirit of mutual co-operation, but at times it may be necessary to consult a sex therapist or counsellor specially trained to understand sexual problems.

Your doctor may be able to refer you to a special 'marital therapy' unit attached to a local hospital, but many GPs are ignorant or unwilling to make use of these scarce facilities. Relate (formerly the National Marriage Guidance

Council) does offer marital or sex therapy in some areas – your local branch is listed under *Marriage Guidance* or *Relate* in the telephone directory – or you can get its address from the national headquarters. The Family Planning Association can also advise about getting help locally.

Doctors rarely initiate a discussion about how an illness or medical procedure will affect sexuality, so you will have to introduce this topic yourself. Find out when you can resume sexual relations. Ask which activities you can resume and when. Be *very* specific in your questions and insist on explicit answers.

I accompanied my partner to the hospital where he was to have a prostate biopsy. The doctor gave a rapid-fire list of instructions on self-care for the days and weeks following surgery. When he mentioned sex, he said, 'Sex, the same.' I stopped him and asked, 'Do you mean abstain from sex the same number of days as the previous instruction, *or the same as usual, or what?' 'Oh, two days' was the reply.*

As instructed, we obediently abstained. When the two days were up we were eager to resume lovemaking. Proceeding in a gingerly fashion, we were gratified to find everything in good working order and had a lovely time. The following day, we began to feel turned on and started playing around. I was masturbating him with my hand, whereupon we were shocked to see a stream of bright red blood shoot forth from his penis. Since we had not yet heard the good news that the biopsy was negative, we were particularly frightened and upset. We rang the hospital and spoke to a nurse who finally reached the doctor and relayed his new instructions to us. No sex for two weeks! Either he had misstated the original instruction, or he was changing it based on changed circumstances. When my partner returned for his follow-up visit, the young doctor was terribly embarrassed, as much out of surprise that we were 'so active' at our age as for his error. [this woman and her partner are both in their late forties]

A nurse tells of a woman in her seventies who seemed inexplicably depressed after being told she could go home following a successful colostomy.* The staff had been impressed with the closeness between this woman and her husband and were surprised at her lack of anticipation about going home. Finally, she confided to the nurse, 'I'm not the same as I was.' She was concerned that the operation would make her unable to have sexual relations. Neither the doctor nor any of the nurses had reassured her or her husband that they could have sexual relations, assuming they were 'too old' to care about sexuality.

Also ask your doctor how prescribed drugs will affect your sexuality. For example, anti-depressant and anti-anxiety drugs may either increase or

*See Cancer chapter for a description of colostomy (p. 470).

decrease your usual level of sexual desire. Some anti-hypertension medications interfere with blood entering the penis, causing problems with erection. Without exception, all drugs have a variety of effects in addition to the effect intended. Since pharmacists frequently know more than doctors about the effects of drugs, you may want to ask a pharmacist. See *The British Medical Association Guide to Medicines and Drugs* (Dorling Kindersley).

Residents of nursing homes may have somewhat changed sexual needs due to illness or frailty, yet most still have sexual needs. Many nursing homes do not allow residents sexual privacy. All of us need privacy regardless of whether we are part of a couple, a single person, or whether we are heterosexual or lesbian.

RESUMING SEX AFTER A HEART ATTACK

After a heart attack, fear of having another may cause people to delay sexual activity. Yet the incidence of death occurring during intercourse is less than 0.3 per cent.[30]

Be sure your doctor understands your interest in resuming sexual activity as soon as you safely can. People who have had a heart attack are usually able to have sex two to four weeks afterward, while bypass patients may reach this point in one to three weeks after they leave hospital.[31] People who have been in the hospital for ten days, and have had a treadmill test, can have sex on the first day home, because a treadmill test is more strenuous than sex. If you can climb two flights of stairs without chest pain, palpitations, or shortness of breath, you can engage in lovemaking safely. If you suffer from angina, you may be able to take a nitroglycerin pill for the pain before lovemaking and then proceed.

Wait one to three hours after eating a full meal. Digesting your food takes an increased amount of blood. Your heart would have to work harder to provide blood during sex.

If you experience angina or pains in the jaw, neck, chest, or stomach, shortness of breath, and rapid or irregular heartbeats, tell your partner, rest, and take medicine if prescribed. When the symptoms disappear, you can resume sexual activity. If the symptoms do not stop, or if they start again, you need to get medical help.

After Surgery

Our culture trains us to believe that 'bodily perfection' is a prerequisite for good sex.* If a part of your body has been surgically removed, you need time to

*See *The New Our Bodies, Ourselves* for a more extensive discussion and bibliography on sex and disability.

come to terms with the changes in order to feel ready to be sexual again. A partner's attitude is of prime importance in helping you to complete the healing process and regain sexual intimacy.

When I came home from the hospital after my mastectomy, my husband literally had to force me to remove my blouse before we made love. My scar did not turn him off, as I was afraid it would, and our lovemaking was good, and healing.

Some hospitals offer counselling to their patients after surgery; this has proved helpful to many people in the past,[32] especially to women who have had mastectomies or who must wear appliances as a result of ostomy surgery. The Mastectomy Association can provide support and counselling from women who have themselves had the operation.

I 'practised' talking about my breast surgery with two of my best friends because I didn't see how I could tell a man I wasn't intimate with; yet how would I ever get that far if I didn't tell him? Saying the words helped me get familiar with the language I would be comfortable using. Then I did meet a man, and when I managed to tell him, he was very easy about it. I think I was more nervous than I needed to be, because afterwards it seemed to fall into place so easily. He likes me for me!

Conclusion

In 1979, Betty Friedan said we must 'create new patterns of intimacy and growth, love, and work in the third of life that most women now hope to enjoy . . . after fifty'.[33] We have the experience and wisdom to manage changes, problems, and losses, and to find ways to continue to meet our needs for pleasure. We are in a position to refine and enhance what we already know. We have learned to both give and receive, and to appreciate the fleeting moment and its pleasures. Our sexual selves become more integrated with our emotional and spiritual selves. We know how to value ourselves and our intimate loved ones and we can share our bodies as it best suits our desires. As long as we want it, sex can be a part of our lives.

NOTES

[1] Lance Morrow, 'Women and Aging'. *Time*, Vol. III, No. 17, 24 April 1978, p. 99.

[2] Ivor Felstein, *Sex in Later Life*. London: Penguin Books, 1973.

[3] Bernard Starr and Marcella Weiner, *Starr-Weiner Report*. New York: Stein & Day, 1981, p. 35.

[4] Timothy H. Brubaker, *Later Life Families*.

SAFER SEX GUIDELINES FOR WOMEN AT RISK FOR AIDS TRANSMISSION

If you believe that you or your sex partner(s) may be infected with the AIDS virus or HIV-positive, or you aren't sure, avoid sexual activity that involves contact with blood, semen, urine, faeces, and, possibly, vaginal secretions. Saliva and tears do not transmit the virus. Remember that a high proportion of HIV-positive people in the UK have become infected through the use of shared needles by drug users. *Unprotected* sexual contact with an infected person is dangerous.

Specific Guidelines for Sexual Activity

Safer (low risk)
Hugging, cuddling, massage, playing with nipples
Masturbation (solo or mutual)
Social (dry) kissing
Body-to-body rubbing
Body kissing
Sexual fantasies
Any other sexual activity that could not involve exchange of body fluids
Sex toys, if not shared

Medium Risk
Vaginal intercourse with a condom
Anal intercourse with a condom
Oral sex (fellatio/blow jobs/cunnilingus) man–woman or woman–woman with a condom
Hand/finger-to-genital contact without a latex or rubber glove (e.g. vaginal or anal penetration with fingers)
Wet kissing
Sex play involving urination (external only)

High Risk
Vaginal intercourse without a condom
Anal intercourse (but with a *strong* condom and plenty of water-based lubricant [not oil or vaseline] the risk may be reduced)
Semen, urine or faeces in the mouth or vagina
Shared sex toys
Rimming (oral–anal contact)
Fisting (hand in rectum or vagina)
Fellatio/blow jobs without a condom
Any type of blood contact (including menstrual blood)

For a full discussion of the risks and precautions see *Women and the AIDS Crisis* by Diane Richardson (Pandora), the British Medical Association booklet *AIDS and You*, current leaflets and publications of the Health Education Authority and the Terrence Higgins Trust.

Reducing the Risk

Remembering that the virus can be present undetected for months or even years, it is important to take the precautions outlined above with *any* new sexual partner, until you can be sure about his/her state of health, lifestyle and sexual habits. He/she has an equal right to know about yours. These are difficult questions to introduce, but as long as women and men are reluctant to ask them, or don't take precautions, AIDS will spread. If you have *any* doubts about the truthfulness of a partner, apply the rules of safer sex.

Here is a brief rundown to amplify these rules:

Condoms: laboratory studies do show that condoms, correctly used, can block the transmission of the HIV virus. A small quantity of spermicide inside the tip of the condom can increase both partners' pleasure – but too much can cause the condom to slip off.

Withdrawal before or shortly after ejaculation reduces the risk of the condom slipping off.

Spermicides, especially those containing nonoxynol-9, can kill the AIDS virus, so as an extra precaution they can be used by those who aren't allergic to them. If one brand causes an itch or rash when applied to a test area inside your wrist, try another.

Broken skin – cuts, scratches, grazes, hangnails – increases the likelihood of blood-to-blood contact, and rubber or latex gloves or finger-stalls in hand–genital or hand–anal contact reduce the chances of passing on the virus in this way.

REMEMBER THAT CONDOMS, GLOVES, SPERMICIDES OR ANY OTHER BARRIER MAY ENABLE YOU TO HAVE *SAFER* SEX – BUT NO ONE CAN CLAIM THAT THEY PREVENT THE TRANSMISSION OF HIV IN EVERY POSS-IBLE CIRCUMSTANCE. AND – NEVER SHARE NEEDLES. (SOME WOMEN THINK IT'S OK TO HAVE UNPROTECTED SEX WITH A NEEDLE DRUG USER BECAUSE THEY ARE NOT SHARING THE NEEDLES. THIS IS NOT TRUE.)

The Department of Health Helpline is on 0800-567123 (confidential advice and counselling). Ring 0800-555777 for free AIDS leaflets.

For books on AIDS see list at the end of Books and Publications (below).

Information on AIDS can be obtained from the Healthline telephone service on 01-981 2717. An operator on 01-980 4848 is available between 2 p.m. and 10 p.m. daily to play you tapes on specific health topics. If telephoning from outside London, dial 0345-581151 and you'll be charged local rates.

Beverly Hills, Cal. Sage Publications, Inc., 1985, pp. 36–45.

[5]This idea appeared in *Feminine Forever* by Robert Wilson, New York: M. Evans & Co., Inc., 1966 and was common in many magazine articles a decade ago. See Menopause chapter.

[6]Starr and Weiner, op. cit.; and Edward Brecher, *Love, Sex and Aging*. Boston: Little, Brown & Co., 1984.

[7]Ewald Busse and Eric Pfeiffer, eds., *Behavior and Adaptation in Later Life*. Boston: Little, Brown & Co., 1968.

[8]Reported in Jane Porcino, *Growing Older, Getting Better: A Handbook for Women in Later Life*. Reading, Mass.: Addison-Wesley Pub. Co., 1983, p. 15.

[9]Joan Cohen, Karen Coburn and Joan Pearlman, *Hitting Our Stride: Good News About Women in Their Middle Years*. New York: Delacorte Press, 1980, p. 168.

[10]In 1979, 36.9 per cent of older women were married compared with 74.6 per cent of older men. US Bureau of the Census, Current Population Reports, Series P-23, No. 59 and Series P-20, No. 349.

[11]Women's Studies Program and Policy Center, *Older Women: The Economics of Aging*. Washington, DC: George Washington University, 1980.

[12]Monica Kehoe, 'Lesbians over Sixty: A Triply Invisible Minority', in Monica Kehoe, ed., *Historical, Literary and Erotic Aspects of Lesbianism*. New York: Haworth Publications, Inc., 1986.

[13]Personal communication from Sarah F. Pearlman, a therapist specializing in counselling couples.

[14]Marcy Adelman, as reported in JoAnn Loulan, *Lesbian Sex*. San Francisco: Spinsters, Ink., 1984, pp. 194–5.

[15]William Masters and Virginia Johnson, 'Human Sexual Response in the Aging Female', in Bernice Neugarten, ed., *Middle*

Age and Aging. Chicago: University of Chicago Press, 1968, pp. 260–70.

[16]Masters and Johnson, *Human Sexual Response*. Boston: Little, Brown & Co., 1966.

[17]Wendy Sanford et al., 'Sexuality', in Boston Women's Health Book Collective, *The New Our Bodies, Ourselves*. London: Penguin, 1989, and earlier editions, as well as other feminist writing on sexuality. See Anne Koedt, 'The Myth of the Vaginal Orgasm' in *Liberation Now: Writings from the Women's Liberation Movement*. New York: Dell, 1971, pp. 311–20.

[18]Alice Ladas, Beverly Whipple and John Perry, *The G Spot*. New York: Dell, 1982. The G spot is the name given to a part of the anterior wall of the vagina which may be especially sensitive to stimulation.

[19]L. Zussman, S. Zussman, R. Sunley and E. Bjornson, 'Sexual Response after Hysterectomy-Oophorectomy: Recent Studies and Reconsideration of Psychogenesis'. *American Journal of Obstetrics and Gynecology*, Vol. 140, No. 7, 1 August 1981, pp. 725–9.

[20]Boston Women's Health Book Collective, op. cit.; and F. Bellview and L. Richter, *Understanding Human Sexual Inadequacy*. Boston: Bantam Books, 1970, p. 196.

[21]Susanne Morgan, *Coping with Hysterectomy*. New York: Dial Press, 1982, p. 163.

[22]Personal communication, Myrna Lewis, co-author of *Sex After Forty*.

[23]G. I. Dyer et al., 'Dose-Related Changes in Vaginal Cytology After Topical Conjugated Equine Oestrogens'. *British Medical Journal*, Vol. 284, 13 March 1982, p. 789.

[24]Robert Butler and Myrna Lewis, *Sex After Sixty*. New York: Harper & Row, 1976, p. 156.

[25]Masters and Johnson, *Human Sexual Inadequacy*. Boston: Little, Brown & Co., 1970, p. 323.

[26]Masters and Johnson, 'Human Sexual Response in the Aging Male', in Neugarten, ed., op. cit., pp. 227–8.

[27]Thomas P. Hackett, *Sexual Activity in the Elderly*. Clinical Perspectives on Aging, No. 4. Philadelphia: Wyeth Laboratories; Dr Irwin Goldstein of the N.E. Reproductive Center, University Hospital, Boston, quoted in *The Boston Globe*, 22 September 1985, p. 34.

[28]Barry Komisarik and Beverly Whipple, 'Evidence that Vaginal Stimulation in Women Suppresses Experimentally Induced Finger Pain'. Paper presented at June 1984 conference in Boston, Society for the Scientific Study of Sex.

[29]Masters and Johnson, 'Human Sexual Response in the Aging Male', in Neugarten, ed., op. cit., pp. 148–53.

[30]Lee Scheingold and Nathaniel Wagner, *Sound Sex and the Aging Heart*. New York: Pyramid Books, 1975, p. 82; Herman Hellerstein and Emanuel Friedman, 'Sexual Activity and the Post-coronary Patient'. *Archives of Internal Medicine*, Vol. 125, 1970, pp. 987–99.

[31]'Sex and Heart Disease', 1983. Available from American Heart Association, National Center, 7320 Greenville Ave., Dallas, TX 75231.

[32]Mary Reid Gloeckner, 'Partner Reaction Following Ostomy Surgery'. *Journal of Sex and Marital Therapy*, Vol. 9, No. 3, Fall 1983, pp. 182–90.

[33]Betty Friedan, 'Feminism Takes a New Turn'. *The New York Times Magazine*, 18 November 1979, p. 102.

BOOKS AND PUBLICATIONS

Sheila Kitzinger, *Woman's Experience of Sex*. London: Dorling Kindersley, 1983.

'Sexuality', Unit 4 of the 'Changing Experience of Women' course. Milton Keynes: Open University Educational Enterprises.

Shere Hite, *The Hite Report*. London: Summit Books/Hamlyn, 1977.

Helen S. Kaplan, *The New Sex Therapy*, Vols. 1 and 2. Eastbourne: Bailliere Tindall, 1975 and 1980.

Fred Belliveau and Lin Richter, *Understanding Human Sexual Inadequacy*. London: Hodder & Stoughton, 1971. A shortened version of Masters and Johnson sex therapy study.

Ruth Brecher and Edward Brecher (eds.), *An Analysis of Human Sexual Response*. London: Panther, 1971.

Christine Sandford, *Enjoy Sex in the Middle Years*. London: Macdonald Optima, 1983.

Bisexual Lives. Off Pink Publishing, 1988.

Stephanie Norris and Emma Read, *Out in the Open: People Talking About Being Gay or Bisexual*. London: Pan, 1985.

Anne Hooper, *Women and Sex*. London: Sheldon, 1987.

AIDS

Michael W. Adler (ed.), *The ABC of AIDS*. London: British Medical Association, 1987. Articles from the *British Medical Journal* covering symptoms, treatment, counselling and control.

Nigel Hawkes, *AIDS*. London: Franklin Watts, 1987.

Dr V. G. Daniels, *AIDS*. Northampton: Cambridge Medical Publications, 1986.

Peter Gordon and Louise Mitchell, *Safer Sex: A New Look at Sexual Pleasure*. London: Faber & Faber, 1988.

Diane Richardson, *Women and the AIDS Crisis*. London: Pandora Press, 1987.

Health Education Authority, *AIDS and You*. Free from local health education units.

8
Birth Control for Women in Midlife

Women continue to need up-to-date, reliable contraceptive information until they are sure they are well past their fertile years. This brief discussion of birth control is meant to highlight special contraception issues that affect women in midlife.

If you do not already have a basic familiarity with reproductive anatomy and birth control and would like to, we encourage you to turn to other resources, such as the Birth Control and Anatomy chapters in *The New Our Bodies, Ourselves*,[1] for more comprehensive information. A woman doctor at a Health Centre or Family Planning Clinic is another good source of instruction and contraceptive services. In general, health workers who specialize in family planning are more thorough and knowledgeable than most gynaecologists and will take much more time with each woman.

Women who are sexually active with men must continue to use birth control until they are past menopause. Middle-aged women often look forward to being free of the need for birth control, yet they may stop believing in their fertility before it is reliably at an end. As early as our late thirties or early forties, our periods may become quite irregular, and those of us who are sexually active with a male partner may worry about whether a missed period means a pregnancy. Keeping track of the patterns in our menstrual cycles and paying attention to other body changes we experience can help us to distinguish them from signs of pregnancy. It can help us to talk with other women who are going through or have gone through the menopause and to become familiar with the signs (see Menopause chapter). Women sometimes ovulate months or even over a year after menstruation appears to have stopped. If you are certain you do not want to become pregnant, it is crucial to continue contraception until two years past the last menstrual period (one year if you are over fifty). It is certainly no less true at midlife that control of our fertility is essential to control over the rest of our lives.

Choosing a Birth-Control Method

Choosing a birth-control method is a very personal matter. We must weigh a lot of factors in making a decision. Each method's safety and effectiveness should be taken into consideration. Unfortunately, no contraceptive exists with is 100 per cent effective and 100 per cent safe. The most accepted measure of effectiveness is the failure rate – the number of pregnancies per 100 women using the contraceptive for one year, most often the first year, as in the chart below. In evaluating a contraceptive's effectiveness for any group of women, it is important to know the failure rate for typical users (usually called the actual or use-failure rate) and the failure rate when a method is used carefully and consistently (sometimes called the theoretical failure rate).[2] Actual failure rates are strongly influenced by age, education, and socio-economic status. Women under twenty-two are much more likely to experience contraceptive failure than women thirty and over. With barrier methods, very young women have failure rates 17 to 22 per cent higher than women thirty and over.[3] Because older women are more likely to have the experience and confidence to use a method carefully and consistently, the theoretical failure rate may actually be lower.

First Year Failure Rates of Selected Birth-Control Methods[5]

Method	*Lowest Observed Failure Rate*	*Failure Rate in Typical Users*
Combined oestrogen and progestogen birth-control pills	0.5%	2.0%
Progestogen-only pill	1.0%	2.5%
IUD	1.5%	5.0%
Diaphragm	2.0%	19.0 %
Cervical cap	2.0%	13.0%
Condom	2.0%	10.0%
Foams, creams, jellies, and vaginal suppositories	3.0 to 5.0%	18.0%
Contraceptive sponge	9.0 to 11.0%	10.0 to 20.0%

A variety of studies in the United States and Great Britain have shown diaphragm failure rates ranging from a low of 2 to a high of 23 pregnancies per 100 women per year. The fact that a large study involving more than 70,000 months of diaphragm use reported a pregnancy rate of 2 per 100 women per year illustrates the high theoretical effectiveness of a properly fitted diaphragm when used regularly with a spermicide by a conscientious woman. On the other hand, a pregnancy rate of 12 to 19 per 100 women per year illustrates the wide discrepancy possible between theoretic- and use-effectiveness of the diaphragm. Some feel that a failure rate of 2 or 3 per 100 women per year is a sound reflection of the overall effectiveness for married women who are long-term users of a properly fitted diaphragm.[4]

The Pill and the IUD

By their middle years, many women have found a birth-control method which they consider convenient and effective. It may come as a nasty shock to many of them, then, to discover that two of the most popular methods, the Pill and IUD (intrauterine device), pose special hazards to middle-aged women.

Oral contraceptives (or birth-control pills) contain one or a combination of artificial hormones which prevent pregnancy by suppressing ovulation. **Women over thirty-five and women over thirty who smoke are strongly advised *not to use* the Pill because of the increased risk of heart attack and stroke.** The Pill has been the most frequently used and the most effective method of reversible birth control. Even so, one million fewer women in Britain are using the Pill compared with the mid-1970s because of growing awareness of its hazards and risks. Pill use in the US also declined in the late 1970s from a high of 10 million to 6 million users. Since then, we have witnessed a 'reselling of the Pill',[6] part of a new effort on the part of drug companies and population-control 'experts' to convince the public that the Pill is no longer risky and may even be beneficial. Yet there were five hundred Pill-related deaths in the US as late as 1982, when the number of prescriptions dispensed had climbed back up to 8.5 million.[7]

As a woman gets older, she is more likely to have a Pill-related heart attack or stroke. One study found that among women thirty to thirty-five years old who take oral contraceptives, the risk of a fatal heart attack is almost three times as great as for women who do not. For women forty to forty-four years old, the risk is almost five times as great.[8] Health risks on the progestogen-only pill are probably less, but the chances of developing ovarian cysts may be greater. Recent research also suggests that women already at risk of developing cervical cancer *may* have a higher incidence of this if they have used progestogen in the Pill – but this needs further investigation. (See Rose Shapiro, *Contraception*, 1987, pp. 108, 122, 125–6, 138.)

The risk of heart disease and stroke for Pill users increases with age:

Age	Cases of Heart Disease or Stroke
Under 25	4 per 100,000
25 to 34	13 per 100,000
35 and over	54 per 100,000[9]

Smoking while on the Pill is dangerous for women of any age. Women age forty to forty-nine who use the Pill and smoke have fifteen times as many fatal coronary and circulatory disorders as women who do neither, and thirty-nine times the risk of acute myocardial infarction (heart attack).[10] If no women thirty-five and over used the Pill, deaths from Pill use would be reduced by over one half. If, in addition, no smokers used the Pill, Pill-related deaths per year would be reduced from five hundred to seventy.[11]

Birth-control pills can cause a number of unintended effects and complications of varying degrees of severity. These effects may range from discomforts such as nausea, weight gain, depression, and increased susceptibility to urinary-tract and yeast infections to serious and potentially life-threatening complications[12] such as the following:

- Blood clots
- Heart attack and stroke
- Liver tumours
- Sickle-cell anaemia
- High blood pressure
- Gallbladder disease
- Malignant melanoma (a type of skin cancer)[13]

It is dangerous for a woman at any age to use the Pill if she already has any of the above conditions, a history of bile-flow blockage during pregnancy, or a past leg injury. Pill use is discouraged as well within four weeks of any surgical procedure. Also, women with diabetes are advised to avoid the Pill.

An estimated 9,400 women in the US are hospitalized each year as a result of diseases brought about by use of the Pill. Heart disease, stroke, and deep vein and pulmonary embolism are the main causes of such hospitalizations. Any woman who takes the Pill should see a family planning doctor at least once a year for a complete well-woman gynaecological exam, including a heart and blood-pressure examination. Women in their thirties should consider discontinuing use of the Pill as early as possible.

Some women who have intercourse very infrequently may be tempted to use the 'morning-after pill' as birth control. This is not advisable because of the very high amount of hormones in this pill and the dangers associated with them, especially for women over forty (or heavy smokers over thirty). Never use the 'morning-after pill' without supervision from an experienced doctor or other health-care practitioner. The post-coital pill should be available at FP clinics or pregnancy advisory services, and some GPs may prescribe it.*

---

*Two long-term injectable contraceptives are available – DepoProvera and Noristerat. Both are progestogen contraceptives. Since 1984 DepoProvera has been licensed for use over long periods in any 'appropriate' circumstances, and feminist groups have campaigned against the use of this form of contraceptive which, it is claimed, is often administered to poor and ethnic minority women without their full knowledge and consent.

The IUD is a small plastic or copper device designed to be inserted through the vagina into the uterus and left in place indefinitely. It is not known exactly how the IUD works. The most widely accepted theory is that the IUD causes an inflammation or chronic low-grade infection in the uterus. This causes the body to produce a higher number of white cells, which may hinder the buildup of the uterine lining, thus preventing implantation.[14] This does not preclude the possibility of conception, however, and may increase the risk of ectopic or 'tubal' pregnancy (outside the uterus), a life-threatening condition.[15]

Because of increasing numbers of lawsuits (and probably increasing evidence of IUD-related infections), American manufacturers of most IUDs have voluntarily stopped selling them. By early 1986, virtually all IUDs had been removed from the market in the United States, but they are still fitted in the UK.[16]

The other most serious risk of the IUD is that it will perforate the uterus and travel partially or completely through the uterine wall. This is a serious emergency requiring immediate medical attention.

If the IUD has been your chosen mode of contraception and you plan to continue using it, it is critical to have regular examinations to check on the condition of the uterus around it, especially as you approach menopause, or if you experience increased bleeding. Any pelvic pain also needs to be evaluated immediately. Aspirin and antibiotics may interfere with the IUD's effectiveness so use an additional method of birth control when you take these.

The IUD and pregnancy constitute a potentially dangerous combination. If you have an IUD in place and you become pregnant, have the IUD removed *whether or not* you intend to continue the pregnancy. If you remove the IUD, your chances of miscarriage are about 25 per cent, while if you do not have it removed, the chance of miscarriage rises to 50 per cent. If you do not remove it, you run the risk of an infected miscarriage, sometimes called a septic abortion. In extreme cases, this can cause the death of the woman as well as the foetus, and in most cases it is serious enough to require hospitalization. Women with IUDs should check out every missed period to be sure they are not pregnant or having a septic abortion. Of course, missing periods is fairly usual in the years prior to menopause, so this is yet another reason that the IUD is not a desirable method of contraception for women in midlife.

Possible health risks are the same as those of other hormonal methods – but research over a long period will be needed to determine these. The same applies to progestogen *implants* – small capsules placed under the skin with the progestogen released over a period of five years. Another method of releasing progestogen is the vaginal contraceptive ring, worn for three months but removable for intercourse if you want to become pregnant. For a fuller discussion of these and all other contraceptive methods see *Contraception: A Practical and Political Guide* (details below).

Barrier Methods

The diaphragm and other barrier methods are the birth-control practices most often recommended for women in midlife. See *The New Our Bodies, Ourselves* and *Contraception: A Practical and Political Guide* (listed below), for detailed descriptions, pictures, and diagrams. In our thirties, forties, and fifties, many of us find that we use barrier methods more successfully than when we were younger because we have grown more knowledgeable and comfortable with our bodies over the years. We more often have the confidence and assertiveness to *use* whatever birth-control method we select. For those of us who feel less comfortable with our bodies than we would like, using a vaginal barrier method is an opportunity to expand our self-knowledge and sexual confidence. Also, for women experiencing vaginal dryness, an increasingly common problem at midlife, contraceptive foam, cream, or jelly can provide additional lubrication. For women who are not in a long-term sexual relationship, barrier methods are advantageous because they do not have to be in place all the time. Barrier methods also provide some protection against sexually transmitted diseases (see p. 159 for notes on the role of spermicides in the prevention of transmission of the AIDS virus).

When the diaphragm is fitted properly and its use taught carefully, it can be up to 98 per cent effective when used with spermicidal cream or jelly.[17] There is a tenfold difference in failure rate between typical users and those who receive thorough instruction.[18] Choose a doctor or clinic that allows enough time for you to practise inserting and removing the diaphragm several times. Too many practitioners omit this crucial step.

Two recent studies implicated the diaphragm as a risk factor for women who suffer from recurrent urinary infections.[19] Pelvic conditions such as a pro-lapsed uterus, a bladder that protrudes through the vaginal wall (called a cystocele), or any other openings in the vagina (called fistulas) are somewhat more common in midlife. If you have any of these conditions you may not be able to use the diaphragm, the cervical cap, or the contraceptive sponge. However, your partner can use a condom, and you can add foam for additional protection. Some women find it convenient to purchase and keep a supply of condoms to offer to a partner who may not have one available. *Used together, the condom and contraceptive foam offer almost 100 per cent effectiveness and no dangerous side effects.*

Toxic Shock Syndrome (TSS)

As women in midlife, we are apparently less susceptible to TSS, but we are not entirely free of risk either. TSS is a rare but serious disease (see *The New Our Bodies, Ourselves* for more information), which primarily strikes menstruating women under thirty who are using tampons, especially high-absorbency tampons. However, a number of cases have been related to post-surgical complications or to use of barrier contraceptives, especially the contraceptive sponge, during menstruation, or to leaving a contraceptive in place for much longer than the recommended amount of time.

Every woman should be aware of the symptoms of TSS:

- A high fever, usually over 102 degrees
- Vomiting
- Diarrhoea
- A sudden drop in blood pressure, which may lead to shock
- A sunburnlike rash

If you have these symptoms, remove the tampon or contraceptive at once and get medical attention immediately.

Birth Control Without Contraceptives

Abstinence is not the only alternative to the Pill, the IUD, or barrier methods. Sex without intercourse is an important birth-control option when we do not have access to safe and effective contraception, as well as an important variation in lovemaking. Fertility observation, or 'natural birth control', involves learning from an experienced teacher to monitor and understand the hormonal changes in our bodies by observing the amount and quality of vaginal discharge, noting changes in the texture and position of the cervix, and keeping track of body temperature. In the years approaching menopause, however, menstrual cycles are apt to be erratic, making fertility observation ineffective as birth control.* However, it can be a useful and interesting – even exciting – tool for monitoring premenopausal hormonal changes, and for women who are trying to get pregnant at midlife.

Sterilization

Sterilization, a *permanent and usually irreversible* method of birth control through surgery, is now widely available, and for married couples over thirty, it is the most commonly used method of contraception.[20] Sterilization is a highly reliable method of birth control; the theoretical and actual failure rate for both tubal ligation (sterilization of the woman) and vasectomy (sterilization of the man) is 0.4 per cent.

*Younger women with regular cycles may be able to monitor their fertility in this way accurately enough to use this as a birth-control method.

A growing number of women and men in midlife choose sterilization because they are very sure they will not want to have more children. However, too many women still choose sterilization without adequate information and in desperation over the limited safety and effectiveness of other contraceptive methods. There is a deplorable history of sterilization abuse in the United Kingdom against middle-aged women, poor women, black and Asian women, and women who speak a language other than English. Primarily as a result of pressure from minority and women's groups in the US, regulations were enacted in March 1979 to protect women obtaining federally funded sterilizations.[21] In Britain, women's groups and some sympathetic doctors have mounted campaigns against this type of sterilization abuse. **Hysterectomy – removal of the uterus – is major surgery, and should not be considered a method of birth control or sterilization.** (See the Hysterectomy and Oophorectomy chapter for more information.) However, too many women, especially non-English-speaking women, are not adequately informed of either the permanence of sterilization or its possible risks and side effects.[22]

The well-known gynaecologist, Wendy Savage, specifically warns women that they should not consent to a hysterectomy or sterilization procedure immediately after childbirth. At least six months should elapse between having a baby and considering an irreversible procedure, to give time for considered reflection of the implications, she believes.

STERILIZATION PROCEDURES

Tubal ligation, popularly called 'tying the tubes', blocks the woman's fallopian tubes so that eggs cannot pass through them into the uterus. It may be done either abdominally or vaginally, often through a laparoscope (see p. 416). Serious complications are rare and the death rate is low (3.6 deaths per 100,000 procedures) compared with other surgery. The risk of death is greater when general anaesthesia is used.[23] The skill of both the anaesthetist and the surgeon is very important; be sure to inquire about the number of tubal ligations the surgeon has performed. Complications of laparoscopic sterilization may include puncturing of the intestine, bowel burns (with cauterization), perforation, haemorrhage, infection, and cardiac arrest. Some women experience a postlaparoscopic syndrome including heavy irregular bleeding and increased menstrual pain, which may create the need for repeated D&Cs or, in some cases, lead to hysterectomies.[24]

Vasectomy, or male sterilization, is a much simpler and less expensive procedure with fewer possible complications than female sterilization. It can be done in an Outpatient Clinic in half an hour under local anaesthesia. However, a vasectomy is not immediately effective, so use another means of birth control for the first fifteen days after the procedure or until after ten ejaculations. Tests should then be done on samples of semen.[25] The man is considered sterile after two negative sperm counts.

Missed Periods and Pregnancy Scares

If you miss a period when you are not trying to get pregnant, consider whether it is a sign of pregnancy or a sign of menopause (see p. 194). If you continue to be uncertain, it is important to have a pregnancy test early, so you can begin antenatal care if you decide to have a child, or make plans for an early abortion if you decide to terminate the pregnancy. If your periods have become irregular, you may want to wait until you have skipped two months before testing, but do not wait until a third month or you will not be able to have a less traumatic first-trimester abortion.

Many of the commonly used pregnancy laboratory tests cannot distinguish the hormonal changes of pregnancy from those of menopause; one test that can is a blood test called the Beta Subunit. This test is rarely available in the United Kingdom.

Abortion

Middle-aged women who are routinely in good health have no special medical problems associated with abortion. A thorough medical history should be taken *before* an abortion and the doctor should check for certain conditions. For example, fibroid tumours or a bladder that protrudes into the vagina may necessitate performing the abortion in a hospital.

According to the 1967 and later Acts, abortion is available on the NHS, but for many women the choice has to be a private abortion arranged through the British Pregnancy Advisory Service or the Pregnancy Advisory Service (see Organizations) or other private bodies. Abortion is a vital option in controlling our fertility – and, therefore, our lives. Whether or not abortion is any one woman's personal choice, safe, legal, and accessible abortion must continue to be available to all women who choose it. As the generation that fought for reproductive freedom, today's middle-aged women recognize the threat anti-choice forces pose to the progress of women in every walk of life. Entering our post-reproductive years does not weaken our resolve to defend the right to choice and control over our bodies for ourselves, our daughters, and future generations of women.

NOTES

[1]Boston Women's Health Book Collective, *The New Our Bodies, Ourselves*. London: Penguin, 1989.

[2]Robert A. Hatcher et al., *Contraceptive Technology: 1986–1987, 13th Revised Edition*. New York: Irvington Publishers, 1986, p. 101.

[3]Howard W. Ory, *Making Choices: Evaluating the Health Risks and Benefits of Birth Control Methods*, 1983. The Alan Guttmacher Institute, 1360 Park Avenue South, New York, NY 10010.

[4]Stephen L. Corson et al., *Fertility Control*. Boston: Little, Brown & Co., 1985, p. 225.

[5]Hatcher et al., op. cit., 13th Revised Edition, p. 102.

[6]Alice Wolfson, 'The Reselling of the Pill'. *Second Opinion*, Coalition for the Medical Rights of Women, June–July 1983.

[7]'Special Report: The Pill After 25 Years'. *Contraceptive Technology Update*, Vol. 6, No. 1, January 1985, pp. 1–3.

[8]Dennis Slone et al., 'Risk of Myocardial Infarction in Relation to Current and Discontinued Use of Oral Contraceptives'. *The New England Journal of Medicine*, Vol. 305, No. 8, 20 August 1981, pp. 420–4.

[9]Ory, op. cit., p. 43.

[10]Charles H. Hennekens et al., 'Oral Contraceptive Use, Cigarette Smoking and Myocardial Infarction'. *British Journal of Family Planning*, Vol. 5, 1979, pp. 66–7.

[11]Ory, op. cit., p. 42.

[12]'New Studies of Malignant Melanoma, Gallbladder and Heart Disease Help Further Define Pill Risk'. *International Family Planning Perspectives*, Vol. 8, No. 2, June 1982, pp. 76–8; and Dennis Slone, op. cit.

[13]Boston Women's Health Book Collective, op. cit., Chapter 15.

[14]Boston Women's Health Book Collective, op. cit., Chapter 15.

[15]Boston Women's Health Book Collective, op. cit., Chapter 15.

[16]Bernard M. Kaye et al., 'Long-Term Safety and Use-Effectiveness of Intra-Uterine Devices'. *Fertility and Sterility*, Vol. 28, No. 9, September 1977, pp. 937–42.

[17]Mary Lane et al., 'Successful Use of the Diaphragm and Jelly in a Young Population: Report of a Clinical Study'. *Family Planning Perspectives*, Vol. 8, No. 2, 1976, pp. 81–6.

[18]Robert A. Hatcher et al., *Contraceptive Technology: 1984–1985: 12th Revised Edition*. New York: Irvington Publishers, 1985, p. 108.

[19]Betsy Foxman and Ralph R. Frerichs, 'Epidemiology of Urinary Tract Infection: Diaphragm Use and Sexual Intercourse'. *American Journal of Public Health*, Vol. 75, No. 11, November 1985, pp. 1308–13; and Larianne Gillespie, 'The Diaphragm: An Accomplice in Recurrent Urinary Infections'. *Urology*, Vol. 24, No. 1, July 1984, pp. 25–30, quoted in Kathleen O'Brien, 'Lifestyle Factors and Urinary Tract Infections'. *The Network News*, Vol. 12, No. 1, January–February 1987.

[20]Boston Women's Health Book Collective, Chapter 15.

[21]See *The New Our Bodies, Ourselves* for more information and for resources on sterilization abuse.

[22]See *The New Our Bodies, Ourselves*, Chapters 15–16, for details and for organizations working on this issue.

[23]Hatcher et al., op. cit., 13th Revised Edition, p. 287.

[24]Boston Women's Health Book Collective, Chapter 15.

[25]Hatcher et al., op. cit., 12th Revised Edition, p. 213.

BOOKS AND PUBLICATIONS

John Guillebaud, *Contraception – Your Questions Answered*. Edinburgh: Churchill Livingstone, 1986.

Nancy Loudon (ed.), *Handbook of Family Planning*. Edinburgh: Churchill Livingstone, 1985.

Hilary Homans (ed.), *The Sexual Politics of Reproduction*. Aldershot: Gower, 1985.

The Boston Women's Health Book Collective, *The New Our Bodies, Ourselves*. London: Penguin, 1989.

Rose Shapiro, *Contraception: A Practical and Political Guide*. London: Virago Press, 1987.

The Family Planning Association. Leaflets from Book Centre, 27–35 Mortimer Street, London W1N 7RJ.

Kaye Wellings and Angela Mills, 'Contraceptive Trends'. *British Medical Journal*, Vol. 289, 13 October 1984, pp. 939–40.

Wendy Savage, 'Abortion, Sterilization and Contraception'. *Medicine in Society*, Vol. 7, No. 1, 1982, pp. 6–12.

E. Billings, *The Billings Method*. London: Allen Lane, 1981. Natural birth control.

9
Childbearing in Midlife

More women today are choosing to have children in their middle years. Because we live longer and stay healthier longer, we can concentrate on other areas of our lives in our young adult years, and still choose parenthood even into our forties. Despite some of the added pressures of the middle years, such as more stressful and challenging jobs, new relationships, and ageing parents, older women often have more experience at balancing life's demands.*

I'm forty-three and becoming aware of the issues of old age, as I help my baby start his life. The advantage of having my children at thirty-five and forty-three is that I know myself; I knew I really wanted children. I know some things about what I need, what contributions I can make in addition to raising the children. I've made a commitment to photography and have a number of projects that I'm working on or looking forward to. Some of them are about lesbian family life.

At times I do feel a bit out of sync – with friends my age whose children are grown up, with friends who have children the age of mine who are ten or fifteen years younger than I; or when I feel myself hitting my stride in photography and need to move at a slower pace partly because of the family commitments.

I've noticed that when I'm with friends in their fifties and sixties I envy their clean, quiet rooms. I tell myself, I've had this before and some day again this will be mine. I'm grateful to be intimately in touch with the stages and cycles of life. I asked the babies, 'Is this too abstract?' They said, 'Ba, Ba, Ba, Ba.'

The best thing in my life is the joy of actually having a child. Eleven years ago when I was pregnant with my son, my marriage was in such a terrible state I almost had an abortion because I couldn't envision living my life with that much dissension. My husband wasn't supportive of me and so I assumed he wouldn't be supportive of a child either. A sister had even made all the arrangements. Then the morning the abortion was scheduled, I decided not to have it, because I was thirty-four and I thought, I may not have the opportunity to become pregnant again. And with all the

*For a discussion of the pros and cons of having a baby at any age, see A Child: Your Choice (listed below).

pressures and difficulties I have faced, some of my greatest joys have come from being a mother. The doctors referred to me as an 'elderly prima', which made me laugh. I was healthy as a horse.

What saved my sanity when I was bringing up my youngster alone was that my mother lived next door to me. I never had to concern myself with finding a baby-sitter. My mother, like so many black grandmothers and aunts, provided care without my asking her and I could work whatever hours I was asked to work. In fact, my son came home once and asked me what a baby-sitter was. [a forty-five-year-old woman]

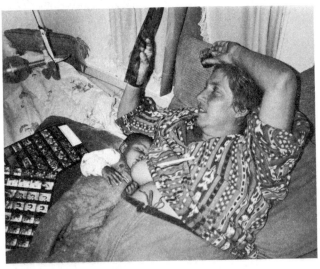

For me, having children in my forties while bringing up two stepchildren seemed natural and appropriate. My age seemed irrelevant to me and to my husband, though sometimes it seemed to concern others when they found out. What is it like now to be fifty-eight and have a sixteen- and eighteen-year-old? Well, we do worry about getting it together for their college and our retirement, but other than that we don't feel very deviant and our kids don't seem to mind having 'older parents'. At least they don't seem to have much to say about it.

I was a forty-one-year-old first-time mother married to a fifty-three-year-old father of three children. In what some called an 'advanced maturity' marriage, we needed time to be alone together as well as time to spend with our newborn, as well as time for his children from his former marriage and time for our dependent parents.

The difficulty of orchestrating all this with time alone for spiritual stretching and meditating seemed to increase with age. The demands on our energy and creativity were titanic. We felt we needed a minimum of one evening out per week and one weekend away alone together every six weeks because we would be sixty and seventy before there would be an 'empty nest'.

We might have managed this if we had forfeited privacy and hired living-in help, or had not moved when our newborn was a year old, leaving a network of friends built up during our adult years. Our marriage did not survive the stress. Paying attention to time alone and time together is a major challenge in combining midlife childbearing and midlife marriage.

Conception and Midlife Fertility

Women who plan a pregnancy in their thirties or forties may worry if they do not conceive right away. Some women's bodies continue to produce eggs regularly up until menopause, while other women in their thirties gradually begin to produce fewer eggs, and thus have fewer opportunities for conception. The reduced fertility of women over thirty compared with younger women may be partly attributable to less frequent intercourse among longer-married couples.[1] So it is wise to be patient and allow enough time and opportunity for conception before assuming that there is a fertility problem.

Infertility is usually defined as the inability to conceive after a year or more of sexual intercourse without contraception.[2] One study found that it takes an average of 3.8 months for women ages thirty-five to forty-five to conceive, compared with about 2 months for women ages fifteen to twenty-four.[3] Medical and lay media reports that exaggerate the degree to which fertility decreases with age have contributed to women's worries about their fertility.[4]

Infertility is becoming increasingly common at all ages due to environmental hazards and pelvic infections resulting from sexually transmitted diseases (STDs) and/or IUDs. If you have been trying to conceive for more than a year, you may want to read some of the feminist literature on infertility and new reproductive technologies (see below) before going to see your GP for a referral to a clinic.

If you have taken a long time to conceive, you may be at risk for the 'medicalization' of your pregnancy and birth. Doctors sometimes intervene unnecessarily in midlife pregnancies with procedures such as Caesareans in order to 'safeguard' the pregnancy of a woman who has taken a long time to conceive.[5] This is a concern because every medical intervention brings its own set of risks and complications. In considering the risks of midlife pregnancy, we must keep in mind that low fertility is a problem of conception, not of pregnancy. Once we are pregnant, we do not need to be treated a special way because we took a long time conceiving. However, a history of repeated miscarriages may require exercising special care during pregnancy.

Childbearing for Women in Midlife

A major change over the past ten years has been the extension of women's 'fertility deadline' from the early thirties to the early forties. What has brought about this change? Several factors stand out:

- Improved health and extended longevity of women
- Reliable birth control
- The women's movement, which has encouraged us to decide for ourselves whether and when we will have children
- More sophisticated antenatal testing and the availability of legal abortion
- New research which shows that some of the earlier assumptions and concerns about pregnancy and age have been incorrect or overstated

Phyllis Kernoff Mansfield, a health educator at Pennsylvania State University, has challenged established beliefs about maternal age and risk during pregnancy. Mansfield examined all the studies ever published in the United States that relate the age of the mother to seven pregnancy complications. She found in her review of the literature that the vast majority of studies published before 1970 did not pass the simplest tests for methodological soundness. The most glaring deficiency was the lack of a control group; that is, no comparison was made between older and younger women. The 'problems' of older women were simply assumed to be related to their age, without accounting for other factors such as fertility history, general health, or number of previous pregnancies. Mansfield's research revealed that when other factors were held constant, only Caesarean sections showed a definite increase in risk with age – and a Caesarean is not a complication but an intervention. Mansfield and her associates concluded that the general health and nutritional habits of the mother had far more influence than age on the outcome of a pregnancy.[6]

A 1982 report from the National Center for Health Statistics concluded that contemporary women who first became pregnant in their thirties and forties have good results because they do not have a history of delayed childbearing due to pregnancy-related problems.[7] These women have *chosen* to begin childbearing in their thirties and forties when they have found the right partner, when their job or career is going well – when they feel ready.

Other studies have also found that some of the risks formerly associated with childbearing in midlife have on more careful examination turned out to be associated with diseases or chronic conditions.[8] As we get older, we are at higher risk of developing such chronic diseases as diabetes, hypertension, and heart disease, as well as fibroid tumours, endometriosis, and scarring from operations and infections in the pelvic area, all of which can complicate conception and pregnancy. But these conditions affect only a relatively small number of women and do not warrant intervention in the majority of pregnancies in healthy older women. **Older women who do not have such conditions have no higher risk of a difficult pregnancy than younger women.** The following is a list of factors that can complicate pregnancy and childbirth:

- Toxaemia, or the presence of toxic substances in the blood, can lead to a much more serious condition called eclampsia, which in turn leads to convulsions and coma. Research has found the risk of this disease to be associated not with age, but with diabetes.[9] Diabetes is also linked to many other pregnancy and childbirth complications.
- Unnecessary Caesareans. Doctors tend to intervene more readily in a prolonged labour when the mother is over thirty-five. They perform Caesarean sections more often and use painkillers and anaesthetics sooner and in greater amounts. The use of anaesthetics during childbirth has been associated with low blood pressure in the mother and respiratory problems in the newborn. And if a woman is apprehensive that she will have a difficult delivery because she is older, she may be more easily influenced to accept or to ask for drugs.[10]

My doctor was certain that my slow labour meant I had a 'sluggish uterus', which he thought typical of older women. He was already preparing for a Caesarean when I went into the second stage. I later found out that my mother and sister had had similar labours. It was a family pattern. [a fifty-eight-year-old woman reporting on a first childbirth at forty]

- Low birth weight tends to be a problem affecting babies born to the youngest (teenage) and the oldest (over thirty-five) mothers, but in the years since 1970, low birth weight has declined as a problem for the oldest mothers. The evidence suggests that the older mothers of today are more highly educated and more likely to be well informed about pregnancy, nutrition, and exercise. They are more highly motivated to take good care of themselves and to seek antenatal care; therefore they are more likely to have heavier, healthier babies.[11]
- Socio-economic status, not age of the mother, is the most significant factor in predicting infant mortality in the UK. Women who have higher incomes have better access to a wide choice of good antenatal care and a wider choice of facilities. They can more easily purchase the additional food and vitamins they need during pregnancy. Recent funding cuts in the Health Service and Social Security threaten to deepen the shocking disparity between the middle class and the poor in infant mortality and to slow the decline in the national infant-mortality rate[12] that was evident in the 1970s.

- Maternal and infant mortality are more likely to be related to disease than to age. In one study, two-thirds of maternal deaths reported were among black women with hypertension[13] (more common in black women than white women). Cardiovascular disease in the mother, not her age, is the factor that most increases the risk of infant mortality.[14] A recent study eliminated those with hypertension from the study sample and found that healthy black women over thirty-five had successful outcomes in pregnancy and birth.[15]
- Placental haemorrhage and other complications of the placenta have been linked to cardiovascular diseases such as hypertension.[16]
- Down's syndrome is sometimes associated with the age of the mother. However, recent research suggests that the age of the father's sperm, not his nor his partner's own biological age, plays a role in one kind of Down's syndrome,[17] and another kind of Down's syndrome is hereditary – the age of neither partner is a factor.

The risk of bearing a child with Down's syndrome, a form of mental retardation in varying degrees of severity, increases gradually with each year of age, rather than rising sharply at five-year intervals, the way the conventional mode of reporting would lead us to believe. Thus, it is helpful for women to see the figures year by year. We do not dramatically increase the risk when we reach 'magic numbers' in age such as thirty-five or forty.[18]

Tables such as this one will need to be revised to account for the age of the father's sperm. This table was compiled prior to the widespread use of amniocentesis. The rates are much lower now.[19]

Estimated Rates of Down's Syndrome in Live Births by One-Year Maternal-Age Intervals, Based on Upstate New York Birth Certificate Data[20]

Maternal Age	Number of Down's Syndrome Babies per Number of Live Births	Maternal Age	Number of Down's Syndrome Babies per Number of Live Births
(20)	(1/1923)	37	1/225
(25)	(1/1205)	38	1/177
30	1/885	39	1/139
31	1/826	40	1/109
32	1/725	41	1/85
33	1/592	42	1/67
34	1/465	43	1/53
35	1/365	44	1/41
36	1/287	45	1/32

Nutrition

Everything in the Ageing and Well-being chapter deserves double emphasis if you are pregnant. Stay away from smoking, alcohol,[21] and drugs, and some people feel you should also avoid caffeine. See *The New Our Bodies, Ourselves* for a more in-depth discussion of the effects of harmful substances on pregnancy. While age itself is not a risk, the chances of developing a chronic disease increase with age. Taking care of yourself often prevents disease, thus improving the outlook for a healthy pregnancy.

It is essential that you eat nutritiously while you are pregnant. Unfortunately, most obstetrician-gynaecologists know little about nutrition and pregnancy, so you may want to talk to a nutritionist.

A SUGGESTED DAILY DIET FOR PREGNANCY[22]

1. A pint of milk (whole, skim, buttermilk) or milk equivalents (cheese, yogurt, cottage cheese) is recommended in the UK, but in the US a quart. Once we are over thirty-five, our bodies do not absorb calcium and protein as well as when we were younger (see Eating Well chapter).
2. Two to four servings of meat, fish, poultry, cheese, tofu, eggs, or nut-grain-bean-dairy combinations for protein. If you do not drink at least one pint of milk a day (or eat its equivalent in milk products), add additional protein foods.
3. A serving of fresh, leafy green vegetables – spinach, dark leaf lettuce, broccoli, cabbage, Swiss chard, kale, alfalfa sprouts, or collard, mustard, or beet greens.
4. One or two vitamin-C-rich foods – potato with the skin, grapefruit, orange, melon, green pepper, cabbage, strawberries, fruit, orange juice.
5. A yellow or orange vegetable or fruit for vitamin A.
6. Four to five slices of whole-grain bread, pancakes, tortillas, or a serving of whole-grain cereal or pasta. Use wheat germ and brewer's yeast to fortify other foods.
7. Moderate amounts of butter, margarine, vegetable oil. (You need some fat in your diet, but in controlled amounts.)
8. Salt to taste. (Avoid table salt and foods and drinks with needless sodium.)
9. Six to eight glasses of liquid – fruit and vegetable juices, water, and herb teas. Avoid sugar-sweetened juices and colas.
10. For snacks, choose dried fruits, nuts, sunflower seeds, popcorn.

Eating well will ensure that you and your baby will be able to meet the demands of pregnancy, labour, and childbirth, and help ensure that your baby

will have an adequate birth weight. Low-birth-weight babies are more susceptible to complications at birth. Eating well also lowers the risk of complications
such as anaemia and toxaemia, and reduces the risk of mental retardation in
your baby. During pregnancy your body stores fats and fluids you will need if
you breastfeed. Older women are a little more likely to have twins, creating an
extra need for nourishment (an additional 100 grams of protein per day is
recommended).[23]

In the past, doctors put a great deal of emphasis on gaining as little weight as
possible during pregnancy. Pregnancy, however, *increases* your body's need
for calories and protein; *it is not the time to diet*.[24] Monitor your weight to avoid a
sudden increase in weight. This can be a sign of toxaemia. It is best to eat as
healthfully as you can and let your weight take care of itself. If you are eligible,
make sure that you claim any social security benefit (see p. 264).

PHYSICAL ACTIVITY AND EXERCISE

Staying active is an important part of good antenatal care. You can swim, run,
walk, dance, do yoga, whatever feels comfortable and does not tire you out too
much. Doctors sometimes advise pregnant women not to 'overdo it'. They
may be even more cautious with older pregnant women. Such advice can cause
stress to women who are accustomed to exercise. It is important to keep up
exercise at your accustomed level. If you have been sedentary, find ways to
move more, beginning with walking and gentle exercise.

*I noticed that although I was one of the oldest women in my antenatal exercise class,
I was in much better physical condition than the majority. Perhaps my regular
swimming and dancing made the difference. Clearly, one's emotional/physical
condition rather than one's age is most important.* [a forty-one-year-old woman]

The pelvic floor exercises (see p. 124 for description and instructions) can
help during pregnancy to strengthen the muscles in the pelvic area, which can
make the entire delivery process easier. See below for books on exercise during
pregnancy and childbirth-preparation exercises.

GETTING SUPPORT

At any age, we want our pregnancy to include solid emotional support from our
partners, friends, and families. That support can be especially important as we
press through the maze of medical decisions and pressures that often
accompany a midlife pregnancy. We may also be dealing with stressful
situations, such as older children going through a turbulent adolescence or

ageing parents depending on us for support; we may have demanding jobs or careers; we may be worried about how pregnancy will change a relationship. Talking with other women often can be an important source of support.

When I first learned that I was pregnant, I was delighted, joyful, excited. And I assumed that people close to me would share my joy. Not so. My mother, my teenage daughter, and my closest woman friend openly disapproved because I was unmarried. However, there were others – my sister, a close older woman friend and mentor, a male counsellor, and other old friends who were happy for me. It was really important to my well-being to have warm support from people around me during my pregnancy. My antenatal exercise classes, besides preparing my body for giving birth, also serve as an open forum for sharing concerns, thoughts, and resources with other pregnant women. It's always such a relief to suddenly step into a room where everyone is pregnant. The feelings of isolation immediately vanish. [a divorced woman in her forties]

An important source of support during pregnancy is a sympathetic doctor, antenatal clinic or midwife who will view you and your pregnancy as normal and healthy, while carefully monitoring any special medical conditions you may have. Books like *Where to be Born* (see below) will make it easier to choose a hospital or midwife likely to provide the sort of care you want, and you can get up-to-date information through the Women's Health and Reproductive Rights Information Centre (see Organizations).

ANTENATAL TESTING

Antenatal tests such as ultrasound, amniocentesis, and chorionic villi sampling offer older women the option of choosing motherhood by reducing their risk of bearing a child with certain congenital disorders. However, several writers on midlife parenthood have observed that the process of testing, waiting for test results to come back, and deciding on a course of action delays a woman's or a couple's emotional commitment to the pregnancy,[25] in addition to raising several difficult moral and ethical issues that each woman must consider carefully. For women, the right to reproductive choice is central to all other rights in life. As legislators seek to reduce the number of weeks of a pregnancy at which termination is allowed, the right to end a pregnancy because of foetal abnormality may be seriously eroded.

I felt I had to make the decision, before we knew the results, that if we got a diagnosis of Down's I would have an abortion. We talked to a genetics counsellor before the test. She was very helpful – all the medical support staff were helpful; they made all the difference in my thinking of it as a positive thing we were doing. [a thirty-eight-year-old first-time mother]

I chose not to have an 'amnio' because, after much soul-searching, I decided that I would be open to having a Down's child. My personal experience with adults who have Down's syndrome is that they are among the most loving people around. Though Down's children take more care, work, and commitment, they can develop into contributing creative adults. They play a very humanizing role in our society. [a forty-one-year-old woman with a long-delayed second pregnancy]

Because of my age, I was considered a high-risk pregnancy, but I did not consider myself one. I was healthy and ate well and had a good family history. At this point in my life I wanted a child very much and felt prepared to accept whatever happened in terms of [the baby's] health. I also had had a miscarriage and felt the risk of another miscarriage, though slight, with amniocentesis, was great enough to warrant not having any unnecessary intervention. [a thirty-eight-year-old woman]

At present women under thirty-five are not usually offered antenatal testing unless there is a history of foetal abnormality. If you are offered a routine test, there is no point in having it if you are not prepared to consider termination in any circumstances, since there is some small risk to the foetus.

ULTRASOUND

Ultrasound is used for one or more of the following: to help pinpoint the exact location and position of the foetus; to help determine the age and size of the foetus; and to check for structural abnormalities in the foetus. It uses intermittent high-frequency sound waves to create pictures of the body's inner organs by measuring the length of time it takes for an echo to be returned.

If you have an ultrasound test, you will be asked to drink several glasses of water just before the procedure is done. A technician will run a transducer, a hand-held instrument resembling a microphone, over your abdomen. A computer then translates the echoes picked up by the transducer into pictures of the foetus on a video screen. The pictures are then 'read' by a radiologist. The results are usually available in a matter of hours.

Though ultrasound appears to be one of the safest tests and can provide important information, its long-term effects are still unknown. Doctors sometimes want to use ultrasound to test for twins. Consider whether you really need to have this information early in your pregnancy. Because of possible, though unproven, risks, organizations like AIMS (Association for Improvements in the Maternity Services, see Organizations) have campaigned against its routine use. In the UK it is common for ultrasound to be used at several intervals during a pregnancy. Perhaps if you are doubtful about it you might accept the test once, and, if all is normal, refuse to be tested further.

AMNIOCENTESIS

Amniocentesis can detect approximately eighty chromosomal abnormalities as well as certain biochemical and metabolic disorders; it is most often used to test for Down's syndrome. Amniocentesis does not detect every possible disorder and is not a guarantee of a healthy infant.

The test involves withdrawing a small amount of fluid from the amniotic sac by way of a large needle and is usually performed between the fifteenth and sixteenth weeks of pregnancy, when there is enough amniotic fluid to give an adequate sample but the least risk of damaging the foetus. It takes approximately four weeks to obtain results.

The risk of miscarriage associated with the test is estimated at between one in 250 and one in 66 procedures, depending on the skill of the doctor.[26] There is also the risk of damage to the foetus: women have reported a variety of problems, including damaged, missing, or underdeveloped limbs, dating from approximately the time of the test.[27]

For women over forty, the chance of finding a defect is greater than the risk of miscarriage. Between ages thirty-five and forty, the odds are about even, and under age thirty-five, the risk of miscarriage is greater than the chance of finding a problem.[28]

A major drawback of amniocentesis is that it must be done too late in the pregnancy to allow for abortion during the first trimester. When you add on the four-week waiting period, it would be not much earlier than twenty weeks into the pregnancy, and may be as late as twenty-four weeks, before a woman could make a decision. If she chooses abortion, an instillation (saline or prostaglandin) procedure would have to be done.

CHORIONIC VILLI SAMPLING

Chorionic villi sampling is a new alternative to amniocentesis which can detect chromosomal and other genetic abnormalities between the eighth and tenth weeks of pregnancy. The chorion, the tissue that grows around the developing embryo, eventually becomes the placenta. Scientists in China discovered that the tiny projections, called villi, which cover the chorion have a genetic composition similar to the embryo. By analysing these villi, genetic information about the foetus may be obtained. To perform the test, a doctor inserts a catheter through the vagina and into the uterus, guided by ultrasound equipment. A small sample of the villi is then aspirated and tested immediately. At present this technique is not available in many parts of the country, and its safety is under review. There is also some question about its accuracy. Its advantage over amniocentesis, of course, is that CV sampling can be done much earlier in a pregnancy.

Alternatives to Midlife Childbearing

As menopause approaches, some women speak of an urge to become pregnant before it is 'too late'. One woman, divorced when her first child was young, and approaching her fortieth birthday, spoke of her wish to have another baby.

My son is sixteen and I suddenly have a strong urge to have a baby. I still want a family with children in it. I wonder if I'm really wanting a baby or if I just want to be part of a family, and it feels like a baby would give me that.

If you decide that having a child of your own is not central to your wish for a family, you may want to explore alternatives such as communal living or foster parenthood.

Before the 1970s adoption was commonly seen as a solution to the problem. Now, however, it is virtually impossible to adopt a baby, and the children available for adoption tend to be older, with physical or mental handicaps. Efforts are always made by the adoption agencies to place children with parents of similar ethnic backgrounds; 'transracial' adoptions, popular some years ago, having given rise to many difficulties for children and parents. Adoption bodies – local authority or voluntary – are more concerned about the needs of the children than those of would-be parents, and you can expect to be subjected to a long 'vetting' process before being accepted as a suitable person, or couple, to adopt a child. See below for useful information books on adoption.

Being a mother is wonderful. It's exhausting, challenging, fulfilling. I feel complete. There's no more of this nagging feeling that there's something missing in my life. I feel like I'm home. But she's a real challenge of a person to be with. Our cultures are different. We're very different people. Yet we've definitely made a bond. She wants very much to be close but at the same time she is testing a lot. She hits or bites or teases. She wants her way and has a hard time with no's. In the beginning she was more into pleasing but I think that she came from a strict environment and this is a much more permissive, loving environment. It's been hard for her to adjust to the change and it's been hard for me to get stronger in setting limits. But she's happy and I feel very lucky to have found such a lively and caring soul, too. Just a real good person. She's a challenge, she tests every area where I'm weak. It's good for me! We're both growing a lot in the process. [a woman in her forties who adopted a four-year-old child]

NOTES

[1]A. F. Guttmacher, 'Factors Affecting Normal Expectancy of Conception'. *Journal of the American Medical Association*, Vol. 161, 1956, pp. 855–60.

[2]Boston Women's Health Book Collective, *The New Our Bodies, Ourselves*. London: Penguin, 1989.

[3]Guttmacher, op. cit.

[4]Alan H. DeCherney and Gertrud S. Berkowitz, 'Female Fecundity and Age'. An editorial in *The New England Journal of Medicine*, Vol. 306, No. 7, pp. 424–6; Bayard Webster, 'Study Finds Female Fertility Drops Sharply After Age of 31'. *The New York Times*, 18 February 1982.

[5]Phyllis Kernoff Mansfield, *Pregnancy for Older Women: Assessing the Medical Risks*. New York: Praeger, 1986.

[6]Ibid.; see also Donna Kirz, 'Advanced Maternal Age: The Mature Gravida'. *American Journal of Obstetrics and Gynecology*, Vol. 152, 1985, pp. 7–12. The author criticizes obstetricians' use of pejorative language to describe a middle-aged pregnant woman.

[7]S. J. Ventura, 'Trends in First Births to Older Mothers, 1970–1979'. National Center for Health Statistics, *Monthly Vital Statistics Report*, Vol. 31, No. 2, Supp. (2); DHHS Pub. No. (PHS) 82-1120, Public Health Service, Hyattsville, Md., May 1982.

[8]David A. Grimes and Gail K. Gross, 'Pregnancy Outcomes in Black Women Age 35 and Older'. *Obstetrics and Gynecology*, Vol. 58, No. 5, November 1981, pp. 614–20.

[9]Mansfield, op. cit.

[10]Mansfield, op. cit.

[11]Ventura, op. cit.

[12]C. Arden Miller, 'Infant Mortality in the US'. *Scientific American*, Vol. 253, No. 1, July 1985, pp. 31–7.

[13]E. O. Horger and A. R. Smythe, 'Pregnancy in Women over Forty'. *Obstetrics and Gynecology*, Vol. 49, 1977, pp. 257–61.

[14]K. R. Niswander and M. Gordon, *The Women and Their Pregnancies*. DHEW Publication (NIH) 73-379, Public Health Service, Washington, DC.

[15]Grimes and Gross, op. cit.

[16]P. Kajanoja and O. Widholm, 'Pregnancy and Delivery of Women Aged 40 and Over'. *Obstetrics and Gynecology*, Vol. 51, 1978, pp. 47–51; and Mansfield, op. cit.

[17]L. S. Penrose, 'Paternal Age in Mongolism'. *Lancet*, Vol. 1, 1962, p. 1101. See also, Patricia A. Martin-DeLeon and Mary B. Williams, 'Sexual Behavior and Down Syndrome: The Biological Mechanism'. *American Journal of Medical Genetics*, Vol. 2, 1987, pp. 693–700.

[18]Pamela Daniels and Kathy Weingarten, *Sooner or Later: The Timing of Parenthood in Adult Lives*. New York: Norton, 1983, p. 186.

[19]Judith Blackfield Cohen, *Parenthood After 30? A Practical Guide to Personal Choice*. Lexington, Mass.: D.C. Heath & Co./Lexington Books, 1985.

[20]Daniels and Weingarten, op. cit., p. 186.

[21]Z. Stein and J. Kline, 'Smoking, Alcohol and Reproduction'. *American Journal of Public Health*, Vol. 73, 1983, pp. 1154–6.

[22]Boston Women's Health Book Collective, op. cit.

[23]J. A. Pritchard and P. C. MacDonald, *Williams Obstetrics*, 16th ed. New York: Appleton-Century Crofts, 1976, p. 531.

[24]Boston Women's Health Book Collective, op. cit.

[25]Daniels and Weingarten, op. cit.; and Barbara Katz Rothman, *The Tentative Pregnancy: Prenatal Diagnosis and the Future of Motherhood*. New York: Viking, 1986.

[26]Santa Fe Health Education Project, 'What Is Amniocentesis? *Health Letter*, Vol. 4, No. 10.

[27]Barbara Katz Rothman, personal communication.

[28]Rayna Rapp, 'XYLO: A True Story', in Rita Arditti, Renate Duelli Klein and Shelley Minden, eds., *Test Tube Women*. Boston: Pandora Press, Routledge & Kegan Paul, 1984.

BOOKS AND PUBLICATIONS

Jean Shapiro, *A Child: Your Choice*. London: Pandora Press, 1987. Assesses the pros and cons of having a baby at any age.

Catherine Boyd and Lea Sellers, *The British Way of Birth*. London: Pan, 1982.

Where to be Born. The Debate and the Evidence. NPEU, Radcliffe Infirmary, Oxford.

Sheila Kitzinger and John A. Davies (eds.), *The Place of Birth*. Oxford: Oxford Medical Publications, 1978.

Ann Oakley, *The Captured Womb: History of the Medical Care of Pregnant Women*. Oxford: Basil Blackwell, 1985.

Yvonne Bostock and Maggie Jones, *Now or Never? Having a Baby Later in Life*. Wellingborough: Thorsons, 1987.

The Boston Women's Health Book Collective, *The New Our Bodies, Ourselves*. London: Penguin, 1989.

S. Borg and J. Lasker, *When Pregnancy Fails: Coping with Miscarriage, Stillbirth and Infant Death*. London: Routledge & Kegan Paul, 1982.

Naomi Pfeffer and Anne Woollett, *Experience of Infertility*. London: Virago Press, 1983.

Robert M. L. Winston, *Infertility: A Sympathetic Approach*. London: Macdonald Optima, 1987.

Mary Anderson, *Pregnancy After 30*. London: Faber & Faber, 1984.

Ann Oakley, *Miscarriage*. London: Fontana Paperbacks, March 1984.

Health Education Authority, *Pregnancy Book*. Free illustrated handbook from antenatal clinics.

British Association for Adoption and Fostering, *Adopting a Child*. BAAF also produces other useful booklets and leaflets – see Organizations.

10
The Menopause: Entering Our Third Age

Most of us remember our first menstrual period. We may remember who told us about menstruation, or, if we were not prepared, we remember the shock of our first period. Just as there was a time for our periods to start, there is a time for them to stop. Yet few of us are ever prepared for menopause. We hope this chapter will help change that.

The generation of women approaching the menopause today has had more choices about reproduction than did their mothers and grandmothers. Whatever choices we have made about contraception and childbearing in our lives, menopause means the end of our choices about fertility. To the extent that women's lives can be described by fertility, there are three stages: childhood until puberty; the years when we are able to bear children; and the 'third age',[1] the years past menopause.[2] We are, however, more than our fertility and have much to offer throughout our lives regardless of our decisions about reproduction.

While females of some species remain fertile throughout their lives, women live past the end of fertility and truly have a 'change of life'. As we go through this change, some of us mourn the end of childbearing potential, while many celebrate entering an age of freedom from the concern about pregnancy.

When we are defined as sex objects and breeders, and valued only while young, we may fear the menopause as a symbol of the approach of a demeaned old age. We are then vulnerable to societal myths that after the menopause we are past our prime. Consider the irony of Sandra Day O'Connor referring to herself as 'over the hill' because she was past menopause when appointed as the first woman justice of the US Supreme Court. With the increase in longevity, our 'third age' can be as much as half our lives and can be a time of activity and productivity.

An American woman, Elizabeth Freeman, started a business when she was sixty-four years old. She writes:

What a burst of energy women experience as they leave menopause. Putting together a newsletter for an organization called the Older Women's Network (OWN) in the

1970s made me aware of the outpouring of poetry, fiction and thoughts of midlife and older women in all parts of the country. I'm continually impressed and excited by the energy and creativity of older women. At the same time I realized the dearth of publishers available to them. I wanted to print the work of older, feminist women. Using the word 'crone', which, though generally derogatory in our society, originally meant 'wise old woman', I conceived of a name for my publishing house. Adding the OWN (Older Women's Network), Crones' Own Press came into being. To me this period of my life has been most exciting and creative.

Menopause is a natural event, but doctors developed, and some still perpetuate, the medical myth that menopausal women suffer a crisis or a 'deficiency disease'[3] for which treatment is needed. The myth still persists, fed by drug company advertising and by ridicule from comedians, that we are difficult to live with at the menopause.

Researchers are only now beginning to study what affects women's experiences of the menopause. Cultural patterns and attitudes may have an influence on these experiences. Yewoubdar Beyene compared the social status of older women, nutrition, and attitudes toward childbearing and menopause of both Mayan and rural Greek women. She found that Mayan women look forward to menopause, eat a diet high in carbohydrates and calcium, but no meat or dairy products, and do not report hot flushes. Rural Greek women report more anxiety about menopause and growing older, eat a diet more like ours than like the Mayan, but although they report hot flushes, they do not seek medical intervention.[4]

The Santa Fe Health Education Project reports that the dominant culture in the United States may be more powerful than its subcultures in shaping the experience of menopause: 'Our experience in giving menopause workshops for over eight years to groups of Hispanic, Native American, and other women of a range of ages, economic backgrounds, geographic locations, and professions has led us to the conclusion that the experience of menopause cross-culturally in the United States is much more the same than it is different.' This probably obtains in 'multi-ethnic' Britain, too.

Most women go through 'the change', as the menopause is often called, with few problems and go on with their lives. Some women, however, do have a very difficult time. Those who feel isolated and friendless, without others to share their experience, may be unprepared and therefore susceptible to fears and misinformation about menopause. Women are often blamed and are told that their attitudes about themselves are the cause of their problems. It is important to acknowledge, however, that some women who are prepared for menopause, who have support, and are happy with their choices may still experience discomfort as their hormone levels are changing.

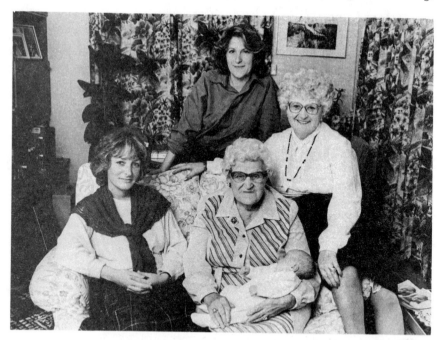

New feminist research shows that many women learn to care for others first and only later to care for themselves.[5] Menopause is a time when, if we have not already done so, we should learn to take good care of ourselves.

This time is a rebirth of sorts, an incredible opportunity to rediscover who I am as a human being. The truth is that I have a very long life ahead, and now I can choose how I am going to experience it and what I'm going to do. It's exciting to be making a journey in response to myself rather than in response to the values placed upon me. [a forty-two-year-old woman]

What is the Menopause?

The word 'menopause' is used in a variety of ways. Popularly, the 'menopause' is used to describe the many years when our bodies are changing from menstrual cycles to a non-cyclic stage. More precisely, menopause is defined as the date of our final period. The medical literature distinguishes three time periods: premenopausal, perimenopausal (when we may notice changes), and postmenopausal (after periods have ceased); it describes the first two together as the climacteric. While the average age at the time of the final menstrual period is between ages fifty and fifty-one, the range is very broad – the menopause may occur between the late thirties and the late fifties. We do not know that we have had that final period and reached the menopause until a year without periods has passed. The common folk expression 'change of life' (often condensed to 'the change') is a good term to describe the entire process, which takes perhaps twenty years – ten years before and ten years after the cessation of menses (periods).

Signs of the Menopause

'Symptoms' is not an appropriate word to describe changes at menopause. A symptom is a change due to disease, while the menopause is not a disease. Three 'signs' are clearly associated with menopause: cessation of periods, vaginal changes, and hot flushes. Cessation of periods is the only sign experienced by all women. Wrinkles and greying hair, which happen to both women and men as a function of the normal ageing process, are not caused by the menopause. Likewise, irritability, which is frequently listed as a 'symptom' of the menopause, may occur at any time in our lives and may also occur as we get older and react to age discrimination, which is so evident in our society today.

Some doctors attribute much of what happens to a woman at midlife to the menopause, sometimes overlooking what might be symptoms of gallbladder disease, hypertension, and other serious conditions.[6] For example, profuse sweating, fatigue, and vaginal itching may be symptoms of diabetes;[7] headaches and dizziness may be symptoms of disease.

Because doctors are often not aware that it is normal for women's experiences of the menopause to vary widely, they often treat the normal signs of the menopause as illness. Rather than offering help in managing those changes which become severe and annoying, they are quick to offer drugs (especially hormones) or, sometimes, hysterectomy. The emphasis of this chapter is on the self-help approaches women have found to deal with menopausal discomforts and to avoid drugs and surgery.

A few years ago this chapter would have been the place for a discussion of doctors' misuse and overuse of oestrogens for women at and following the menopause. In the late 1970s and early 1980s, the risks of oestrogen therapy for the menopause were widely publicized so its use in the United States dropped and then levelled off. Now in the 1980s, both in the UK and the US, we are again seeing a surge in prescriptions – oestrogen or a combination of oestrogen and progesterone. Some doctors still prescribe hormones when they may not be necessary so the discussion of whether to take them or not is still relevant. Since most drug companies that sell hormones and doctors who prescribe them are now basing their recommendations for hormones almost entirely on a campaign of fear of broken bones, **the discussion of hormones has been placed in the Osteoporosis chapter**, pages 355–61.

The myth that women go mad at the menopause persists despite research showing that women are *less* likely to experience mental illness at midlife than in other years. Some women do report temporary depression during the perimenopausal stage when hormone levels are fluctuating and readjusting. While this depression does not happen to many women, the few who do experience it need to know it will most likely pass after menstruation ceases, with the coming of the menopause.[8]

I searched for the truth about the menopause but what I found didn't help me. All the books I read and all the people I talked with told me it was nothing at all. Some said, 'Think positively and don't gain weight.' Others said, 'It's all in the culture.' I had to validate my own experience. No one would acknowledge or could explain why I had a hard time whenever my hormones shifted. I thought I was going mad at thirteen, I was depressed when I was pregnant, and I had unexplained depression and mood changes for the nine years between the ages of forty-five and fifty-four when my periods were changing. I was raising a daughter alone but I lived with people who were supportive and I tried everything: oestrogen for two years, jogging, massage therapy, a women's support group, homoeopathic remedies. They helped a little but not enough. I even tried an antidepressant, which did not help either, and caused me to gain twenty-five pounds. Once my periods stopped, I not only had an absence of depression but had a lightness and buoyancy, a state of being positively happy. I am fine now but I feel I lost a decade of my life. [a fifty-six-year-old woman]

HORMONE REPLACEMENT THERAPY

The recent upsurge of interest in HRT in Britain is discussed in the Osteoporosis chapter. It is important to note that there are now groups of doctors and organizations who are trying to promote HRT for all but a small group of women who have medical conditions which clearly put them at risk, claiming that women on HRT feel better, look younger, have no problems with vaginal dryness or hot flushes. The last two conditions can indeed be treated with HRT; the question of 'well-being' is more subjective. Although HRT, as at present administered, is claimed to be perfectly safe, there are many possible risks to its use and even a group such as the Amarant Trust, which favours HRT for every middle-aged or older woman, has to admit in its literature that there is still need for research on a possible link between hormone therapy and breast cancer.

Some of us may experience premenstrual changes for the first time: swollen, tender breasts, water retention, and some tension or anxiety. Women who have had these and other discomforts severe enough to be considered premenstrual syndrome (PMS) can look forward to relief from their discomforts.* As periods stop and hormone cycles level out, so will PMS. This process may take several years. Even women with only minor water retention and breast tenderness may still be aware of some cycling in their bodies after their periods cease. Those women who suffer from underlying depression in addition to PMS may find their symptoms a little worse during this time. After the menopause, PMS will subside, but they still may have to cope with the underlying depression.[9]

CHANGES IN MENSTRUAL PATTERNS

Our bodies may require years before our well-established pattern of periods stops completely. Some women do not experience menstrual-cycle changes before their periods stop; but most experience some changes in the length, amount, and frequency of menstrual flow, often starting in their forties and sometimes their thirties.

The chart on pages 196–7 shows the hormonal patterns that result in varying patterns of flow. The heavy period (heavy bleeding or menorrhagia) is the most annoying and worrying. Sometimes the flow is so heavy that a tampon can be flooded out of the vagina and even heavy pads cannot contain it. We may feel faint momentarily. We may fear or be embarrassed by so much blood. Heavy periods are common but subside as the oestrogen level drops.

As a primary school teacher I found it almost impossible to deal with the situation. I had to retire to the loo in the middle of lessons to clean myself up and change my pad. It got so bad that I felt nervous about taking my turn at break duty. In the end I had to take three weeks' sick leave, as the period just went on and on. But that was the very last period I had! [a fifty-four-year-old woman]

Women have found helpful things to do to control heavy bleeding, such as eating a healthy diet, taking vitamin A in limited quantities, and getting plenty of rest. Also, it is best to avoid alcohol, strenuous activity such as swimming or jogging when the period is beginning, and aspirin and other drugs that slow

---

*PMS can sometimes be alleviated by a low-salt diet or other dietary changes, natural diuretics, aspirin, and acupuncture. Vitamin B_6, calcium with vitamin D, and magnesium may help relieve PMS. Some women have found essential fatty acids (specifically linseed oil and/or evening primrose oil), along with some zinc, vitamin C, and vitamin B complex, very helpful. For a discussion on PMS see *Seeing Red* by Laws, Hey and Eagan (Hutchinson); and *The New Our Bodies, Ourselves* (Penguin).

down blood clotting. Some women report that their periods seemed to be under better control after using techniques such as acupuncture and meditation combined with visualizing a compact uterus. Self-help techniques require months of learning about and observing our bodies' patterns and changes. This is part of the process of taking care of ourselves.

Sometimes the periods become so extended and so close together that we seem to be having one continuous period. You should report repeated heavy and continuous periods to your doctor and may want to undergo tests to assess the state of the lining of the uterus. Beware of pressure to have surgery for bleeding (see Hysterectomy and Oophorectomy chapter). There are other options. Though heavy bleeding is inconvenient, embarrassing, and scary, the only real health hazard (once a biopsy rules out malignancy) is iron deficiency (anaemia). Have your haemoglobin checked and eat iron-rich foods. Take iron supplements, if recommended, but not unless you are actually anaemic.

Progesterone is a hormone secreted by the ovaries, adrenals, and placenta. It is responsible for the changes in the uterine lining in the second half of the menstrual cycle, for development of the maternal placenta after implantation, and development of the breast glands.

Progestin or *Progestogen* are terms for any natural or synthetic hormonal substance which produces effects similar to those produced by progesterone.

Usually the word 'progesterone' is used for the body's hormone and 'progestogen' for any substance which has the same effects on the body as progesterone. The words, however, are sometimes used interchangeably.

One medical approach to the heavy bleeding caused by the body's prolonged oestrogen or reduced progesterone production is the use of a progestogen. When used at the very beginning of a period, progestogens cause the lining of the uterus to slough off more completely than in previous cycles. The next period may be lighter because the lining has not built up so thickly. Progestogens may also be used to interrupt prolonged oestrogen production, stimulate a period, and start a new cycle. Some women decide to try small doses of an oral progestogen for a very short time, or sporadically, depending on the pattern of their periods. Beware of large doses or injections that stay in the body for several months. Progestogens do not alleviate all bleeding problems. IUDs impregnated with a progestogen have all the dangers of IUDs plus longer exposure to the progestogen.

The occasional 'missed' period can be worrying to women who are heterosexually active and fear they might be pregnant. In spite of scanty periods you can still be fertile, so keep using contraceptives for two years after the final period (see Birth Control for Women in Midlife chapter, p. 163). Become familiar with your pattern by charting your periods and noting other body changes which differ from those of pregnancy.

Pregnancy	*Menopause*
Missed period	Missed period
May have other signs such as:	May have other signs such as:
Nausea	Hot flushes
Tender breasts	Vaginal dryness

Many women have reported occasional bleeding after they thought their menstrual periods had finally stopped. We now know that stress can affect the level of reproductive hormones in the body. At a menopause workshop, two women reported experiencing some bleeding long after the cessation of their menses. Each started flowing when she took a sick parent to a hospital emergency department.

Prolonged bleeding or more than a few brief episodes of bleeding after the menopause may be a symptom of cancer, and should be checked by your doctor. Most NHS doctors would not offer a hysterectomy unless there is a confirmed diagnosis that warrants it. Private doctors may be less cautious (see Hysterectomy and Oophorectomy chapter).

VAGINAL CHANGES

As we age, there is a tendency for the skin and mucous membranes in various parts of our bodies to become drier. To help with this condition add moisture to the air in your house and drink four pints of fluid each day. The vaginal membranes become thinner, hold less moisture, lubricate more slowly. Even walking may be uncomfortable. Some women also suffer dry eyes, and some a loss of saliva. For some women vaginal dryness is an early sign of the menopause; others do not experience it until many years later, and many never do. Little research has been done on this subject but data from the first surveys of a large number of women to find out how many are bothered by vaginal dryness should be available shortly.[10]

Some prescription and over-the-counter drugs can cause dryness. Antihistamines, for example, dry other tissues as well as nasal tissues. Do not use douches, sprays, and coloured or perfumed toilet paper and soaps, which can irritate the tissues of the vulva. If itchiness develops, avoid scratching, which can irritate the delicate tissues and lead to infections and further problems. Prescription ointments are available to help the itchiness.

Hot Flushes

It was a freezing December night when I lay in bed, dreading to get up and go down a long cold hall to an even colder bathroom. Then I had a hot flush, and, all of a sudden, it was very easy to leave my warm bed! For the rest of the winter I used my nighttime hot flushes this way. My friends laughed when I told them that hot flushes are not all bad! [a fifty-nine-year-old woman]

Many of us had flushes during pregnancy or experienced something resembling hot flushes at other times – the red face of blushing or the increased heartbeat and sweating during times of great stress. In folk wisdom and humour, hot flushes are the sign most commonly associated with the menopause.

Sometimes our flushing is interpreted as blushing or being flustered. Since sweating from a hot flush reveals age and menstrual status, both of which are supposed to be secrets, we may be subjected to jokes and embarrassed reactions. Also, many older women were taught that 'Ladies don't sweat!' Fortunately we are speaking up, supporting each other, and changing many of these attitudes.

Surveys report that anywhere from 47 to 85 per cent of women will experience hot flushes.[11] Some women never experience hot flushes at all. In one study of one thousand women, 470 had hot flushes but only 155 (15.5 per cent of the total) reported that they were bothered by them.[12]

For most, a hot flush means nothing more than a transient sensation of warmth. Many women report their hot flushes are not unpleasant, may even be pleasant, and as in the above example, useful. Some women experience waves of heat and drenching sweats, often followed by chills; some experience chills first. The flushes are often preceded by a brief aura, a sense of the coming flush. Feelings of tension, heart palpitations, anxiety, and nausea may also accompany hot flushes or may precede and be relieved by the hot flush.

Hot flushes can begin when menstrual cycles are still regular or when they are becoming irregular. Typically, they continue for less than a year after the final menstrual period; however, for some women they persist for five, ten, or even more years.[13] In some instances, hot flushes first begin many years after the menopause. Although they usually last a few minutes, the duration of some hot flushes may be shorter or longer. Their frequency also varies. Hot flushes may occur once a month, or once an hour, or several times an hour. They can

Patterns of Natural Hormone Levels and Their Effects on Menstrual Periods

	Oestrogen Level	Ovulation
MENSTRUAL YEARS	Usual cyclic pattern. More oestrogen than progesterone before ovulation	Egg produced. Both oestrogen and progesterone drop at ovulation, then rise
PREGNANCY	Oestrogen level increases after fertilization and during pregnancy	Egg produced and fertilized
PERIMENOPAUSAL YEARS	Usual cyclic pattern and level	Egg produced
Hormone levels may fluctuate from one period to the next causing variations in cycles and in periods. Some cycles may be ovulatory (an egg produced and some cycles may be anovulatory (no egg produced). Oestrogen levels may drop gradually so that periods diminish gradually, may drop suddenly so that periods stop suddenly, may fluctuate so that the flow is heavier, lighter, or skips some months	Less oestrogen	Egg may or may not be produced
	Even less oestrogen	No egg produced
	Prolonged oestrogen	Probably no egg produced
POSTMENOPAUSAL YEARS	Low oestrogen; no cyclic pattern (some oestrogen is still produced)	No egg produced

Progesterone Level	Effect on Endometrial Lining	Effect on Period
Usual cyclic pattern. More progesterone than oestrogen after ovulation	Oestrogen builds up lining. Progesterone causes lining to slough off	Usual period
Level increases during pregnancy	Endometrium builds up to provide environment for embryo to develop	No period
Usual cyclic pattern and level	Usual cyclic pattern	Usual period
Less progesterone	Thin uterine lining	Period may be lighter in flow or last fewer days
Even less progesterone	Thinner uterine lining	No period
Less progesterone	Irregular or thick lining. May not slough off completely or evenly. Portion may remain during the next cycle	One period may start, stop, and start again. Period may be longer and heavier and clotting may be present
Even less progesterone; no cyclic pattern (production of progesterone virtually ceases)	Thin uterine lining. No cyclic changes	No period

occur any time day or night, though one study reports they are more frequent between 6 and 8 a.m. and again between 6 and 10 p.m.[14] Each woman has her own pattern.

At age fifty I skipped a period and had hot flushes at night for the first time during the month I was on jury duty. I got my period the day after I finished jury duty and didn't have another hot flush for six more months. [a fifty-five-year-old woman]

We have few clues as to who is most likely to get hot flushes, how intense they might be, or how long the hot flushes might last. Generally the body gradually adjusts to the lower level of oestrogen, and for most women the hot flushes stop.[15]

Many women report that their hot flushes are most disturbing at night when they are awakened and may have to change their nightclothes and sheets due to drenching sweats. The loss of sleep over many nights can cause fatigue, irritability, and feelings of inability to cope similar to depression (see 'Dealing with Insomnia', in Habits Worth Changing chapter, p. 55).

Women whose ovaries are removed before the menopause, resulting in a sudden drop in oestrogen levels, may experience intense hot flushes often beginning immediately after surgery, and vaginal dryness at an earlier age. Hot flushes occur more frequently and severely in these women (especially for about six months after surgery) than they do in women who go through natural menopause.[16] The ovaries continue to produce oestrogen after the menopause so a woman may begin to experience hot flushes if she has her ovaries removed after her periods have already stopped.

During a hot flush, the blood vessels most commonly expand (dilate) and blood flow to the skin increases. Though the skin temperature often rises from four to eight degrees F. during a hot flush, and the sensation is one of heat or blushing, the internal body temperature actually falls.[17] This occurs because the body eliminates heat through increased blood flow to the skin and by sweating. The dilation can clear a stuffy nose, and the rush of blood to the surface can cause dizziness, reddening, and crawly feelings on the skin. The increased heartbeat that often occurs with a hot flush may be accompanied by a feeling of anxiety. Some women experience chills and tingling skin when the blood vessels narrow (constrict).

Since my studio apartment had a patio door, I could easily step outside to cool off when I felt a hot flush coming. I felt shut in and constricted when that source of relief wasn't present in other settings. [a fifty-three-year-old woman]

At my first unexpected hot flushes I was afraid. I had in mind that hot flushes involved a loss of control, but when I paid close attention, I felt half in a dream state, flushed and physically lightheaded. Actually, it seemed like an altered state of consciousness, which wasn't that unfamiliar to me, because I meditate. But I can see that for many women it would be a new experience, one they'd fear and try to suppress. [a forty-two-year-old woman]

Only in recent years have researchers begun to study what causes hot flushes. Their occurrence is related to a decline in oestrogen levels. However, something else is probably involved in triggering each hot-flush episode. Some researchers speculate that the hypothalamus (the part of the brain which regulates body temperature) is involved in a hot flush, perhaps through the release of some substance which triggers the hot flush. They are looking at the ways hormones interact with the temperature-regulating system.[18]

Doctors and researchers would gain much by listening carefully both to the descriptions that women give of their sensations of hot flushes and to the techniques women have found to minimize and relieve their discomforts. We hope that a better understanding of the mechanism of hot flushes will lead to new approaches and self-help techniques for relief rather than just to new drugs.

Self-Help for Hot Flushes

KEEP TRACK

Chart your hot flushes in relationship to your menstrual periods and other events to see if you can find a pattern. The more you know about yourself, the better you'll be able to manage your hot flushes and the better you will feel.

From ages fifty-one to fifty-three I missed many periods. Whenever I missed periods I had hot flushes; the months I had periods I had no hot flushes. I began to see a pattern and could predict what to expect. [a fifty-five-year-old woman]

KEEP HEALTHY

Some women have found that caffeine (coffee, tea, cola drinks, chocolate), alcohol, sugar, spicy foods, hot soups, hot drinks, and very large meals may trigger hot flushes. Eat sensibly.

Some women find that vitamin E minimizes or eliminates hot flushes. Vitamin E is found in vegetable oils (wheat germ, corn, and soy-bean), wheat and rice germ, legumes, corn, and almonds. Egg yolks contain vitamin E but also contain very high levels of cholesterol. If you take a supplement, start with 25 milligrams per day and find your effective level by increasing gradually up to, but not more than, 400 IUs per day. Avoid it if you are taking digitalis or are diabetic. Take only water-soluble vitamin E if you have high blood pressure. Some find adding 25 mg of B complex to be helpful.

Many women report more hot flushes at times of stress. Try the methods described in Disarming Stress (p. 21) to relax. If hot flushes disturb your sleep at night, take naps and meditate to avoid fatigue.

KEEP COOL

Dress in layers. Clothes made of natural fibres may be more comfortable than those made of synthetic materials. When you feel a hot flush starting, take off some clothes. Go to a cooler spot, stand by an open window. Relax, take a few deep breaths. There is no reason to feel embarrassed. Fan yourself with whatever is at hand or collect fans to match your wardrobe as our great-grandmothers did. Drink something cool. Place something cool where it feels best – on the wrists, temples, forehead. Shower. Visualize yourself in a cool place such as sitting by a lake with a cool breeze blowing. Lower the thermostat, get a cooler, an electric fan, or an air conditioner. Before bed, put a cup of table salt in a tub of warm water; lie in it until the water cools; rinse with cold water and go straight to bed.[19] If you have a bedmate get a dual-control electric blanket.

USING HERBS

Over the years women of many cultures have used herbs for menopausal complaints. The following information was compiled by the Santa Fe Health Education Project with help from Amadea Morningstar (nutritionist), Chavela Esparza (herbalist), and Gregorita Rodriguez (curandera-healer). See below for other books on using herbs.

Some herbs can be toxic in large quantities, so if you are not familiar with a herb, obtain more information, preferably from someone with experience in their use. Use herbs with caution and start taking them in moderate amounts. Read labels carefully. You can save money and be assured of purity and freshness by growing your own.

Herbs are available from herbalists, health-food stores, herb stores, some Asian shops, and country markets. They come in different forms – dried for making teas, or powdered in capsules. Dried herbs may be fresher than capsules. Some people prefer the capsules because not all herbs are soluble in water and it is easier to swallow a capsule than to brew tea. Allow two to six weeks to feel the herbs' effects; do not expect immediate relief.

The most commonly used herbs for complaints of the menopause include black cohosh, damiana, dong quai, cramp bark, ginseng, golden seal (used in England), licorice root, red raspberry leaves, sarsaparilla and spearmint (*yerba buena*). These are traditionally taken as teas. Herb mixtures for the menopause available in capsules in health-food stores may contain false unicorn, blessed thistle, and squaw vine.

Ginseng and black cohosh contain natural oestrogen, so precautions about oestrogen therapy apply to them also. Ginseng is also not advised for women with high blood pressure or diabetes. Dong quai is also called female ginseng.

The following are herbal tea recipes. Try one for six weeks to see if it helps before trying another. Different combinations of herbs work best for different people.

1. A tea made from the following three American herbs: skunk weed, snake broom, and lizard tail (*yerba de zorrillo, escoba de la vibora,* and *yerba del manso*). Bring half a gallon of water to a boil. Add two tablespoons of the dried leaves of each herb (or a quarter of a cup of each of the fresh plants – leaves, stem, and roots). Boil two to three minutes. Set aside, covered, for ten minutes. Strain. Drink a cup three times a day. (These herbs may be difficult to find in the UK.)

2. A tea brewed in the same way from two tablespoons of alfalfa seeds to a pint of water. Drink three times a day with lemon. For economy, the same seeds may be used for a second brewing.

3. A tea brewed from an ounce of wild or sweet marjoram in a pint of hot (not boiling) water. Cover. When cool, strain and add a large glass of port wine. Take one tablespoon before meals, three times a day.

4. A tea brewed from two parts each of motherwort and red sage, and one part each of tansy, pennyroyal, and skullcap. Take one-half teaspoon in a little lukewarm water before meals three times a day.

5. A tea brewed from black cohosh, sweet flag, licorice root, star root (*Aletris farinosa*), black haw, cramp bark (*Viburnum opulus*), squaw weed (false valerian), and motherwort. Take one cup during the day with a meal.

6. Gotu Kola is a high-mineral herb. Drink one cup of tea in the morning for energy before breakfast. This is not recommended for women with overactive (hyper) thyroids.

Especially for Anxiety and/or Insomnia

1. A cup of tea per day brewed from a rounded teaspoon of any one of the following herbs: camomile, spearmint, rosemary, skullcap, passion flower (*Passiflora incarnata*), tilia flowers.

2. A tea brewed from a mixture of catnip, valerian, camomile, skullcap, lady slipper, and peppermint.

3. Sleeping on a pillow stuffed with dried hops.

KEEP TALKING

Break the taboos against the menopause. Stay comfortable by letting people know when you are having a hot flush and reaffirm that it is nothing to be ashamed of. Use positive, not demeaning, humour. Tell household members or co-workers what is happening.

I never felt that I should suffer hot flashes in silence, so my husband and kids called me 'Flash'. When I told my husband it was the first anniversary of my last period he said, 'Congratulations, Flash. You've done it.' So we went out to dinner and celebrated that night. [a fifty-one-year-old American woman]

Talking with others, sharing our experiences and feelings, acquiring knowledge about how our bodies are changing, and giving each other support eases our 'change of life'. A group of women coming together in a menopause self-help group or workshop to learn from one another, in a respectful, informative, and supportive setting, can effectively counteract fears and uncertainties with support and information. Much of the material in this section comes from women who have shared their experiences and their wisdom. An indispensable resource is *Menopause: A Positive Approach* by Rosetta Reitz, a pioneer in menopause self-help groups. By talking with other women we will continue to discover and exchange new self-help methods.

*Rondel**

Now that I am fifty-six
Come and celebrate with me.

What happens to song and sex
Now that I am fifty-six?

They dance, but differently.
Death and distance in the mix;
Now that I am fifty-six
Come and celebrate with me.

MURIEL RUKEYSER

*'Rondel' by Muriel Rukeyser, from *Breaking Open*. New York: Random House, 1973, p. 18.

NOTES

[1] So-called by the French and Portuguese according to Betty Friedan, 'Changing Sex Roles: Vital Aging', in Robert N. Butler and Herbert P. Gleason, eds., *Productive Aging: Enhancing Vitality in Later Life*. New York: Springer Publishing Co., 1985, p. 93.

[2] In ancient times women in the three ages were called nymphs, maidens, and crones. See Barbara Walker, *The Crone: Women of Age, Wisdom and Power*. New York: Harper & Row, 1985.

[3] Frances B. McCrea, 'The Politics of Menopause: The "Discovery" of a Deficiency Disease'. *Social Problems*, Vol. 31, No. 1, October 1983, pp. 111–23.

[4] Yewoubdar Beyene, 'Cultural Significance and Physiological Manifestations of Menopause: A Biocultural Analysis'. *Culture, Medicine and Psychiatry*, Vol 10, No. 1, March 1986, pp. 10–17.

[5] Carol Gilligan, *In a Different Voice: Psychological Theory and Women's Development*. Cambridge, Mass.: Harvard University Press, 1982.

[6] Catherine DeLorey, 'Health Care and Midlife Women', in Grace Baruch and Jeanne Brooks-Gunn, eds., *Women in Midlife*. New York: Plenum Press, 1984, pp. 277–301.

[7] Jane Porcino, *Growing Older, Getting Better*. Reading, Mass.: Addison-Wesley Publishing Co., 1983, p. 277.

[8] John B. McKinlay, Sonja M. McKinlay and Donald Brambilla, 'The Relative Contributions of Endocrine Changes and Social Circumstances to Depression in Mid-Aged Women', in Mary Roth Walsh, ed., *The Psychology of Women: On-Going Debates*. New Haven: Yale University Press, 1987.

[9] Information on PMS at the menopause from a conversation with Michelle Harrison, M.D.

[10] Sonja M. McKinlay and John McKinlay, New England Research Institute, 9 Galen Street, Watertown, MA 02172.

[11] Sonja M. McKinlay and M. Jeffreys, 'The Menopausal Syndrome'. *British Journal of Preventive & Social Medicine*, Vol. 28, 1974, pp. 108–15; and Bernice L. Neugarten and R. J. Kraines, 'Menopausal Symptoms in Women of Various Ages'. *Psychosomatic Medicine*, Vol. 27, 1965, pp. 266–73.

[12] Jane Haliburton, personal communication about research in progress.

[13] Fredi Kronenberg, unpublished data.

[14] Ann M. Voda, *Menopause – Me and You*. Salt Lake City: University of Utah College of Nursing, 1984, pp. 7–8.

[15] R. Don Gambrell, Jr, and Ann L. Hyatt, 'Benefits and Risks of Estrogen Replacement Therapy in the Menopause'. *Delaware Medical Journal*, Vol. 56, No. 4, April 1984, p. 20.

[16] S. Chakravarti et al., 'Endocrine Changes and Symptomatology After Oophorectomy in Premenopausal Women'. *British Journal of Obstetrics & Gynaecology*, Vol. 84, 1977, pp. 769–75.

[17] I. V. Tataryn et al., 'Post-menopausal Hot Flashes: A Disorder of Thermoregulation'. *Maturitas*, Vol. 2, 1980, pp. 101–7.

[18] Fredi Kronenberg et al., 'Menopausal Hot Flashes: Thermoregulatory, Cardiovascular, and Circulating Catecholamine and LH Changes'. *Maturitas*, Vol. 6, 1984, pp. 31–43.

[19] Gregorita Rodriguez, Santa Fe, New Mexico.

BOOKS AND PUBLICATIONS

Rosetta Reitz, *Menopause: A Positive Approach*. London: George Allen & Unwin, 1985.

Dr Barbara Evans, *Life Change*. London: Pan, 1979.

Anne Dickson and Nikki Henriques, *Menopause: The Woman's View*. Wellingborough: Thorsons, 1987.

Dr Caroline M. Shreeve, *Overcoming the Menopause Naturally*. London: Arrow, 1986.

Jean Coope, *Your Menopause Questions*. London: Family Doctor Publications/British Medical Association, 1981.

Judi Fairlie, Jane Nelson and Ruth Popples, *Menopause: A Time for Positive Change*. Poole: Blandford Press, 1988 (and see Books and Publications at the end of Osteoporosis chapter).

11
Relationships in Middle and Later Life*

Women value relationships. For us middle-aged and older women, especially, concern for inter-personal relationships has been a central theme of our lives. Most of us have worked hard to reach out to others, to express feelings of caring and attachment, and to be helpful when friends and family members are troubled. Throughout our lives our 'people skills' have helped us get through some of the tough times.

As we move into the later decades of our lives, however, nearly all of us experience losses or changes in many of our most important relationships. When this happens, we fear the loneliness of being 'unattached' and the emptiness of not being needed or valued. Many of us from traditional backgrounds were raised on homilies like 'Blood is thicker than water' and taught to avoid sharing confidences with 'outsiders'. Yet long-lived women frequently survive all of their close family members. Though we grieve for the loss of relationships we can never replace, we *can* overcome loneliness and isolation by reweaving and changing family relationships, nurturing old and new friendships, and especially by reaching out to other women to form new connections for support and intimate friendships. Our middle and later years can be a time of expanding choices and opportunities.

Extending our Families

This chapter speaks about extending, rather than extended, families, to emphasize our active role in expanding the conventional definition of family. Most women who have lived their younger adult years in a nuclear family with children extend their definition of family to include partners of children and, of

*In this chapter we talk about many different life situations. We recognize and even celebrate our diversity as women. We have included in the chapter some material on relatively uncommon situations to extend to women the full range of alternatives that are available to all of us in our middle and later years. We hope this approach will raise consciousness and encourage women to unite across barriers of generation, race, class, and sexual preference that have divided us in the past.

course, grandchildren. Particularly in our middle and later years, we may also begin to think of our closest friends as a kind of extended family.

Family is important throughout our lives as a source of intimacy and connection. Whether we choose a family similar to or different from the one we grew up in, most of us continue to value the love, acceptance, and intimacy of family life.

Being the centre of a family network goes right on for us anyway, even though the children don't live at home any more. I am still embedded in family. Different people need me and us for different reasons. I've taken on my husband's family as well as my own, and he's taken on mine. I have two children by my first husband and my former mother-in-law is still living. My husband has three children and two of them have families of their own. Also my stepmother and stepfather, the second spouse of each of my parents, are still living and I, for various reasons, am their most responsible child. We have a stable happy marriage and my husband is a doctor, so we attract whoever is ailing. And we are both in the 'support business', it's just how we are emotionally. [a fifty-seven-year-old woman]

I have two sisters who live upstairs. People are always surprised that we get along so well, living in the same house. My sisters never go out without coming by to ask me if they can get me anything. We weren't always like that. We were too busy with our own lives. Now we try hard to help each other. [a seventy-year-old woman, widowed]

Living with Loss

During our middle years, most of us first become aware of signs of advancing age in our parents, aunts, and uncles. We are shocked! These are not the elderly relatives of our grandparents' generation, but the stalwart adults who formed the strong, dependable landscape of our youth. Can it be possible that they are slowing down and needing help from *us?* This process can be a frightening reminder of our own mortality.

My father and all his family died in their late fifties. So, does that mean I have only four more years? I don't really feel morbid about it, but I live with a different perspective. [a fifty-five-year-old woman]

It suddenly hit me last year when my father died, having lived to the ripe old age of ninety-three, that I was now the oldest living member of my family. When you get into your middle years, as long as you can say, 'My father or my mother . . . this or

*that', as long as you are still somebody's daughter, then you can't be that old.
Somehow I can't see myself as the matriarch of the family.* [a fifty-nine-year-old
woman]

*It's scary not to have any parents or grandparents or any relatives except for one
sister. I miss the unconditional love and caring – the free caring of someone calling
not because they want me to serve on some committee but because they just want to
know how I am. I get a little of that from my twelve-year-old daughter. I wish I had
more kindness coming my way. I wish I weren't alone so much.* [a fifty-year-old
married woman who works on crafts at home]

FRIENDS AS FAMILY[1]

For all of us, irrespective of marital status or sexual preference, women friends
provide the support and continuity that enable us to enjoy new challenges and
cope with the changes and losses we face in the second half of life. With this
awareness, growing numbers of us are learning to regard our friendships as
lifelong relationships to be worked at and cared for 'just like family'. For those
of us who grew up thinking of other women as our competitors, or as less
interesting or less valuable than men, it has been rewarding to share our lives
and our histories in women's groups and discover that women are, in fact,
terrific.

*I am lucky enough to be part of a women's group. Without that group I don't think I
could have survived these last few years. My husband left me – he'd been having an
affair with a younger woman for years, and all his colleagues and friends knew about
it, but I never heard anything. It was my friends who gave me support: put me in
touch with a good woman solicitor and a counsellor who had helped one of them;
made sure to keep an eye on me between meetings of the group; phoned me just for a
chat when they knew I was feeling low. And since the divorce several of these women
have introduced me to new circles of friends – women and men – and I've even gone
on holiday with one of them and her children. I only hope that none of my friends
have to go through what I had to – but if one of them did, I hope I'd be able to give the
same sort of loving support.* [a woman in her fifties]

Many of us are accustomed to forming primary emotional links with a man.
But even when we live in a traditional way with a male partner, there is a high
statistical likelihood that we will grow old in the company of other women. The
divorce rate is rising and most married women outlive their partners.

Because I was widowed young (in my early thirties), I had a series of short- and long-

term relationships with men near my own age over the next twenty years that met my sexual needs pretty well. However, they did not always meet my emotional needs for closeness on a daily basis; they were not live-in arrangements, and in fact, more often than not, the man lived in another part of the country. In my fifties, I became aware that even the sexual aspects of this type of relationship were not as satisfying as they had been, as my now middle-aged partner's sexual needs and problems often required that my attention be diverted from my own. At about the same time, a new friendship with another woman developed, with almost daily contact, and I recognized that the closeness and affection it was providing on a regular basis were meeting deeper emotional needs than the more sporadic sex offered by men my own age. [a fifty-four-year-old woman]

It's extremely important for women growing older to have a circle of women friends; there's no other way to guard against the inevitable loneliness. [a woman in her eighties]

If we have been used to forming our closest bonds with family members and others within an ethnically homogeneous community, we may be more comfortable having our most intimate friendships with those of similar background. However, it can be a pleasant surprise at times to find a kindred spirit in a more diverse setting.

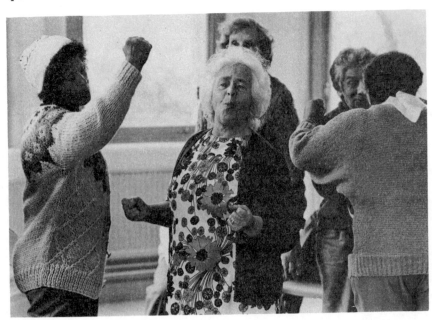

I have often been shy about making new friends, but I am learning to reach out. I have just made a new friend. Though I am Jewish and she is Methodist, we share so many things in our life experiences that we could almost have been twins. Our ideas about the spirit, about religion, about life are so similar. We even share the experience of being estranged from our own children. We have helped one another and have found in one another sisters, extended family, friends for life. [a fifty-five-year-old woman]

Freda Rebelsky, an expert on adult development, observes, 'So many good friendships start at times of our lives when we feel the most need for someone else to understand our pain. . . . From that we can develop the kinds of friendships that lead to lots of laughter, lots of joy, lots of sharing, and lots of growth.'[2]

I still have friends from way back, as well as some I've made recently through Pensioners' Link. My older friends are black women, like me. At Pensioners' Link there are older women and men from several other communities, and we all get on wonderfully well. We not only enjoy serious discussions and political campaigns, but we have loads of fun, too. I wish that some of my older friends could be persuaded to come along too – it's just a question of taking the plunge. [a seventy-year-old woman]

Some of my friends got together and gave me a surprise party for my seventieth birthday. They invited my children and grandchildren, a few people I hadn't seen for years (I don't know how they rustled them up), some of my neighbours, too. We had a wonderful time – lovely food and drink; someone took pictures I'll treasure; and above all, everyone had a chance to mix and talk and enjoy themselves. Everyone who could lingered on, because they were having such a good time. I'd never have thought of organizing such a thing myself.

For those of us who have brought up families, being a mother was probably one of our most absorbing, time-consuming, and demanding relationships. We become parents in part because of our own needs to bond with others and to find fulfilment and meaning. Yet once our children are grown up and leave home, we must accept the fact that the daily caregiving part of mothering is done and trust our children to take care of themselves, while we go on to take care of ourselves.

When we have meaningful work and other relationships outside the home – plans and goals to look forward to and other anchors for our identity and self-esteem – it becomes easier to let children go and to relish the freedom and opportunity of the next stage.[3] If we turn the concern and energy that we had directed toward our children toward meeting new possibilities, we can be happy and positive about the future, and as a bonus we give our children an optimistic view of growing older.

For some of us, the end of the caregiving years of mothering can present as much of a challenge and be as emotionally demanding as becoming a parent for the first time.[4] Some of us have to work at relinquishing control over our children's choices and giving up the dailiness of the relationship with them.

The way I get on with my kids is to realize that their lives are theirs and mine is mine. So I've learned to leave them alone to make their own decisions. When I was having trouble letting go of my youngest, my oldest daughter helped me. I now let them live their own lives. Actually, that's been my philosophy all along. I felt I had to prepare them to be on their own and make their own way. So I can't cry when they finally get to the point of doing what I had planned for them all along, can I? [a sixty-eight-year-old woman]

I really missed my children when they moved away but you have to 'divorce' your children. One way I got over longing for my children was to think about the relationship I had with my mother when I was my children's age. I, too, had wanted freedom and control over my own life. Back then I didn't want to be with my mother all the time. I had my own friends. When I finally recognized this, the longing disappeared and I didn't worry any more. It's an act of love to want your children to live their own lives. [a sixty-five-year-old woman]

Others of us look forward to the time our parenting obligations will be fulfilled.

I had a lot of worries when my daughter was growing up in the 1960s. Like so many others, she was a school dropout and it was very difficult to stand by and see her apparently wasting her talents and abilities. But I hung on, and of course the storms passed, and she's made a good career for herself and I'm now a very happy grandmother. We help each other out in lots of ways, but we don't live in each other's pockets. I enjoy the independence, and she does, too. [a woman in her sixties]

Having children return home or make new demands for support and nurturing after they have left home and been on their own is a prevalent concern of middle-aged women today. Though we may now feel ready to begin a new life of our own, there is always the possibility that we may be called upon to share our resources once more.

My son's marriage broke up and he's come back home to live, bringing his two young children with him. I'd been really looking forward to having some time of my own on my own. But he needs someone to care for the children, and unless and until he can find someone else to do this, and somewhere to live that he can afford, I feel I'm stuck. The children are lovely and we all get on very well, but there are times when I feel a bit resentful that people depend on me so much. [A sixty-five-year-old woman]

Some parents find it possible to live with adult children, and sometimes grandchildren, but the transition from the mother/child relationship to one of independent and mutually respectful adults is a very difficult one, and may not be possible for everyone. It requires willingness to compromise, clarity about individual as well as family goals and values, and the weathering of crises. It is also easier if housing is adequate (see Chapter 12).

At the other extreme, some adolescent and adult children may want to put the maximum possible distance between themselves and their parent(s). It is natural to grieve if your child does not wish to see you or be close. Don't add to your feelings of rejection and loss by perceiving this situation as a personal failure, however. Try to remain warm, understanding, and open to communication while keeping busy with your own life. Chances are that once your child feels more secure in her or his independence, she or he will once again want to be in touch with you. There is little you can do but accept the fact that your child, for whatever reasons, does not want to be close for the time being. Sometimes the closer we have been to a child, the more extreme is the need for separation.

I decided that if my daughter did not want to communicate with me, I would respect her wishes; that in doing so, she would learn that I am indeed a separate person and might become curious about this person who is separate, who respects her, and who is no longer 'available mother'. And that this separation would help me grow as well as help her grow. [a fifty-three-year-old woman]

Barring serious financial, emotional, or health problems, the parent-child relationship, which was based on dependency, should now be based on mutuality: mutual recognition of each other as separate personalities, mutual respect, and mutual helping.

There may be times when a mother finds herself in need of help from her children. Many women are particularly reluctant to accept help from children even when freely offered.

My son is a doctor but it took me a long time to recognize his skills. I continued to think of him as my little Johnny – messy, awkward, and uncertain. Then some of my friends became his patients and were constantly praising him. I began to see him in a different way, began to ask him questions about my health and to seek his advice. Now I go to one of the doctors in his health centre, and my son takes care of me by consulting with my doctor. [a sixty-eight-year-old woman]

My daughter is always buying me something, even if I need it like a hole in the head. She wants me to look good. She always notices if I don't wear it. My daughter wants to give me something. She wants to take care of me. I think she would like it better if I were more dependent. [a sixty-eight-year-old woman]

Though it is hard for us to give up our role as the helping or caring person within the family, it may help to think of receiving help as part of the mutual exchange of family caring.

I really don't like being dependent on my children, but what can I do? I have to face reality. I'm sure they know that for many years they were dependent on me. I really tried hard to help them, protect them, give them a good education. I suppose it's my time to receive help from them. [a woman in her seventies]

When I was between jobs, my son emptied out his bank account and sent it to me for my birthday. He wrote, 'This is for you to use as an interest-free loan. You'll pay me back when you are able to.' I hadn't asked for help, but somehow he got the idea. It made me feel that all that nurturing and caring had made an impression. [a fifty-nine-year-old woman]

Becoming a Mother-in-Law

Mothers-in-law have been the target of jokes and derision. These woman-hating barbs reflect the low regard in which older women are held in our society. The conventional rivalry between a woman and her daughter-in-law, supposedly competitors for the attention of the man, epitomizes the very essence of the generation barrier between women that this book seeks to change.

It is eye-opening to look at the two roles of grandmother and mother-in-law together. It is evident how little the stereotypes conform to reality. After all, the sweet, loving, gentle soul that a grandmother is supposed to be and the critical, interfering busybody that is the caricature of a mother-in-law are often the same woman.

Mothers-in-law have traditionally been advised to 'mind their own business'. This can be in practice a very difficult prescription, because for so many years, your child *was* your business. Yet once your child is grown up, and certainly once she or he is in a serious relationship, you are not expected to offer help unless it is requested, or advice unless it is sought. The in-law relationship is one in which we have no choice at all. Perhaps that is part of its difficulty. Whether we like our son- or daughter-in-law, his or her parents, and the other in-law relatives is almost a matter of chance. We must suspend judgment and simply accept the mate that our child has chosen. This is a way to show love and respect for your child.

It is difficult to see your child make a choice that you disapprove of or consider harmful. It is particularly hard if the choice means that your child will live far away from you, either geographically or emotionally, by choosing a lifestyle which is very different from yours.

The best part of our trip to Australia was getting to know our son-in-law. He and I took long walks on the beach, had breakfast together, and visited with his mother, who told me all about him as a young boy. When he took us sailing for a week, his skills and interest were apparent.

There had been problems between us before, but I approached this trip with a positive attitude. I travelled 6,000 miles to discover that my son-in-law was very lovable. I should have known, since my daughter had been telling me so for years. [a woman in her sixties]

You have had some twenty or more years to transmit your values to your child. The entire family relationship will be strengthened if you can trust that your child has absorbed those values. It would probably help both of you to let your child know that you still love her or him and want to maintain a caring relationship, whether you approve of the chosen partner or not. Resist the temptation to say 'I told you so' if their relationship does not work out. Your child and maybe even the former partner may need your continued support. They will feel freer to turn to you if they have not been made to feel defensive.

As if being a mother-in-law were not difficult enough in itself, many of us now have the additional confusion of being a 'something-or-other' to our child's live-in lover. Perhaps a new title would change the whole view of this difficult relationship. Perhaps, just as we talk of love relationships and love children, we should also speak of mothers-in-love.

In traditional cultures, the roles and obligations of the parents of an engaged or married couple are formally defined. Today, however, it may take time to recognize a relationship as serious and lasting. Without guidelines to tell us what our role is during the courtship's progression, we may feel at a loss in determining where we fit in the couple's life.

I did find it difficult at first to accept my son's girlfriend. I still don't know why, although they live together and she's pregnant, they've decided against marriage. Her mother has been pressuring them to 'do the right thing' and of course it's alienated them from her. I just have to accept that that's the way they've decided to live, and there's nothing I can do about it. If they're happy, that's the important thing. I wouldn't do anything to cause a break between them and me. [a fifty-five-year-old woman]

Some of us who considered ourselves open-minded and 'modern' have surprised our children and even ourselves by being upset over the non-traditional and unexpected choices our grown-up children may make. We may discover that we unconsciously harboured a fantasy of a partner from a similar religious or cultural background, reflecting a wish to have our children carry on our family traditions into the future. If this happens, or if our children choose not to marry and have children at all, or simply delay these choices,[5] we may find ourselves feeling anxious, guilty, and wondering what we have done wrong.

The issue of children who delay having children or choose not to have them may be a major part of the dilemma for parents of those who choose a partner of the same sex. This can be a problem even for parents who *can* accept their child's sexual preference. There are also many other issues that come up for parents of a gay or lesbian child. Parents' Enquiry (see Organizations) offers help and support to parents of gay and lesbian teenagers and adults.

Our favourite in-law is our daughter's woman friend. They have lived together happily for over four years, and are an important part of all family gatherings. I have found this new member of our family particularly sensitive to both the joys and sorrows in my life. I feel most comfortable to just drop in on them and to share the experiences of their life – but also, to know they want to share my feelings, too. [a sixty-two-year-old woman]

Becoming a Grandmother

One cannot deny the pleasurable feeling of self-renewal that is experienced by grandparents. To see a new generation coming, perhaps carrying on our features, talents, or idiosyncrasies, is most fascinating.

Being a grandmother is one of the great experiences of life, especially today, when we don't take the miracle for granted. There is no question that having a grandchild come to visit is demanding physically, mentally, and emotionally, especially when the grandmother is also working. Our three-year-old granddaughter has just left after a four-week visit. As the wildflowers in the juice glass fade, I try to decide which of the twenty-one crayon and watercolour pictures to keep taped to the banister. I rescue a 1950 miniature trailer truck her father used to play with from under the bed and hear her say proudly, 'I'm bigging!' I see the world anew through her eyes and hope I'm still bigging too. [a woman in her seventies]

Some women look forward to having a less stressful relationship with their grandchildren than they did with their children, especially if they were too busy or too unsure of themselves to have fully enjoyed the early years of their children. Women whose economic conditions have improved over the years may take special pleasure in indulging their grandchildren in ways that they

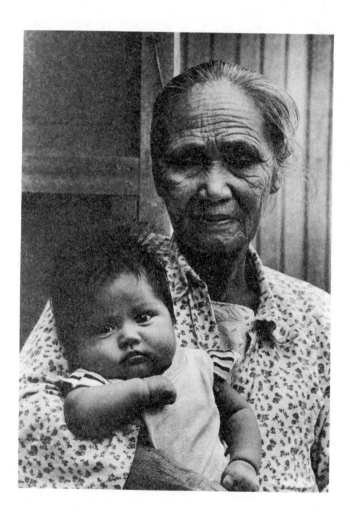

were not able to with their own children. Unfortunately, this can become a source of friction, so be sure to discuss treats and presents with your own child in advance.

A new stage in the mother-in-law relationship often follows the birth or adoption of our first grandchild. At that time we become more like colleagues or peers to our daughters or daughters-in-law, and can relate to each other as one mother to another. While we may be able to be closer to them than we were in the earlier honeymoon-couple/in-law phase, it is important to continue to respect the autonomy of our adult children, as well as their authority as parents.

In our culture, which is still too much in the grips of the adoration of youth, becoming a grandmother often bears a stigma for a still-youthful woman.

When my daughter rang me to tell me I was now a grandmother, I was not in the least elated. I had recently remarried and was seeing myself as a young, passionate lover. I didn't want to think of myself as a grandmother. That was because of the picture I had of my own grandmother – a fussy, domineering, and strict woman who took care of us when my mother worked. I think when my daughter first informed me of the birth of my grandchild I felt I couldn't fulfil the role expected of me. And I didn't want to. I finally made my own decision about our relationship but sometimes I feel guilty that I'm not a good enough grandmother. [a woman in her fifties]

Today's grandmothers want to define for themselves the specific relationship they have with their grandchildren. Few grandmothers want to baby-sit regularly or be responsible for child care. Most women resist the stereotype of the 'doormat' grandmother, always there when anyone needs her.

I have an unwritten understanding with my children: I do not baby-sit my grandchildren. I entertain them. I invite them. I think baby-sitting damages the relationship. They know when I'm with them I'm there because I want to be and because I enjoy their company. And I invite them on that basis too. I don't want to be considered a baby-sitter because that's not the relationship I want to establish with my grandchildren. [a seventy-four-year-old woman]

Some women, however, view grandchildren differently.

I'm going to do my first stint of grandchild care for my nine-month-old grandchild this summer. My daughter is signed up for a four-day course. I really love children and I think it will be fun. I'm looking forward to it. I'm a little narked that her husband isn't doing it, but I'm really staying out of that. And it's nice to do something concrete for my oldest daughter. She's just consistently very giving and thoughtful. [a fifty-year-old woman]

Some women care for grandchildren because of the illness, incapacity, or death of the child's parents. Often when we do this we have many mixed feelings and need support. Other grandparents experience anguish at losing contact with their grandchildren after the parents have been divorced or separated. It is important to realize that such things happen and to build good relationships with our children's partners. If you cannot work things out with your child's former partner, it can help to have the advice and support of an organization involved with grandparents' rights. See Organizations (The National Association of Grandparents).

Some women find it easier to ask their older grandchildren for help or companionship than they do their own children. Conversely a grandparent may offer help in a way that complements what parents can do, or that fits better with what a young person wants.

When one of my grandsons got himself into a jam with jobs during his last year at school and couldn't make it home to dinner, I invited him to come and have dinner with me. I would set my dinner hour to accommodate the time when he could make it because I thought it was unhealthy for him to be skipping meals.

I don't feel hesitant about asking them to do things that I don't have the strength to do. My sixteen-year-old grandson is very strong and if I have a piece of shrubbery I can't uproot, I phone him and ask him, and he does it. Sometimes I pay them, especially if it is a special skill that they should be paid for. My other grandson services my car and I pay him for it, but when I need someone to pick me up at the airport, he comes and meets me and picks me up and, of course, I don't pay him for that.

I have a very easy relationship with my grandchildren now. I hope that they consider me as a friend and not as an authority figure. That's what I aim for. I'm not the kind of grandmother who needs cosseting. [a seventy-four-year-old woman]

My two sets of grandchildren live at opposite ends of the country and the only time they see each other is when they come to stay with me. I think it's important that they get to know their 'extended family', and although it's a bit of a squash to fit them all into my little bungalow, the pleasure they – and I – get from these visits makes it worthwhile. [a woman of seventy-two]

Partners and Lovers

Some of us have stayed married for decades to partners who remain as dear to us as they were when we first fell in love. We can enjoy our joint achievements with no interruptions in our later years.

I am sixty-eight years old and have been married to the same man for almost forty-three years. In earlier periods we had more ups and downs, preoccupied as we were with the ambitions and pressures of work, child raising, and developing our identities as separate persons. We are more capable now of appreciating one another and have a more relaxed and confident view of ourselves and a greater sense of gratitude and contentment that we have each other. I think we have come to have a kind of pride in each other, in the kind of person we each have become.

From the beginning of our much-valued marriage, we agreed that we would each gather gifts of knowledge, skills, and a wide variety of disciplines to bring to our relationship so that it would prosper and serve as a measure of our own growth.

After forty-six years we have learned that we cannot change each other and that it is not weakness but rather strength to be willing to adapt. We have also learned that it is a myth that one member of a long-term relationship is always dominant while the other is a follower. Over the long years, we have taken turns at being leader, in both good times and bad.

Today, as we near our seventies, our daily lives are rich in shared experience and in appreciation of the many aspects of human love. We are both lucky and skilful in maintaining our sexuality as a happy resource in friendship and communication.

For many women, the demands of raising a family have meant delaying or holding back our individual aspirations. After the children are grown up, however, the husband's life outside the family often continues as before, while the wife may face a total redefinition of all her roles, even if she has been employed continuously outside the home – but especially if she has not. Most households are arranged around the personality or the employment needs of the husband and the developmental needs of the children. The changes we women go through inevitably make waves in our relationships and challenge us to rework our ways of living with our partners. Some men are flexible, secure, and caring enough to understand and accept the required adjustments, but in many relationships a period of renegotiation may be needed.

My husband didn't like it when I got a studio away from the house to do my art work, but I did it. I don't ask permission any more. When I want to go somewhere, I say, 'I'm going,' not 'Is it all right if I go?' I'm going to travel for a month by myself. That would have been inconceivable ten years ago. So this has been a long slow process of changing myself and my marriage. At first, we had a lot of fights and arguments and we started to say, 'Let's call it quits.' But somehow the love kept it going and we decided to go to a counsellor. After a while, my husband began to appreciate some of my changes. One of the nice things about ageing is that after so many years of coping you begin to see that problems aren't insurmountable. You know you've solved them before and so you can see the light at the end of the tunnel. We have finally learned to accept each other as we are. If the positives outweigh the negatives in a relationship, then it is worth saving. No relationship is a bed of roses. [a fifty-seven-year-old woman]

My husband worked on a car assembly line more than forty years. Sometimes he worked double and triple shifts during the good times. He provided well for me and our six children and all the kids went to college. We had money in the bank and looked forward to the time when he could come home and relax. We never dreamed this would cause any problems, but it did. For about a year after he retired we fussed and quarrelled. Then, even though I hadn't worked since my youngest was in nursery school, I went out and got a job as a saleswoman in a department store in town. He resented that – wanted to know who would cook and keep the house. I said, 'You can.' The biggest surprise was that he learned to cook. Every day when I come home he has dinner on the table. We have learned to enjoy each other's company and we are both happy with our new life. [a sixty-eight-year-old woman]

When partners carry out the tasks of marriage and family building as 'shoulds', putting aside their own needs for growth and development, unmet needs and resentments fill the void left by the children's departure. These may have begun to surface during the children's adolescence. Partners in long-standing marriages need to have individual and shared goals to keep themselves and the relationship vital. A challenge of midlife marriage is to develop new goals once the family-building stage is completed.

There are so many aspects to a marriage: love, children in common, mutual friends, common interests – each a thread that keeps a marriage together. Sometimes only one or two of these threads have remained unbroken, yet the partners are reluctant to separate. Often the transition of grown-up children starting a life of their own, or the sudden understanding that an unsatisfactory marriage will forever prevent us from achieving our life goals, becomes the needed push toward the dissolution of a long-standing partnership.

After twenty years of marriage my husband and I decided to divorce. We had got along badly for many years and whatever was left of our relationship was finished long before we made this decision. The one thing that was hard to give up was our group of friends. We engaged in a very active social life and actually had fun going out often in social groups. Our friends were astounded – many people called us the 'golden' couple, always happy and having fun. They never dreamed my husband was an alcoholic – though still successful in his work – and his drinking and affairs with other women corroded our family life. [a forty-five-year-old woman]

Women who initiate a divorce themselves may feel the exhilaration of a new beginning, or at least the energy of acting on long-repressed feelings. That energy can give us the courage to face the changes of marital separation.

All my life I'd played second fiddle and had seen my role as having to put up with anything he handed me. The more I submitted to him, the more violent he got. In the end I had to get out and I stayed in a Women's Aid hostel for a while. There I got a lot of help and support and after a while I was able to find a small flat and live by myself for the first time in my life – it was wonderful. Now I'm getting legal aid to sort out my divorce. I feel as if life is beginning again – at fifty-three.

My husband came home drunk night after night. The children were terrified of him. We often were so short of money by the end of the week that I had to ask my sister for help just to keep going. Then one day I asked myself 'Why am I putting up with all this? I've been telling myself that the children need a father, but what kind of a father have they got?' I knew he wouldn't change. So I made my plans carefully. My mother in the North knew my situation and had been begging me to get out and bring the children to live in her large, half-empty house. I lined up a job for myself in the town where she lives, and when everything was fixed up we simply took off. The divorce is through now; my ex-husband has simply washed his hands of us and we're all settled and happy. [a forty-three-year-old woman]

Breaking up a marriage is rarely an impulsive decision for women, and often it is preceded by years of gradual preparation. Preparation for financial self-sufficiency can be a significant step toward emotional readiness to withstand the pain of separation and the challenge of being on your own.

I did try to keep my marriage going. I went to Marriage Guidance, but my husband simply refused to come along so I really got nowhere. He just wouldn't accept that we needed help or that anything was actually wrong, despite the fact that we scarcely spoke to one another and hadn't slept together for years. The children had left home very early because of the hostile atmosphere between us. Even when I finally decided to consult a solicitor about a divorce my husband didn't really react. I realize that there's something quite wrong with him – depression or something – but you can't force a person to get help, and I just couldn't spend the rest of my life as I'd spent the last ten years. [a forty-eight-year-old woman]

When it is our partner who initiates the breakup of a marriage or a long-term relationship, the feelings of pain and rejection can be especially devastating, especially if he or she has left us for a younger lover.

I'm so bitter – I sometimes feel like totally destroying him. I gave twenty-five years to this marriage – making sacrifices, taking care of the children, taking his shit. Now he's with this girl young enough to be his daughter. I have been in therapy for a year trying to cope with it. It's helped me handle my anger. Yet I feel exploited. He took my youth, my beauty – he destroyed that. My innocence, too. I long for that sometimes. [a fifty-year-old woman]

Divorce

Divorce is having
all your teeth out one by one.
First the incisors wear down dull
as your grandfather's carving knife,
then the eye teeth go blind
lose their dogged bite.
The molars cease to grind out love
and then the judge excises
the impacted wisdom of the wedding
and you bleed and bleed.

JANE BAILEY-BLOOD STRETE

I had never allowed myself to face the possibility of divorce. I was so fearful at the thought of being on my own. I was in shock, briefly, and then I was sad, frightened, and lonely. For six months I believed I could get my husband to come back. Finally I began to accept what had happened and to look ahead to my own future.

I got my former husband to share in the care of our youngest son so I could go back to university. Then I lived with a group of older people; that created a new home for me and helped me to feel less lonely.

Today I am living on my own as a single person in a city 300 miles from my former home and building a new life. I see myself as a dependent person acting independently. I'm a risk-taker, that's what's helped me make the changes I've made. [a sixty-year-old woman]

The breakup of a marriage, however devastating it may seem, carries with it the potential for a new life. With age, we grow in maturity, experience, and confidence, qualities which have a beauty and power to attract in their own right. Best of all, these are qualities that reflect how we feel about ourselves and do not depend on the perception of others.

Widowhood or Loss of a Partner

Since women usually live longer than men and are often younger than their mates, widowhood is the experience of the majority of married women. One woman in two in the United Kingdom is a widow by the age of sixty-five, while only one man in six is a widower.[6]

My youngest son had just decided not to stay in college. I remember driving along thinking that now my husband and I could begin to plan for our old age. When I got home I got a call about my husband. He died suddenly just as I was about to turn fifty-eight. [a seventy-eight-year-old woman]

The experience of widowhood varies according to the time of life in which it occurs. If you have lived with a partner happily for four or five decades, and perhaps raised a family together, your grief may be tempered by an awareness of the good fortune you shared together. Yet, if you are in your seventies or eighties and in failing health yourself, you may have less emotional and physical energy to rebuild your life as a single woman. Women who are widowed young often are devastated by the shock and overwhelmed with the responsibility of bringing up children on their own, yet the younger you are the more likely you are eventually to recover from your grief.

Many recently widowed women report that they imagine their partner is still there and catch themselves starting to talk to him or her. They worry that they are losing their minds. However, this is not unusual behaviour in the early months of widowhood. It may seem inconceivable to many a recently widowed woman that she can ever find happiness again, or comfort, or even peace of mind by herself or with a new love. Gone is the companionship, the sexuality, the economic partnership, the intimacy of many years. Some of these pieces of the lost relationship will never be replaced; for others perhaps only a pale substitute can be found.

I think I'm still depressed. I don't think I've got over it – after twenty years I still feel his presence. When I lost my husband I cried and cried even though I had a lot of support. People would talk to me, try to reason with me – still I just wanted to die. But then always my mind would come back to 'I have three sons who still need me. I can't just die.' [a sixty-five-year-old woman]

In the last four years I have come from the depths of despair to feeling that life is good and that there still is a reason and a need for me to be in this world. At the beginning I continued to live because I felt my children had been through enough and they didn't need any more grief. It took a long time before I started to live for myself. I functioned extremely well most of the time (everyone always said how well I coped) but felt like I was just going through the motions, waiting for my husband to come home. [a woman in her fifties]

Particularly stressful is loss of a partner in a relationship that was not publicly acknowledged. If you have lost a lover and few of your friends and acquaintances knew of the relationship, you may feel quite alone with your grief, and have to carry on without the usual social supports that are mobilized for the widow. Even if you have been open about your relationship, friends may not fully appreciate the depth of your loss.

Recently I went on holiday with friends who had been friends also with my deceased partner-in-life. A guest arrived with slides of earlier holidays, including pictures of my lover.

I objected that if I had been a man who had been recently widowed, they surely would have asked if I would object to showing the pictures. One friend responded that she wanted very much to see them. She blanched when I suggested that she might feel differently after the death of her husband. Clearly, she thought that my relationship to Karen differed from her marriage; she evidently also thought my love differed from her friendship with Karen only by degree. Heterosexuals really do not understand what lesbians feel for their partners, even when they know us well. All of these friends had known Karen and me as lovers and had sent me bereavement condolences when Karen died.*

For a few women, the death of a spouse is a relief from a relationship that they may have wanted to leave earlier but for one reason or another were not able to do so. This situation can also be painful, as we grieve for the kind of relationship we might have hoped for when we first married.

For years I stayed in a marriage with an abusive husband because I was always afraid to divorce for economic reasons. After all, where was I to go and how would I be able to support myself? I did miss him for the year following his death. I never minded taking care of him while he was ill. After all, he was family. But I did resent all of the earlier years when he was so dominating and critical. Being a widow is my first freedom. I have a good relationship with my children and with my brothers and sisters. I have friends of long standing. I don't mind being alone at all. No one shouts at me . . . I do what I want. [a seventy-eight-year-old woman]

It is not uncommon for recently widowed women to continue to receive

*Excerpted from an unpublished manuscript by Carolyn Ruth Swift.

guidance from their husbands, in dreams, in daydreams, in convictions that 'this is just what he would want me to do'. Women who were accustomed to relying on a husband, who have not had a lot of experience making their own decisions, may need time to accept that the ideas they are willing to trust, the advice they consider wise, come from themselves.

I still have dreams – not as often as I did when Bill first died – that he is giving me advice on how to do things. And it is always good advice; I listen to it. If I am ever undecided about something, he seems to come in my dreams and tell me what to do. [a sixty-seven-year-old woman, five years after the death of her husband]

Once a woman experiences some of the satisfactions of doing things for herself, she may begin to realize that she has many of the abilities she formerly ascribed to her husband.

Getting more education or a better-paying job is part and parcel of this process for many widows. Yet some women are reluctant to assume their independence and to feel the possibility of being active and powerful, as if managing for themselves would be disloyal or would diminish the importance of their past relationship.

Eventually, widows must restructure their lives as single women. We appreciate old friends who continue to call, to invite us and include us in their lives, but we may be disappointed in some who maintain the Noah's Ark system in social life: couples only. These friends may simply be afraid to confront the widow's grief. By avoiding her they can deny the possibility that death could disrupt their own relationship.[7] For a fuller discussion of the emotional and practical adjustments to be faced by widowed, divorced and separated women, see *On Your Own* (listed below).

While well-meaning friends and family may tell a widow to make new friends, find new interests, and create a new life for herself, many recently widowed women may need at first to reminisce about the past relationship, relive its good moments, hold on to the sense of the continuing presence of the lost spouse. If the relationship was a deep and involving one, then a widow's new life must be made out of parts of the old, and some of these parts must now be retrieved from the ended relationship. This is a way that many widows preserve the continuity of their lives.

My children, family, and many friends have been extremely supportive. Contrary to the experiences of many widows, the friends who are couples and who were friends of my husband and myself have continued to include me in their social lives. For the first two years or so it was usually too painful and I preferred not to spend too much time with them, but they were persistent and continued to invite me. In the last several months I have felt more comfortable and it is easier and even pleasant to join them sometimes. Most of my other social life is with women friends and family. I haven't 'dated' at all but feel that if the opportunity arises I am ready to consider a new relationship. [a fifty-two-year-old woman]

Married friends, children, and relatives usually find themselves inadequate to the task of comforting a recent widow. Once the apparent emergency and the immediate needs are past, the widow is expected to pick up her own life and take care of herself. This is the time when the grieving person tends to feel most abandoned and helpless. But our lifetime habit of forming friendships and creating extended emotional 'networks' contributes, according to researchers, to women's greater ability to survive after widowhood.[8]

Only someone who has actually been through the same experience can fully appreciate and meet the continuing needs of a grieving widow. This is why various kinds of organizations of widows – both the ones that deal with practical matters such as coping with money problems and the ones that focus more on emotional issues – have been growing (see Organizations).[9] Being part of a group of women dealing with loss helps us understand that grief is appropriate and normal. In such groups we can feel freer than we do among family and friends to expose the depth of our pain and loss, knowing that we will be understood.

Being Single

Contrary to the prevailing stereotypes, a recent study of fifty single women aged from sixty-five to the mid-nineties found that those women who had never married were as embedded in relationships and social networks as women who were presently, or had been, married. For many women, the world of work was an important source of friends, but in retirement many went on to initiate new friendships with neighbours or members of organizations to which they belonged. Families were also a significant source of important relationships, especially siblings.[10]

These women understand the importance of friendship; they have had the lifelong habit of reaching out to other women and the freedom to do so. Women who have been single all their lives are probably less likely than married women to go through midlife upheavals.

Older single women we spoke to expressed satisfaction with their lives and their choices.

Single? I feel great about what I've seen and what I've passed up. I haven't missed a thing. I have a good many friends. Most of my closest friends have been married, a few single. I made matches but not for myself, even though I did have three different engagement rings which they never would take back. I eluded all attempts to marry. If I had my life to live over again I think I would marry – it's nice to have children. But being single has given me a lot of freedom to do what I want when I want. I help others solve problems, rather than have my own. My relationships have grown richer. My friends and I appreciate each other more. Many of us are still around and we've gone through a lot together. Today, we have a little more in material comfort than we started out with and we have friendships that have lasted a lifetime. [a seventy-two-year-old woman]

In generations past, marriage was the norm for women, and the main concern of their families. Not to marry was to be an outsider. Singleness was a stigma.

I come from quite a poor background. I was the only girl I knew who went to university, went on to get a teaching qualification and finally became headmistress of a famous school. You'd think my family and friends would see me more as a successful woman than as 'the one who never got married'. But I know that's what they think about me. [a forty-five-year-old woman]

Often it is only in the middle years, when the supply of potential mates is dwindling and it becomes clear that one's life-style is firmly established, that women admit to themselves that they have made a choice and that they are happy with it.[11] Some women for whom sexuality has not been a priority may have truly preferred to be celibate. Others have guarded their personal freedom by making their sexual lives, with men or with women, a small and perhaps temporary part of their lives. Whatever the reason, once the choice is recognized and accepted, it opens up new possibilities for security and comfort. Buying a house, deciding on a new geographical location, joining resources with other women in business or leisure, and providing for old age all complete the life of the single woman.

In later years, loneliness and isolation can be a serious problem for older women who have outlived their friends, spouses, or partners. If you are feeling isolated, if your neighbourhood has changed and you find you no longer know many people, senior citizens' clubs can be good places to find new activities and to meet people.

I was a bit shy about going to a Pensioners' Link meeting, but a friend insisted on taking me along. Everyone was very friendly, and in no time I found myself on a committee organizing coach trips and theatre visits. It was such a change from sitting moping in my flat. [a seventy-year-old woman]

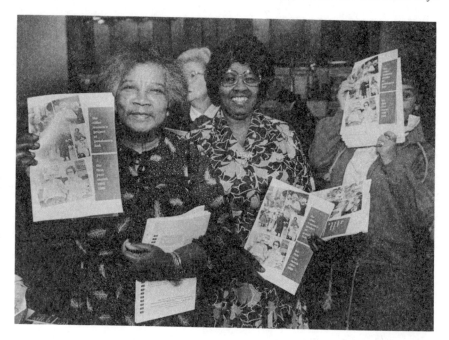

You can't just sit and wait for someone to come to you. They won't. Let's face it, old people are easy to forget, not through any fault of their own but because everyone is so busy these days. Young people don't have the time to sit around and talk. So we have to make more of an effort ourselves. I phone my family even if they don't call me. I know some people who just sit around all alone and then get fed up if nobody calls them. They've got the telephone right there and probably have more time than a lot of people to make the calls and keep in touch. [a woman in her seventies]

For women who've been divorced or widowed after a long marriage, it is not easy to begin again. Perhaps you have spent most of your adult life within a family where you had to expend little energy to maintain comfortable contact with close friends. Close association with your family and your husband's family and with friends who also socialize in couples may have met all your social needs. Now you have to become more assertive in reaching out to others.

I needed a new social life. With older couples, you begin to feel you don't belong with them any more. I looked for single people to be with because they understood my problems. After my divorce I wanted to talk about the hurt and disappointment, but my married friends didn't want to hear about it. Perhaps they didn't want to acknowledge that it could happen to them too. So we grew apart.

I had a girlfriend who was a widow. She said, 'You can't just sit at home.' We Latin people love to dance and go to parties, so she took me to a party at her church for widowed people. When I protested that I was not a widow, she said, 'Who cares?' At first, it was a mixed group of mostly widowed people. Recently, more divorced people have joined the group. [a sixty-year-old woman]

New Partners

Many women are eager to find a new partner, if not immediately after their marriages end, certainly at some point thereafter. This is when the insecurities of ageing, of changing values, and of confused expectations come into play. It is perhaps useful to consider that we are not starting over from the beginning, but from where we are right now. The search for love, companionship, and new friendships may take us down some roads we never thought we'd take. Many women try new activities such as amateur theatre, adult education, or political-action groups that suit their talents, interests, and time schedules. Although it's a bit like entering a sweepstake (the odds for finding true love may not be so good), the fun of new activities and sometimes curiosity about who is 'out there' can be very energizing. Consider reaching out beyond your usual circle. You may find new friends who are appropriate to the new person you are in process of becoming.

I want someone like myself, with some education, but not so clever that I would bore him, someone I could get along with. I almost married again. I met someone who took the time to get to know me. I was unhappy and he lifted me out of my unhappiness. He made me feel that I deserved love and respect when I had been feeling that I was 'finished' in my forties, an old bag. I was afraid that I would end up living in a bedsitter or having to move in with one of my kids, so I was going to marry him. But he was old-fashioned. He wanted to do things a way that I used to like, but that I don't want any more. He didn't want me to work after we were married or to own my own house. We couldn't seem to agree on anything so the relationship fizzled out. But he did me the big favour of making me feel valuable, that I was a mature, beautiful woman, even though I was no longer young. [a fifty-nine-year-old woman]

Some women find someone they care about enough to risk a second marriage. Remarriage can be challenging, yet experience and maturity can make it an easier adjustment than it was the first time.

My present husband is more supportive and less critical than my first husband. We're very different and that makes this marriage astonishing and full of surprises. If we'd married young the differences between us would have overwhelmed us. In middle age the differences are sort of a lark – they're intriguing. Here's this person who has to watch football. In my twenties I would have felt quite critical because I would have thought it reflected on me and my taste in men, but when you're fully formed in your middle years it doesn't bother you. Instead the differences between you keep the relationship surprising and fresh. [a fifty-seven-year-old woman]

LESBIAN PARTNERSHIPS

Over the years, some women who were thought to be single have in fact been in discreet lifelong relationships with other women, which for reasons of public opinion had to be kept secret. Though the social strictures are less severe than formerly, many women are still understandably reluctant to make their sexual preference known. For other women, however, the relaxation of social attitudes has provided a liberating atmosphere in which to exercise new options. Some women, after years as wives and mothers, turn to a lesbian relationship and become part of a community of women. Whether our friendships with women will also include sexuality is a matter of very personal preference, but knowing that there is such a possibility can be very liberating.

I feel so lucky to have the choice in this period of women's liberation to leave behind society's negative attitude about women and instead be a woman-identified woman. How rich we are in wisdom, experience, talents, and skills! I believe we have within us the necessary balance to turn the society around and I am a part of that movement! [a woman in her fifties]

Around the age of forty, I began realizing that I was sexually attracted to women, but I continued to go out with men until I fell in love with a woman at age forty-five and began a long-term relationship. I was married for sixteen years and have two adult children. I am now in a relationship with a West Indian woman which has presented me, as a Jewish woman, with numerous challenges in terms of cultural and racial differences.

I feel that my life would be far more limiting if I were still heterosexual and erotically dependent on men. I find traditional men of my age sexist, controlling, patronizing, and unable to express emotion . . . qualities which are unattractive and boring.

Although the stigma and restrictions of homosexuality certainly affect me, I love being a lesbian. I love the companionship of women and a life-style where my relationships are primarily with women. [a woman in her fifties]

The advantage of such a 'coming out' is the existence of a ready-made supportive community which the new lesbian can enter. Yet, as the following experience shows, acceptance may take a while.

After twenty-five years as wife and mother, the label I heard when I first mingled with lesbians was that I was not a real lesbian. I didn't understand – after all, wasn't I in love with another woman? I was confused and intrigued at the same time that lesbians expected me to be strong, self-supporting, with a place out there in the world. No one was interested in the passive, unopinionated woman I had been who knew how to use her body seductively for attraction and approval. I had to learn how to be with lesbians – to develop my knowledge and creativity at a deeper level than I had ever before been challenged to do.

Now I realize that I was still acting like a privileged heterosexual princess. Even though lesbians depend emotionally on others, they are usually self-supporting. I had never been trained to be that and I still expected, on some level, that someone would take care of me. I am grateful for the lesbian community's higher expectations. I have discovered a lot of inner strength and know now that I can be financially, emotionally, and mentally self-supporting, and that is freedom! [a fifty-four-year-old woman]

There are, of course, risks in changing sexual orientation. Those who are close and dear to us may find the change too drastic and withdraw, or refuse to accept our newfound selves, friends, or lovers.

Sadly, I've met quite a few family problems. Christmas is one of them. My son and his wife usually invite me. Last year they did, as usual, but didn't include Sandra. I said I wanted her to come too, but they wouldn't have it. I think they couldn't face up to the situation as it really is. They don't see her as 'family' or even as they would if I had a male partner. So of course I didn't go. I'm very sorry about it, because it's meant I'm cut off from my grandchildren as long as their parents won't recognize Sandra's existence. [a woman in her fifties]

I remember the morning I greeted my friend of twenty years with the usual hug and kiss, then sat her down to tell her I had become a lesbian. She listened as we talked for hours, and told me she didn't understand at all, but would remain my friend. When she got up to go, and I approached her for a goodbye hug, she put out her hand at arm's length and said, 'I cannot hug you anymore.' That really hurt. [a fifty-four-year-old woman]

If we come from a social world where women and men mingle, we may long for the comfort and security of social acceptance. We may be fortunate in carrying some friends over from former days, but they, too, now lack our experience. Realizing that we may lose old friends both compels and enables us to embrace a concept of 'family' which includes a larger community. Maintaining relationships is an important value of the lesbian community and women who formerly were lovers often remain close and supportive friends.

The lesbian community that we see at women's dances, at concerts, in bars, often seems to have found the key to eternal youth. Already disoriented in many ways, an older woman new to lesbian life may miss the companionship of women her own age. In some large cities, organizations specifically for older lesbians (and gay men) can help you meet other women your age. It is important to find a balance between former friends and new friends who are lesbians, even if you find yourself among women your daughter's age. Changing your sexual preference can make you feel insecure for a while, and you will need other lesbians for support. It is a rare old friend who can talk with you about your new self-discovery without questioning your choice or feeling threatened by it.

As lesbians, we have sharpened our wits and shaped our viewpoints on discrimination and the struggle for survival. We are drawn, as are many women, to the fight for women's rights over our bodies, for our rights not to be abused sexually, emotionally, or physically, for the restoration of health to the earth, for peace and a decent standard of living all over the world, and for the rights of those of our loved ones most vulnerable: children and the frail elderly. For some of us the work is never done as long as we feel the pinch of discrimination in our own lives. [a fifty-six-year-old woman]

Living in a Community

It is important for women at any age to overcome the notion that we are somehow incomplete if we are not married or involved in a long-standing sexual relationship. The middle and later years can be a time to achieve a balance between companionship and solitude. It can help to stop thinking of our unpartnered state as aloneness, and to think of ourselves instead as moving into a life community. We have many choices to make in this new way of life. How big a community feels comfortable, and whom do you want to include in it? Do you want to consider a group-living situation? Do you want to see friends more often? Think about what you like to do and which of your friends would enjoy sharing that activity with you. Reaching out to other women in similar circumstances to yours can be a good source of new friendships. Women's and senior citizens' organizations, community activist groups, adult education classes, and exercise and recreational activities are just a few of the many ways to meet new friends.

If you find yourself excited about a new creative pursuit or political agenda, you may find as you join groups or classes that you meet new people who share your passion, a wonderful basis for new friendships. We are never too old to begin new friendships.

NOTES

[1]Heading borrowed from a book of the same title by Karen Lindsey, Boston: Beacon Press, 1981.

[2]Freda Rebelsky, 'Friends: Who Needs Them? Part II', a lecture reprinted in *The Community Church News*, 565 Boylston St, Boston, MA 02116, November 1986.

[3]Lillian B. Rubin, *Women of a Certain Age: The Midlife Search for Self*. New York: Harper & Row, 1979.

[4]Zenith Henkin Gross, *And You Thought It Was Over: Mothers and Their Adult Children*. New York: St Martin's Press, 1985.

[5]Susan Christian, 'Grandparent Anxiety'. *Modern Maturity*, December 1983–January 1984, pp. 32–5.

[6]Figures from Cruse (see Organizations).

[7]Phyllis R. Silverman, *Helping Women Cope with Grief*. Beverly Hills, Cal.: Sage Publications, 1981.

[8]Knud Helsing, Moyses Szklo and George W. Comstock, 'Factors Associated with Mortality After Widowhood'. *American Journal of Public Health*, Vol. 71, 1981, pp. 802–9.

[9]Phyllis R. Silverman, *Widow to Widow*. New York: Springer, 1985; and Silverman, op. cit.

[10]Barbara Levy Simon, *Never Married Women*. Philadelphia: Temple University Press, 1987.

[11]Nancy L. Peterson, *The Ever-Single Woman: Life Without Marriage*. New York: Morrow, 1982.

BOOKS AND PUBLICATIONS

Jean Shapiro, *On Your Own: A Practical Guide to Independent Living*. London: Pandora Press, 1985.

Consumers Association, *Divorce: Legal Procedures and Financial Facts*.

Maggie Scarf, *Intimate Partners: Patterns in Love and Marriage*. London: Century Publishing Co. Ltd, 1988.

Robert Morley, *Intimate Strangers*. London: Family Welfare Association, 1984.

Relate (the National Marriage Guidance Council), *Marriage Guidance*. Quarterly journal.

Ellen Malos (ed.), *The Politics of Housework*. New York: Schocken, 1980. This anthology includes the groundbreaking article of that same title by Pat Mainardi.

12
Housing Alternatives and Living Arrangements

For many women their home has been the centre of their lives. Even those whose chief interests have been focused on outside activities and work have felt the need for the secure base that satisfactory housing provides – and this need often increases as we age. If our present living conditions are good, we may be loath to consider a change; if they're poor or below standard, the time may have come when we're in a position to move to something better.

In this chapter we'll be considering the options, but, because the subject is a vast one and detailed information on every aspect is available elsewhere, the aim will be to steer readers in the direction of that detailed help.

Staying Put

Those who have been forced to move house several times already will know how stressful, time-consuming and costly it can be.

'Never again' is how I felt after all the hassles of our move ten years ago. But the children have left home now and we're rattling around in our big house. We really ought to move to something smaller before we're too old to cope with another change. [a fifty-seven-year-old woman]

There are advantages in staying where you are. If you are able to accommodate your children and their families and your friends on visits now, consider what would happen if you moved to a smaller house or flat. Moving is expensive, too, and any advantage gained by settling for a smaller place may be offset by the agents' fees, legal charges, movers' charges, new furnishings, etc., involved. If you are in rented accommodation there will still be a number of inescapable expenses. Location is important, too. As we get older, a familiar neighbourhood and old friends matter more to us.

I thought a move to a country cottage we'd seen on holiday would be wonderful. We hadn't reckoned with the isolation in winter, the difficulty in making contact with neighbours, and the great distance from the nearest hospital. The cottage certainly is lovely, but I still hanker for my suburban house, so near to the shops and entertainments and the many friends we left behind. [a woman in her sixties]

Even if you are not starry-eyed about a move to the country, the seaside, or an area where house prices or rents are lower, a reduced income in retirement or redundancy may force you to consider moving. But before taking drastic action, look at the options that may be available to you to enable you to stay where you are. These are outlined in *Using Your Home as Capital* from Age Concern (see below) and a free Age Concern leaflet (No. 12) *Raising an Income from Your Home*.[1] Both these publications do make the point, however, that it's essential to seek legal and financial advice about any particular scheme involving 'home income plans' and 'home reversion schemes', because there can be problems which you should fully understand before committing yourself. Age Concern issues a special warning for those who are receiving means-tested social security benefit such as income support or housing benefit, because the weekly income from a home income plan can affect entitlement, and you could lose some or all of your benefit.

Rather than move I decided to take in a lodger. I didn't want to make it impossible to have my grandson to stay in the school holidays, so I approached the local Polytechnic's Accommodation Officer and she fixed me up with a student who's only there during term-time. Since then I've had a succession of young women students, and we've mostly got on very well together. Even if there are problems, you only commit yourself for a year – and if they were really bad, the Accommodation office would sort things out. [a fifty-eight-year-old woman]

Many older people find that maintaining their house or flat in good condition is an impossible burden.

I could manage to look after the house but after my husband died the garden was far too much for me. Through an ad in the local paper I found an elderly man who loved gardening but lives in a flat. He comes in regularly and grows his own vegetables in my garden and keeps the rest under control. This keeps us both happy. [a seventy-year-old woman]

Financial help *may* be available – though 'cuts' in the 1980s have drastically curtailed the help formerly given by local authorities. Age Concern's leaflet No. 13, *Elderly Home Owners – Sources of Financial Help With Repairs* (free, see below), outlines possible ways of getting help for improvements and repairs, including a 'maturity' loan from a building society, and the special housing agency services available in some parts of the country which will help you find sources of funding.

Housing Benefit

The statutory scheme which provides help with rent and rates is called Housing Benefit. There were drastic changes to this scheme and to the supplementary benefit scheme (now called 'Income Support') in April 1988. Both these schemes involve a form of means-testing in which income and savings are assessed. People with capital under £8,000 (1988 figures) are eligible for housing benefit. Entitlement may be difficult to work out, but Age Concern leaflet No. 17, *Housing Benefit*, and No. 16, *Income Support and Housing Benefit: Income and Savings/Capital*, should help. All Age Concern leaflets are updated if regulations change.

When the 'poll tax' replaces the rating scheme in 1990 (earlier in Scotland) people may find themselves at a disadvantage in some areas, while in others residents may pay less than under the old method. See local newspapers for the way in which you will be affected. It is intended that everyone shall be liable for at least 20 per cent of the tax, which may mean that those not paying rates before 1990 will then be liable.

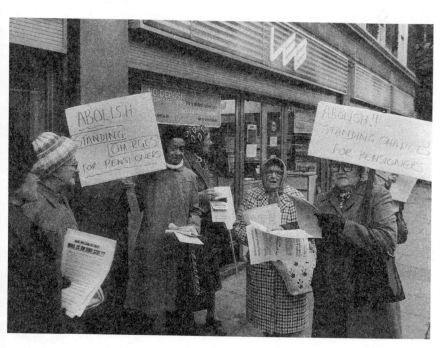

THE 1988 HOUSING ACT

As part of its overall drive towards privatization, the government has introduced a number of 'reforms' affecting the rights of people who *rent* their accommodation – whether from the local authority, a housing association or a private landlord. This Act is only part of the plan – to follow will be a Housing and Local Government Bill, which will prevent local councils subsidizing their tenants' rents from the rates. As the housing campaign group Shelter says, the idea must be to force rents up so high than council tenants will 'think twice before voting to stay with the council, under the Change of Landlord proposals in this (1988) Act, or under voluntary transfer initiatives'.

Since January 1989 landlords have been able to let on the basis of so-called *assured* tenure, and the related *assured shorthold* tenure (both limiting protection against rent increases and possible eviction). The legislation applies to new tenancies: landlords in general won't be able legally to tamper with the protection offered under the 1977 Rent Act to those who were tenants before 15 January 1989. However, Shelter believes that these existing tenants will be much more vulnerable to harassment and threats of illegal eviction, and that it will become extremely difficult for those in rented housing to move to a new area in search of a job since they would find greatly increased rents operative once they left their 'protected' dwelling.

The Act can affect anyone not owning her own home, and essential reading for anyone in this position is *The Housing Act 1988*, a Shelter Guide, price £2.50 from Shelter (see Organizations). If you can't afford to buy it, ask for it in your public library reference section or Citizens' Advice Bureau. Shelter publications keep abreast of all new legislation affecting housing and attempt to explain in simple terms what amount to extremely complicated legal enactments.

Living Alone Versus Living with Others

One important decision to make is whether you want to live alone or with others. For some of us, the thought of having to accommodate the timetables, moods, habits, and needs of others may be a deterrent to shared housing. This may be especially true if we have often done that in the past – for parents, partners, roommates, spouses, and children.

I like living alone. It's peaceful. There's nobody to boss me around. The hardest time for me was when my husband first went to the hospital. We were married thirty-three years and did everything together. Work, too. He was a fine carpenter and we had an antiques business. His doctor told me I couldn't live alone, but I told him since I was a little girl someone has always told me what to do. Then, after my husband died, I was almost crazy, but I got hold of myself, and I mended a rocking chair that was in such bad condition that he had said he'd never fix it. Well, I did – and I sold it for £35.00! So I found out I could get along alone. And that was twenty years ago and I'm still at it. At seventy-six, I work as much as I want to, and I do get out and see people – but only when I feel like it. I even helped fix my own roof last summer!

I like quiet – I don't like silence, there is a difference – and depending on how I am feeling, I may have the radio or telly on even if I am not paying attention, because it is too silent otherwise. In talking with others, I gather that this is not at all unusual. I do miss sharing a home with someone and yet I must say that I also really like the fact that I have a wonderful home which I have put together by myself. I like being able to do what I want when I want. [a woman in her fifties]

People are always asking me why I don't have a telephone. Well, I don't need one! I have so many friends here, and I can always walk down the road and use my neighbour's phone if I have to. And besides – I still ride my bicycle whenever I want. One of my friends and I cook dinner together almost every night, either at her house or mine. And sometimes we go out to eat. I'm a very lucky person! [a seventy-seven-year-old woman]

Still, many of us find that no matter how active we are, how full our social or professional lives, living alone can be painful.

In spite of supportive children and a large circle of friends, I really don't like the idea that I may be living alone for the rest of my life. I even tried having a dog, but the disadvantages and limits to my freedom outweighed the joy of having her there to greet me as I opened my door. She is now romping happily on a farm, while I am often lonely and wondering what's next for me. [a woman in her fifties]

One of the reasons I opt for shared living in some form is that it can provide a balance which most of us need: privacy along with an opportunity for informal companionship. I even like the adjustments I have to make when my pattern comes in conflict with others. There is great satisfaction in learning to agree and work together in running our joint enterprise. I've found that a sense of being at home is a realizable goal. It may be greatly different from the home we grew up in or that we had when we were on our own, but it can have as much validity as those other homes. [a woman in her seventies]

Sharing a Home

We've already seen how one woman increased her income sufficiently by taking in students to enable her to stay in her own home. Another way of sharing expenses is to invite someone to move in with you, or to move in with her, or find somewhere together.

When my marriage broke up, the relationship of an old friend of mine also came to an end when the man she had been living with for eight years battered her. We decided to buy a flat together since neither of us had enough money to do so independently, and rent for a two-bedroom flat was too expensive. After much argument we managed to convince a building society to give us a 100 per cent mortgage – the society apparently felt two women were a bigger risk than a married couple! – but even so all we could afford was an East London maisonette requiring a lot of work. The roof leaked so badly that part of the hall ceiling eventually fell in; there was dry rot throughout and every room had virtually to be gutted. Neither of us had ever done DIY before, but we got stuck in. The builder did the structural work, we did the rest, including the plastering! Sometimes it was a desperately hard slog at nights and weekends, but both of us, for the first time in years, felt in control and ultimately became pretty competent – to the builder's astonishment. He'd never seen women plaster walls! It has taken six years to create a beautiful, comfortable environment which we're both very proud of and enjoy sharing. Initially we had thought we'd sell the flat when it was done up and try to buy separate flats with the profits. But now we find our living arrangements too congenial to change. My friend has established a loving relationship with a man thirteen years younger than she is, and I, too, enjoy a caring, if less involved, relationship with another man. Numerous friends come and marvel at our 'accomplishments' and we find ourselves giving advice on how to sand or plaster to our male, as well as female, friends. Given the security of our home life, we've both managed to reconstruct/find challenging and, to a degree, rewarding jobs. [a forty-two-year-old woman]

As we get older, some of us become 'set in our ways' and find it very difficult to adapt to another person's life-style, however much we may like this individual as a person. The same applies when an older woman thinks of moving to live with relatives. However, it's always wise to avoid selling a house or flat if possible – best to try out the new arrangement before committing yourself.

My friend Betty and I were widowed around the same time. We each had a house that was too big for us alone, so we decided to sell Betty's house and she would move into mine. I'm sorry to say that it didn't work. Betty felt all the time that although she was paying her share, and in fact we'd been careful to work out the finances beforehand, she was in my house and couldn't feel free to do things the way she wanted. She kept deferring to me and that made me feel guilty and uncomfortable because I knew she really resented it. In the end we had to decide to split up, and the awful thing was that because house prices had risen in the two years she'd been in my house, she couldn't afford to buy a decent place of her own. We're still picking up the pieces – I've had to help her out with money, which has made things difficult for me. I'd never have believed we could have got into such a mess. [a woman in her sixties]

What Makes Shared Living Work

The most important factor in the success of shared living arrangements is the willingness of all parties to change and compromise.

Living involves changes. Shared living is no exception. I have seen many changes both in situations and in the people who have shared them. I like it that way. Static living can be a bore. [a seventy-eight-year-old woman]

Another factor is respect and consideration of the desires, responsibilities, and needs of each person involved. Does one housemate have a child who is away at school but still living at home during part of the year? Or does one invite grandchildren for school holidays? Do any of you have frail or elderly relatives who may need temporary care? How will your prospective house-mate(s) react to a short visit from a friend or lover (old or new), or an extended visit by an adult daughter or son who returns to the nest after a broken relationship or a lost job? Though no one can foresee the future, such issues should be clarified as much as possible before, not after, people decide to share a home.

If you are thinking of sharing a home with your parents or adult children, you should ask yourself some hard questions. Can you co-exist as adults, or are there still unresolved power struggles between you? Are you – or they – flexible enough to adapt to new dynamics, new roles? As with any other group living situation, mutually agreed upon ground rules and periodic re-evaluation will help establish an equitable distribution of responsibilities and resources.

Such 'extended family' arrangements are more common among those ethnic groups whose traditions are far removed from the current British perception of single-family living that makes the enforced sharing of the home with two or more generations unacceptable to many families. Housing shortages, high rents and the huge increases in house prices and mortgages have forced many of us to share cramped accommodation with our adult children or other relatives while they wait – sometimes in vain – to move to somewhere of their own. The resulting tensions can be difficult to resolve, partly because we do have these fixed ideas that everyone should expect to be able to move away from parents once she's an adult, or at any rate when she forms a relationship – but largely because our small houses and flats aren't suited to the numbers of people involved. Perhaps we need to re-think, not only introducing practical ways in which this relative overcrowding can become more bearable, but seeing some of the positive advantages we could enjoy in terms of companionship, mutual help and closeness.

My Asian friends don't understand my attitude, and I'm beginning to change. When my daughter got married I was dismayed that the young couple had to move in with us. But the lady next door positively revels in the presence of her daughter, her son-in-law and baby grandchild who are sharing the home. The two women are at home all day and share everything – cooking, baby-care, shopping. I can see it makes life much easier. [a woman in her fifties]

SELECTING A HOUSEMATE

How we go about finding someone to live with can vary with our individual circumstances. Some of us are lucky enough to have a close friend or relative with whom we can share a home.

My daughter insisted that I come and live with her when my husband left me. We gave it a lot of thought and I said I would, provided I could sell my flat and pay for some alterations to be made to her house so that my two rooms would be self-contained. We also set up some ground rules about baby-sitting, helping each other out in various ways, maintaining both contact and privacy and so on. Everyone, myself included, was rather apprehensive – but it's worked. We only break the 'privacy' rule when someone is ill, and then the support we give each other is wonderful. It would be much more difficult if we lived at a distance. [a woman in her fifties]

Or we may start out with a temporary arrangement and find it so successful it becomes permanent.

I met a teacher at the institution where I did volunteer work who was urgently looking for a flat. She moved in temporarily with my father and me. She was helpful in doing things for my father that I didn't have time for, such as watching football with him or taking him for a ride. I in turn would get the meals. After my father died we just kept living together. For twenty years my housemate and I have had very separate but compatible lives. Financially she is better off than I am. It would be difficult for me to live alone on my shrinking pension. We still split everything right down the middle, except that she always had a car and I had household furnishings. I eat at home and entertain more than she and we often don't have lunch or dinner together, but we split everything. I became a 'member' of her family, an adopted sister. When I have been hesitant to spend my more limited money, she will say 'I think you should do it' and will provide the funds.

Whatever happens, happens, but after twenty years of being sharers, I would expect us to stay together. In my will I leave everything to her. [a seventy-two-year-old woman]

If there is no one in your circle who is interested in shared living and if you have never advertised for a housemate before, you may want to get some help. In addition to informal or private arrangements, specific home-sharing options may exist in your area. Check with women's centres, social-service agencies and pensioner centres. Check also with your church, synagogue, YWCA, or other community agency or university or college housing offices. If you think you will have difficulty choosing, checking references or saying no to someone, a social worker or some other neutral third party can serve as a mediator. This will give you time and support as you decide upon this important step.

Getting a Mortgage

If you are near to or past retirement age, there may be some difficulty in securing a mortgage if you decide to buy a house or flat, and you are unlikely to be able to repay the loan plus interest over such a long period as twenty-five years, which is the more common period offered to younger people. This may mean that your monthly repayments could be rather high. Don't forget, too, that they may fluctuate as interest rates change, as they have done frequently in recent years.

Shop around – high street building societies and banks are the most common sources of loans, but it is sometimes possible to get a loan from a private source through a solicitor. All the major building societies and banks issue leaflets describing their terms.

In the event that you have some difficulty in securing a mortgage, a recognized mortgage broker may help – select someone from the lists of the British Insurance Brokers Association.

At present the Inland Revenue allows tax relief on the interest payable on a mortgage: this could change.

See Money Matters chapter for books and publications.

Sheltered Housing

With the increase in the numbers of older people in the population, both local authorities and the voluntary organizations have stepped up provision of sheltered housing schemes, with bungalows or flats specially equipped for older people, warden services and communal facilities. Private enterprise has also stepped into this lucrative market, offering various schemes, some involving straightforward purchase, others some form of deferred payment. Before considering a commercial scheme you should find out what is available for rent from a local authority and what schemes are offered by a voluntary society. It's essential to be very cautious in inspecting both the property and the terms offered. Age Concern's leaflet No. 24, *Housing Schemes for Elderly People Where a Capital Sum is Required*, and their booklet *A Buyer's Guide to Sheltered Housing*[2] provide basic information and no one should consider sheltered housing without consulting one, or, preferably, both of these publications. Each contains lists of some of the voluntary agencies and commercial companies providing sheltered housing, but the point is made that there is no substitute for personal inspection and a close examination of possible commitments and snags. When considering a possible move for any reason, it's a good idea to look as far ahead as possible – to visualize future needs, not just those of the moment. Become informed about what's available *before* you need it. Try to arrange a short-term stay. Once your house is sold

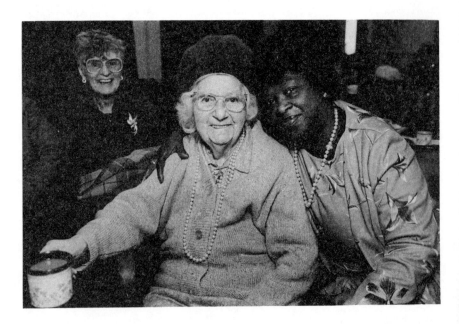

and furniture dispersed, it can be hard to go back to your former life-style. For a discussion of residential and nursing home accommodation see Chapter 17.

MAINTAINING YOUR HOME

Basic repairs and maintenance methods are described in *On Your Own* (see below) and any public library will provide a variety of do-it-yourself books. In some areas – mostly inner cities – youth groups under titles such as Pensioners' Link or Task Force provide the services of amateur painters, decorators and handypersons to help pensioners unable to afford commercial rates. Ask at your Social Services Department or Volunteer Bureau if this service is operating in your area. It's sometimes possible to arrange a 'skills exchange' with another pensioner – you provide her or him with a service you can perform in return for help with household repairs. An Age Concern local group could put you in touch with this and other sources of help.

COMMUNAL LIVING

Getting together with like-minded people to buy and share a large house seems an attractive option, but in Britain 'communes' have never been popular, and many have proved unsuccessful. Perhaps there's something in the saying that the British prefer to 'keep themselves to themselves', however inconvenient and expensive this may be. But the intermixing of the newer ethnic groups who may be more open to extended family and community-based living alternatives may revitalize the traditional sense of community for everyone in the UK, and may change the overemphasis on privacy that can lead to isolation for older women. Women in the Older Feminists' Network have been trying to set up communal houses and the Community Resources Centre has a publication, *A Directory of Christian Communities and Groups* (see below). *Communes Network* lists communes in the UK (see below).

Housing Co-operatives

An option for women who live in privately rented, council or housing association accommodation, or their own home, and who would prefer to have greater control over their dwelling or rid themselves of mortgage and repair worries may consider the advantages of co-operative housing.

This is a system whereby a group of people get together to take charge of the design, upkeep and repair of the homes they live in. This takes control away from a landlord; enables the group to ensure that the housing is kept in good

CHEAPER BY THE DOZEN BY BETTY DEXTER

When people hear that I live with eleven other people, they raise their eyebrows and ask, 'You're fifty-eight, why do you want to live like a hippie?' 'How do you stand the noise?' 'Don't you want privacy?' 'Do you have a lock on your bedroom door?'

I really don't know where to begin – the image of group living, in so many minds, is one of chaos, dirt, nightly orgies, and deafening stereos. Our house has none of these. We are a multigenerational group of adults who want to save money and who believe that community is healthier than aloneness. Otherwise, we are the same as the rest of the world: we like our home clean; we want love, not one-night stands; and we enjoy solitude as well as festivity.

Where my life greatly differs from that of most single women my age is in the area of responsibility. I do not want to pay for, insure, repair, polish, paint, tend, display, or worry about a house and its furnishings. But I want to live well. To me that means not only comfort and good food but stimulation and fun. Group living provides all of these and much more. I'm not living barricaded behind multiple locks because I fear unfamiliar steps outside my door. My social life is based on a bunch of people doing things together. In our house there are joggers, music and art lovers, and sports fans. Some people love board games while others retire to their rooms with a new book. I and two others are theatre buffs. But most important, all of these pursuits are guilt-free because the time for them is not stolen from our duties.

How do we run a sixteen-room house and still have lots of leisure? Organization. It's not a perfect world and sometimes people slack off, but on the whole this is the grand plan:

Decision-making:
Everybody attends house meetings twice a month.

Food shopping:
Rotation (two persons every six weeks).

Cooking:
Everyone makes her or his own breakfast and lunch. Twice a month each member cooks dinner for the group and cleans up afterward.

Kitchen cleaning:
Rotation (one person every twelve weeks; the job takes three hours).

Painting:
Everyone paints her or his own room. We have a once-a-year painting party at which everybody paints the common areas.

Other jobs, such as accounting and paying bills, cleaning bathrooms and living/dining/guest rooms, and performing minor repairs, are done by those who choose them. If a person gets sick of some job, he or she asks for a change and somebody swaps. When people leave, jobs are rearranged so nobody ends up, as the average housewife does, doing the same old jobs for a lifetime. If you have a bad back, you never have to lift a heavy window. If you're hopeless at maths, forget it, the bill payer will struggle with the bank statements.

At present my jobs are cleaning the living and dining rooms and washing the house linens. I usually devote Saturday morning to these chores. Besides that, I cook two big dinners monthly and in exchange I get twenty-two free evenings in which I come home, put my feet up, and wait for the dinner gong. I make two trips to the supermarket every sixth week. About four times a year I do kitchen cleanup.

There! The drudgery's finished; now let's talk about other aspects of group living.

1. One's mindset

If you're a woman who is upset if the house does not reflect *your* taste, then you'll have to decide whether that's important in the great scheme of things. If it is, then don't move into a group house where the common rooms belong to everybody and are dioramas of diversity. This was a stumbling block for me. I now confine my decorating efforts to my own bedroom. If you haven't missed an issue of *House and Garden* for years, think about this, because you don't want to be apologizing for your home.

2. One's role

In my first group experiment, I took in to live with me two young men who had been orphaned early in life. (I had lost custody of my own ten-year-old son just three months earlier.) Of course at the time I didn't see any connection, but shortly thereafter I found I couldn't say the things that needed to be said to make the house run well. I was too sorry for motherless boys during that period.

3. One's openness to change

I think you have to let go. Admit there is more than one way to wash lettuce; try exotic dishes you'd never make for yourself; go along with the gang to a 'far-out' film. (I'll bet next year you won't even call it far-out.)

But finally, best of all, if a middle-aged woman stays alert and tuned in, she can become a star in *Group Living*, the only soap opera I know that runs seven days a week all year round without repeats or commercials.

repair; and means that the group can work together to improve their environment and the community in general.

Much work, research and consideration is required before setting up a housing co-operative. The National Federation of Housing Co-operatives (see Organizations) has a number of information leaflets (send s.a.e.) and suggests further sources of information. Local inquiries about Housing Co-ops or Tenant Management Co-ops can be arranged; how to get in touch with organizations which help set up co-ops (the leaflets give addresses covering different parts of the UK); how to let the National Federation know that you're interested, because they can offer a lot of help and advice.

At the time of writing it appears that no 'women-only' co-ops have been set up, but there are one or two mixed-sex pensioners' co-ops.

A housing co-operative for black members can be contacted at the Spitalfields Housing Co-operative (see Organizations) or through local organizations such as the Black Women's Centre in Brixton (see Organizations).

NOTES

[1]All the Age Concern leaflets mentioned in this chapter are obtainable from Age Concern England, Information and Policy Department, Bernard Sunley House, 60 Pitcairn Road, Mitcham, Surrey CR4 3LL. Send a stamped 9-inch self-addressed envelope marked with the name and number of the factsheet you require. Single copies are free. Price list for Age Concern books.

[2]*A Buyer's Guide to Sheltered Housing* (Age Concern).

BOOKS AND PUBLICATIONS

Consumers Association, *Which? way to buy, sell and move house*. London: Hodder & Stoughton Ltd, revised reprint November 1988.

Buying a Flat: don't buy a lifetime of problems as well. Booklet produced annually, available from the Surveyors' Bookshop, Royal Institute of Chartered Surveyors, 12 Great George Street, London SW1.

Your Housing in Retirement. Mitcham: Age Concern.

Jean Shapiro, *On Your Own: A Practical Guide to Independent Living*. London: Pandora Press, 1985.

A Directory of Christian Communities and Groups. Available from the Community Resources Centre (see Organizations).

Communes Network Magazine. Available from Redfield, Winslow, Bucks. MK18 3LZ.

13
Work and Retirement

Nothing gives a human being more sense of achievement than the satisfaction derived from useful and socially-valued work whether paid or not, within or without the home. Women's dual role of home-maker and worker outside the home has been blamed – not least by women themselves – for stress-related illness, juvenile delinquency (remember the latch-key kids?) and marital breakdown. Yet researchers have consistently come up with the fact that when child-care arrangements are good, working conditions satisfactory and the work properly rewarded, the satisfactions greatly outweigh the disadvantages.[1] For many women, earning their own money, and working alongside others, banish the undermining sense of isolation and dependence upon a partner and children that can lead to depression and a loss of sense of self-worth. For older women, in particular, care of partner and home just aren't enough. The implications of under-employment and being 'past it' are intolerable.

Today in the United Kingdom 42 per cent of all women are in full- or part-time employment.[2] It's impossible to quantify the percentage of women who are 'housewives': even if we subtract the economically active and, for instance, students, the remaining female population would still include self-employed women, child-minders and so on.

But women continue to fill the poorly-paid jobs – their average pay is 74.8 per cent of the average man's. Women from the ethnic minorities earn, on average, even less.[3] Out of a total 'working population' of 27.2 millions in 1987, 2.8 millions were registered as unemployed* – but there was a continuing growth in female employment, part-time work and self-employment, a fact which reinforces the finding that it is in the low-paid sector that women most easily find work.[4] Older women, though, especially those nearing retirement, have not shared in this rise in employment.[5] This is particularly the case for

---

*Official methods of computing unemployment figures are constantly changing – usually in ways which result in the figures being 'better' than they actually are. Thus, adjustments are made so that people on training schemes (which may or may not lead to regular employment in the future) are not counted as unemployed. If they, and other groups (including some part-time women workers) were added to the official figures, these would be much higher.

Pakistani/Bangladeshi women, whose employment rate is exceptionally low, while, conversely, older women of West Indian and Guyanese origin have high rates of employment, compared with others in the age-group.[6]

What about women in 'managerial' jobs? Out of all the 'managers' in employment in the UK, only 11 per cent are women – 6 per cent full-time and 5 per cent part-time. This is in complete contrast to the figures for 'catering, cleaning, hairdressing and other personal services' where women constitute 21 per cent of full-time workers in these jobs and 54 per cent part-time, and 'secretarial' where a total of 75 per cent are women.[7]

Many women – particularly older women – complain that, despite all the provisions of Equal Opportunities legislation, they are discriminated against in employment. This may be subtle – for instance, a woman aspiring to a

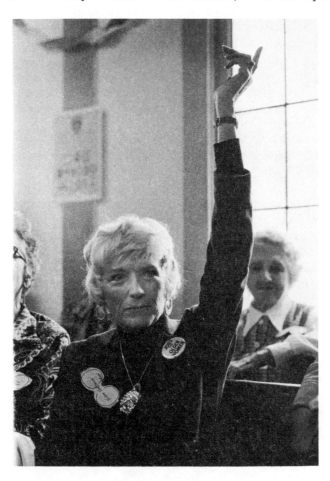

UNFAIR PRACTICE?

If you think you are being discriminated against

- raise the question with your employer or trade union
- if that fails seek advice from the Advisory, Conciliation and Arbitration Service (ACAS) or the Equal Opportunities Commission
- if you are still unable to reach agreement with your employer, you can go to an industrial tribunal
- if you are taking or contemplate taking your case to an industrial tribunal, the EOC may give you assistance. This is free and includes advice, helping to settle the dispute, arranging for the help of a solicitor or counsel
- remember that if you are taking the case to an industrial tribunal you must present your complaint to the tribunal within three months from the time the action complained of was done

- if your case concerns unequal pay, you may complain to the industrial tribunal at any time
- if your case concerns discrimination in employment on racial grounds contact the Commission for Racial Equality, which will give you the address of your regional office where you can discuss your case and receive backing.

Your regional ACAS address can be found at your public library, employment office or Citizens' Advice Bureau. The EOC leaflet *Equal Pay for Women* lists all regional offices of ACAS.

For the addresses of the EOC and CRE see Public and Professional Advisory Organizations (p. 582).

managerial job will probably have gone through the secretarial mill first, while a man will seldom be expected to have shorthand, typing and word-processing skills as part of his qualification for the job. Promotion of a valuable and knowledgeable secretary may be delayed because she is so useful to her boss that he doesn't want to lose her. A part-time woman worker's advancement can be blocked because job-sharing is inconvenient to the employer – though in fact, two half-time workers are often more productive than one full-time one.[8]

It's instructive to read just what the legislation can achieve and if you are in doubt about your rights, ask the Equal Opportunities Commission for their publications catalogue. Of particular interest to older women is the report in the leaflet *Sex Discrimination Decisions No. 9: The Case of Price v Civil Service Commission* – an outline of the case of a woman who had had a break from work for child care, and age barriers were used to prevent her returning to work in her previous job. However, the EOC claims that after the age of about forty-five, age bar affects women and men more or less equally. In the US, advocates

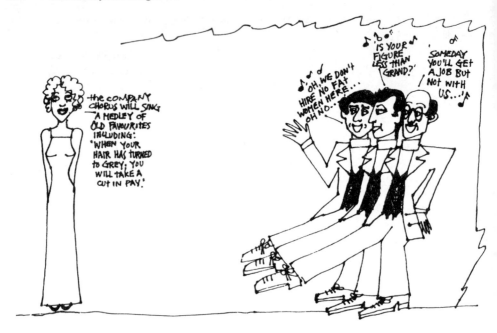

for older women have found that age bar affects women earlier than men and a combination of ageism and sexism stifles women's advancement in their prime years.

Women and the Unions

Although the trade union movement has played a key role in improving the pay and conditions of employees in general, some have been less than progressive in the field of women's employment. Think of women trade union leaders and most people will come up with only one name – Brenda Dean – though most trade unions with a proportion of women members do have one or two women on their executive committees. The TUC officially encourages the participation of women, but many local branches, meeting as they do at inconvenient hours, don't adapt themselves to the needs of their women members who have young children to feed and care for after leaving the workplace. It would be a great step forward if, as in some branches of the National Union of Journalists, members who have child-care responsibilities were helped to attend committee meetings by having their child-minding costs paid from branch funds. Until women are fully represented at all levels of the trade union movement their particular needs and concerns will not be met.

GETTING BACK TO WORK

Some women have managed to hang on to their original jobs – with some breaks for the birth and care of children – and others, without children, have worked all their adult lives. Both groups have probably suffered from the poor educational opportunities and low aspirations current in their youth. But someone who has little work experience and no formal qualifications is even more disadvantaged.

I left school at fifteen and got a job in an office. I learnt typing at an evening class and landed up as a copy typist. I got married at nineteen and spent more than twenty years looking after my home and three children. Now I'm 'free' at last – but for what? When people ask me what I do, I still have to say I'm just a housewife. Of course I want to do something more with my life, but I feel I've nothing to offer and I just wouldn't know where to start looking for a job. [a woman in her forties]

So what are the chances of a return to work for women in their forties or older? In our work- and success-orientated society it is difficult for a woman who has always put her caring role first to believe that she has any potential for 'real' achievement in the outside world. Many older women may never have had the education and training needed for a satisfying and well-rewarded job in their youth, and the years at home may have eroded their confidence and self-esteem. What hope is there for middle-aged women who want to retrain or re-enter the job market?

No one pretends that it's easy for an older woman to summon up the courage and confidence to look at herself and her potential and then go out and take advantage of the limited opportunities that do exist for getting qualifications and experience.

For a start, if you've ever had any training or experience, think about building on that. If you've been a typist, think of attending an evening class to brush up your skills and to learn word-processing. Then, go for a routine job that won't be too demanding, and once you've got your confidence back, try for a change that will provide you with something more interesting. If you worked in a shop, think about a part-time job with a small local business to start with. Examples of women who built on past experience and made a success of their return-to-work are given in *On Your Own* (see below).

But perhaps you want to try something completely different and you don't know exactly *what*. Maybe, too, it's more a question of reclaiming confidence than of brushing up a skill. You might then consider one of the many, but not too well publicized, courses run by further education colleges and polytechnics under titles such as *New Opportunities for Women, Wider Opportunities for*

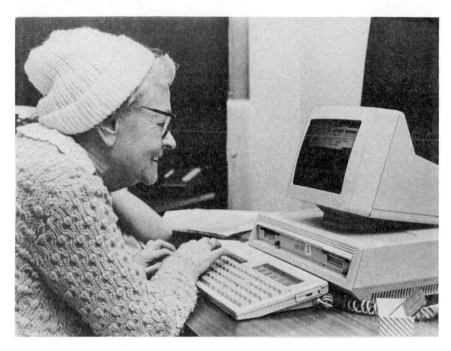

Women, *Fresh Start*, and *New Horizons*. Some are short, full-time and intensive, others evening classes held over a longer period. Inquire at your local college or from the Educational Guidance Service for Adults (inquire at your public library or education office). The aim of these courses is to help participants choose a suitable field of study or employment and get them accustomed to the routines of educational and working life.

TOPS – the Training Opportunities Scheme – is intended for people who have been out of full-time education for at least two years and want either to change their jobs or re-enter the job market. You can get information from the Job Centre or Shop or the Employment Office; sometimes people on a TOPS course are eligible for grants to meet part of the cost of travel, etc. TOPS training includes various types of skills and lasts for up to one year.

Another source of help is the Open University: it doesn't only offer degree courses, but a wide range of 'brush-up' courses in vocational subjects. If you *are* interested in working for a degree, the OU welcomes 'mature' students for its distance-learning courses which are combined with radio and TV programmes, local tutored groups and summer schools. You have to be dedicated and hard-working to stay the pace, but hundreds of older women have succeeded in getting their degrees (a satisfaction in itself) and in re-entering the world of work in a new capacity.

'Matures' are often welcomed by other higher education institutions, and if you have some relevant experience or qualification, and can show that you're capable of sustained academic work, age shouldn't be an insuperable barrier. If you've never had a Local Education Authority grant before, you should be eligible for one on the scale offered to mature students. Ask the LEA office about your entitlement once you've been accepted for a degree course. Other grants are normally discretionary, and with tight education budgets in recent years they aren't easily come by.

Whatever you decide to do about getting training or looking for employment, a useful introduction can be a good carers guide. *Equal Opportunities* (see below) is excellent. It covers practically every imaginable job or career, tells you what educational qualifications will be needed, where to train (if applicable), what the job entails, what sort of person it suits, prospects for late entry and part-time work, and lists further sources of information.

I was trained as a teacher, but that was years back. Organization and methods have changed so much since then. But luckily my subject was science and despite cutbacks, science teachers are still in demand. I took my courage in my hands and applied for a part-time job in a small local school. I was amazed to get it. For the first year I had to work really hard keeping just a few steps ahead of my pupils, but eventually all that study plus my firm base of knowledge paid off. I was offered a full-time post when the other science teacher retired. Our exam results are excellent and I find the whole atmosphere most satisfying. I could so easily have felt defeated by my apparently out-of-date qualifications. You've got to be bold. [a woman of fifty-one]

WORKING FOR YOURSELF

I left school at fifteen without any qualifications and got an office job – I was an errand-girl really, and it was just a way of earning a bit of money till I got married. I married at eighteen and had four children, quite far apart. So now I'm middle-aged, the children have left home and I'm completely without the sort of skills and experience I'd need for someone to offer me a job. But because we were so hard up when the kids were little, I had to make all our own clothes, and I used to go round the posh shops looking at what they were selling. Then I'd buy similar fabric and copy them. I got so good at making really unusual toddlers' outfits that friends asked me to make some for them. That was the start of my business – though I didn't realize it at the time. Now I've got a friend working with me keeping my accounts, another who does the cutting out, and we've developed a mail-order business offering a few popular lines. There's been some hassle on the way, but we make quite a good profit and we've had no help from anyone but ourselves. It's really satisfying. [a forty-seven-year-old woman]

Actually there are now several schemes aimed at helping people start their own businesses. Under the Enterprise Allowance Scheme you get not only help and advice but a weekly payment to help you over the first year – but unfortunately this scheme applies only to people who have been unemployed or receiving income support for at least eight weeks before application. Full details are set out in *Be Your Own Boss* (see below). There are other schemes for people setting up businesses in rural areas, and it's worth inquiring about local possibilities at your nearest office of the Department of Employment. Be warned, though. A high percentage of new businesses fail; so you must do your homework thoroughly, make use of skills and experience you already have, listen to advice, and tread cautiously. If you have no business experience, look for a local class on 'Running Your Own Business' – some education authorities provide these.

Retirement

In the United Kingdom the official retirement age for women is sixty – sixty-five for men. This is one of the lingering statutory forms of discrimination, and many women would like to see a compromise: retirement for all at sixty-three, for instance. Better still, why not adopt the system that is successful elsewhere – earlier retirement for those of both sexes who want it, but job security for those in their later sixties or seventies who prefer to keep on working and are capable of doing so?

Objections range from the difficulty of adapting the social security and pensions system to the fallacy that older people take jobs from the younger to the widespread belief, reinforced by ancient prejudice and employers' attitudes, that once you're over sixty or sixty-five you're suddenly enfeebled, incapable and fit for the scrapheap. This is despite everyone's daily experience: we all know active, productive septuagenarians; and if 'retirement age' were applicable to everyone, many prominent politicians, lawyers, artists and writers would also be pensioned off and forgotten.

The day after my sixtieth birthday I had to retire. I worked up to that Friday, and I was a key member of my team; on the Monday I was apparently 'past it'. The boss (a few years older than me, incidentally) found it difficult to replace me and after a couple of months I was called back. I was put on to a 'consultant' basis so that no precedent was set, but at sixty-five I did have to go. The crazy thing is that I still feel perfectly capable of doing the job. I'm finding the adjustment to idleness very difficult. [a sixty-six-year-old woman]

This woman was in an interesting and rewarding job. But many who have worked at boring or degrading jobs out of necessity wouldn't want to stay in their workplace for a day beyond the date when they qualify for retirement pension.

I've gone out to work for the last twenty years and I'm sick of it. All my life I've been short of money, short of time, ground down because of the demands made of me. I know I'll find it difficult to manage on my pension – but how wonderful to be able to see more of my grandchildren, spend more time exploring my neighbourhood, reading and studying. I would have retired several years ago if I could have afforded to. [a fifty-nine-year-old woman]

KEEPING ACTIVE

Whether you wanted to retire or not, the sudden break from the daily routine in which the demands of work were paramount can represent the kind of 'life change' that triggers depression. Ideally, you would have been making positive plans, some years earlier. By all means take a holiday or a breathing-space in which to think more concretely about your future – but after those first few weeks of catching up with things and people you've neglected, it's time to put a long-term retirement plan into action. If you're a healthy sixty-year-old, you could have at least twenty years before you.

I found myself bored and drifting. I couldn't spin out the domestic jobs to fill each day; I just wasn't into spending hours cooking up gourmet meals or doing useless embroidery. I felt so low that I couldn't even summon up the energy to go for the weekend walks I'd always enjoyed. That made me feel lower still. Then suddenly a friend called on my help. She had to go into hospital and there was no one to look after her handicapped daughter. I moved in to their house for a few weeks, until my friend was out of hospital and fully recovered. I'd felt so much better doing something useful, the very next week I volunteered to help at a local MENCAP branch. I now have a rota of mentally-handicapped young people whom I visit or take out on various activities to give their parents a break. Volunteering for something like that does something for both parties – helper and helped. [a sixty-three-year-old woman]

Running a job and a home I simply had no time to study. I missed out on higher education, but I always yearned to learn another language. I decided that when I retired I'd find a local class and really get down to learning German. I started at an adult education centre, from scratch. When I'd acquired a basic knowledge of the language, I went on to do a more advanced course at a further education college and eventually did A-level German. Was I pleased to get a good pass! Friends ask me what good it is, what's the use of it? I can't even afford to go on holiday to a German-

speaking country. But I do have a German penfriend; and anyway, it's the
satisfaction of achievement that counts. Now I'm doing a Spanish language course.
When I reach A-level standard with that it will open up a new world of literature to
me, as the German has. You're never too old to learn. [a woman in her sixties]

It was this belief that learning well into old age is possible that inspired the
University of the Third Age movement in France and which has now spread to
the United Kingdom. There are no entrance qualifications and no exams; no
'teachers', and a low annual fee enables members to study a great variety of
subjects, under the leadership of 'co-ordinators' who are also students like
themselves, but who have a greater depth of knowledge of their particular
subject. In London the U3A has around a thousand members and flourishing
branches are based on a number of other cities (see Organizations).

In recent years there have been crippling cutbacks in the adult education
centres run by Local Education Authorities, but many classes still remain and
fees for pensioners are usually on a reduced scale. At evening or afternoon
classes you can attend keep-fit groups for the over-sixties, local history study
groups, learn a variety of crafts and brush up on old skills. Further education
colleges and polytechnics also offer suitable classes. Your public library
usually has literature and a programme or prospectus covering these institutions – most of which start classes in September or October each year.

Work and retirement are two areas where we must expand choices for
women of all ages. We must fight sex, age, and other types of discrimination
and join together in women's organizations, labour unions, senior citizens'
advocacy organizations to fight the gender gap in earnings and to enforce our
right to decide when and whether we want to retire. We want retirement to
mean that we have chosen to leave paid work for something else, and not
survival on a pittance because we are no longer welcome at work. To
accomplish all this we must keep informed and connected with movements for
equal rights in the workplace. See below for names of publications that can
help you fight for your rights and keep in touch with the struggle around the
world.

NOTES

[1] Grace Baruch and Rosalind Barnett, *Life-prints: New Patterns of Love and Work.* New York: McGraw Hill, 1983; and Lillian B. Rubin, *Women of a Certain Age: the Mid-life Search for Self.* New York: Harper & Row, 1981.

[2] Equal Opportunities Commission, 1987 figures.

[3] Equal Opportunities Commission, *Women and Men in Britain: a Statistical Profile.* London: HMSO, July 1987, p. 30.

[4] Ibid., p. 30.

[5]Ibid., p. 31.

[6]Ibid., p. 31.

[7]Ibid., p. 32.

[8]Information from New Ways to Work (see Organizations).

BOOKS AND PUBLICATIONS

Action for Jobs, *Be Your Own Boss*. Free booklet from Job Centres, Equal Opportunities Commission, etc.

Jean Shapiro, *On Your Own: A Practical Guide to Independent Living*. London: Pandora Press, 1985.

Maggie Steel and Zita Thornton, *Women Can Return to Work*. Wellingborough: Thorsons/Grapevine, 1988.

Deborah Fowler, *The Woman's Guide to Starting Your Own Business*. Wellingborough: Thorsons/Grapevine, 1988.

Anna Alston and Ruth Miller, *Equal Opportunities: Careers Guide for Women and Men*. London: Penguin, 1987.

Ann Oakley, *Housewife*. London: Penguin, 1976.

Ann Oakley, *Sociology of Housework*. Oxford: Blackwell, 1984.

Ann Oakley, *Taking it Like a Woman: Autobiography of a Feminist*. London: Fontana, 1984.

14
Money Matters: The Economics of Ageing for Women

In no section of the community is the gap between rich and poor or North and South more obvious than in the age-group sixty plus – and it is in this group that a majority are women. While some (who have their own or their husbands' occupational pensions to provide a good standard of living, and several holidays a year) may share in the 'affluent society', there are many others living in poor circumstances, inadequate housing and rundown neighbourhoods. They, and not the comfortably-off, are the ones whose poor diet is criticized by the medical profession and government ministers; they can't afford any kind of leisure activity and dread any unexpected expenditure for fuel, new clothing or household repairs.* Since on average women live longer than men, widows and older divorced women form a high proportion of these older women.

As we've seen, discrimination in education and at work have meant that women now at retirement age have always been disadvantaged and have had no opportunity to build up an independent 'nest egg' to help them in their old age. Older women in particular are often badly hit following divorce. Difficult as it may be for a young woman with children to supplement any financial support ordered by the court from the former husband, someone over fifty who may have few marketable skills is even worse off. She has probably been out of employment for twenty or thirty years, retraining opportunities for someone so near to official retirement age are practically non-existent – and most employers just don't want to know. The great shake-up of the 1988 changes in social security and the whole benefit system has discriminated even more sharply against older people – and on the whole, that means women.

It's not possible here to outline the whole social security system – it would take a whole book to do that; anyone wanting a complete rundown should consult the Family Welfare Association book listed below. But there are numerous government leaflets which cover all aspects of payment and benefit

---

*Official methods for computing 'low income' statistics are criticized in the Fourth Report of the Social Services Committee of the House of Commons (1988). Poverty is now re-defined – family rather than individual income being taken into account. According to the statistics, there were 9,380,000 persons living at or below the supplementary benefit level in 1985.

and you can find these at your local social security office, public library or Citizens' Advice Bureau. To help you select those that may apply to you, a list of some of these free leaflets is included at the end of this chapter.

Tax Problems

The government department responsible for direct taxation (income tax) is the Inland Revenue, whose local office should deal with your tax affairs. Despite their bad name, local tax officials are often quite helpful in sorting out problems, so make an appointment at the local office before seeking other advice. The tax year runs from 6 April in one year to 5 April the following. The annual Budget (March) outlines the proposals for the following year. In 1990 everyone, including married women, will be responsible for filling in their tax return and paying tax – until then husbands were responsible for paying some of their wife's tax and completing her return with his, though the majority of married women workers, like others, had their PAYE deducted by their employers.

Which? (the Consumers Association magazine) publishes a useful guide to filling in your tax return in their May issue each year, and the Consumers Association book listed below should be in your public library. Make sure you get the current edition.

If you're over sixty-five make sure you claim Age Allowance on your tax form – if your income is below a set amount you're entitled to this, and if it's slightly above the limit, you will be entitled to an allowance on a lower scale.

Working Out a Budget

Everyone has her own way of budgeting. This is one system:

I get my pensions monthly – the OAP and one from my old job. At the beginning of each month I note the inescapable payments coming up – rates (which I pay on the monthly instalments system), gas and electricity (ditto). My mortgage is paid off already. Then I bank a fixed sum each month for clothes replacements, clothes repairs and dry cleaning, and draw from this account when I need to. I save for household repairs and replacements by paying a fixed monthly sum into the building society, so that, with luck, when a big expenditure comes up, I can draw enough to cover it. This system of regular payments means that I just forget about these sums and know that what I actually have in my purse or bank account is for everyday spending on food, books and entertainments. [a sixty-three-year-old woman]

RETIREMENT PENSIONS

In its general drive toward privatization, the government has sought to devise new ways of making us 'stand on our own two feet'. The State Earnings Related Pension Scheme (SERPS), in which employees earning more than £2,132 per annum (1988–9 figure) contribute to their future pension through their National Insurance contributions, has proved too costly for the government, so in 1988 it changed the way contributions and the amount of pension ultimately received are calculated. Employees are now allowed to pay less toward SERPS by 'contracting out' through Private Pension Payments, or employers' own schemes. This means that the government gives you a rebate on what you and your employer pay in National Insurance contributions.

The press is now full of advertising for private schemes, and information about the benefits and possible snags can be gleaned from getting the various leaflets and booklets available from insurance companies and banks. The whole system is very complicated and the best run-down for the ordinary reader available at the time of writing is a comprehensive article published in *Which?* magazine (August 1988). Your public library ought to have file copies of *Which?*

For general information on pensions the Society of Pensions Consultants, the Company Pensions Information Centre (see Organizations) can be useful. The Occupational Pensions Advisory Service gives advice on company schemes. And for general information on pensions, in addition to the leaflets listed on pages 264 and 283, ring:

Freeline Social Security 0800 666555

To find out your SERPS entitlement to date and what your future SERPS pension is likely to be, fill in leaflet NP38 'Your future pension' available from the local social security office.

And another:

I'm rather bad with money and now that I've got so little I've resorted to a rather old-fashioned method – but it works for me. I draw my pension weekly, and when I get it I divide the money up between a lot of tins and jars – so much for rent, so much for gas, so much for the insurance payment and so on. Whatever's left in my purse is for food and other necessities. I know there's the risk of a break-in, but I do hide these tins away and in any case, most of the time there's very little in them! I think if I had a bank or post office account I'd tend to overspend. Of course on my low income I can't save. I don't know what I'll do when the Poll Tax comes in – obviously I'll get a reduction, but I don't pay rates now because of my low income, and how I'll find that extra beats me. [a sixty-nine-year-old woman]

Or:

I don't have a system. Or perhaps you'd call it a rough-and-ready one. At the beginning of the year I work out just how much all my housing, heating, self-employed taxation, rates, holidays and similar costs like insurance are going to come to over the year. It invariably leaves about a quarter of my income (after tax) for day-to-day expenses. So I bank all my money, pay for all those items by cheque or credit card and regard the one quarter as current spending money – clothes, food, small extras. I'd recommend this only to someone whose income is fairly good, and rising with inflation, and who, like me, gets into a muddle if she tries to keep too closely to a detailed budget. [a forty-six-year-old woman]

What About Your Savings?

Even though you may not be able to save in retirement, you are probably able to save *for* retirement if you're in work. Here's where the fixed savings plans, carried out on an individual basis through paying into a building society or bank deposit account a regular monthly or quarterly sum, or by taking out one of the many new schemes for personal pensions, could help you. Get all the information you can about these plans, by reading the financial pages of the 'quality' newspapers, picking up leaflets from high street banks and building societies. Get advice from professionals, but remember to check whether they have a financial interest in the advice they offer you. Try to assess the advantages and disadvantages of various schemes. The Consumers Association book listed below offers helpful advice on choosing the scheme most suited to your needs.

When it comes to considering actually spending your savings once you've retired – be cautious, too. You may want to know just how long your money will last, given the increased longevity of women, and here the table prepared for the original (American) edition of this book could be useful (see p. 262).

For more information on managing your money, see *On Your Own* (Books and Publications), but bear in mind that with the 1988 legislation, figures will have changed.

Taking Action

You won't have needed convincing from the information given in this chapter and in the previous one that women – especially older women – are at a disadvantage financially as well as in many other ways. So what can you do about it?

On a personal basis: you can ensure that you get your rights at work and social

HOW LONG WILL YOUR MONEY LAST?

Percentage of Savings You Can Withdraw Annually and for How Many Years

	Number of Years Your Money Will Last				
Percentage of savings you can withdraw annually	@ 5% interest	@ 6%	@ 7%	@ 8%	@ 9%
5%	Forever				
6%	35 yrs	Forever			
7%	24 yrs	32 yrs	Forever		
8%	19 yrs	22 yrs	30 yrs	Forever	
9%	15 yrs	18 yrs	21 yrs	27 yrs	Forever
10%	13 yrs	14 yrs	16 yrs	20 yrs	25 yrs

Figures are approximate; annual compounding is assumed; inflation is not considered.

CONCESSIONS AND SERVICES

Anyone of pensionable age should take advantage of the various extras that may be available such as:

Free chiropody
Free or reduced-rate local travel (not available everywhere and possibly under threat in the future)
Railcards, available to over-sixties for travel by train at reduced rates (make sure you travel at the right time to get maximum benefit from special offers, Away-days, etc.). A higher rate card enables you to travel anywhere in the British Isles, the lower rate is for day-trips.
Hairdressing at reduced rates on some days

Dry-cleaning at reduced rates on some days
Meals-on-Wheels, if cooking or shopping are difficult (ask your GP or social worker)
Free transport to hospital appointments (arrange with Outpatients' Department)
Free or cheap entry to local amenities such as swimming pools
Cheap matinee prices at cinemas and some theatres
Reduced-rate tickets for museums, art galleries, stately homes, exhibitions, etc.
When requesting reduced rates, produce your pension book, bus pass or other means of proving that you qualify

*For instance, if you are earning 5% on your capital, and you withdraw 7% annually, your money will last 24 years. If you withdraw the same, or a lesser, per cent than you are earning, you will not use up your money.

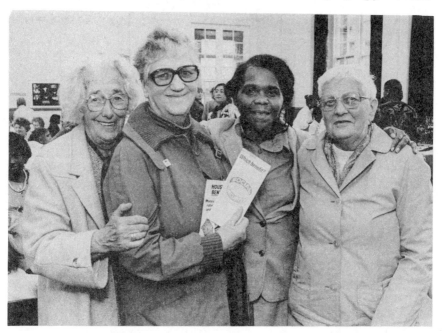

security benefits by making use of the machinery that does exist through the Equal Opportunities legislation, the social security system, etc. If you're in doubt about rights and entitlements, ask at the Citizens' Advice Bureau. Pick up leaflets from there and the local social security office. Talk to the librarian at your public library who will steer you toward useful books. Consult the local Law Centre if it exists. Ask Rights of Women, the Equal Opportunities Commission, the Commission for Racial Equality and – if it hasn't been axed through local government spending restrictions – your council's Women's Committee for help and advice.

Working with others: join a political party with whose aims you broadly agree, participate in their meetings and activities and campaign with them for better conditions for older women and pensioners. Join your trade union, if you're eligible, and support or initiate campaigns for the improvement of women's pay and conditions. Join a pensioners' organization (see Organizations: Pensioners' Link, the National Federation of Pensioners' Organizations, etc.). Work with other organizations not specifically geared to the needs of older women, but where you could be effective in calling attention to the needs of older women and in initiating action (The Women's Institutes, Townswomen's Guild, Co-operative Women's Guild).

The changes in the social security system, entitlement to Housing Benefit and general erosion of the Welfare State upon which so many of us expected to rely in our later years, were implemented in 1988, following the 1987 general election. It seems that unless we, as older women, join with all those groups and individuals opposed to the cuts and changes, we can expect the existing 'I'm all right, Jill' situation to last beyond the next election. The consequences to ourselves and the generation that will follow would be disastrous.

So write to or lobby your MP – s/he does take note of what constituents say. Remember that older people are constituting a larger and larger proportion of the population and hence of voters, and there's a limit to the disillusion and alienation from current policies that we will suffer; just as MPs, who will press our point of view, will gain strength and encouragement if they are assured of our support.

BOOKS AND PUBLICATIONS

Family Welfare Association, *Guide to the Social Services*. Annual publication – consult reference section of local library.

Consumers Association, *The Which? Book of Saving and Investing*. London: Hodder, 1989.

Ruth Lister and Beth Lakhani (eds.), *National Welfare Benefits Handbook*. Child Poverty Action Group.

Jean Shapiro, *On Your Own: A Practical Guide to Independent Living*. London: Pandora Press, 1985.

Perrie Crowshaw, *Money Matters – A Practical Handbook for Women*. London: Macdonald Optima, 1988. Covers pensions, benefits, differences between treatment of women and men, etc.

Government leaflets covering all aspects of social security payments and benefits:

NI 244	Statutory Sick Pay – check your rights
NI 16	Sickness benefit
NI 16A	Invalidity benefit
IR 41	Unemployment benefit

NI 51	Widows
NI 95	Divorced women
NI 230	Occupational pensioners over age sixty
NP 32	Your retirement pension
NI 92	Earning extra pension by cancelling your retirement
NP 32B	Retirement benefits for married women
CH 11	Child benefit
NI 14	Guardian's allowance
N 2	Industrial diseases
NI 205	Attendance allowance
NI 212	Disability allowance
NI 225	Vehicle allowance
MPL 152	War widows and dependants' allowance
SB 20	A Technical Guide to Income Support

(others may be needed in special circumstances)

15
Caregiving*

Caregiving is a Woman's Issue

Caregiving has traditionally been a woman's role. Women have always cared for dependent members of the family and community – infants, children, the infirm, the handicapped, and the frail elderly. Societal pressures and expectations have trained generation after generation of women to put others' needs before their own. In the US women constitute 71 per cent of family caregivers;[1] they are 'the invisible laborers without whom neither the health system nor the patient could survive'.[2]

It is imperative for all of us to take a hard look at the unthinking way women are simply handed the job of taking care of whatever dependent person happens to be in their home or even outside their immediate home and family. I have a forty-five-year-old daughter who has been disabled by an obscure form of epilepsy since birth. When she is not institutionalized I take care of her and when she is, I am constantly doing errands to make her stay in the hospital more bearable. With a great deal of prodding from her professionals, my daughter is trying to be more independent at last. My mother lived to be ninety-eight, the last twenty-one years of her life as a widow. I became her principal caregiver in my early forties. Now my husband suffers from memory loss and has been diagnosed as having Alzheimer's disease. Again I am the principal carer. I have given this kind of care without questioning it since the beginning of my marriage. [a sixty-six-year-old woman]

I've had a lot of experience in caring for old people – first my grandmother and then my father. When both had died, I volunteered to help at a day centre and luncheon club for pensioners. I think the professionals looked at me with some suspicion at

---

*Though we are focusing on the unpaid carer here, we do not wish to dismiss the work of paid carers in hospitals, nursing homes, and private homes. Paid carers also are predominantly women, and are underpaid and undervalued in society and in the institutions where they work. We feel that recognition of the importance of caregiving will contribute to better quality of life for all carers, paid and unpaid, and those they care for.

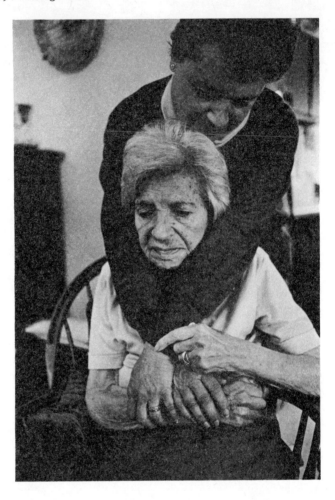

first, but I'm now accepted by them – and, more importantly, by the old people, who've given me much more than I've given them. [a fifty-five-year-old woman]

Caregiving Wives

Remember the poem that says, 'Grow old along with me, the best is yet to be?' Unfortunately, many couples plan their retirement years with this in mind only to have their dreams end in a nightmare when one partner becomes disabled or chronically ill – a victim of Parkinson's disease, Alzheimer's disease, a stroke, or cancer.

I'm glad now that we did so much travelling before my husband became ill. I try to think of those times now and relive them. We had so many things planned for after the children had grown, but that's not the way it turned out for us. Because of my husband's illness, we never go anywhere. We're caged in, the two of us. [a woman in her seventies]

A familiar pattern is that when a man becomes ill or disabled, his doctor will send him home, commenting that he is lucky to have a wonderful wife to care for him. When the same thing happens to a woman, however, the doctor will often recommend a nursing home. (In some cases, men *are* caregivers for their wives, and of course those who are certainly deserve the same relief and support argued here for women.) As medical science prolongs lives, women, who are frequently younger than their husbands, and also tend to live longer, will more and more often find themselves facing the difficult task of caring for their husbands.

I cry a lot because I never thought it would be this way. I didn't expect to be mopping up the bathroom, changing him, doing constant washing. I was taking care of babies at twenty; now I'm taking care of my husband.[3]

Wives usually have no special preparation for caregiving, and little choice about offering it. In many communities, when a husband needs constant care, the only alternative is a nursing home. Many women prefer to keep their husbands at home when faced with this alternative,[4] feeling that the separation would break the vow 'Till death do us part'. Also, both husband and wife may recoil from a nursing home because of horror stories heard from family, friends, and the media. Both partners may want to remain together without realizing what a physical and emotional strain will eventually be placed on the wife.

Caregiving wives carry a heavy emotional load. They often have no one to tell them how well they are doing or how to do the job better, and no one to help when a difficult situation arises. They usually put aside their own lives and aspirations to give their husbands' needs top priority. On top of all of this, they may have their own physical ailments, which may be aggravated by the work they have to do.

I'm seventy-three years old and use a walking frame. Last year I had a hip replacement. My husband is a paraplegic. When I'm helping him in the bathroom, I have to get into positions that hurt my hip. He doesn't want anyone else to help him.

Carers often talk about being isolated, of losing companionship and social contacts. Friends and family who are upset by seeing changes in the husband tend to stay away. Sons and daughters – especially sons, who may see their own future in their father's illness and be unable to face it – may have difficulty coping with the new situation. Sons and daughters may also view their mother as the one who always holds things together, and may continue to expect her to hold this role in the family despite the change in circumstances.[5]

People tell me that he deserves all the care I can give him because he's such a nice person and was always so good to me. Well, I'm a nice person and have always been good to him – what do I deserve? [a seventy-three-year-old woman]

Wives feel isolated as carers because they have lost the support of their husbands – often the one with whom they had their closest relationship. This is especially the case when a husband is mentally impaired, since the wife has then essentially lost the man she married. He is still alive, but their relationship, with its shared memories, humour, hopes, and dreams, slips away as his illness progresses. Some carers in these circumstances experience apathy,

'Your husband is lucky to have you to take care of him at home, Mrs Jacobs.'

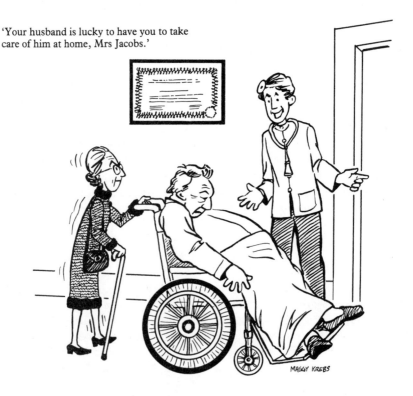

nervousness, irritability, a decrease in vitality and mental energy, and a prevailing sense of depression. Many husbands are aware of the burden that their illness has created for their wives, saying, 'This illness has been as much my wife's as it has been mine.'[6]

Caregiving may mean taking over affairs that the husband took care of before. Such a change in roles may cause anger, pain, conflicts, and confusions for *both* husband and wife, adding even more stresses to an already stressful situation. In a marriage, spouses often act as loving fathers or mothers to one another during times of stress, uncertainty, or illness. When the husband becomes so ill that he cannot share in making decisions, the wife's sole responsibility becomes permanent.

He was such an intelligent man, an engineer, used to giving orders. Now he has no memory, I have to tell him what to wear and what to do, and he resents it. He doesn't really know who I am. For the first year or so he thought I was a housekeeper; now he must realize that I belong with him. If he had a moment of clarity and saw what has happened to him and to us, he would want to die. It would have been a blessing if he had died in the hospital. [a sixty-eight-year-old woman, with an eighty-one-year-old husband]

Wives may feel guilty if at times they wish for their husband's or a parent's death and resent the continuing need for care. For those women who have stayed married despite unhappy marriages, caregiving is even harder. To all the other stresses are added resentment over wasted years and dislike of their husbands.

Some wives caring for husbands are helping an elderly parent at the same time. The parent may not be able to understand the extent of care that the son-in-law requires and thus resent the time that the daughter gives to him, or the husband may resent time devoted to caring for the parent. Obviously the woman cannot divide herself in two to care for both equally, yet she may feel guilty over the conflicting demands. This situation places extraordinary stress on the carer.

Daughters as Carers

We live in a time when many of us are fortunate enough to see our parents live until they are quite old. The challenge of longevity is that older parents may need our help, not just occasionally, but on a continuing basis and at a time when we ourselves are getting older. It is not uncommon today to hear of a seventy-year-old woman who is concerned about and responsible for her ninety-year-old mother.

Those of us who take on caring for parents often have to make major adjustments. Both carer and parents lose freedom and privacy and may have to give up or defer plans for the future. It is not easy for either the daughter or the parent; both feel resentment and frustration. Carers often feel caught between their parents' needs and their own. Women who still have children at home feel the additional squeeze of being 'sandwiched' between generations.[7]

Most carers have very little understanding at first of what the job will entail. Many agree to take care of a parent when she or he is still somewhat self-sufficient, and are unprepared for what happens when the picture changes.

I decided I would take care of my father when he could still stay by himself and get snacks. But by the time he actually came to me (only a few weeks after I made the original decision) he was partially paralysed and needed help doing everything. [a woman in her late thirties with two preschool children]

My father had a heart attack and my parents came to live with us when we still had children at home. Then my mother had a series of strokes. She died when my oldest was eighteen. I would really tell anyone in that situation not to try to care for parents in your home – to make other arrangements, have your family life less disrupted and better balanced. It was a very difficult period. My father was very nervous from his illness. He was a helpless person who was taught that the woman did everything. [a woman in her sixties]

Helping an older parent stay in his or her own home often requires extensive logistics and support systems.

I help my eighty-eight-year-old disoriented mother stay in her own flat through a system of phone calls and hired help coming in four times a day. They give my mother her meals, bathe her, and dress her in the morning and help her get ready for bed at 10 p.m. I've accident-proofed the flat and constantly modify the support system as my mother's condition changes. I drive fifty-eight miles round trip to do the washing, the shopping, and pay the bills. In effect, I run two households and I also have a full-time job. This is a ten-year-old routine that is demanding but has worked for us both up to now. [a fifty-seven-year-old woman]

Despite the difficulties, however, keeping a parent in her or his own house may be preferable from the standpoint of preserving both the parent's and the daughter's independence.

Elderly parents often expect their daughters – rarely their sons – to care for them. Parents may not approve of their daughter's working (or of her involvement in outside activities if she does not have a paid job), as these take up time that parents may feel belongs to them.

My mother, a courageous, proud immigrant woman, always looked to me for her primary emotional support. My brothers were devoted to her but she rejected a good deal of what they offered because traditionally daughters are expected to be the primary carers. When I returned to college while my children were growing up, my mother was often hostile toward my pursuits, making my visits with her very uncomfortable. However, when I graduated, she insisted upon having her picture taken with me after the ceremony – a frail eighty-eight-year-old immigrant lady with a face full of pride posing with her daughter, the college graduate. It was a moment of pride for us both. [a woman in her forties]

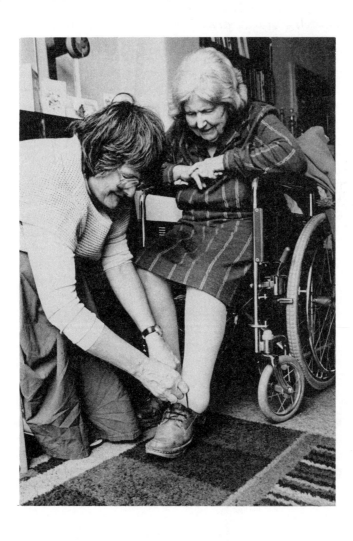

Some parents believe that women belong in the home and that taking care of parents is a logical extension of that. Many daughters place themselves in the caring role in their own minds, subjecting themselves to internal as well as external pressures. Their brothers, husbands, and male friends do not feel the same pressures. Most men are able to separate themselves both physically and emotionally from their parents, and experience less guilt about doing so.[8]

I live near my parents and take care of them. I do the shopping, cooking, cleaning; you name it and I do it. My sainted brother lives in Scotland. Once a year he flies down, takes them out for dinner and a show, then he's off again for another year. My parents think he's great and I get all the complaints. [a woman in her forties]

In traditional families, if the sons provide financial help, mend a broken door, visit, call, or send flowers at the appropriate times, then they are 'good sons' and meet their parents' expectations. Although it is rare, some men do care for parents; when they do they are usually not torn by the same conflicts as women. Most often, sons expect to hire help or delegate other people (fill in wife, sister, aunt, some female relation) to do the actual caregiving.[9]

My brother does most of the work of co-ordinating home care and medical appointments for my parents. We try to share the calling, errands, and visiting as much as possible, but I am a divorced parent with a full-time job, including some evening meetings, while he is married, without children at home. Though his job is also demanding, he has more time and energy to give at this point in our lives. When I hear some of the horror stories other women tell, I feel lucky that my brother is so responsible. [a forty-five-year-old woman]

Daughters may feel a nagging guilt over putting their own needs first. Some parents find it scary or difficult to make new friends and to be in new social situations, and thus rely heavily on their daughters to meet all of their needs.

My mother is eighty-two and needs assistance because she is partly deaf and has severe cataracts. She lives alone and spends most of her time by herself. She is nervous but very independent and I wouldn't consider a nursing home or an old age home for her. She is in fine health otherwise, but really needs a little more companionship. I don't have a lot of time to spend with her, since I work full time and have two children at home. She refused any help that I could get and will not go to a group in her church or join a senior citizens' centre. She wants me to be there. [a forty-eight-year-old woman]

I usually phone my mother every day to check on her. Sometimes I get busy and a day or two will go by and I forget to call. The calls are repetitious, we don't have much to say – she usually complains a lot. But what really riles me is that when I miss a day she calls me and starts out with 'I thought your index finger was broken and you couldn't use a phone – how are you?' I can feel the hair on my body rise, but I ignore the moment and just say, 'How are you?' [a fifty-five-year-old woman]

My grandmother lived to be almost one hundred and two years old, and my mother cared for her until she was ninety-seven and had to go into a nursing home. Now my mother obviously feels it is her turn, which it is. I am the real problem here, for I have led a very active life and cannot seem to adjust to this demanding and devastating situation. I do not know what to hope for and am almost overcome with the inevitable guilt at my resentment and anger. I have no one to talk to. [a seventy-two-year-old woman]

Some of us may have parents who were never happy or content with life. To maintain a sense of balance and sanity, we have to face the fact that we may not be able to make them happy and that their unhappiness is not our fault.

People who have lost eyesight, hearing, or mobility and are undergoing a lot of pain have legitimate reasons for being unhappy. Parents may also be angry about not being able to do things for themselves. It's important to recognize that they aren't angry at you, just as you aren't angry at them; it is what has happened to them that is the source of the anger.

If we have unhappy childhood memories of parents and believe that they wronged us we may feel resentful and angry at having to care for them.

My mother left me when I was two and my father moved us into his parents' house. My grandmother actually brought me up and I loved her. I rarely saw my father – he ran around and was not part of my life. After I had children, he and his new wife grew close to us because of the grandchildren. Now he's a widower and sick, so he moved in with us eight years ago. Our children are grown up and we finally had the house to ourselves, but now he's here. We have no privacy. He expects me to wait on him. He was a lousy father, but I can't throw him out. He has no money and where would he go? Inside I'm angry at him and I resent him all the time. [a fifty-six-year-old woman]

Some of us may feel that we *want* to be the caregiver of a parent or close relative.

My aunt was still very active into her nineties. I felt as though she was almost like my mother. But she kept having these little 'occlusions' – the blood wasn't getting through the arteries to the brain and she would pass out. Finally the doctor said she could never be left alone again. So I took care of her at home for five and a half years. I made the garden for her and cooked the best food in the world for her. She had taught me how to cook. She was a dear wonderful person. She gradually got worse. When she couldn't go down the stairs, I would carry huge pots of flowers to show her because she loved plants and flowers so much. She gradually got weaker and weaker until one day she said, 'I'm just all tired out.' She was just like a clock that had run down. And I was with her. So I felt that I had done all I could. I really loved her more by the time she died. It was a hard job but I'm glad I was able to do it. I feel very good about it. [a single woman in her fifties]

My mother never had any joy, only hard work and struggle. I tried to make it up to her, to do things for her and give her things, and felt guilty because I couldn't take away the old pains and troubles or make her into a happy person. But at least I was able to take care of her in her old age. I have no guilt about that. And she died at home, in my house, where I could say goodbye to her in my own way and in my own place. That was five years ago, and as I get older I see more and more of my mother in myself, and that's okay because she was a wonderful woman and I love her. [a woman in her fifties]

Sometimes siblings rekindle old wounds and feelings when discussing how and who should help care for the parents. You hear statements like 'You were always Mum's favourite', or 'You always got what you wanted, so you take care of them now'.

We feel helpless as we watch elderly parents become more dependent and frailer. We may be afraid and sad, fearing our parents' death or our own old age. Deep inside we still think of our parents as dependable and strong, the way we saw them when we were children; and the child inside us still wants it that way. We may still want their approval and their wise, loving care.

I take care of my mother, who is physically well but has no memory and is disoriented. Several years ago my oldest daughter went into the hospital for a biopsy. I made arrangements for someone to care for my mother and I told her where I was going. For one moment she understood and said, 'I hope everything goes well', then she lapsed back into her usual state, and I wanted to cry. I realized that I wanted my mother; I wanted her to comfort me and tell me it would be all right like she did when I was a child. But she's like a child now and I'm her mother. [a fifty-eight-year-old woman]

Role reversal is one of the hardest aspects of being a carer. No one wants to think of her parents as incapable of making decisions. A healthier relationship will be maintained if you can take on caregiving responsibility without thinking of the parent as a child.

It is difficult for caregivers to find time for themselves. Most try to maintain their family obligations and perform well at their jobs, but may overlook their own personal needs, especially time for fun, exercise, and relaxation. The logistics of getting help for the dependent parent may seem so overwhelming that it doesn't feel worth it. It is not surprising that caregivers often develop physical manifestations of emotional stress.

Three years ago my father had a stroke. He and my mother wanted to stay in their home, but my mother was really too frail to look after him – he was partially paralysed. In the end it seemed best to move them both to my house. Now both of them are virtually helpless. I've had to give up my job. I do draw Attendance Allowance on their behalf but it doesn't compensate me for my loss of earning and promotion prospects, let alone for all the worry and sheer hard work. They are now both so demanding that I can't get anyone to stay with them to enable me to get out – so apart from doing the weekly shopping, when my husband takes over for a couple of hours, I'm a prisoner in my own home. The constant, almost twenty-four-hours-a-day caring for them is getting me desperate. Yet somehow I can't wash my hands of them and get them taken into a geriatric hospital. But if I collapse, I'll have to. [a fifty-four-year-old woman]

No one should have to give up her own life or risk her health to the degree described by this and other women who care for family members at home. Family caregivers need a variety of support and respite services. We must get together and fight for universal availability of such services, and for the funding to keep them going, so that we can keep going. The 'Care in the Community' system in this country increasingly depends on the in-home carer and threatens to move even further in this direction. More nursing-home beds are needed nationwide as well as much better social security benefits for those in residential homes, but many family caregivers want to keep their family member at home, and they need help to do so.

Some of us have been able to turn to friends and relatives for help that should be forthcoming from the NHS and local Social Services.

For many years after my mother's death, my father and I shared a house. The landlady lived upstairs with her elderly mother, who also needed someone to be around. So the landlady and I alternated taking weekends off. Both parents would leave the back door open so they could be in touch. I also had a temporary 'lodger', who was helpful in doing things with my father such as watching TV or taking him to football matches. I in turn would get the meals.

After my father died, my housemate and I just kept living together [see p. 240]. We each have had some illnesses and have recently developed a bond that has a different dimension. Now that we need each other, we do more things together, and our caring has grown. We still have our usual disagreements but we learned how to resolve them long ago.

The landlady and a friend who bought a share of the house are both older than we are. I heard one of them fall at 3 a.m. and we took her to the hospital. We shop for them often and they feed the cat for us, and vice versa. I tell one of them when I will be coming in late and she keeps the spotlight on until I'm home. There's a reciprocal feeling of caring. [a seventy-two-year-old single woman who has lived with her friend for twenty years]

Some women who have met through Pensioners' Link help each other out on a regular basis. Sometimes one whose sight is failing teams up with another member with a different disability – the first woman enjoys being read to while the second needs help in cooking. It's an idea that could spread through such groups – a version of 'skills exchange' which enables older people to give and receive help and maintain their feelings of usefulness and self-respect.

In the United States one branch of the Older Women's League had an enthusiastic response from members willing to respond to SOS calls from fellow-members with help such as acting as substitute carers or lending sick-room equipment.[10]

Caring is Stressful

Though each carer has her own set of problems and her own ways of coping – and sometimes falling apart – all carers experience emotional, physical, or economic stress, and sometimes all three. All experience feelings of frustration and isolation. To add to these stresses, many carers are the only breadwinners in the family. Some hold demanding jobs outside the home in addition to the demanding jobs of caregiving.

I've been caring for my father for over eight years. The first few years were good ones. He'd been a chef and contributed to the family by making all our meals. Now he is blind, confined to a wheelchair, and needs a lot of help. I am a special education teacher and love my work. I have hired a woman to stay with my father during the day, but from the moment I come into the house at 4 p.m. until he goes to bed around 8, I am the one who gives him all the care. I get up with him several times a night and I get up at 6 a.m. and get him ready for the day. One day my neighbour told me that if I really loved my father I'd leave my job and stay at home to care for him. I was angry and hurt and asked her if she would have told me that if I were a man. My work is very important to me and it keeps me sane. [a fifty-seven-year-old woman]

'WOMAN'S WORK' – BALANCING OUR JOBS WITH DEMAND FOR CARING BY PAULA BROWN DORESS

Most of us Americans over forty can remember when women in traditionally 'female' occupations – schoolteachers, nurses, airline stewardesses, telephone operators – were not allowed to keep their jobs once they married. Others, especially poor women and black women, were expected to remain employed after marriage. Today, 50 per cent of married women work in paid employment, compared with 4 per cent at the turn of the century, and we think of such restrictions as archaic. Yet the demands of the women's movement for child care and maternity leave[1] have been ignored in this country, forcing women to give up their jobs in the early child-raising years. In countries where women have these options, their pay relative to men's is higher.[2] In our middle and later years, we may have to care for an older or infirm family member. When this happens, we fall even further behind men in our careers and retirement benefits.

Employed women who care for ill or older persons or a disabled child need day-care services and flexible working hours just as parents of young children do. These policies would cut down on absenteeism and be a strong selling point for attracting new employees. A 1982 survey found that 44 per cent of women who cared for a parent were also employed, and many caregivers rearranged work schedules or reduced their hours. Some even had to quit their jobs.[3]

What can employers do? A survey conducted by The Travelers Insurance Companies found that 28 per cent of their employees over thirty spent 10.2 hours per week caring for older relatives and friends and 8 per cent devoted 35 hours per week! They found that many employed workers need a variety of support services, ranging from information and referral to flexible scheduling and adult-care programmes. As a result, the company is exploring ways of providing information and support to those employees to prevent stress, exhaustion, and loss of productivity.[4] As women, we should not have to choose between family responsibilities and a satisfying work life.

[1] Boston Women's Health Book Collective, *Ourselves and Our Children*. New York: Random House, 1978; and Margaret O'Brien Steinfels, *Who's Minding the Children? The History and Politics of Day Care in America*. New York: Simon & Schuster, 1973.

[2] Sylvia Hewlett, *A Lesser Life: The Myth of Women's Liberation in America*. New York: Morrow, 1986.

[3] National Center for Health Services Research, quoted in Older Women's League press release, 'Family Caregivers – A Fact Sheet'. November 1986.

[4] Glenn Collins, 'Many in Work Force Care for Elderly Kin'. *The New York Times*, 6 January 1986, p. B5.

One third of carers are in fair to poor health themselves.[11] If you find yourself frequently feeling unwell, don't excuse it by saying, 'Well, I had a bad night', or, 'The weather is damp'. Take time off to go for a checkup from your doctor. Explain not only your symptoms but also your role as a caregiver so that she or he fully understands the stresses you are under. Beware of a doctor who dismisses your concerns or feels that the answer to all your aches and pains is a tranquillizer – which will make you feel groggy and only add to your problems. If your blood pressure is high – a common symptom among overworked carers – your body is sending you an important message. You have to learn how to reduce your stress level to help bring down your blood pressure. (See Hypertension, Heart Disease, and Stroke chapter and the section on stress management in Ageing and Well-being chapter.) Carers also often experience nausea, fatigue, and difficulty in sleeping. If your doctor has determined that you don't have an underlying medical problem, you'll want to go beyond the medical community to get help and relief.

Self-Help and Support Groups

Those of us who are carers have found self-help and support groups a valuable source of comfort, advice, and understanding. Among other things, sharing experiences provides a safety valve for pent-up anger and frustration.

I need someone out there who will listen to me and not say, 'But they're old, they need you.' I already know that. I have eighty-two-year-old parents; my father is in a nursing home getting along pretty well, but my mother is another story which would take too long to tell. I feel sometimes as if I'm handling things pretty well, but some days I want to pack my suitcase and leave forever! [a woman in her fifties]

These groups offer a supportive and non-judgmental atmosphere where members can openly express their innermost fears, discuss problems, and share coping skills. Joint problem solving is far better than what most of us can do on our own, especially because it's often difficult to keep a perspective on problems when you're alone.

For the first time, only recently, after attending a self-help group, I was able to really hear my daughter when she offered to come home and stay with her father for a week or two so I could get away. [a sixty-six-year-old woman]

Members share their knowledge of community resources and services. New members often say, 'It's great to learn I'm not alone. All of you understand what I'm going through.'

In Britain, the Association of Carers (see Organizations) has a central office which offers help and advice and above all will put carers in touch with local groups. Anyone needing contact with others in the same position should make every effort to attend local meetings, or, at the very least, keep in telephone contact with the group. Members can help each other out in crises or on a regular basis.

Anyone caring at home for an old person or for someone with a disability should be in touch with her Social Services Department. Social workers ought to be able to arrange for home helps – though local government cuts may have resulted in shorter hours of help being available than in the past; they can also arrange for the loan or supply of disability aids, adaptations to the home (ramps, handrails, bathing aids, etc.). Many carers and the people they care for don't know about the range of help offered locally, and struggle on without services and equipment that would make life a great deal easier for both. Over-stretched social work departments are unfortunately often unable to go out and seek the people who need their help, so it is up to the carer and her GP to ensure that they are receiving all the support to which they are entitled. No one pretends that the installation of a wheelchair ramp or a bath rail will solve all the carer's problems, but anything that makes life a little easier is worth asking for.

Local women's organizations and churches are often sources of volunteer help – for the single-handed carer someone able to take over her job one evening a week while she gets out of the house may be a sanity-saver.

Planning Ahead

Ideally, families should plan ahead for various crises before they actually happen. Even though you can't anticipate everything, everyone in the family should have a turn to voice her or his feelings without the pressure of an imminent emergency. It is best to do this when your parents are still living active, independent lives, and are in relatively good health. Preplanning takes effort and thought on the part of everyone in the family, but can prevent irreversible or long-lasting errors of judgment, such as selling a house or furniture in the midst of a crisis and regretting it later. Though sisters and brothers who live far away can be part of the dialogue through phone calls or letters, it's best when a whole family can get together.

My brothers and I sat down one night with our mother and decided who would do what to care for her. My two brothers and I have been sharing the care of our mother for several years now. Mother is eighty-five and lives in a retirement estate that is convenient to all of us. I do her food and clothes shopping and the washing, and sometimes my sisters-in-law help me. One brother handles the financial matters, pays the bills and so on, and the other brother takes her to the doctor, gets her medicines, and watches over her health. My brothers and I and our spouses meet for dinner once a week and then visit our mother. We all enjoy getting together – it keeps us close as a family. Mother enjoys having us all as guests once a week. So far it's worked out well for us. [a fifty-eight-year-old woman]

Of course, preplanning doesn't mean making firm promises that can't be kept. Sometimes out of love and with the best intentions, we say, 'I'll never put you in a home', or announce some other 'never' regarding something we have no control over. These 'nevers' may come back to haunt us. Since nobody has a crystal ball, none of us knows what the family situation will be in several years or even several months. Nevertheless, we can try to plan for a range of contingencies.

Planning discussions should be open and loving, with no secret pacts between family members. Unfortunately, even talking about caring for a parent can cause hard feelings and bitterness among brothers and sisters. If your family meetings deteriorate into fighting and recrimination, or if it has always been difficult for your family to communicate well, you may want to ask a third party, such as a social worker or member of the clergy, to join you. This person should be someone everyone respects and will listen to. It is ideal if she or he has had experience with the problems you are discussing. An understanding outsider can dispel family hostility, keep the discussion going in a productive way, and allow everyone to voice feelings and opinions.

Preplanning is easier to write and talk about than to put into practice because most people do not want to discuss growing old or getting sick. When parents are healthy and leading active lives, we may feel uncomfortable bringing up what we think of as a morbid subject. Try putting it this way: 'Mum and Dad, we hope that you have many more healthy years. We'd like to talk together about what could happen in the future and ask what you would like us to do in the event of disability or illness. Do you have any plans that you'd like to discuss with us? We want to do what is best and what you think would be right for you.' Parents may be thankful that you took the initiative.

HELPING PEOPLE WE CARE FOR TO MANAGE MONEY

Whether or not any long-range planning has been done, there may come a time when an ill or confused person is managing financial affairs so poorly that it becomes necessary to intervene. Deciding when this should happen may not be easy. Some people live their entire lives missing appointments, losing keys, and paying bills only after they get threatening notices. Nearly everyone occasionally forgets a meeting, gets locked out, neglects a bill, or leaves the burner on under the kettle. However, a developing pattern of such habits in someone who has not previously had them is a sign of trouble. People who suffer from disorientation, memory loss, or other conditions that make their handling of money erratic and unreliable may dissipate assets, become victim to frauds and swindles, or be threatened with eviction or have their electricity supply turned off. Families or other caregivers must step in to prevent such a person from harming himself or herself further.

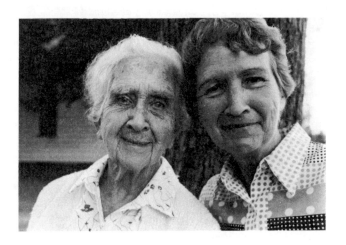

I hadn't heard from my aunt for some time, so I tried to phone her. I found she'd been cut off. She hadn't answered letters. So I decided to visit her – she lives hundreds of miles away. I was terribly shocked when she finally let me in after I'd rung the bell, hammered on the door, and she eventually recognized my voice. She was living in filth and chaos. The flat was full of old papers, rotting food and empty tins. She'd always been an independent person and she just wouldn't admit that she needed my help. However, I did persuade her to let me deal with the bills that had piled up – she actually had quite a bit of money in the bank, more than enough to meet them and get her phone re-connected. I cleaned and tidied the place, and talked to a neighbour who agreed to keep an eye on her, despite previous rejections of offers of help. And I arranged for a home help to come in twice a week. Actually I really believe she'd be better off in a residential home. But I don't think anyone has the right to force an old person to relinquish her 'independence'. Her doctor knows about her, so do the social services – so if things get too bad, someone will be around to take action. I just can't take responsibility at this distance and with a family and job to think of. But that doesn't stop me worrying and feeling a bit guilty. [a fifty-four-year-old woman]

It is important not to do more than the situation really requires. A person who needs help with paying rent or utility bills may still be perfectly capable of shopping and paying for her or his own groceries and toiletries. Your help should be designed to recognize and support a person's abilities as well as compensate for weaknesses.

If the person being cared for should become mentally incompetent, the caregiver can act in her or his name if a 'power of attorney' has been set up in advance.

Remember that in some cases confusion and memory problems may be reversible, so assistance may not have to be permanent.

If a person is certified by her or his doctor as being incapable because of mental disorder of administering their assets and their property, the Court of Protection can take control of them for her or him. Anyone can apply to the court for appointment as 'receiver' of the property, although the court gives preference to close relatives. Being a 'receiver' is rather like being a 'trustee', and the mentally infirm person loses almost all control over his property and affairs. MIND (see Organizations) can suggest suitable reading and will offer advice through their legal officer.

If you plan to have a parent or other infirm relative move in with you, consider the financial implications.

Attendance allowance is payable to people who are severely disabled, whether physically or mentally, and require a lot of care. A higher rate is payable to someone who is so disabled that for at least six months he or she has required full-time supervision. To qualify for the lower rate, the person must need either constant day-time *or* constant night-time care. Ask for the combined leaflet and claim form NI 205 at the local social security office or Citizens' Advice Bureau.

Invalid care allowance is payable to people of working age who cannot work because they have to stay at home to look after a severely disabled person. (Until quite recently married women did not qualify for this, as they were deemed to be at home anyway!) Ask for leaflet NI 212 if you think that you qualify – there's an 'earnings rule' that means that you can earn a small weekly sum by working outside the home (up to £12 in 1988) and still qualify.

Mobility allowance is available for people under sixty-six who are unable, or virtually unable, to walk because of physical disability. Anyone aged sixty-five when she claims has to prove that she could have qualified before that age. Once entitled, the person can receive the allowance up to age seventy-five if the conditions remain the same. Leaflet NI 211 is the one to ask for, together with leaflet NI 1243, which deals with direct payment of the allowance to a bank or building society account. The aim behind this allowance is to enable people unable to walk to pay for transport. It is tax-free.

The *Motability* scheme is run by a voluntary organization set up to enable recipients of Mobility allowance to obtain a car. Further information from Motability, Boundary House, 91–93 Charterhouse Street, London EC1M 6BT (tel: 01-153 1221).

All the above schemes are additional to the Retirement Pension to which women sixty and over and men sixty-five and over are entitled. A number of leaflets cover pensions information – NP 32 is general, NP 32B (covers married women) and FB6 (*Retiring?*) are basic. An additional retirement pension for people over eighty is payable to those who are not receiving a National Insurance retirement pension or whose benefit is less than £24.75 a week (1988 figures). Information: leaflet NI 184.

The general leaflet NP 32 gives up-to-date information on the state earnings-related pension scheme, which is being gradually modified. It will probably not apply to an elderly person who has retired some time ago, so the person you are caring for is unlikely to be affected. She may, however, have been employed before 1948, when the present pension system was introduced, and *National Insurance Contributions and Retirement Pensions Up to 1948*, an Age Concern factsheet (No. 20), explains her position (see Age Concern leaflets and factsheets, Organizations). Those who have retired more recently should get Age Concern factsheet No. 22 – *National Insurance Contributions and Retirement Pensions 1975 Onwards*.

People being cared for 'in the community' – that means, probably, being cared for by a female relative – are as entitled as any other elderly persons to the various services and concessions available to senior citizens – see page 262. As a carer, your problem may be to get them to a day-care centre, the hairdresser offering cheap rates, and the outings offered by voluntary organizations. Here your local branch of Age Concern (sometimes called the Old People's Welfare Committee) can offer help.

One concession that is particularly valuable to *carers* is known as Respite Care. Your first inquiry should be at the local Social Services Department, which should be running a scheme which enables carers to take a break or a holiday while the person they're caring for is offered a bed in a residential home. Unfortunately there are waiting lists, so try to apply well in advance; and, as in every other area of social services provision, central government cuts have made inroads into what local authorities can provide. A residential home offers general supervision, but not actual nursing. The Association of Crossroads Care Attendant Schemes (see Organizations) may advise. Their schemes operate in over seventy areas.

Some voluntary organizations are associated with nursing homes and residential homes that offer short breaks to carers. The Citizens' Advice Bureau will have a list of local and national voluntary organizations, as will the local Council for Voluntary Service or Age Concern. You could also look in the Yellow Pages of the telephone directory under *Nurses and Nursing* or *Residential and Retirement Homes*. Cancer sufferers and those who care for them are offered respite care in some nursing homes run by Marie Curie Cancer Care. Write with self-addressed, stamped envelope to 28 Belgrave Square, London SW1.

A computerized booking system that links elderly or disabled people with vacancies in around five hundred private homes is offered by Care Home Holidays. Write for a brochure to Care Home Holidays Ltd, Wern Manor, Porthmadog, Gwynedd LL49 9SH. And there's a voluntary agency, Counsel and Care for the Elderly, 131 Middlesex Street, London E1 7IE which is a good source of information about homes they've inspected, as is Grace Link, Upper Chambers, 7 Derby Street, Leek, Staffs. Of course any privately-run home is going to be costly, but to some carers it may be worth doing without a holiday away from home themselves to pay for a week or two of care for their relative, while they get a much-needed break for relaxation.

Taking a Break (free to carers) is an excellent booklet with full information on day care, home nurses and facilities available to relieve pressure on carers. One chapter, 'Your Concerns About Taking a Break', helps carers cope with feelings of guilt about getting away from their responsibilities for a while. Published by the Health Education Authority with the King's Fund, it's available from Taking a Break, Newcastle-Upon-Tyne NE85 2AQ.

Working for Change

Since 1979 there's been a gradual shifting of responsibility from central and local government to the so-called 'community'. In the guise of running down bleak and punitive institutions, making the care of the elderly and disabled people more humane, with 'the family' taking responsibility for its members, in sickness as in health, many old people as well as those suffering from mental illness have been denied admission to, or discharged from, institutional care. No one would defend the sort of conditions that the media and court cases have exposed, where old or mentally-frail people are ill-treated or neglected, but government has not taken real responsibility for improving these conditions. It has preferred to return to 'Victorian' values in care, knowing that, somehow or other, the majority of relatives (usually women) will have to shoulder the burden.

As we've seen earlier (pp. 263–4) it's only through united political action that the system can be changed. The Association of Carers (see Organizations) not only presses for help in relieving individual cases of distress and hardship, but is beginning to form a powerful lobby on behalf of carers and the cared-for.

Anyone with a family member to look after should contact the Association, contact her MP and make her voice heard. Our population is ageing – we ourselves will need care in our later years. Do we want to become burdens on our own families or suffer the indignity of total dependence on others?

NOTES

[1]National Center for Health Services Research, 1982 survey, quoted in the Older Women's League press release 'Family Caregivers – A Fact Sheet', November 1986.

[2]Elinor Polansky, 'Take Him Home, Mrs Smith'. *Healthright*, Vol. II, No. 2, Winter 1975–6.

[3]Alfred P. Fengler and Nancy Goodrich, 'Wives of Elderly Disabled Men: The Hidden Patients'. *Gerontologist*, Vol. 19, No. 2, 1979, p. 178.

[4]Vanda Colman et al., *Till Death Do Us Part: Caregiving Wives of Severely Disabled Husbands*. Older Women's League, Washington, DC. Grey Paper #7, 1982, p. 4.

[5]Linda Crossman et al., 'Older Women Caring for Disabled Spouses: A Model for Supportive Services'. *Gerontologist*, Vol. 5, 1981, p. 466.

[6]Fengler, op. cit., p. 182.

[7]B. Soldo, 'The Dependency Squeeze on Middle-aged Women'. Paper presented at the meeting of the Secretary's Advisory Committee on Rights and Responsibilities of Women, US Department of HHS, 1980.

[8]Sharon Johnson, 'The Dilemma of the Dutiful Daughter'. *Working Woman*, August 1982, p. 66.

[9]Amy Horowitz, 'Sons and Daughters as Caregivers to Older Parents: Differences of Role Performance and Consequences', pp. 12–16. Paper presented at the 34th annual scientific meeting of the Gerontological Society of America, Toronto, Canada, November 1981 (EDRS ED 216–52).

[10]'Owls Fly to Help'. *OWL Observer*, May–June 1985.

[11]National Center for Health Services Research, op. cit.

BOOKS AND PUBLICATIONS

Dr Chris Phillipson and Patricia Strang, *Health Education and Older People: The Role of Paid Carers*. Newcastle: University of Keele, 1984.

Association of Carers, *Who Cares?* (See Organizations.)

Equal Opportunities Commission 1984, *Carers and Services: A Comparison of Men and Women Caring for Dependent Elderly People*.

Equal Opportunities Commission 1980, *The Experience of Caring for Elderly and Handicapped Dependants*. Survey Report.

Isobel Allen, *Short Stay Residential Care of the Elderly*. London: Policy Studies Institute, 1983.

Melanie Henwood and Malcolm Wicks, *The Forgotten Army: Family Care and Elderly People*. London: Family Policy Studies Centre, December 1984. Briefing paper.

Anna Briggs and Judith Oliver, *Caring: Experiences of Looking After Disabled Relatives*. London: Routledge & Kegan Paul, 1985.

M. Keith Thompson, *Caring for an Elderly Relative: A Guide to Home Care*. London: Macdonald Optima, 1986.

16
Problems in the Medical Care System

The NHS – How We Feel

Women now in their sixties and seventies remember what 'health care' was like before 1948. Many worry that the bad old days may return.

When I was little, if any of us fell ill we were looked after at home – you had to be very bad to be sent to hospital. Mother paid half-a-crown a week into some club and that was supposed to meet medical bills. Doctors charged a bob or two a visit, and most families we knew put off calling the doctor as long as possible. [a seventy-three-year-old woman]

Whatever its faults and failings, the NHS has transformed our lives. Before the NHS came in, you had to be quite well off to get proper medical attention. Hospitals were for the poor and they were run like charities. I was put into hospital when I was seven, and visitors were allowed only once a week. I felt I'd been deserted. Now my grandson has had to spend a week in hospital and his mother was allowed to 'room in' with him all the time. What a difference! [a sixty-eight-year-old woman]

Here are the opinions and experiences of some younger women:

I grew up with the NHS, and I'd defend it to the death. We have an excellent Health Centre near us, with full services from the doctors, nurses, health visitors, chiropodists, the full team. The doctors really care about their patients. They don't get on their high horses if you ask questions and if they're not sure about a diagnosis they don't hesitate to refer you to a consultant. There's always one Health Centre doctor on duty, so they don't use a deputizing service in an out-of-hours emergency – in fact if you're registered at this Health Centre you gradually get to know all the doctors, so there's real continuity. [a fifty-two-year-old woman]

The NHS is A Good Thing, but my experience as a hospital outpatient isn't good. They make appointments for lots of people at the same time, so however early you

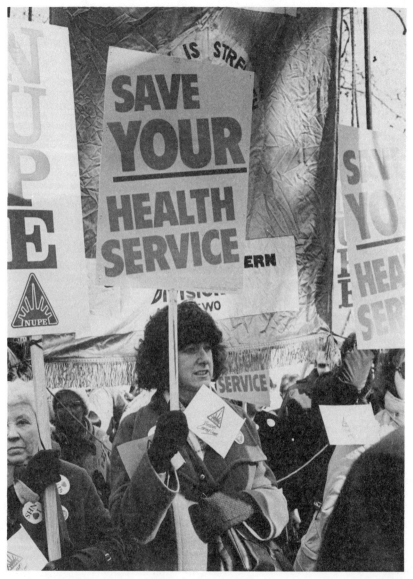

*arrive you may have to wait for hours. My consultant (when I see him) often arrives
late, and I wonder whether he's been involved in an emergency or whether he just
doesn't bother to be on time. Actually I don't see him on every visit, and I find myself
explaining to yet another doctor what my symptoms are. They often don't seem to read
the notes.* [a forty-nine-year-old woman]

My doctor is awful. Whatever the problem, he just seems to dish out pills. I can't change because his is a one-man practice in the village, and the nearest Health Centre is miles away. Fortunately I'm seldom ill – I don't know what I'd do if I was. [a fifty-two-year-old woman]

My outstanding memory of hospital is the wonderful care I had from a night sister. I was in severe pain after a spinal operation and the nights seemed endless. But she gave me support and comfort, drugs when I needed them, and all sorts of little adjustments to my bed and my position that made a difference. I'm so angry that someone like that can be so badly paid by the NHS – she did quite as much for me as a top consultant! [a fifty-year-old woman]

I feel that my woman doctor is a friend. She listens. It's worth waiting for a long time after your appointment is due because you know she's probably giving a lot of time to the patients before me, as she does to me. [a forty-three-year-old woman]

My one experience of going private was interesting. I saw the same consultant as I'd seen at the clinic. There he'd been brusque and apparently uninterested. When I saw him in Harley Street he gave me plenty of time, examined me thoroughly, explained my symptoms and treated me like an intelligent being. It's shocking that the same man can behave so differently in outpatients and in his consulting room. [a sixty-one-year-old woman]

These very mixed experiences of the National Health Service are typical of our relationship with this most popular of the provisions of the (much eroded) Welfare State. The Patients Association (see Organizations) and the many voluntary bodies concerned with different disabilities, conditions, and illnesses are campaigning to see that our good experiences of the NHS become the norm, and that the slide into private medicine, where the treatment you get depends on the size of your bank balance, is stopped in its tracks. And for once, the medical establishment is on our side.

Throughout the 1980s whenever the National Health Service has been under threat or actually under attack, people of every political persuasion have united in defence of the system. It's seen as the greatest achievement of the Welfare State, and, in its early days, the envy of the rest of the world. Despite the erosion of benefits and all the problems of financing and staffing, hospital waiting lists, and general disillusionment with the government's intentions, a majority of the population still makes use of the NHS, and those old enough look back in horror at the bad old days before its existence.

But the system certainly is not what it used to be in the fifties and sixties – various free services have been replaced by partial payments by the consumer for appliances, prostheses and other necessities, for instance. Although the government claims to be spending more on health than ever before, the consumer experiences lengthening waiting lists, premature discharge from hospital, industrial action by health workers who see their standard of living deteriorating, while any increase in salary scales is offset in cuts in patients' services.

In this chapter we can't attempt to outline the whole range of NHS administration and services (particularly as the whole system may be in the process of change). No one can predict, at the time of writing, what the future of the NHS will be.

In February 1989, the government published its White Paper *Putting Patients First*. This programme, seen almost universally as a step on the road to partial privatization of the National Health Service, was presented as a scheme which would offer patients a better service at less cost to the Exchequer, and would give us a freedom of choice about our treatment that had been hitherto lacking.

The following month 100 per cent of the members of the council of the British Medical Association voted down the proposals and decided to mount a campaign against them. Opinion polls had shown similar concern in the general population about what was primarily seen as a cost-cutting exercise; and by-election results, in which the Conservatives appeared to have lost ground, in part because of the threat to the NHS, confirmed the hostility of ordinary people to the proposals.

In these circumstances it's impossible to predict to what extent the White Paper proposals will be implemented, and when. They are, in any case, couched in vague terms and nothing has since been added which really clarifies the situation. However, the proposals can be summarized as follows:

- Self-governing trusts to run some (possibly all?) NHS hospitals independent of district health authorities. These would employ their own staff and negotiate their own rates of pay.
- Patients could opt for treatment in other districts or in the private sector, with 'exchange payments'.
- Tax relief for pensioners taking out private health insurance (this may be implemented in 1990).
- Large GP practices to be allowed to draw up their own budgets, out of which hospital care for patients would have to be 'bought'.
- Health authorities to be reorganized on the model of company boards of directors, local authorities no longer being represented.
- Government funding to be re-allocated, thus ending existing discrimination against the South East.

- Hospitals to be fully computerized under a 'resource management initiative' in which doctors and nurses would take responsibility for budgeting.
- Audit controls to be imposed on doctors, transferring overall responsibility to the Audit Commission, which would see they offered 'value for money'.
- Prescription costs to be monitored with the aim of reducing the drugs bills.
- Changes in consultants' contracts and a new system of merit pay awards.
- One hundred new consultants to be appointed.

The main objections to these proposals are that local, elected, representatives would no longer have any say in the running of local services; and that in any budget system a GP could either refuse to accept a patient whose drugs or hospital bills were likely to eat too deeply into his allowable funds, or might prescribe the cheapest, rather than the most effective treatment, in order to keep within his cash limits. But the whole scheme, as BMA Chairperson Dr John Marks is reported as saying (the *Guardian*, 2 March 1989), would put the clock back to the time when patients were hunted by doctors anxious to increase their income; and doctors who increased their lists would inevitably have less time for individual patients. There would be one service for the rich and articulate, and quite a different one for the poor, unsure about their entitlements and rights. Older people needing frequent care and prescriptions could be 'too expensive' for doctors' budgets.

FUNDING OF THE NHS

Despite government claims that funding of the National Heath Service increases year by year, our experiences as consumers seem to belie these pronouncements. The paradox is that, largely as a result of our improved longevity owing to past improvements in health care, more of us are in greater need of the health services; and as a result of great technological advances more and better treatments are available. Both factors mean that the National Health Service needs far more money in real terms than ever before – and as we enter the 1990s it isn't getting it. Tax cuts and concessions to the well-off mean that there is less money for the NHS, and if the proposals in the 1989 White Paper are passed in Parliament, a two-tier system, one for the rich and one for the poor, will make things even worse.

Community Health Councils

Under the pre-1989 system, each Health District in England and Wales has responsibility for setting up a Community Health Council. Half the CHC's members are appointed by the local authority, one-third by voluntary organizations and the rest by the Regional Health Authority. There seems to be no place for the CHC in the government's reorganization plans. The CHC's job was to assess the adequacy of the local health services and comment on plans for future development. As long as it lasts the CHC is our watchdog and we should make use of it, but like every other aspect of the Health Service it may be under threat.

Family Practitioner Committees, who were responsible for the planning and general management of family practitioner services (doctors, dentists, pharmacists and opticians) in their area, also appear to be under threat. These committees would seem to have no place in the future, and it is not clear to whom complaints about doctors' services may be made. Perhaps now that the GP services may be partly 'privatized', the FPCs may take a different form.

Complaints about Hospital Services

This is another area in which the future is unclear, with the proposed abolition of the District Health Authorities. Formerly, an ultimate appeal could be made to the Health Service Commissioner (Ombudsman). A leaflet *The Health Service Ombudsman for England* should be available at a Citizens' Advice Bureau. For addresses of Health Service Commissioners for Wales and Scotland, consult *Guide to the Social Services* (see below).

Complaints about Doctors

When a complaint was concerned with the clinical judgment of a hospital doctor and the person complaining was dissatisfied with the health authority's reply she could ask for the complaint to be referred to the Regional Medical Officer. It is not yet clear how this would apply in the future. The Health Department's leaflet *Comments, suggestions and complaints about your stay in hospital*, which may need updating, explains the procedures.

Costs and Charges

The National Health Service is available to everyone who lives in Great Britain. The government claims that even when the NHS is reorganized, this will still remain. Visitors from overseas are not covered unless there is a reciprocal arrangement with the health care authorities in their own countries. Most NHS provision remains free, but the principal exceptions are as follows:

- cost of attending a person involved in a road traffic accident and for hospital treatment resulting from a road traffic accident

- cost of private accommodation and treatment in an NHS hospital
- cost of an 'amenity bed' or single room in an NHS hospital
- provision of domestic help or certain aids by the local authority when the patient has the ability to contribute to the cost
- maintenance and incidental costs of persons leaving hospital to go to daytime work while still receiving treatment and accommodation
- prescription drugs or appliances (except for the young and people of pensionable age)
- cost of dentures and spectacles
- cost of dental treatment
- cost of repair or replacement of appliances, etc., broken through negligence

Anyone receiving 'Income Support' may be exempted from some of the above charges.

OPTICAL SERVICES

Eye tests are available from opticians – free in 1988, but no longer free except for children and those on Income Support. Prescriptions may be made up by any optician. The optician may refer a patient to the hospital ophthalmic service if necessary.

DENTAL SERVICES

Anyone wanting to consult a dentist must make sure that before treatment begins she will be receiving it under the NHS. Dental checkups are no longer free, except to claimants in certain groups. Many dentists take private as well as NHS patients. Most adults now have to pay part of the cost of NHS treatment – unless they are expectant mothers, have had a baby in the previous twelve months or are on Income Support. Leaflet D11, from Citizens' Advice Bureaux or public libraries, explains the system.

PRESCRIPTIONS

At the time of writing adults below pensionable age and children over sixteen have to pay for part of the cost of prescription medicines and appliances, unless they are receiving Income Support or Family Credit, are pregnant or have a baby of less than twelve months or are war or service pensioners. Anyone requiring regular items under prescription can purchase a pre-payment certificate costing (1988) £12.50 for four months, £35.00 for a year. An explanatory leaflet is available at large post offices, chemists and doctors' surgeries – ask for form P11.

HEALTH VISITORS AND DISTRICT NURSES

Health Visitors offer health education, advice and support to people of all ages in the community. They work closely with GPs, district nurses and other members of the Primary Health Care team. They are usually based in Health Centres or in a GP's surgery. Much of their work concerns babies and young children and the elderly.

District Nurses are employed by the Health Authority and provide skilled nursing care at the homes of patients in their locality. They are referred to patients by their doctors. Anyone nursing a relative at home should ask for this service to be provided – even if visits can be made only a few times a week for bathing, etc.

DAY CARE CENTRES

In some areas day care centres cater for older or disabled people who are sufficiently mobile to attend them. However, this service is underfunded, and transport to and from the centres may be inadequate. Where the facility exists, it can represent a respite for the carer. The local Social Services department should be approached, if day care seems appropriate.

CHIROPODY

There is a free service for the elderly, expectant mothers, and handicapped people. Ask at the Health Centre or GP's surgery – treatment is provided in clinics or in the patient's home. Non-eligible people must pay for treatment by private chiropodists.

The Private Sector

Most people register with a General Practitioner and expect to get their 'primary care' through her or him. The GP can refer patients to hospital consultants under the NHS, and any treatment or surgery is free of charge, as is hospital accommodation. Problems arise, however, when 'non-urgent' consultations and treatments are suggested. As everyone knows, the result can be a wait of months or possibly years, and meanwhile the patient suffers inconvenience, disability and often, severe pain.

Before considering 'going private' in these circumstances (an option not open to the majority, in any case), it's worth finding out whether treatment under the NHS is available in an area further from home. The College of Health (see Organizations) publishes information about hospitals with shorter-

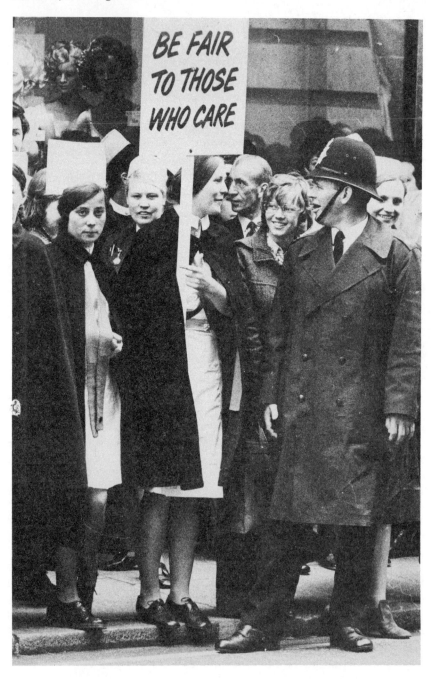

than-average waiting lists. Your doctor may be able to suggest where to go. Of course it can be disrupting and inconvenient for visitors if you're in hospital far from home and it may be hard for you to have no or few visitors, but if this speeds things up for you, you must decide what the trade-offs are and what is important to you.

As part of its privatization drive, the government is keen to encourage those who can afford it to shift to the private sector. Few people can afford the huge cost of surgery and a stay in a private hospital for a major operation, but increasing numbers are joining the various private health insurance schemes which involve regular payments and in return offer cover for private consultations, treatment, surgery, hospital stays and other medical expenses. Depending on the person's age and medical history, payments in the event of illness or surgery cover all or part of the cost.

Is it worth joining a scheme? The advantages of private treatment are a) you can see the consultant of your or your GP's choice; b) you can make appointments to suit your convenience; c) you can have non-urgent treatment at a hospital or at a time chosen by you; d) you can have a private hospital room or one shared with perhaps one other person; but the main reason for choosing private treatment is that you can 'jump the NHS queue'. This, of course, has an erosive effect on the NHS: as an increasing number of people join private plans, privatization of the NHS is hastened.

Whether this is ethical or not depends on the way you see things. The more people opt out, the more medical and other services are directed away from the NHS. If you feel that it's up to everyone who believes in the NHS to stick by it, at the same time working through local organizations and local pressure as well as through the ballot box to improve the service, you'll resist the pressure to go private, even if you can afford it. You'll be aware that jumping the queue, as a private patient, will probably mean that an NHS patient has to wait even longer for treatment. Of course it's not easy, if you're in great pain and need a hip replacement, and you have the funds to pay for treatment, to wait your turn. But most people just don't have that option. And the good news is that, if there's a real emergency (as defined by doctors, of course) the NHS still provides the best of all possible treatments. (In fact, it sometimes happens that a private hospital can't cope with serious conditions and shifts patients to an NHS hospital for the special care and expertise available only from that hospital.)

It may not be possible to get the benefits from private health insurance if you are elderly, or have a 'bad' medical history, but if you want to find out about costs and provision of services the following are the three major private medical health insurance organizations:

• The British United Provident Association (BUPA)

- Private Patients Plan (PPP)
- Western Provident Association

For addresses see Organizations.

Changing Your Doctor

You may not be in a position to make use of private health care or may not wish to do so. But you may be dissatisfied with your present GP for a number of reasons – perhaps you'd prefer to be registered with a woman doctor, or the GP may treat you brusquely, or you just don't 'get on'. Many women don't realize that they do have a choice (though in some rural districts this may be limited). In most practices there's at least one woman doctor. You can ask to see her if you feel embarrassed about a particular problem being dealt with by the male doctor you're registered with. But if you're dissatisfied with the treatment you've received in the practice generally, you may register with another doctor or practice (providing they will accept you) without confronting your present GP if you'd prefer not to. You may either obtain your present GP's consent, or send your medical card to the Family Practitioner Committee for your area (if it still exists) stating that you wish to transfer to another doctor. It's necessary to make sure that the new doctor agrees to accept you on her or his list, of course, especially if the White Paper plans go ahead – there may be problems if your drugs or treatment bite too far into their budget. If you don't nominate the new GP, you will be entitled to choose one fourteen days after the FPC has received your card. GPs, too, have the right to ask for your removal from their list at seven days' notice. Perhaps this will happen more often if in the future a GP is on a budget. If you can't find a doctor willing to put you on her or his list, as of 1988–9 the FPC could assign you to a doctor. The FPC's address is available at a main post office or public library if you can't find it in the telephone directory. If a new system applies, machinery for such changes will have to be provided.

EMERGENCY TREATMENT

If you're away from home, or aren't yet registered with a GP, any available NHS doctor is obliged to treat you in case of accident or emergency.

MENTAL ILLNESS

The NHS is responsible for mental health services just as it is for other health problems. A GP who believes that a patient needs investigation and treatment can refer her to the psychiatric department of a general hospital or to a psychiatric hospital.

I spent some weeks in a psychiatric ward. I've never had such a terrible experience! In the end I discharged myself, because I was getting no real treatment, no exercise, lousy food, no occupational therapy. I've had more constructive help with my problems from my women friends. [a fifty-five-year-old woman]

Most patients who are admitted to psychiatric units go voluntarily – 'informal admission'. But for a minority who are unwilling or unable to accept care and treatment the Mental Health Act of 1983 provides for compulsory admission and detention, based on two medical recommendations – one normally being a doctor who knows the patient, the other a specialist. The period of detention can be up to twenty-eight days. In an emergency a patient can be admitted for seventy-two hours on one medical application (this is popularly known as 'sectioning') but if within the seventy-two hours a second medical opinion is added, the period of compulsion is extended to twenty-eight days. For full information about compulsory detention under the Mental Health Act, discharge and patients' rights, see pages 72–7 of *Guide to the Social Services*, and/or contact MIND (see Organizations).

BOOKS AND PUBLICATIONS

Family Welfare Association, *Guide to the Social Services*.

The Boston Women's Health Book Collective, *The New Our Bodies, Ourselves*. London: Penguin, 1989.

David Widgery, *The National Health – a Radical Perspective*. London: The Hogarth Press, 1988.

Health Education Authority, *Health and Older People: Attitudes Towards Health in Older Age and Towards Caring for Older People*. Free leaflet.

Age Concern, *Your Rights*. Booklet revised annually – telephone Age Concern for details.

College of Health, *Guide to Hospital Waiting Lists*, 1989. Regularly updated list of hospitals where there is little or no delay in admission.

17
Residential and Nursing Homes

This chapter assumes that dignity, quality health care, and control over one's own life are basic human rights. This chapter also assumes that a residential or nursing home can be a good choice for some individuals and their caregivers. One's own or a family member's home can be more isolating than a nursing home.

That night I tossed and turned and I couldn't sleep. I felt so bad that my daughter couldn't go out with her husband because they didn't want to leave me alone. So I made up my mind that I would go into a home. And they tried to talk me out of it, but I said, 'In a home I'll be with people my own age and we'll have things to talk about together.' So, I've been here almost four years and I haven't been sorry. [a woman in her nineties]

My mother benefited from the mental stimulation of being surrounded by a lot of different people and activities which could never have been achieved in her own home. She was able to make new friends she never would have met had she lived alone in her flat with a series of hired caregivers. I am sure the quality of her life during those years, although by no means ideal, was much better than it had been in those lonely and sick years before her collapse.[1]

After my husband had a devastating stroke, everything in my life other than that stopped. He was in hospitals, then in nursing homes, and then I took him home against everybody's advice. I felt like I was retired from life. It seemed as though the world deserted us. I used to say, 'I'll never put my husband in an institution again. Home is the best place for him.' But I was wrong. I really was wrong because there was very little contact with others and no diversions for him at home. [a woman in her sixties]

One reason so many of us react negatively to 'homes' is that serious problems *do* exist in some. Even 'better' homes that provide a clean, safe environment and competent basic medical services may infantilize and dehumanize residents, ignoring their needs and desires for choice, control, privacy, and meaningful lives. All of these problems are part of our society's tendency to write off older people and people with disabilities, whether or not they reside in nursing homes.

The solution to these problems lies in action. Successful nursing home placement, care, and reform require information, planning, and maximum consumer/family involvement; in other words, a sense of control.

It's never too late – or too early – to start learning about nursing homes. Although only 5 per cent of people over sixty-five are in institutions[2] we must recognize that alternatives to family-based care are essential. In the rapidly growing over-eighty-five age-group nearly 25 per cent require care. Negative attitudes only reinforce the imperfections of those alternatives and paralyse our ability to help ourselves.

It is particularly important for women to understand as much as possible about nursing and residential homes. Women outnumber men as nursing home residents, as primary caregivers who may help others to make nursing home decisions and adjustments, and as workers in the homes. Most (71 per cent) nursing home residents in the US are women, and the percentages increase by age-group: 6 per cent of all residents are women under sixty-five; 10 per cent are women sixty-five to seventy-four; 26 per cent are women seventy-five to eighty-four; 29 per cent are women over eighty-five.[3]

Furthermore, the number of poor older women is growing rapidly. Their poverty (often a lifetime's worth) increases their chances of poor health and of a need for long-term care. We must stretch the feminist ideals of empowerment, action, hope, co-operation, and respect to them – to us.

Residential or Nursing Home?

In the UK most homes for elderly people are of the residential type. An old or disabled person requiring ongoing medical care and nursing is not generally accepted into a residential home, nor is able to stay there if she becomes really infirm. She then has to move either to a nursing home (in the private sector) or to hospital, probably in a 'geriatric' ward.

With the ever-increasing number of older people in the community, and the inability of many local authorities to expand their services because of financial constraints, private enterprise has leapt in to fill the gap, mostly in the provision of *residential* homes. Throughout the 1970s periodic media reports of bad conditions in both council-run and private homes led to the legislation which now requires local authorities to register and regularly inspect all the residential and nursing homes in their area. Guidelines for acceptable practice have been issued, and the authorities are empowered to close down homes that don't meet basic requirements. However, in the mid-1980s, when these

Questions to keep in mind as you determine whether you – or a family member or friend – need residential care:

What kinds of services are needed and how many are available in your community? Health Visitor care, home helps, personal care, district nurses, Meals on Wheels, communal meals, and respite care are some of the services to look for. However, it is usually difficult to find quality in-home assistance, especially for evenings, nights, and weekends. Most workers do their best, but their salaries, benefits, professional prestige, training, and supervision are often inadequate. Consider what you would do if helpers left, arrived late, got sick, or went on holiday.

What can you afford? Will National Insurance pay for the home care you need? Are there other allowances available on a sliding fee scale?

What financial or other assistance can your family, friends, and neighbours realistically provide? The answer should be fair to both caregivers and the people they're helping. An exhausted caregiver helps no one.

What is your housing situation? If you are living in a high-crime area, or if your home needs numerous or extensive repairs, or if you simply feel isolated, a move of some sort may be wise. Again, a residential home is only one option to consider if you decide you should change your living situation. It's hard to move from a home you love; but the further in advance you can plan for it, the better you will be able to cope.

powers were supposedly in place, a series of media articles and TV documentaries showed that all was by no means well. Old people were still being poorly fed, neglected, or actually exposed to physical abuse in some of the homes that had apparently been passed as adequate by the inspectors.

Part of the problem is the system of social security benefits. Obviously the great majority of old people are unable to find the large fees charged by private nursing or residential homes. Social security, therefore, contributes to the fees on a sliding scale which means that if the resident's capital is less than a specified amount, her costs are paid to the home from her income support benefit and pension, leaving her with a modest sum for 'pocket money'. It is clearly tempting for unscrupulous proprietors to take all they can get from social security and not return value for money: they can cut costs of staffing, food, laundry and amenities and add to their profits by pocketing the difference between the sums they actually receive and their outgoings.

When considering admittance to a residential or nursing home, therefore, it's crucial for the woman herself or her relatives to satisfy themselves that conditions are acceptable. Essential reading is the free leaflet issued by Age Concern – ask for Factsheet No. 29 *Finding Residential and Nursing Home Accommodation* and send a large stamped, self-addressed envelope (see Organizations). Age Concern also publishes a book *At Home in a Home* (see below). And in consultation with Help the Aged, an organization, Care Home Consultants, which has large numbers of private home proprietors as its members, has compiled a full directory of registered residential and nursing homes which it has inspected and graded (see below).

CHOOSING A HOME

1. Decide where the home should be. Near family (who may move) or friends, and in the locality you know? In a beautiful part of the country, with the danger of isolation?

2. What is available? Ask local Social Services for a list of registered homes – there may be a vacancy in one of their own.

   Counsel and Care for the Elderly can advise about homes they've inspected, as can GRACE (see Organizations). Find out about waiting lists.

3. Narrow down your choice to about three places. Visit each and check out their facilities in line with the suggestions on page 302.

4. Check finances. The Department of Social Security will subsidize the cost of residential or nursing home care through Income Support, provided your capital is less than £6,000 (1988 figure). Some local health authorities pay for beds in private *nursing* homes to which patients can be discharged from hospital, but this is rare. The official limits for residential home care fees in 1988 were £130 per week (£147 in London) so if your home costs more, you will have to pay the difference. The limits for elderly people in nursing homes were £185–£230 depending on degree of disability and location (see Age Concern's Factsheet No. 11: *Income Support for Residential Care and Nursing Homes*).

5. Find out what your chosen home's policy is if you fall ill. If you have to go into hospital, your room should be reserved for you unless you will definitely need full-time nursing in the future. A residential home should be able to cope with minor illnesses and disabilities, including incontinence.

Required reading the above may be, but nothing can be a substitute for a personal visit. The Centre for Policy on Ageing[4] suggests that a number of questions should be asked of staff and residents, including some about the suitability of the home for your or your relative's particular needs. Find out about:

- Activities and interests catered for
- Involvement with the local community
- Independence and freedom
- Number and quality of rules and regulations
- Degree of privacy
- Security for personal documents and possessions
- Medical care – can the resident have her own GP?
- How much personal furniture, etc. is allowed

And, of course, try to check just how much choice there is in diet, and whether fresh fruit and vegetables are regularly included in menus.

A Residential Homes checklist produced by the College of Health (see Organizations) will help make sure you've asked all the right questions.

The Centre for Policy on Ageing suggests very firmly that there should be a trial period of, say, six weeks before a resident should commit herself to a permanent stay.[5] This means that it would be unwise to sell or give up the tenancy of your home until you're quite sure you want to stay. If this causes financial problems, social security should help.

Although the quality of staff in a residential home is very important, qualified nurses aren't necessarily required, nor, indeed, are they always the best people to run these homes. 'Nurses tend to organize things on medical lines, and that can result in the greatest danger for old people – over-dependence. It's better for an old person to take two hours to dress herself, with someone pottering about while she's doing it, than to be dressed in ten minutes flat and then conducted to the lounge to sit inactive for the rest of the day.'[6]

As we've seen, most old people never need to go into a 'home', but some will need to move first into residential and then into nursing care. Others who have stayed at home as long as possible – making use of all the appropriate social services available to them through their local authority as well as the care of family and neighbours – may still have to be admitted to a nursing home or hospital ward.

Difficult Conditions in Nursing Homes

'Medicalization' is an unfortunate fact of life in nursing homes. Set up to be like hospitals – although they are called 'homes' – nursing homes' medical orientation encourages a narrow approach to residents' well-being. Loneliness, confusion, depression, and behaviour problems resulting from a lack of

RESIDENTIAL HOME RESIDENTS: THE EXPERTS ON QUALITY CARE

In *A Consumer Perspective on Quality Care: The Residents' Point of View*, published by the National Citizens' Coalition for Nursing Home Reform, residential home residents around the United States were asked to discuss and define quality care. The 457 participating residents said that choices in and control over their lives were the most important factors. They also pointed out the need for:

- Positive staff attitudes and relationships with residents
- Adequate wages and other rewards for staff
- A wide variety of activities

- Food that is fresh, tasty, and varied to reflect ethnic differences and individual needs
- Explicit, workable channels for problem resolution (accompanied by love and understanding)
- Safety of the environment
- Maximum possible independence for residents
- Strong, enforced regulations
- Resident participation in policy making and quality control, both in their own facilities and at state and federal levels
- An active, concerned, informed administrator
- Community involvement

freedom and meaningful activity are addressed medically (if at all). Drugs are too often the first choice, rather than the last resort, in dealing with what are often sane reactions to an impossible situation. Doctors have the final say, even as to whether or not a 'patient' can receive visitors. The medical model requires efficiency and hierarchy. Because it cannot incorporate the chaos of individuality and assertiveness, it treats 'patients' as cases instead of as people and rewards those who conform.

LOSS OF AUTONOMY

The medical, institutional approach fosters regimentation and loss of privacy and autonomy. Most residents must share rooms, follow schedules, and accept a preplanned menu. Activities offered are often limited to the large-group, lowest-common-denominator type. Negative attitudes among staff and a lack of resources rarely allow for excitement, or choice. Also, because passivity is built into the medical approach, even kind and caring staff members tend to overprotect. Too much help takes away a resident's right to risk, experience, and learn.

Three groups from the same home were asked to complete a puzzle. One group was assisted by staff members. A second group was left to itself. A third received less help than the first group, more than the second. Result: those who received the most help thought the puzzle most difficult. The less help received, the easier the puzzle seemed.[7]

Lack of control over daily life has serious consequences for residents' well-being, in a vicious cycle of increasing dependence.[8] Residents themselves identified choice and control as key components of quality care in an American nationwide research project.[9]

I make my own bed. It's a small thing but it's important. I've seen those people who think they can't do anything. Sometimes their families or the staff don't take the time to encourage them or teach them. Soon they can't do anything for themselves. Any little thing you can do for yourself helps keep you going. [a seventy-year-old woman]

Sometimes, nursing homes can rise above their limitations and rescue residents from a medically dictated oblivion.

When [my mother] collapsed, her doctor advised me to find a nursing home 'for her to die in'. . . . As soon as she arrived at the nursing home, their doctor stopped all treatment: the tranquillizers, IVs, catheters. The dentist replaced her dentures. . . . The physical therapist had her up in a wheelchair and doing exercises, and the attendants and I started feeding her. Within two months, she was walking and talking. She lived for another four years as an active, loving, thinking, feeling individual, not the 'vegetable' her doctor had predicted she would be.[10]

ABUSE

An increasing problem inside and outside nursing homes is abuse and neglect. Within an institution, staff members are usually the guilty parties. Outside, family members are most often involved. The problem often stems from a history of abuse, including alcohol or drug abuse – for example, parents who abused their children may later find themselves victims; a nurse's aide who abuses alcohol or takes drugs may find it hard to maintain caring behaviour.

In addition, both family carers and nursing home staff often feel frustrated, isolated, and under stress. In a home caregiving situation, a single carer may be responsible twenty-four hours a day. Nursing home staff are often underpaid, overworked, and inadequately trained and supervised. These conditions increase the likelihood of abuse.

A universally accepted definition of abuse and neglect has yet to be formulated. Most of us would agree that physical assault, from a pinch or slap to a severe beating, is abuse, as are physical carelessness and intentional cruelty, such as bathing someone in dangerously hot water. We could probably also agree on a definition of verbal abuse, and that treatment resulting in malnutrition, bedsores, infections, and other physical problems constitutes the worst kind of neglect. These are the more obvious problems, addressed to some extent by laws and regulations.

LESS OBVIOUS PROBLEMS

Other common problems in nursing homes are less dramatic but no less damaging. They are difficult to detect, and prejudiced attitudes toward older people with disabilities may blind us to their seriousness. For example:

- **Overmedication,** or inappropriate medication, may be intentional, an attempt to control a resident's behaviour. It may be the result of ignorance about the effects of medication on older people. Or it may occur because the nursing home's drug-monitoring systems are inadequate. In any case, this is very dangerous.
- **Physical restraints** may help some people to sit up and even participate safely in activities, but they should be used judiciously and removed or changed periodically. Improper use or overuse can cause pain, prevent needed exercise, and otherwise inhibit physical and mental rehabilitation. In addition, residents may not be able to express their discomfort.
- **Verbal indignities** can be harmful even when not extreme. A statement that doesn't sound threatening to a visitor may terrify a resident. A patronizing tone and low expectations may create or reinforce confusion, depression, and dependence.

I encouraged the residents to talk, but no one spoke. To get the discussion started, I asked one interested-looking resident to read a proclamation of independence written by another group of residents. The activities director quickly said, 'Oh, she can't read.' But the resident took the paper and read it to the group.[11]

- **Subtle, daily neglect** gradually wears residents down and may lead to withdrawal or apathy.

No one was cruel, but I just wasn't very happy. Then, after the new administration started, little things started going right again and so did my spirit. Hot coffee, crisp toast, medication that comes at about the same time each day, and fewer clothes lost in the laundry – it made all the difference. [a woman in her eighties]

- **Financial exploitation** can take many forms. Family members, acquaintances, or nursing home staff or administrators may steal cash, property, or other assets outright. They may pressure the older person for gifts. Or they may deprive the older person of control over her or his resources.
- **Inadequate rewards and training** affect all staff, even the most caring and competent, and reflect the low status of nursing home residents. High turnover and unprofessional behaviour are too often the result.

Another area of concern is the potential for easy spreading of infectious diseases. Some facilities don't take appropriate precautions. Others are so overcautious that residents lose access to visitors and activities both inside and outside the home in return for only a marginal improvement in safety.

Making the Decision

This section mainly addresses long-term rather than short-term placements. However, it is worthwhile to resist the impulse to assume that a stay will be long-term and to try to keep your options open (see Housing Alternatives chapter).

Many, if not most residential or nursing home decisions are made in the midst of a crisis. But prospective residents and carers who prepare in advance retain more control of the process and cope better with the strong feelings evoked by such a major transition. The likelihood of a waiting list adds to the importance of advance planning. All of us, even those who are healthy, should make our wishes known to loved ones in advance. Or, as carers, we can sensitively approach the subject before our loved one becomes incapacitated or we become exhausted.

My brother can't seem to handle what he calls the 'sin' of abandoning Ma to strangers, but he lives 600 miles away. I'm the one who has to deal with the day-to-day problems, and I've run out of patience, energy, and understanding. My health, my job, and my other relationships have all been affected. I've just about lost my sense of humour, which always got me through the roughest days. [a woman in her sixties]

Decision-making should involve the prospective resident to the greatest degree possible. Even confused people can respond to carers' attempts to communicate lovingly the realities of a difficult situation. Avoiding the topic or misleading the prospective resident – even if intended as kindness – can have a devastating effect on morale.

How is it? Don't even ask. I was living by myself. My husband died many years ago.

Four months ago my son came down to visit me and said, 'Ma, I'm taking you home with me.' He did take me to his home for one night, but the next day he brought me here and dropped me off. I've only seen him once since then. [a ninety-year-old woman]

Involvement in the decision, on the other hand, can have quite the opposite effect.

My mother was lonely and miserable, but would not even talk about moving. As her health deteriorated, my sister and I knew we had to look at homes that would accept her. The dishonesty of a paid companion finally shook her sufficiently, and I'm sure made her feel so helpless that she was willing to look at the places we had screened. Our preference was a small place, but she chose a larger one, hoping to have a greater selection of bridge partners! She selected her clothes and those few belongings one is allowed to take. It seemed a pathetic end. Yet this was not the end. She is now in many respects more alert and interested and in constant contact with people. [a fifty-six-year-old woman]

Remember that a residential or nursing home is only one of many options. Sometimes it is the right choice; sometimes it isn't. The more you plan for the *possibility* of living in a home, the better you will be able to control the move if you need to make it.

The Transition

A comfortable transition from a private residence into a home is important to a resident's well-being. The decision-making process and the choice of a home are only the beginning. You should also consider:

- **Planning for the disposition of personal belongings.** Most residential homes allow you to bring a few possessions, and some will store a few valuables. What do you want to have with you? What do you want to leave behind? What would you like to give to loved ones? What can you sell? Do you want to keep anything in storage – especially in the event that your stay in the home is short?
- **Thinking ahead about adjustments you will have to make.** You will probably have to get used to one or more roommates, a large group of people in close proximity, a loss of privacy, and having a daily schedule set for you. Many residents do make good adjustments; humour, a spirit of compromise, and self-confidence can help. Think about ways to retain as much independence as possible.

Once you're in the home, you can do a few things right away to hasten your adjustment:

- **Get to know the staff and their procedures.** This applies to both residents and their families and friends. You will feel comfortable more quickly, retain more control, and get more satisfaction if you know who handles complaints. For example, do you tell the dietician, the nurse, the cook, the matron, or a residents' committee if you have a problem with the food?
- **Encourage family and friends' visits.** Having someone stay with you on your first day is especially helpful.

I stayed with my mother for most of her first day. Together we got to know the home, met the staff and learned their names, found out about schedules and procedures, and visited several residents. We set up her room and had lunch together. When I had to leave, we both felt sad, but we had both expected it to be much worse. [a forty-two-year-old woman]

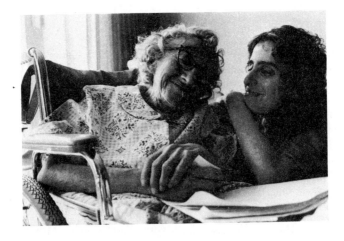

Visits will keep your morale high, provide you with mental stimulation, and ensure better care for you and others. Do your best to make visits pleasant. If family and friends fail to visit, don't blame yourself. Some people feel so distressed by a hospital or nursing home, anticipating physical and emotional discomfort, that they are literally unable to visit.

Family and friends who don't know how to create an enjoyable visit, especially if their loved one finds communication difficult, should ask for help. Nursing home staff or other experienced people may have suggestions. Many people have solved difficult communication problems in spite of overwhelming odds against them.

RIGHTS OF RESIDENTS

When the 1984 Registered Homes Act was in its early stages, the Centre for Policy on Ageing was asked to produce a code of practice for home owners and proprietors. This code, *Home Life*, is intended to be a guideline both for inspectors and managers or owners. It sets out the rights of residents and what sort of care they can expect. But unfortunately the Act did not make these guidelines mandatory – therefore they don't *have* to be followed, and every local authority can set its own standards.

An even greater deficiency is that the guidelines are not necessarily followed by local authority homes, who can set their own standards and make their own rules.

The code lists a number of ideals:

- **Quality of Life** – the right to lead the sort of life the resident prefers.
- **Dignity** – the right to privacy, courtesy and respect.
- **Autonomy** – the right to freedom and self-determination within the limits necessary in communal life.
- **Individuality** – especially important for people from ethnic groups.
- **Quality of Experience** – freedom to come and go; the right to form relationships with others.
- **Responsible Risks** – the right not to be overprotected and to make one's own decisions about possibly 'risky' activities.

If you feel that you as a resident or that someone who is a resident is not being given these rights, you should complain to the person responsible for running the home in the first instance; then to the responsible local authority's Social Services department; then to an old people's welfare organization such as Age Concern or Help the Aged, who can offer advice. The local press, local councillors and your MP can initiate action, and this has sometimes proved very effective. Protests and complaints are most likely to result in action if you get together with other residents or relatives who may have had similar experiences. There is always strength in numbers.

Remember that the 'guidelines' say that complaints should be dealt with quickly and effectively by those in charge, and justified grievances remedied.

Under the 1984 Act's Regulations, an authorized person must be allowed to interview a resident in private – so she must be given the opportunity to speak freely to a relative, friend, doctor, social worker or solicitor without the presence of staff. Complaints about the professional conduct of doctors or nurses should be referred to the General Medical Council (see Public and Professional Advisory Organizations) or the UK Central Council for Nursing, Midwifery and Health Visiting or the appropriate National Board for Nursing. If a nursing home bed is subsidized by the Department of Health, ask for advice from the Community Health Council about making a complaint.

*Mama awakened, and I put her hand on my head, our code for showing her it was I.
She is completely deaf and almost blind. 'Oh, dear child!' she said with a delighted
smile of recognition. 'It's my youngest!' I took her hand and moved it up and down in
a vertical signal to 'nod' yes, and gave her a big hug and kiss. Her fragile warm
hands took one of my big strong cold hands and rubbed it lovingly. I thought to
myself, 'How lucky I am to be receiving all this caring love!'* [a sixty-three-year-old
woman]

If you are a family member who feels guilty about placing your loved one in a
home – and most do – try not to withdraw from the situation. Keep visiting as
often as you can. Nursing home staff who advise you to stay away because the
resident 'gets too upset' are looking for a short-term solution or trying to save
themselves work. In the long run, visiting almost always pays off and makes
both families and residents feel better.

Talking with others in similar situations can also help. A few nursing homes
and communities sponsor family support groups. If none exists, consider
starting one. Nursing home staff or self-help groups may be able to make
specific suggestions for dealing both with your emotions and with any anger a
resident may feel. Above all, remember that you are a human being, too, with
legitimate time, financial, and other constraints. Self-sacrifice almost always
leads to resentment and that helps no one, least of all the person for whom the
sacrifice is made.

NOTES

[1]Mickey Spencer, 'Nursing Homes', *Broomstick: A Bimonthly National Magazine by, for, &
about Women over Forty*, Vol. 8, No. 4, July–
August 1986.

[2]1986 figures quoted by Jean Shapiro, 'A Place
to Call Home', *Good Housekeeping*, May 1986,
p. 105.

[3]National Center for Health Statistics (US)
based on a 1982 survey.

[4]Centre for Policy on Ageing, *Home Life: A
Code of Practice for Residential Care*.

[5]Ibid.

[6]Deirdre Wynne-Harley of the Centre for
Policy on Ageing, quoted by Jean Shapiro, 'A
Place to Call Home', *Good Housekeeping*, May
1986, p. 106.

[7]From *Investigative Newsletter Institutions/
Alternatives*, Vol. 7, No. 9, September 1984, p.
12.

[8]This point is documented in various articles
and books, notably Ellen Langer, *Psychology of
Control*. Beverly Hills, Ca: Sage Publications,
1983.

[9]'A Consumer Perspective on Quality Care:
The Residents' Point of View'. National
Citizens' Coalition for Nursing Home Reform
(NCCNHR), a study of quality care with 457
resident participants.

[10]Spencer, op. cit.

[11]Personal communication, staff member,
LIFE, Woburn, Mass.

BOOKS AND PUBLICATIONS

Pat Young, *At Home in a Home*. Mitcham: Age Concern.

Centre for Policy on Ageing, *Home Life: A*

Code of Practice for Residential Care – Working Party Report, May 1984.

The Good Care Homes Guide. London: Help the Aged/Longman Group, 1988.

18
Joint and Muscle Pain, Arthritis and Rheumatic Disorders

My left leg hurt all the time, down the outside, across the foot, behind the knee. My hip joint ached mightily. I thought, 'What do you expect, over sixty?' But it turned out a nerve in my spine was being pressed – and there were things I could do to hurt less. [a woman in her sixties]

As we grow older, we may experience aches in our joints and muscles. We may fear pain and immobility as a result of these conditions. It is important that neither we nor our doctors dismiss pains and aches as inevitable signs of age. We should not assume discomfort is normal and so neglect preventable and correctable conditions.

As we age, our spines may change shape in response to stresses placed on them. Bony growths, called spurs, may limit joint motion. The soft tissues that stabilize the joints can become inflamed by overuse or strain. Arthritis can attack our joints. Muscles may weaken or become tight with disuse, tension, and postural habits, making it hard, for example, to look back when we drive or to hook a bra. What hurts and what shows up on X-rays don't always go together. As we understand the environmental and life-style factors that affect our joints, we can find ways to stay supple and comfortable.

A joint is formed where two bones meet. It is surrounded by a capsule of soft tissue lined with a synovial membrane that produces a rich fluid. This fluid lubricates the cartilage-covered bone ends as they move against each other. The cartilage absorbs shocks, protects the ends of the bones, and receives nourishment only through exercise. Ligaments, which attach bone to bone, and tendons, which attach muscle to bone, keep bones stable while permitting them to move. Bursae, small, pillowlike sacs lined with synovial membrane, cushion the movement of muscle over bone, or of one muscle over another.

Inflammation is an indication that the body is attempting to heal and repair injured tissue. Injury can result from many causes, including a blow, strain, overuse, or reactions to foreign substances or anything the body interprets as foreign. The symptoms of inflammation can be local pain, heat, redness, swelling, or general discomfort, including headaches and weakness.

Pain may arise from:

- *Overuse* – stressing joints or soft tissues by repetitive motions, such as hammering
- *Underuse* – not moving enough, resulting in stiffness and limiting mobility of the joint
- *Incorrect use* – habitually moving in ways inappropriate for the way the body is made, such as holding the phone to one ear with a raised shoulder
- *Reactions to stress* – habitual tension in the muscles can create muscle spasm and pain
- *The pain-spasm-pain cycle* – pain causes further tightening or spasms in other muscles, creating still more pain
- *Inflammation* – in the joints (arthritis), tendons (tenosynovitis or tendonitis), bursae (bursitis), muscles, or blood vessels
- *Changes in bone shape* – pressing on nerves and causing other strains

Prevention of Joint Pain

To prevent joint problems, and to prevent reinjury or disability from them, you can:

1. Keep muscles strong with exercise and flexible with gentle stretching.
2. Reduce muscle tension. Regularly use relaxation techniques, such as systematically tensing and relaxing groups of muscles from head to toe, meditating, and getting massages.
3. Deal with difficulties in movement as soon as you notice them. Be alert to any difficulty you may have in performing daily activities, to pain where you never had it before, and to changes in the ease and range of your motion. For example, if you have trouble climbing stairs, your knees, hips, or front thigh muscles (quadriceps) may need attention.

I noticed in exercise class that I had pain when performing certain motions with my arms – my shoulders would not let me do things I had always done before. I wish I had paid attention to the slight signs earlier. Now I've lost quite a lot of shoulder motion. [a sixty-one-year-old woman]

4. Try to manage your weight. Being very heavy stresses the joints.
5. Use good body mechanics. This means using the body in ways that minimize joint stress. Use the largest and strongest joint for any given task – for example, push with your hips or thighs instead of with your hands.
6. Wear comfortable shoes. Foot problems can affect the whole body. Wobbling on high or thin heels creates strain on the knees, hips, and back as these joints try to stabilize the body when the feet can't do the job.

Home Care for Sprains, Mild Injuries and Inflammation, and Joint and Muscle Pain

Pain in joints and soft tissues often respond to home care and will heal in two to six weeks given rest, hot or cold compresses, and time. Rest gives the body a chance to make repairs and helps reduce inflammation, but too much bed rest for back pain caused by muscle or ligament strain may result in loss of muscle strength.[1] You may want to immobilize the joint with a sling, splint, or corset. Once or twice a day, move resting joints through their normal range of motion, because inflammation can make tissues stick together and become hard and tight ('frozen'). Heat relaxes muscles, while cold reduces swelling and inflammation, and can ease muscles in spasm.

WHEN TO USE HEAT AND WHEN TO USE ICE[2]

If there is swelling and warmth from inflammation in the joint or muscle, ice packs or ice massages (passing ice over the painful area, without pressure, for twenty minutes) is generally more beneficial for reducing swelling, inflammation, and pain.

When the main problem is stiffness and there is no swelling, moist heat – such as a shower or bath, wet compresses, or a wet washcloth placed between the skin and a plastic-covered heating pad – is more effective than dry heat. Guard against scalding or burning.

When an area is sore and painful and an application of heat does not bring relief, it is likely that an ice pack will.

For trauma to a joint, such as twisting an ankle or a knee, the best treatment is ice to decrease swelling and bruising.

If you 'pull' your back muscles while exercising, the pain felt afterward is usually caused by a spasm in the muscle. It may be more comforting to apply heat at first. However, if you do not get good relief with heat, ice packs or ice massage can often be beneficial.

The treatment that gives the greatest relief is best for you.

SIGNS OF FURTHER PROBLEMS

The following symptoms require more complete investigation.[3] **Contact your doctor if:**

- your temperature is over 100°F
- you feel numbness or tingling
- the pain runs down the back of your leg to your foot or down your arm to your finger
- the pain persists or is very bad

- you can't use the joint
- you have severe pain and swelling in one or more joints
- you have trouble in the same joint on both sides
- you have stiffness that lasts more than one hour after waking up
- you feel weak, fatigued, or generally unwell
- you have lumps under the skin, particularly near the elbow

Managing Long-Term Pain

I've really learned to listen to my body. All my life I wasn't listening. My mind was too ambitious. But now, if I don't feel good one day and can't do anything, I say the hell with it and wait. If you say, 'I'll do it tomorrow,' somehow tomorrow comes. [a seventy-five-year-old woman]

Living with pain is physically and emotionally stressful. Work with a physiotherapist may be essential to reduce pain but you may also have to use drugs before you can try the following important self-help programme.

EXERCISE

When in pain we tend to tighten muscles and move less (the pain-spasm-pain cycle), so even a few gently performed small movements can have an astonishing effect and lead to larger pain-free movements. Even those confined to a wheelchair or bed will find exercise helpful. Mobility and strength do not develop in a straight line; remember that you will have bad days as well as good days.

Every morning and before I go to bed I do bicycling on my back, knee-chest stretches, leg lifts, and turn my head. When I rest I practise breathing from my diaphragm instead of my chest. I work on posture and thigh muscles by bending my knees and sliding my back up and down against the wall. [a seventy-five-year-old woman]

Listen to your body. Exercise gently and slowly, with relaxation between repetitions, only as much as is comfortable, up to but not beyond the point of pain. Increase exercise very slowly. One or two rest days a week may help. You may even need to begin exercising in the supportive environment of warmed water.

When my body seemed stiff beyond repair because of the pain-spasm-pain cycle, I used water to support me as I turned my head from side to side or slowly walked back and forth in the pool. Small changes gradually led to larger ones. Now I swim a half-mile. [a sixty-one-year-old woman]

I won a victory over arthritis in my fifties. I was acting in a mime troupe and walking got so painful I was crying as I was walking with the pain in my hip. A surgeon suggested surgery, but I refused. I started using a whirlpool and doing exercises in a swimming pool for a year, three times a day. I was so successful that at fifty-eight I learned to ski. [a fifty-nine-year-old woman]

I'm always stiff when I get up in the morning. Then I stand in a hot shower, and I'm okay for the rest of the day. [an eighty-five-year-old woman]

I don't like to use dishwashers. I like to do dishes by hand in hot water. The water feels so friendly to my hands. [a seventy-eight year-old woman]

The Adult Education Centre in your area may offer exercise classes for people with joint problems and the teacher can suggest exercises to perform in water.

The Feldenkrais method and Alexander technique (see Moving for Health chapter) realign our bodies and show people how to move with less effort. Yoga has helped many people with arthritis.[4] Like any other exercise, yoga must be modified to suit you.

I came to yoga in my fifties when my mother was dying. I couldn't sleep because I would see her dying face. All my pains got worse. When I read a book on yoga, I could feel that my body was full of tension. I got a record, took a course, and grew more supple. When I saw my osteopath, he was astounded at how flexible I had become.

But my yoga teacher insisted that I could do a shoulder stand, which I knew was not right for me. Against my better judgment I tried it and injured my neck. I had to wear a collar until it healed. [a seventy-five-year-old woman]

REST AND ENERGY CONSERVATION

Pain is exhausting, and feels worse when you are tired. You need to find the right balance between exercise and rest, and to avoid tiring yourself by learning to conserve energy.

Plan rest times into your day. Plan workspaces so you do not waste steps. Sit to work instead of standing, use gadgets that avoid straining your joints, and plan restful tasks between more energetic ones. Your body will tell you when you've done too much.

I thought I had done everything right in planning a small party. I bought most things, made others on three different days. The day of the party, I felt good and ran around a lot instead of resting. The next morning I could not get out of bed. Everything hurt. It took a week to get over it. [a sixty-one-year-old woman]

Only by trial and error can you discover the balance between rest and activity best for you.

I told my doctor I had tickets for a show, but I was in such pain how could I go? He asked, 'If you stay at home, will the pain go away? So why not go?' And that did a lot for me. I went. I had to stand against the wall from time to time, but I went, and I kept going. Once, when I felt like giving up, the same doctor said, 'If you don't keep active, you'll end your days in a wheelchair.' That shook me. I put a fancy scarf around my neck collar and I went out. [a seventy-five-year-old woman]

DEALING WITH STRESS

Emotional or physical stress seems to increase pain, perhaps by suppressing endorphins, the body's natural painkillers. Try to limit the effects of the stress you cannot avoid. Exercise, relaxation techniques, and daily meditation are all useful methods for increasing endorphins.[5]

SEX

Sex can help to reduce pain. For helpful suggestions on sex when you or your partner has pain or limited mobility, see the Sexuality chapter.

SELF-HELP GROUPS

Self-help groups make it possible to exchange ideas for managing back and joint pains and rheumatic disorders, to share experiences, and to give and get support. The nearest branch of the Arthritis and Rheumatism Council, Arthritis Care or the Back Pain Association (see Organizations) or a local hospital may know of a group – or you can start one yourself. Managing these disorders requires a lot of support. An important resource in coping with pain is the ability to ask for help.

My husband said to me, 'Don't be a baby.' I was terribly hurt. I was hysterical. He doesn't know how much pain I'm in. But my group knows. [a woman in her sixties]

EXPLORING WHAT IS AVAILABLE IN YOUR COMMUNITY

Massage, acupuncture, meditation and other relaxation techniques, visualization (making mental images of the way you want to be), and hypnosis have helped many people. Myotherapy (pressing on spots in the body that send pain to other parts) may relieve muscle spasms.[6] Acupressure, a form of massage that includes pressure on acupuncture points, has been a help to many.

During an acupressure massage, the masseuse found a very sore spot on my back. When she pressed it for a while, some of the pain on my right side went away. Now, if my right side pains me when I am walking, I just reach around and press the sore spot and the pain goes away. That's a wonderful trick to know. [a sixty-five-year-old woman]

Some people find similar relief after treatment by an osteopath practising cranial osteopathy (a gentle, non-manipulating form of treatment). This is a method whereby gentle pressure is applied to strategic spots (usually on the spine) rather than the more vigorous movements usually associated with osteopaths. Those practising this method have usually had special training beyond the usual four-year course. Unfortunately, it isn't always successful.

DRUGS

Drugs are often prescribed to break the pain-spasm-pain cycle and to reduce inflammation. Aspirin is useful because it relieves both pain and inflammation. Diazepam (Valium), however, is potentially addictive and is frequently misused and overused. See page 335 for a summary of anti-inflammatory and other drugs. Recent research suggests that fish oil taken in liquid or capsule form lubricates the joints.

Common Joint Problems

FOOT PROBLEMS

It is important to take special care of our feet, since the entire body depends on them for mobility and stability. Much foot discomfort comes from the restrictive styles of women's shoes, which are rarely designed for comfort and health. High heels force our weight on to the metatarsal joints in the ball of the foot, distort our walking gait and posture, and strain other joints, including the back and neck. Pointed-toe shoes can push the big toe out of its normal position and place pressure on the joint, causing bunions. Instead of being a modern version of Chinese footbinding, women's shoes should provide the same level of comfort as good men's shoes. Try them sometime. You'll be amazed at the toe room.

A comfortable shoe should outline the shape of the foot – broad in front with rounded toes, heel wide enough to distribute weight, and with room enough for the top of the foot.[7] It should have plenty of room for the toes to wiggle, and thick crepe or soft rubber soles and heels. Sandals and properly shaped shoes give the foot room to spread.

I have found a style of flat sandals with built-in supports that keeps me pain-free. I wear them all the time. On the rare occasions, such as a wedding, when I feel I must wear another style of shoe, I change my shoes in the ladies' room so I wear the less comfortable shoes for the shortest time. [a fifty-four-year-old woman]

Check the bottoms of your shoes. If they are worn down unevenly, that can be an early sign of a problem. Repair your shoes frequently, because walking around in unevenly worn shoes can produce strain on your knees and back. If you have pain on top of your feet where laces tie, choose shoes with more than two shoelace holes on each side and loosen the laces over the painful area.

As we grow older, our toenails may be harder to cut. They may become horny, we may have difficulty reaching them, or our hands may not have sufficient strength to work the clippers. Try large clippers with long handles and a spring. Cut nails straight across a little at a time. Ask for help. You might want to exchange pedicures and foot rubs with a friend. Remember that NHS chiropody is free to pensioners. The chiropodist will cut toenails regularly.

If you need moulded shoe inserts (orthotics) but have flexible feet (feet with very loose joints), be sure the orthotics are moulded without your weight on them but with your foot supported in the correct position.[8] People with flexible feet are often more comfortable in shoes with very flexible soles.

Flat feet may cause more pain as you get older. Exercise and well-fitting shoes, perhaps with arch supports, will make your feet and legs more comfortable.

If your second toe is longer than your big toe, you have a Venus de Milo foot. This sounds nice, but it may contribute to back pain because the long toe changes the way the foot rolls when walking. Padding under the ball of the foot may help.

Bunions (swelling, tenderness, and redness of the big toe joint) do not usually cause pain if we wear comfortable shoes. A tendency to have them may be inherited, but the shoes we wear may also be at fault. If you see a bunion coming, visit a chiropodist or a physiotherapist who specializes in foot problems. An orthotic, or new shoes, can reduce the stress that produces the bunion.

Morton's neuralgia, a condition in which a tender nerve at the base of the third and fourth toes causes tingling and numbness in the middle toes and pain in the ball of the foot, is common among middle-aged women. It can often be relieved by changing to shoes with wide toe room, support for the metatarsal arch, and low heels.

If your foot joints are affected by rheumatoid arthritis, ask your doctor for a specialist referral.

BACK PROBLEMS

Almost everyone has a back problem at one time or another. Most back pain comes from muscle or ligament strain, muscle spasm, sacroiliac joint strain, disc problems, excessive curvature of the spine (kyphosis), or arthritis. Once injured, the back can take several weeks or months to heal.

The backbone, or spine, supports us and lets us twist, bend, and turn. It consists of bones (vertebrae) alternating with flexible units (discs) containing a gel-like centre. The nerves of the spinal cord, which connects brain and body, pass through openings in the vertebrae. When viewed from the back, the spine should appear to divide the body into two equal parts. When viewed from the side, the spine has a characteristic S-curve that helps absorb shocks.

AVOIDING BACK AND NECK PROBLEMS

Observe the basic rule: Don't do anything that causes pain. If something causes pain, stop doing it, and follow the suggestions for home care beginning on page 314.

The suggestions above for preventing and managing pain apply especially to the two most common causes of back pain – back muscle sprains and sacroiliac joint inflammation. The following suggestions may prevent problems, ease the pain you have, and save you from reinjuring or aggravating a bad back or neck. Suggestions marked with a bullet (●) are particularly useful for disc problems.

1. Strengthen your abdominal and back muscles. (See p. 323.) Excessive back sway from weak muscles, a slack or protruding abdomen, and poor posture place severe stress on the muscles and joints of the lower back and can cause pain.
●2. When you sit or stand, try keeping your feet at different levels. Rest one foot on a stool, a book, a bar, or on the floor of the cabinet underneath the sink when washing dishes.
3. If your mattress sags, put a ¾-inch plywood board under it. The best mattress is soft on the top so it contours and supports weight evenly, but

firm enough so it doesn't sag. However, you need to sleep well, and what is comfortably firm to one person may be a bed of nails to another.

●**4.** Don't sleep on your stomach. Sleeping on your stomach is especially bad for neck problems. If you can't sleep any other way, place a pillow under

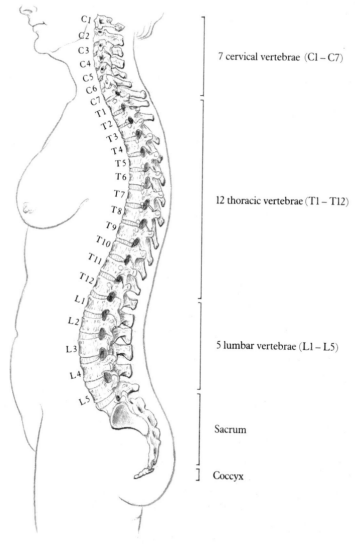

7 cervical vertebrae (C1 – C7)

12 thoracic vertebrae (T1 – T12)

5 lumbar vertebrae (L1 – L5)

Sacrum

Coccyx

THE VERTEBRAL COLUMN (SPINE)

your waist to prevent the sway-back position. If you sleep on your side, place pillows in front of you to support your top shoulder and top knee.

5. If your days are sedentary, get up often and walk around or lie down. While sitting, periodically round and straighten your back or, holding your elbows in opposite hands, twist gently to the right and left.[9] During car travel, stop and walk around every hour. Move around in a train and plane as much as possible and exercise in your seat. Two examples of exercises to be done slowly and gently are stretching alternate arms upwards and lifting one knee at a time toward opposite elbows.

●6. Some positions put more pressure on lower back discs than others. Sitting exerts more pressure than standing, and both more than lying down. When you have to lift an object, don't twist. Lifting and twisting puts four hundred times more pressure on your lumbar spine than lying down.[10] Bending over and lifting can also harm your back. Don't bend at the waist, but instead bend your knees, keep your back straight while lifting, and hold the weight close. If you can't bend your knees that far or need help to get up, support your back by leaning a hand on a nearby solid object, or by resting a forearm on your own thigh. If you need to move furniture with someone, you should be the one in front with your hands behind your back.

7. Change a baby on furniture of comfortable height. Do not bend over. Carry an infant with her back resting on your forearm and her head cradled in your hand. Don't lift children. Let an older child climb on your lap. Some of us can kneel or sit to let an older child climb on our backs to be carried.

8. Carry all objects close to your body *above* waist level. Use a backpack. If carrying shopping bags, divide the load in two so you are balanced. Lighten the load whenever possible.

●9. Don't reach for or lift an object over your head; stand on a stool so that you can keep your elbows bent.[11]

10. Since most chairs do not provide support for the lower back, supply it yourself by folding a towel or sweater 6 to 8 inches wide and about $1\frac{1}{2}$ inches thick in the middle. Put it in the hollow of your back. You can do this at the cinema or while riding in a car.

11. At work and at home, try to use chairs that are adjustable in height, so your feet can be flat on the floor with your knees bent at ninety degrees. Your chair should have an adjustable backrest placed where the back curves most inward. It should be upholstered in a non-slip material and be soft at the edge of the seat so that circulation in the thighs is not cut off. It should have arms whenever possible.

●12. Get up from a chair by sliding to the edge so that your weight is directly above your feet. Don't lean forward, for this increases the pressure on your discs. Use the chair arms to help you, or push with your hands on your thighs to support your back as you straighten up.

13. Share helpful hints with others. You may find it easier to lie on your back in bed to put on shoes and socks. If pulling up the hand brake in a car hurts, it may help to press against the dashboard with the other hand when you do it.

14. If your back hurts, relax in the position that is most comfortable for you.

15. Some people find that sleeping on a special neck pillow helps relieve back and neck pain. Anatomia (see Organizations) supplies neck pillows.

When my back hurts the most comfortable position for me is lying on my back, legs loosely together and raised at right angles at the hips and knees, with my calves and feet on a hassock or chair seat. Sometimes I even put the hassock in bed with me. [a fifty-five-year-old woman]

For most people, specific exercises are essential to help prevent back pain. Exercises that strengthen your back muscles, abdominals, and front thigh muscles (quadriceps) will help protect your spinal discs. Abdominal muscles provide the sole support for the lower lumbar vertebrae and help hold us erect. Women of middle age characteristically have weak abdominals. If your quadriceps are strong, you have less tendency to rely on back muscles to lift you up. If you have repeated bouts of back pain it is wise to invest in a

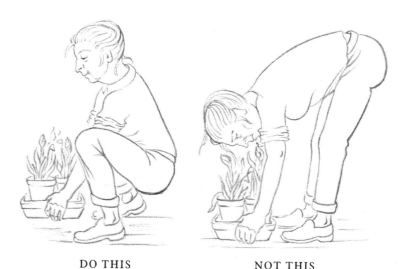

DO THIS   NOT THIS

consultation with a physiotherapist who specializes in back problems for an individualized exercise programme.

While exercise is important, choose sports with care. Warm up and gently stretch your back muscles before doing sports or heavy labour. Some sports are harder on your back than others.[12] Walking and swimming are good, but you may need to select and modify your strokes. The breast and back stroke, for example, arch the back and may cause pain.

Some Special Back Problems

A **herniated disc** occurs when the soft centre inside the disc is forced through the outer casing. This may cause pain when it presses on a nerve. Most likely to herniate are the two lower lumbar discs, which can press on the sciatic nerve. When this happens, the lower back may hurt, followed by pain running down the back or side of the thigh, the outside of the calf, and possibly into the toes. You are most likely to have a herniated disc when you are between thirty and sixty. As we age, our discs dry out, becoming thinner, harder, and less likely to herniate. The majority of people with disc problems do not require surgery but respond partly or completely to conservative, non-surgical treatment. The most common treatment is bed rest, which is very debilitating for older people. Ask for exercises you can do in bed to keep your muscles strong. A sudden severe pain in an older woman is more likely to be a fracture from osteoporosis than a disc problem.

Sometimes, to avoid surgery, chymopapain (the enzyme from papaya used in meat tenderizers) may be injected into the herniated disc. The injection is given only in hospitals, under anaesthesia, and involves risks equal to those of surgery. It is important that the doctor first determine whether you are allergic to the injected material.[13] As with any surgery, always get a second opinion before undergoing the procedure. Long-term follow-up studies comparing surgery and chymopapain indicate that the end results from both procedures are the same.[14]

Vertebrae tend to develop rims of extra bone, called *spurs*, around their edges and on the projections at their rear. While spurs and/or narrowed spaces between vertebrae may combine to press on a nerve, not everyone who has rims and spurs experiences back pain. Stretching exercises, relaxation techniques, and traction may relieve discomfort.

Spinal stenosis is the name for a narrowing of either the spinal canal or the openings for nerve roots in the vertebrae. Appearing mainly in people over fifty, it is now diagnosed more often than before as a source of pain, because it can be seen with the CAT scan. The pain usually increases gradually over time.

Treatment may involve appropriate exercise, anti-inflammatory drugs, a corset or brace, and, as a last resort, surgery.[15]

Scoliosis is a condition in which the spine curves to one side. Mild scoliosis is common in adolescent women and, as we age, can contribute to tight muscles or limited motion and strain on the back. If you have scoliosis, ask your doctor

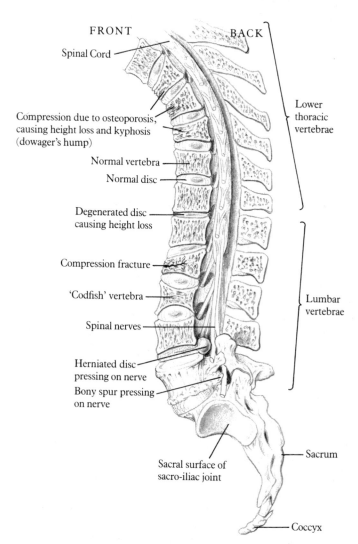

FRONT   BACK

Spinal Cord

Compression due to osteoporosis, causing height loss and kyphosis (dowager's hump)

Lower thoracic vertebrae

Normal vertebra

Normal disc

Degenerated disc causing height loss

Compression fracture

'Codfish' vertebra

Lumbar vertebrae

Spinal nerves

Herniated disc pressing on nerve

Bony spur pressing on nerve

Sacrum

Sacral surface of sacro-iliac joint

Coccyx

DISORDERS OF THE SPINE

about the role it may play in your back pain. Be sure to monitor the degree of curvature, especially after pregnancy, for any change. Chiropractic techniques cannot correct this condition.[16] Deep breathing and exercise can be helpful in counteracting the strain created by scoliosis.

Only 5 per cent of back problems require surgery (laminectomy). A CAT scan may be used for diagnosis. Before surgery, most surgeons perform a myelogram, in which a flow of dye is injected into the space surrounding the spinal cord so that anything that blocks the flow will show up on an X-ray. Unfortunately, it is not a comfortable procedure and may result in severe headaches and backaches for weeks. The discomforts are lessened when water-soluble dyes are used.

I saw many doctors for my leg, back, and hip pain. I liked a woman neurologist best of all because she talked with me for forty-five minutes. She said either I had a disc problem or the openings in my spine might be closing down on my nerves. I had a CAT scan. It was spinal stenosis. The neurologist said that 80 per cent of the people operated on for this problem felt better, but before surgery I would have to have a myelogram. I didn't want to have one. She said there was no hurry to decide. [a woman in her sixties]

Getting Help with Back Problems

What kind of specialist is most likely to help with back pain? An informal survey in the US of former back patients indicates that they were most satisfied with sports medicine practitioners. They also had kind words for rheumatologists. The former back patients received temporary relief from both osteopaths and chiropractors (who cannot prescribe medications), both of whom manipulate the spine; but manipulation is not advisable for herniated discs or sciatica. They found yoga teachers who understand back problems helpful. Physiotherapists helped with massage and taught useful exercises, and occupational therapists showed how to perform daily tasks comfortably. The study indicates that the greatest long-term help came from life-style changes. A practitioner who, regardless of specialty, understands the interaction of bones and soft tissues in movement and encourages changes in daily habits gives the most help.[17] The Back Pain Association can give up-to-date advice (see Organizations).

Other Common Joint Problems

KNEES

Many knee problems really originate in the foot. People who walk are less likely to develop knee problems than joggers or runners. Keep your quadriceps muscles strong because they stabilize the knee. Arthritis and bursitis are also common causes of knee pain.

HIPS

Finding the exact source of pain in the hip is often difficult because the joint is located deep in the body. The pain may come not from the hip but from arthritis of the spine. Pain caused by arthritis of the hip is usually felt in the groin, and may radiate to the area above the knee. Pain felt on the outside of the hips (at the widest part) is usually caused by bursitis and is often most painful when we are climbing steps or rising to a standing position.

STEPPING OUT WITH A STICK

We hurt, we're stiff, we want to get around more in spite of the difficulties – but use a stick? Never! Everyone will think we're old!

But a stick can really help. Problems that severely limit our mobility can often be eased by the proper use of a stick. Like fans, which are so helpful for the hot flushes of the menopause, sticks used to be more fashionable than they are now. Let's make them so again. We can decorate them to match our outfits or save up for an elegant one with fancy carving. We can use a stick to get a seat on the bus, or stamp the floor with it when we want to emphasize a point. A stick can say, 'Don't mess with me' if we choose.

Hold a stick in the hand opposite the sore leg. Your elbow will be at a 120 degree angle if the stick is the right height for you. Step out with the stick and the sore leg at the same time. The stick lessens pressure on the sore leg, resting it and giving it time to heal.

Be sure to have the height and your use of a stick (or crutches) checked by an experienced physiotherapist or nurse. You can cause damage by incorrect use.

SHOULDERS

Pain in a shoulder most often comes from bursitis or tendonitis and is usually the result of repeated motions such as overhead work, throwing, or racquet sports. A progressive loss of motion with some stiffness and pain may be so gradual that we don't notice it until it has become quite serious.[18] 'Frozen shoulder' occurs often in women over fifty. If not cared for, this condition can become permanent. Rest, hot packs, ice massage, and ultrasound treatments from a physiotherapist can prepare the way for passive exercise (someone moves your arm for you) and regular exercise.[19]

NECK

When you sleep, your neck should be supported so that it is in a straight line with your spine. If you awaken with neck pain, the position you slept in may be the cause. For sleeping, fold a hand towel lengthwise to a width of four inches, wrap it around your neck, and pin it with a safety pin.[20] Or try a cervical pillow shaped to fit under and support the neck (see p. 323). Neck pain may also come from vertebrae or disc problems in the spine.

JAW

I suddenly awoke about 4 a.m. with a severe earache. Aspirin kept the pain down, but it hurt to chew. A few days later it became painful to talk or even swallow. A friend who is a dental hygienist had told me about TMJ but I hadn't really paid much attention at the time. Then it dawned on me that this might be my problem. It was. My right jaw joint had slipped out of kilter.

The jaw joints – the temporomandibular joints (TMJ) – work twenty-four hours a day when we eat, talk, yawn, drink, and sleep. They must be synchronized to allow three-way movement: vertical, horizontal, and back-and-forth. When these joints get out of alignment, a wide range of symptoms may present themselves, among them headaches, earaches or ringing in the ears, eye pain or redness, dizziness, lower back pain, neck stiffness, numbness in the limbs, and a clicking sound in the jaw joint.

The causes of TMJ syndrome are diverse and some are not yet known. We do know that poor occlusion, or misalignment of the teeth, and grinding or clenching of teeth under stressful conditions are often causes, as are whiplash or other head injuries, arthritis, and injuries at birth caused by such practices as forceps delivery. Misalignment can be natural, caused by faulty dental work or orthodontics in youth, or caused by other problems such as ill-fitting dentures.

For years physicians and dentists dismissed those with TMJ symptoms, especially women, as complainers. It is now known that jaw joint disorders are very common and often overlooked, particularly among older people.

I'd had headaches for years that sometimes were so bad I really couldn't function. When the dentist did a lot of work, including realigning my teeth, my headaches stopped. When I remarked about my headaches stopping, my dentist said it might be TMJ syndrome – something I'd never heard of. He examined me closely and then made a mouthguard for me to wear at night. [a sixty-three-year-old woman]

TMJ problems should not be ignored. When diagnosed early, TMJ can usually be treated easily. When ignored, misdiagnosed, or mistreated, it can become intractable, forcing sufferers to stop working and socializing. The keys, therefore, are a careful diagnostic work-up done by a physician or dentist who is knowledgeable and sensitive to jaw joint problems, and treatment by an experienced practitioner.

The treatment of TMJ syndrome is controversial, especially in Britain, and is almost as varied as the symptoms and causes. Treatment can include a temporary switch to soft foods, stress management, corrective dental work, physiotherapy, muscle relaxants, and, in rare cases, surgery. However, always get an independent second opinion – perhaps a third – before having surgery or any other irreversible treatment.

TMJ sufferers need to band together in self-help groups and as advocates to get better care from dental and medical groups. Private insurance companies often define TMJ problems as dental problems and, therefore, deny payment under medical insurance policies that do not include dental payments.

ELBOWS

Much used and in a position to be bumped, our elbows are particularly subject to bursitis and tendonitis. Tennis elbow, which can come from any repeated strenuous movement (not just tennis), is a form of tendonitis. A wrist splint made by an occupational therapist to immobilize the wrist muscles that attach at the elbow is more useful than an elbow bandage.[21]

WRISTS

Inflamed or swollen tissues in our wrists may squeeze a nerve as it passes through a tunnel on the underside of the wrist, causing pain in the wrist, prickling, numbness (usually in the thumb and first three fingers) and pains shooting up the arm. This syndrome, called *carpal tunnel syndrome*, is common in women who work in the garment and electronics industries, in food service workers, in cashiers and clerical workers,[22] in typists and word processors, and in some musicians. Discuss with your doctor whether you would benefit from using a wrist splint.[23]

HANDS AND FINGERS

Arthritis affects our fingers in many different ways. (The sign language alphabet is excellent exercise.) Osteoarthritis may enlarge just the joints nearest the fingernail (these enlargements are called Heberden's nodes). These swellings may be painful, but they do not usually interfere with activity and do not require medical consultation.[24] A tendency to have these seems to run in families. Rheumatoid arthritis can affect all of the joints in the hand and wrist, especially the knuckles and middle joints of the fingers, and warrants immediate medical attention. Splinting, cold or heat, and exercise are necessary to keep the fingers from becoming deformed.

Many women complain of pain and swelling in the lower part of the thumb, near the palm.[25] Ice packs are helpful for this. Pictured is one type of splint which rests the sore joint while still permitting movement in the rest of the thumb.

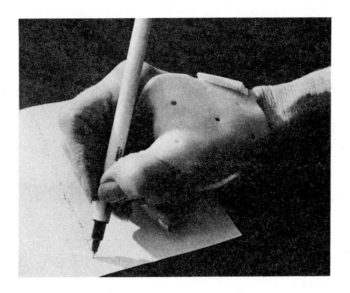

The base of my thumbs hurt for two years. It got so bad that I couldn't write letters. Medications didn't help. An occupational therapist made a small lightweight plastic splint to support and immobilize the base of my thumb so the joint could rest. In two weeks the inflammation was gone. Now I use the splint during stressful activities such as writing and shopping to prevent pain and irritation. [a fifty-year-old woman]

A sixty-four-year-old woman who spends most of her working day typing ran tape from the back of her hand around the thumb joint to her palm to rest her sore joints in the evenings.

Arthritis and Rheumatic Disorders

The word 'arthritis' describes a condition in which a person has inflamed, painful, stiff, and sometimes swollen joints and muscles. 'Rheumatism' is an older word for the same symptoms. There are many conditions that produce these discomforts, however, so if a doctor uses these general terms, ask her or him to be more specific.

By age sixty-five to seventy, about 80 per cent of all women have some arthritic complaint.[26] People who have arthritis and the health workers who work with them are firm in stating: **All arthritis can be helped.** Although people with arthritic disorders require more rest than most others, millions of people with arthritis are living normal, rich, and fruitful lives. Ninety per cent of people with arthritis are employable,[27] although some may need help changing to more appropriate jobs. Only 3 per cent of those with arthritis are seriously disabled,[28] and prevention, self-help, early diagnosis, and new methods of treatment are reducing that percentage. Many react with disbelief at the pain and stiffness which may be the first indicator of arthritis.

GETTING HELP WITH RHEUMATIC DISORDERS

We can find appropriate people to help us when we have arthritis or another rheumatic disorder. We must not assume, as some physicians do, that pain, stiffness, and decreased mobility are inevitable. A thorough examination is essential: ideally a general checkup, including blood tests and heart/lung function evaluation. You may also want to consult a doctor who specializes in joint and tissue diseases (a rheumatologist). A surgeon who specializes in bones (an orthopaedic specialist) is useful for an early consul-tation even if you do not intend to have surgery, but she or he should not be used exclusively. Nurse practitioners are skilled at helping you manage chronic conditions. Chiropodists help with foot care; occupational therapists help adapt equipment for your use; physiotherapists can teach body mechanics and evaluate which exercises are best for you. In addition, many women find relief through the services of acupuncturists and massage therapists.

I refused to consider that anything was wrong with me until I found myself going down the stairs one at a time holding the banister with one hand and the wall with the other. I was only forty-three. [a sixty-one-year-old woman]

Osteoarthritis

The most common form of arthritis is osteoarthritis, called 'wear-and-tear arthritis' or degenerative joint disease (DJD) because of the gradual wearing away of joint cartilage. Although almost all adults past forty show signs of osteoarthritis on X-rays, only 10 per cent of them have any symptoms.[29] So don't worry if an X-ray shows some osteoarthritis; just follow the suggestions for prevention of joint pain (p. 313).

Osteoarthritis is a localized, mechanical problem rather than an illness involving the whole body. It develops earlier in previously injured or stressed joints. Osteoarthritis of the spinal joints is called *spondylosis*. As with all osteoarthritis, pain or stiffness from spondylosis is worst after inactivity and improves as we move around.

Managing osteoarthritis involves combining rest, exercise, and pain relief (including, if necessary, drugs). Sometimes losing weight relieves the pain. Exercises involving gentle stretching of all muscles two or three times a week are helpful in reducing pain and maintaining mobility. Gently stretch frequently during the day to reduce stiffness. When you feel up to it, *slowly* begin an aerobic activity such as walking, swimming, or cycling (if your knees can take it).

Keep warm – people with arthritis are often sensitive to cold, dampness, and changes in barometric pressure, which change the pressure inside the joint.

You may be tempted to move to a drier climate. This does not always help. Try a visit first. Moving can be one of life's most stressful experiences, and the loss of one's friends and familiar environment may be more painful than bad weather or aching joints.

Rheumatoid Arthritis

Rheumatoid arthritis (RA) is an inflammatory illness that affects the whole body. It feels, and is, systemic, like flu. While it may affect many organs, it usually causes most problems in the joints. In RA, the lining of the joint capsule (synovial membrane) becomes severely inflamed, producing enzymes that damage cartilage, bone, and soft tissue, in severe cases destroying the joint.[30]

RA affects three times as many women as men. While it first strikes most often between twenty-five and forty-five, half the women who have it are over fifty years of age. What causes the inflammation is not clear but may involve autoimmunity, in which the body attacks its own cells.

Joints, almost always the same ones on both sides of the body, become painful, stiff, swollen, warm, and tender. Early diagnosis and therapy can do much to prevent the disabling aspects of the disease: of those who start treatment *within twelve months* of the early signs of the disease, 75 per cent will show substantial improvement.[31] Physical and occupational therapy should start early. Unfortunately, people sometimes wait years before seeking treatment, enduring needless suffering and sometimes irreversible damage.

A major US study found some increase in RA at the menopause, but found a particularly high instance of it in women who had had both ovaries removed (bilateral oophorectomy). Something other than oestrogen may be involved, since neither oral contraceptives nor postmenopausal hormones are effective in preventing or treating RA.[32] For this and other reasons, removal of healthy ovaries should be avoided.

People with arthritis do best when they are active participants in managing their disease. Be sure you understand your illness, with its painful flare-ups alternating with good periods, and your consequent emotional ups and downs. You will be the best monitor of your condition.

The progress of this disease is so individual that it is entirely up to me to determine (by listening very hard to my body) what is appropriate, what is too much, when to rest, when to cut back on activities, when to call it quits. This entails constantly reassessing goals, resetting the 'clock' back to zero when I overextend. It is very frustrating but even more so when friends and family pressure me, however subtly. A close friend said to me that the five-hour train trip to visit her is easy. 'After all, you're sitting down all the way.' It gets so hard to always have to explain. [a thirty-eight-year-old woman]

Lupus

Systemic lupus erythematosus (SLE), like rheumatoid arthritis, is considered an autoimmune disease. One mild form of lupus (called discoid lupus) affects only the skin. The inflammatory processes of lupus can attack connective tissue in any organ system, making the disease difficult to diagnose. It was not even recognized as a disease until 1946. Of the 500,000 to 1,000,000 people in the US who have lupus today, 90 per cent are women. About half of the people with lupus will have symptoms similar to the symptoms of rheumatoid arthritis.

Early diagnosis is important to protect the kidneys, and checking kidney function is part of living with the disease. Before the use of corticosteroids, lupus was often fatal within three years. Since corticosteroids tend to drain the body of calcium, people with lupus should pay particular attention to calcium intake. They require even more rest than those with other rheumatic disorders. Although lupus usually strikes during the childbearing years, more women with the disease now survive into middle and old age. One antihypertensive drug, hydralazine hydrochloride (Apresoline), may cause lupuslike symptoms, which cease when the drug is stopped.

Other Rheumatic Disorders

Inflammation that attacks the connective tissues of the body can cause other rheumatic disorders. Two of these disorders are relatively common:

Fibrositis is often called fibromyalgia or myofascial pain syndrome.[33] Symptoms, including aching, pain, stiffness which has persisted for at least three months, sore spots that radiate pain elsewhere when pressed, fatigue, and sleep disorders, may continue for months or years and then taper off. A long-lasting remission is possible. Anti-inflammatory drugs, therapeutic exercise, relaxation techniques, stress management, and physiotherapy can make an enormous difference in the quality of life.

For some months I had been feeling sore, stiff, and tired. I found sore spots on my shoulders, neck, elbows, hips and knees. All my joints hurt. Then my cheekbones began to hurt (no joints there!) and pain in my shins kept me awake. My doctor told me the sheaths of my muscles were inflamed and causing my pain. He prescribed an anti-inflammatory drug and physiotherapy. I was astonished at how limited my movements had become. I began a slow programme of specific exercises, working up to walking and swimming. After ten months I feel much better. The main limitation is that I must avoid fatigue or choose to pay the price in pain. [a sixty-one-year-old woman]

Polymyalgia rheumatica, an inflammation of the small blood vessels that supply the muscles, has been recognized as a disease only since 1969. Appearing often in women over fifty, the average age of onset is seventy. One woman in several hundred experiences this increasingly recognized condition, which causes stiffness and aches. The symptoms of inflammation in the temporal arteries may include headaches on the side of the forehead and sudden severe stiffness in the shoulders and neck, on one side or both. **Inflammation in the temporal arteries must be treated immediately with corticosteroids to prevent blindness.**[34]

Drugs for Rheumatic Disorders

Control of inflammation and pain is essential for the management of rheumatic disorders. Inflammation can be so damaging to the body that even those who dislike taking medication may decide to do so. When necessary, medication can enable us to lead normal lives or even save our lives. (See OTC and Prescription Drugs, p. 52.) Several groups of anti-inflammatory drugs are described below. All of them must be carefully monitored because people react to them in individual ways. What works for one person may not work for another. If one prescribed drug does not agree with or help you, talk with your doctor about others. Patience is necessary to find the drug that works best for you.

Recent research indicates that very high levels of fish oils may have an anti-inflammatory effect.[35] It is not clear, however, that the expensive omega-3 fatty acid supplements now sold by several drug companies contain the effective ingredient. Moreover, high doses, especially if combined with other drugs that retard clotting, such as aspirin, may result in excessive bleeding.[36] Instead of taking expensive unproven supplements, make fish a regular part of your diet. It is high in protein and vitamin D, low in fat and cholesterol, and may possibly have an anti-inflammatory effect.

Anti-inflammatory non-steroidal drugs reduce inflammation and pain. Among these drugs are aspirin, ibuprofen, and many others. All these drugs tend to irritate the stomach, so are best taken after food. Aspirin, the standard against which the other drugs are measured, is the cheapest. When prescribed to control inflammation, it is used in high doses over long periods of time. For some, the amount of aspirin necessary to control inflammation may cause ringing in the ears or other undesirable effects, or may not work at all.

One anti-inflammatory drug, piroxicam (Feldene), which can cause gastrointestinal ulcers and bleeding, was in several countries labelled harmful to people over sixty but was marketed in the US for several years before a warning label was finally added.[37] Opren, another drug once prescribed for arthritis sufferers, is no longer prescribed in the UK.

Serious undesirable effects accompany two other non-steroidal drugs, phenylbutazone (Butazolidin or Butacote) and oxyphenbutazone (Tandcote). These two drugs are dangerous, because on rare occasions they can kill most of the white or red blood cells.[38] Older people cannot replenish these cells so quickly as young people. These drugs also cause fluid retention, which can lead to heart failure in older people.

Some people with rheumatoid arthritis respond well to antimalarial drugs: chloroquine (Avloclor) and hydroxychloroquine (Plaquenil). Because these can cause damage to the retina, possibly resulting in blindness, eye examinations every six months are necessary.

For many of those who have severe rheumatoid arthritis, gold salts or penicillamine can bring dramatic relief. These drugs may actually halt the progression of the disease. However, both treatments also have rare but severe and sometimes fatal effects.

Corticosteroids (hormones obtained from the adrenal gland, most commonly cortisone and prednisone) are appropriate, even lifesaving, treatments for rheumatic disorders. They have severe effects, among them masking symptoms of acute infection, raised blood pressure, slowed healing of injuries, osteoporosis, cataracts, diabetes, water retention, and increased appetite. They can cause fat deposits on the face, shoulders, and abdomen. Never take corticosteroids without supervision; carry a warning card if you do take them. Don't decide on your own to stop or reduce the amount of corticosteroids you are taking even if you feel well.[39] Stopping steroids suddenly or failing to taper off slowly can cause serious problems, even death. Advise any new doctor if you have been under corticosteroid treatment within the past two years.

Cortisone given by injection into a joint affects that joint but not the entire body. Its use should be limited to no more than three injections in the same joint in a year.

Surgery for Rheumatic Disorders

Long-endured pain makes us vulnerable to the hope that surgery may solve the problem. Since speed is rarely a factor in surgery for arthritis, you have time to get other opinions. When joints are so seriously affected that the results are disabling, surgery may be helpful. Arthritis surgery requires special skills and should not be performed by a surgeon who does such operations only occasionally.

For example, surgery can reposition tendons in the hands and feet moved by the bone changes of rheumatoid arthritis, thereby restoring some function in these joints. A synovectomy – removing the inflamed lining of a joint – can provide dramatic pain relief for some years, but the painful symptoms usually return.[40]

You may choose to have a hip or knee replacement if you have severe and worsening pain even when at rest, have great difficulty walking or performing movements such as putting on or removing shoes and stockings, and if other methods have not helped. Over 120,000 hips and knees are replaced each year in the US and the number is rising. The main complications of these procedures are blood clots and infections (but a good hospital for hip replacement will have an infection rate of only 0.5 to 1 per cent – ask). Hip

HIP JOINT BEFORE SURGERY   HIP JOINT AFTER SURGERY

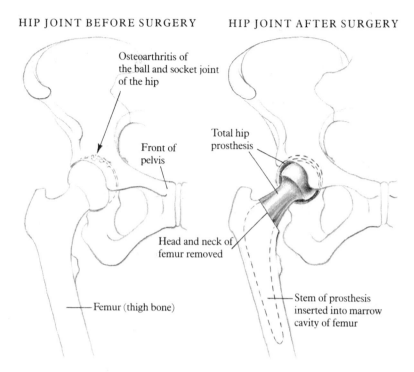

Osteoarthritis of
the ball and socket joint
of the hip

Front of
pelvis

Total hip
prosthesis

Head and neck of
femur removed

Femur (thigh bone)

Stem of prosthesis
inserted into marrow
cavity of femur

replacements are more successful than knee replacements, but both can improve the quality of life. Take time to consider; waiting will not affect the results. Be aware, though, that limping because of hip pain can increase pain and arthritis in the opposite hip. NHS waiting lists for hip replacement operations are scandalously long, forcing many sufferers to seek private surgery.

A hip replacement is a *temporary* solution to a serious problem. The replacement will wear out in ten to fifteen years, but those years may be more mobile and pain-free than without the operation. **No one is too old for a hip replacement,** but those unable to take anaesthesia or who are very heavy may not qualify. Replacements wear out faster under the impact of heavy weight.

A hip replacement has two parts. One, a polished metal ball and stem, attaches to the leg bone nearest the hip (the femur – see illustration). The other attaches to the hip bone and is a socket into which the metal ball fits and moves. A glue or cement similar to Lucite holds these parts on to the bones.

Five years ago I had one hip replaced. I knew that before I left the hospital I would have to learn bed exercises from a physiotherapist, what positions to avoid, how to use the toilet, get into the bath, and manage stairs. I knew I'd be on crutches for three months, then one crutch, then a stick. At first, I needed help getting dressed. I exercised on the floor, but now I swim and walk every day. The hips (I had the other replaced also) are not like my own when they were healthy, but they don't hold me back from anything like when my own were bad. If I knew someone who needed a hip replacement, I'd say, 'Go ahead and do it!' [a seventy-two-year-old woman]

Knee joint replacements wear out faster, have more complications, and a slightly higher infection rate than hip joint replacements. Restriction on weight is important and regular physiotherapy is essential for a satisfactory outcome after the operation. Knee replacements have limited motion, but you should be able to get up from a chair, go up and down stairs, and walk without pain.

I had two hips replaced eight years ago because of osteoarthritis. They've been fine. But my knees also had osteoarthritis, and when I could no longer take walks with my husband, which I like to do, I had them both replaced. I worked very hard at exercising while I was in the hospital. I'm losing some weight now. I take exercise classes and swim. I have a little limitation of motion in my hips and I can't cross my legs any more, but that's not so bad. When I read in bed at night, I'd like to put my knees way up the way I used to, but I can't. But I can walk and do most of the things I want to do. [a sixty-year-old woman]

Two years ago after a very brief examination, an orthopaedic surgeon advised a joint replacement for a knee problem I was having. I sought a second opinion from an arthritis clinic in a teaching hospital. They examined and questioned me for an hour and said I did not need an operation. One corticosteroid shot and their suggestions helped the problem and it hasn't returned. [a seventy-six-year-old woman]

Unproven Remedies

One characteristic of rheumatic disorders is that periods of pain alternate with periods of relief (spontaneous remission). People who experience this may be convinced that whatever they did just before the relief caused the relief, and therefore may easily adopt unproven remedies, thinking they are miracle cures. Many people make money promoting such cures. US *Consumer Reports* estimated in 1979 that for every dollar spent for research in arthritis, $25 was spent on useless or, in some cases, dangerous treatments – nearly $1 billion a year of wasted money. Except for the value of eating fish for their fatty acids, research has not yet confirmed claims that vitamin therapy or dietary changes can help arthritis. Eating well will improve your general health whether or not it has a direct effect on your arthritis.

Some unproven cures may be relatively harmless, such as wearing copper bracelets or observing dietary restrictions that do not interfere with good nutrition. Some, like chemicals that can carry medication through the skin, not only have no value for arthritis, but may cause other problems.[41] Many people take medications that indeed make them feel better, only to pay a terrible price in unhealthy effects later, if they have been unknowingly taking corticosteroids or hormones without supervision and necessary testing. Never take drugs if you don't know what they are, especially if they are provided by someone who does not oversee their use. Ordinary ointments like Ben Gay or Tiger Balm could be helpful because they provide warmth and the rubbing involved in applying them can feel good.

Protecting joints, exercising daily, balancing activity and rest, learning to ask for help, trying different techniques to relieve pain – these add up to changes (often modest, sometimes sweeping) that can help us enjoy life in spite of arthritis and joint pain.

I used to do ceramics, painting, leatherwork. The first time the doctor said 'Stop before the pain starts,' I said, 'You must be crazy. I'm involved in creative work. I have to finish!' It took years before I learned. Later I discovered that flower arranging did not drain my strength and gave me pleasure. It became a new creative outlet for me. I joined a garden club and won several ribbons. [a seventy-five-year-old woman]

NOTES

[1] Richard A. Deyo et al., 'How Many Days of Bed Rest for Acute Lower Back Pain? A Randomized Clinical Trial'. *The New England Journal of Medicine*, Vol. 315, No. 17, 23 October 1986, pp. 1064–70; and Nortin M. Hadler, 'Editorial: Regional Back Pain'. *The New England Journal of Medicine*, Vol. 315, No. 17, 23 October 1986, pp. 1090–2.

[2] Arthritis and Health Resource Center, *Newsletter*, Vol. 1, 1984, p. 2.

[3] Adapted from James F. Fries, *Arthritis: A Comprehensive Guide to Understanding Your Arthritis*, rev. ed. Reading, Mass.: Addison-Wesley, 1986, p. 6.

[4] Mary P. Schatz, 'Yoga Relief for Arthritis'. *Yoga Journal*, Issue 62, May–June 1985, pp. 29–34.

[5] John Hoffman et al., 'Reduced Sympathetic Nervous System Responsivity Associated with the Relaxation Response'. *Science*, Vol. 229, 8 January 1982, pp. 190–2.

[6] Bonnie Prudden, *Myotherapy: Bonnie Prudden's Complete Guide to Pain-Free Living*. Garden City, NY: Doubleday, 1984.

[7] René Cailliet, *Foot and Ankle Pain*, 2nd ed. Philadelphia: F. A. Davis Co., 1983, p. 115.

[8] Personal communication from Bruce Woods, MD.

[9] Suggested by Connie Slater, physiotherapist.

[10] Personal communication from Alf Nachemson, MD.

[11]"Preventing Lower Back Pain'. *Drug Therapy*, December 1982, pp. 97–102. Prepared with the assistance of Dr Bernard Jacob.

[12]Augustus A. White, III, *Your Aching Back*. New York: Bantam Books, 1983, pp. 193–219.

[13]G. Timothy Johnson and Stephen E. Goldfinger, *The Harvard Medical School Health Letter Book*. Cambridge, Mass.: Harvard University Press, 1981, pp. 135–8.

[14]J. Weinstein et al., 'Lumbar Disc Herniation'. *The Journal of Bone and Joint Surgery*, Vol. 68-A, No. 1, January 1986, pp. 43–54.

[15]White, op. cit., pp. 43–5.

[16]Arthur C. Klein and Dava Sobel, *Backache Relief*. New York: Times Books, 1985, p. 32.

[17]Ibid.

[18]Walter R. Sundstrom, 'Painful Shoulders: Diagnosis and Management'. *Geriatrics*, Vol. 38, No. 3, March 1983, p. 91.

[19]Ibid., p. 96. For exercise suggestions, see Kate Lorig and James F. Fries, *The Arthritis Helpbook: What You Can Do for Your Arthritis*, rev. ed. Reading, Mass.: Addison-Wesley, 1986, pp. 49–52.

[20]Fries, op. cit., pp. 192–3.

[21]Personal communication from Jeanne L. Melvin.

[22]"Women's Health'. Report of the PHS Task Force on Women's Health Issues, Vol. I. *Public Health Reports*, Vol. 100, No. 1, January–February 1985, p. 92.

[23]Fries, op. cit., p. 198.

[24]Personal communication from William P. Docken, MD.

[25]Letters to *Broomstick*, Vol. IV, No. 4, July–August 1982, p. 29, and Vol. VI, No. 6, November–December 1984, p. 36.

[26]Jane Porcino, *Growing Older, Getting Better: A Handbook for Women in the Second Half of Life*. Reading, Mass: Addison-Wesley, 1983, p. 248.

[27]Ephraim P. Engleman and Milton Silverman, *The Arthritis Book*. New York: Simon & Schuster, 1980, pp. 144–5.

[28]Ibid., p. 144.

[29]Patricia J. Cooper, ed., *Better Homes and Gardens Women's Health and Medical Guide*. Des Moines, Iowa: Meredith Corp., 1981, p. 639.

[30]Fred G. Kantrowicz, 'Rheumatoid Arthritis'. *Medical Times*, Vol. 110, No. 2, February 1982, p. 73.

[31]Engleman and Silverman, op. cit., p. 20.

[32]Preliminary Results from the Nurses' Health Study, Harvard School of Public Health. *Menopausal Status, Estrogen Use, and Incidence of Rheumatoid Arthritis*, abstract presented at the 110th Annual Meeting of the American Public Health Association, 1982.

[33]Stephen M. Campbell, 'Referred Shoulder Pain'. *Postgraduate Medicine*, Vol. 73, No. 5, May 1983, pp. 193–203.

[34]Fries, op. cit., p. 63.

[35]Tak H. Lee et al., 'Effect of Dietary Enrichment with Eicosapentaenoic and Docosahexaenoic Acids on In Vitro Neutrophil and Monocyte Leukotriene General and Neutrophil Function'. *The New England Journal of Medicine*, Vol. 312, No. 19, 9 May 1985, pp. 1217–24. 'We conclude that diets enriched with fish-oil-derived fatty acids may have anti-inflammatory effects. . . .' See also Summary in Jenny Dusheck, 'Fish, Fatty Acids, and Physiology'. *Science News*, 19 October 1985, pp. 252–4.

[36]"Should You Begin Taking Fish Oil Supplements?' *Tufts University Diet & Nutrition Letter*, Vol. 4, No. 11, January 1987, pp. 1–2.

[37]"Feldene: Canada and Germany Protect Older People Better'. *Health Letter*, Public Citizens' Health Research Group, Vol. 2, No. 4, September–October 1986, pp. 14–15; 'Feldene'. *Health Letter*, Vol. 3, No. 1, January 1987, p. 18.

[38]Fries, op. cit., pp. 106–7; and Cooper, op. cit., p. 636.

[39]Lorig and Fries, op. cit., p. 218.

[40]Engleman and Silverman, op. cit., p. 133.

[41]Annabel Hecht, 'Hocus Pocus as Applied to Arthritis'. *FDA Consumer*, US Dept. of Health and Human Services, September 1980, HHS Pub. No. (FDA) 81-1080.

BOOKS AND PUBLICATIONS

F. Dudley Hart, *Overcoming Arthritis: A Guide to Coping with Stiff or Aching Joints.* London: Macdonald Optima, 1981.

A. Stoddard, *The Back: Relief from Pain.* London: Macdonald Optima, 1979.

C. Quick, *Why Endure Rheumatism and Arthritis?* London: George Allen & Unwin, 1982.

J. T. Scott, *Arthritis and Rheumatism: The Facts.* Oxford: Oxford University Press, 1980.

Michael Jeffries, *Arthritis and You: Answers to Some Common Questions.* Free leaflet from Arthritis Care, 6 Grosvenor Crescent, London SW1X 7ER.

Disabled Living Foundation, *Ideas to Assist Those with Arthritis.* (See Organizations.)

Professor Paul A. Dieppe, *Arthritis.* Wellingborough: British Medical Association/ Thorsons, 1988.

19
Osteoporosis

Lately, osteoporosis is mentioned everywhere we turn – in newspapers, women's magazines, and television talk shows. Advertising promotes 'calcium rich' milk, and articles are published devoted entirely to osteoporosis and its causes and 'cures'.[1] This strange term, which most of us had never heard until fairly recently, has suddenly become a household word.

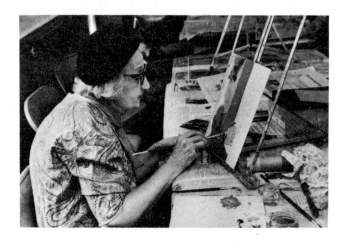

An illustration of a woman with a 'dowager's hump' is used repeatedly as the symbol for osteoporosis. The media blitz is raising our consciousness to the dangers of this 'silent condition' that takes years to weaken our bones, making them vulnerable to breakage in old age. This sudden attention to a major health problem, which had been largely ignored in the past, can help us prepare for a healthy old age.

There is no denying the extent of the problem. Osteoporosis affects over 44,000 British people of all ages suffering from fractured neck of the femur – nearly 35,000 of them women. Women of seventy-five plus are most at risk: 26,000 fractures (1985 figures). One fourth of all white women are affected by the disorder. Osteoporosis is a vital women's health issue because we develop the condition more frequently than men. The condition leads to loss of teeth and wrist fractures, usually starting in our fifties, spinal crush fractures when we are between fifty-five and seventy-five, and hip fractures in our seventies and eighties.[2]

Still, there are some troubling aspects to all the new attention to osteoporosis. Why has this long-time public-health issue suddenly come to the forefront now? Why is osteoporosis being linked to menopause? Why are men who develop osteoporosis being ignored? How can we best cope with the conflicting advice we are given by various experts in medicine, nutrition, and exercise?

Understanding Osteoporosis

Our bones are made up of living cells in a state of constant breakdown and repair. Except for the skin, no other substance in the body has such excellent regenerative powers as bone. As new bone is produced, it is actually laid down on the solid outer shell (cortical bone). Old bone disappears from the softer, less dense substance inside (trabecular bone) where calcium can enter and leave. Normally, our body balances the two processes of building new bone and removing old bone so that our bones remain strong. This continuous building process is called remodelling. When new bone formation no longer keeps up with bone loss, bones begin to thin and weaken.

We lose a certain amount of lean muscle tissue and some bone cells as a natural result of the ageing process, although most of us will not develop osteoporosis. Bone loss starts in women a few years after bone density peaks at about age thirty-five. The loss increases slightly in the four to five years following menopause.[3] There are large differences in the rate and amount of thinning among individuals.[4]

In addition, calcium can be leached out of the bones if the level of calcium in the blood drops below normal. Through an intricate process, the level of calcium in the blood is kept within a very precise, narrow range[5] necessary for muscle contractions, transmission of nerve impulses, and blood clotting. If the level of calcium in the blood is higher than necessary, the body excretes whatever cannot be absorbed.

Osteoporosis is a complex condition that usually takes years to advance to the stage where it can be detected. Many interrelated factors affect the exchange of calcium between the blood and the bones. These factors include the amount of calcium in the diet, how efficiently our bodies absorb it, hormonal balance, and our level of physical activity. Lowered oestrogen level

A GLOSSARY OF BONE CONDITIONS

Osteopaenia: a general term for decreased bone density. Osteopaenia refers to all forms of bone weakness, including osteoporosis and osteomalacia.

Osteoporosis: from 'osteo', referring to bones, and 'porosis', full of holes. In this condition, the actual bone is normal – there is just not enough of it. When osteoporosis exists, certain bones become so thin that they are likely to fracture or become compressed as a result of even a minor fall, or making a bed, or opening a door.

Osteomalacia: the adult form of rickets, a softening and weakening of bones due to vitamin D deficiency. It is caused by poor diet, lack of exposure to sunlight, or the inability of the body to absorb vitamin D. In this condition, bone cells are abnormal and the bones may actually change shape.

after menopause is only one factor – often overemphasized in the mass media and medical literature – that contributes to the development of osteoporosis. We can understand these factors and make changes that will slow bone loss and improve bone remodelling.

For example, when we are young, diet is our chief source of calcium. Vitamin D is often added to babies' milk because it helps the body absorb calcium from the small intestine and also promotes the transportation of calcium into bone. The level of calcium in the blood, in turn, controls the amount of hormone secreted by the parathyroid gland (parathyroid hormone, or PTH). If the level of calcium in the blood decreases, more PTH, which triggers leaching of calcium from the bones, will be produced to correct the deficit in the blood. Other hormones also play a role – normal oestrogen levels protect women from producing too much PTH; cortisone-like products (corticosteroids) can increase PTH production, leading to excessive loss of calcium from the bones.

It is also important to understand how activity, or the lack of it, affects bone strength. Bone mass will increase or decrease according to the demand placed on it. The total amount of calcium in the body increases with exercise, but muscle strength, bone-mineral content, and specific bone mass will vary depending on activity patterns. For example, tennis players have thicker bones in their dominant arms. Demand in an active part of the body will pull bone mineral away from inactive parts. In one study, women aged thirty-five to sixty-five in an aerobic movement programme showed loss of mineral in upper-body bone, which was regained when upper-body resistance exercises were added.[6] Exercise physiologists have known the value of motion and the pull of muscles on bones (not just weight-bearing) since the 1890s, but knowledge is forgotten and the research in one field is not always read by other specialists. (See Moving for Health chapter for a balanced exercise regimen.)

All these factors – reduced activity, reduced calcium absorption in our intestines, and reduced levels of oestrogen to counteract the effects of PTH – result in increased calcium loss as we age.

Symptoms

Seven years ago, I developed a pain up under my right breast and I couldn't imagine what it was. It hurt to move and it hurt to breathe and I ignored it for a little while. Finally it got so bad that I went to the doctor and he ordered X-rays of my back and rib cage. He said, 'Oh, my, your bones are so thin I'm amazed you haven't broken everything you've got.' The vertebrae had thinned and compressed – one was pressing on a nerve which caused the pain in my chest. [a fifty-nine-year-old woman]

Early warning signs of osteoporosis include wrist fracture following a simple fall or blow, and muscle spasms or pain in the back while at rest or while doing routine daily work such as making a bed or picking up an object from the floor. This pain comes on suddenly; most women can recall the exact moment it began. It is often caused by the spontaneous collapsing (a spinal crush fracture) of small sections of the spine that have been severely thinned or weakened. These compression fractures can lead to 'dowager's hump', which shortens the chest area and makes digesting food more difficult. Because compression fractures do not always cause prolonged, severe pain or disability, some women are not aware that they have this condition, although 20 per cent of women do by age seventy.

Loss of height is another early sign of spinal crush fractures and osteoporosis. It would be wise to measure your height routinely. In extreme cases, women can lose as much as eight inches of height, all from the upper half of the body.[7]

Risk Factors and Self-Help

BIOLOGICAL RISK FACTORS

Women are at greater risk of osteoporosis than men because men have 30 per cent more bone mass at age thirty-five than women, and they lose bone more slowly as they age. If you are black, the chances of your developing osteoporosis are rare. Black women have 10 per cent more bone mass than white women, and may have more calcitonin, the hormone that strengthens

MULTIPLE FACTORS AFFECTING
THE CONDITION OF BONE

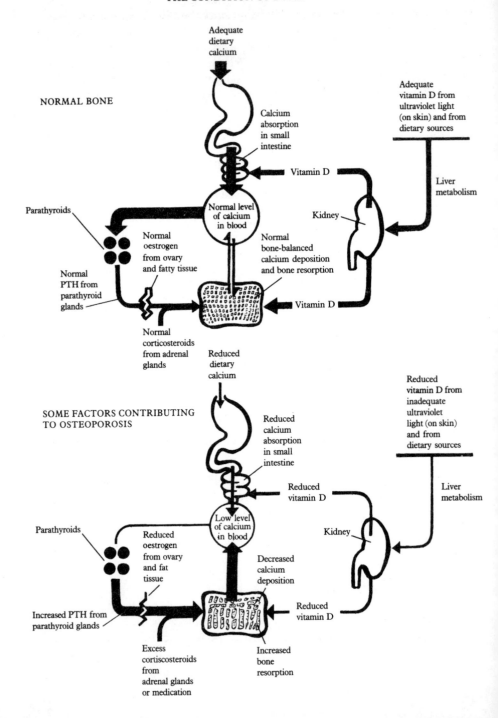

EXTRA CALCIUM?

Doubt was thrown on the efficacy of calcium supplementation in the prevention of osteoporosis in a 1988 paper by British researchers. The evidence about calcium supplements either alone or in combination with other treatments, they state, was contradictory. Skeletal measurements and dietary intake of calcium were determined in 59 healthy postmenopausal women, most of whom were within five years of the menopause. No correlation was found between current intake of calcium and either total calcium in the body or the density of trabecular or cortical bone in the forearm or vertebral trabecular bone. Dietary intake of calcium did not influence the rate of postmenopausal bone loss in the 54 women who completed twelve months of active or placebo treatment. Even when extremes of calcium intake were examined, no difference was found in bone measurement between women with the highest and lowest intakes. This study, the researchers say, suggests that bone density of women in the early menopause is not influenced by the current dietary intake of calcium. (J.C. Stevenson et al., 'Dietary intake of calcium and postmenopausal bone loss', *British Medical Journal*, Vol. 297, 1988, pp. 15–17.)

However, the usefulness of calcium as a dietary supplement was not discounted in guidance issued by the Royal College of Physicians and the Drugs and Therapeutics Bulletin (January 1989). Calling for osteoporosis prevention, particularly through increase in exercise and calcium consumption and reduced alcohol and cigarette consumption, the Royal College did not endorse the use of hormones for *all* women because not enough was known about long-term effects. It is never too late to start eating healthy foods, including adequate calcium (see Eating Well chapter).

bones.[8] If you are of Hispanic, Mediterranean, or Jewish ancestry, the risk seems to fall between the low risk for blacks and the high risk for Northern European white women and Asian women. The fairer your complexion, the greater your risk.

A person's risk of hip fracture doubles approximately every six to seven years, regardless of sex or race. At any age, the risk for white women is approximately double that for men, regardless of race, and also double that for black women. The unusual susceptibility of white women is, thus, not simply due either to sex or race, since there is no clear gender correlation among blacks and no clear race correlation among men. This suggests that there is a similar underlying process which increases fracture risk in all groups as they age, but that this process either begins earlier or presents symptoms earlier in white

FACTORS THAT INCREASE YOUR RISK OF OSTEOPOROSIS

Biological Factors

- Being female
- Having a family history of osteoporosis
- Having Northern European ancestry
- Being thin and short
- Having fair skin and freckles
- Having blonde or reddish-coloured hair
- Early natural menopause
- Childlessness
- Lactose intolerance
- Teenage pregnancy
- Scoliosis

Medical Factors

- Oophorectomy (removal of ovaries)
- Anorexia
- Coeliac disease
- Chronic diarrhoea
- Diabetes
- Kidney or liver disease

- Use of certain prescription and over-the-counter drugs
- Extended bed rest or immobilization
- Surgical removal of part of the stomach or small intestine

Life-Style Factors

- Lack of exercise
- Smoking
- High alcohol intake
- Low-calcium diet
- Vitamin D deficiency
- Prolonged dieting or fasting
- High caffeine intake (over five cups a day)
- High salt intake

Environmental Factors

- Inadequate fluoride level in the water supply
- Living in a northern climate
- Being confined indoors

women.[9] Therefore, if you are white, slender, short, and of Northern European descent, although you cannot change these biological factors, you can make a special effort to prevent osteoporosis by starting early in life, or starting now, to eat a calcium-rich diet, and also by exercising.

In addition, talk to your mother, aunts, and grandmothers to find out whether any of your close relatives have had a dowager's hump, many fractures, or a diagnosis of osteoporosis. There appears to be a slight tendency to inherit the predisposition to osteoporosis, so you need to take special precautions if your relatives have had this condition.

Women who have never had a child or breastfed an infant have missed out on the temporary surges of oestrogen that accompany pregnancy and follow breastfeeding and help protect us against osteoporosis in later life. Although oestrogen levels temporarily drop during lactation and calcium leaves bones to go into milk formation, as soon as you stop breastfeeding your oestrogen level rises again. This helps strengthen the bones in preparation for another pregnancy.[10]

A nutritious diet during pregnancy will help bones get stronger. If you are not on a nutritious diet, pregnancy and breastfeeding can actually draw calcium out of the bones – hence the adage about losing a tooth for each child. Many British women now in their sixties and seventies may have been poorly nourished when pregnant during the Second World War. It was not until 1942 that the need for special rations in pregnancy was recognized. When the mother's own bones are not fully formed, adequate calcium is especially necessary. The adolescent mother can suffer as much as a 10 per cent loss in bone content after four months of breastfeeding.[11] We can't change our own childbearing history, but we hope this information will influence young women to delay pregnancy until their own growth is complete, or, if they become pregnant and breastfeed, to eat wisely. Recommended dietary allowances for pregnant teenagers include a 2500-calorie diet daily, including 76 grams of protein and 1600 milligrams of calcium.[12] We believe a higher intake of calcium, closer to 2000 mg during pregnancy and 2200 mg while breastfeeding, is best for women of any age. In the UK the official Recommended Daily Allowance of Calcium for pregnant and lactating women is 1200 mg daily.

Medical research in the US reports that women experience increased bone loss four to five years following the onset of the menopause.[13] If you have an early natural menopause, before age forty, you are at risk for osteoporosis because the cessation of menstruation causes oestrogen levels to drop.

If you experience diarrhoea, cramps, and wind after drinking milk or eating milk products you may be lactose intolerant – without enough lactose, the enzyme that helps us digest milk properly. If you are lactose intolerant, see page 101 in the Eating Well chapter for good alternative sources of calcium. About 70 per cent of blacks and Asians are lactose intolerant, compared with 15 per cent of the general population. Sixty per cent of American women with osteoporosis are lactose intolerant, compared with 15 per cent of the general population.[14] Note, however, that blacks have a low rate of osteoporosis despite their high rate of lactose intolerance, which shows that other factors are involved.

MEDICAL RISK FACTORS

In addition to biological factors, certain diseases or chronic conditions can make us vulnerable to excessive bone loss. Women with anorexia, for example, may develop osteoporosis as early as age twenty-five – even to the point of having spinal crush fractures, which are usually seen only in elderly women.[15] Extremely strenuous exercise, as a result of which the percentage of body fat drops so low that menstruation stops, can also lead to osteoporosis.

Coeliac disease in childhood (malabsorption of food usually caused by sensitivity to the gluten in wheat) is never completely outgrown, and even if controlled may recur in adults when irritating food is eaten. Chronic diarrhoea caused by ulcerative colitis or Crohn's disease (chronic inflammation or tuberculosis of the small intestine) also prevents the calcium in food from being absorbed.[16]

If you have diabetes, you have to contend with frequent urination, which causes excessive loss of calcium, and high blood acidity, which interferes with the absorption of vitamin D. If you have kidney or liver problems, the calcium in your food is not efficiently absorbed; kidney dialysis adds to calcium deficiency.

Certain surgery can also put you at risk for osteoporosis. Surgical removal of the ovaries, especially before, but even at the time of, the menopause, reduces oestrogen production more rapidly and for a longer period of time than a normal menopause. If you undergo this surgery, you need to take special care to maintain an adequate calcium intake and exercise programme. Many researchers report a high rate of osteoporosis if hormone-replacement therapy isn't started soon after removal of premenopausal ovaries.[17] But we believe that each woman has to decide for herself if she wants hormone-replacement therapy, based on a careful evaluation of her individual situation. For a further discussion of HRT see page 355.

Stomach surgery (a gastric bypass for weight reduction, ulcer removal) and intestinal surgery can also place you at risk for osteoporosis; stomach surgery can lead to insufficient hydrochloric acid, which is necessary for the proper digestion of food before it passes into the small intestine.[18] Calcium can get into the bloodstream only through the small intestines or bones. If there are problems with intestinal absorption, your bones pay the price.

It's also necessary to consider medications often taken for chronic health problems, such as cortisone for severe arthritis, thyroid for hypothyroidism, phenobarbital or phenytoin (Epanutin) for seizures, aluminium-containing antacids for ulcers or heartburn. Exercise and a nutritious diet are a must if you take these drugs, because they all interfere with the body's ability to absorb calcium from food and calcium supplements.

LIFE-STYLE RISK FACTORS

Avoiding osteoporosis isn't as complicated as we are led to believe. Most of us can take immediate steps to slow down bone weakening by changing our daily habits.

Nutrition, for example, plays a major role in preventing and treating osteoporosis. (See the Eating Well chapter for a full discussion of the role of calcium in a balanced diet.) The amount of phosphorus (which aids in the development and maturation of bones)[19] we consume should be equal to the amount of calcium we consume. Most of us, however, probably take in too much phosphorus from eating red meat, processed cheese, baked goods that contain phosphate baking powder, cola and other soft drinks, instant soups and puddings, bread, and phosphate food additives. High amounts of phosphorus are absorbed very efficiently; high amounts of calcium, on the other hand, are absorbed less efficiently. Dried skim milk is very high in phosphorus – each 100 grams of milk contains 950 mg of phosphorus[20] – so if you add powdered milk to soups or casseroles for extra calcium, take care to cut out other unnecessary sources of phosphorus.

We also need magnesium for strong teeth and bones. The amount of magnesium we consume should be at least half the amount of calcium we consume – perhaps equal to it.[21] If magnesium intake is too low, the body is not able to utilize calcium or vitamin D, even if a sufficient amount of those substances is available. There is a rich supply of magnesium in nuts, whole grains, sprouts, beans, fresh vegetables, and fruit.

It's also important that we get enough zinc and manganese, because calcium added to the diet decreases their absorption. Zinc is found in whole-grain breads and cereals, nuts, and seeds. Manganese is found in sunflower seeds, nuts, rice, barley, oats, and blueberries.

Vitamin D is a vital factor in the body's use of calcium. In order for vitamin D to aid in calcium absorption, it has to be converted into a hormone in the liver and in the kidneys. Osteoporosis may occur when the conversion is not taking place, and hence may be a symptom of liver and/or kidney disease. In addition, vitamin D can't be converted to its active hormone form when the blood is too acid due to stress, diabetes, or fasting, or if you have a magnesium deficiency. Certain medications such as anticonvulsants, laxatives, cortisone, and mineral oil can also interfere with the absorption of vitamin D.

A summer holiday in the sun allows us to store vitamin D for prolonged periods of time. Half an hour in the sun with 30 per cent of the body exposed several times a week is fine too. This is especially important if we live in the North, in overcast areas, or are confined indoors. But be sure to avoid excessive exposure to the sun.

Foods rich in vitamin D are egg yolk (if hens are allowed outside), certain fish, fish liver, and butter. Fortunately vitamin D is added to margarines and some milks. Over the age of sixty-five we need 600 to 800 IU daily because our bodies have a decreased capacity to absorb and convert vitamin D as we get older, which may be a significant factor in osteoporosis. You can take a supplement if you dislike dairy products or are lactose intolerant. Supplementary amounts over 1000 IU a day interfere with calcium absorption and, because vitamin D is stored in the body for long periods of time, higher amounts can be toxic.

Prolonged dieting and fasting are common in our society because of its obsession with slenderness. If you habitually eat little, your daily requirements for calcium and related nutrients are not met, so that calcium has to be taken from your bones. Adequate weight and fat tissue offer protection from osteoporosis. The weight on the bones makes them work to produce new bone tissue, and the fat tissue helps to maintain some oestrogen in the body after the menopause. The ovaries continue after the menopause to produce a little oestrogen of the type seen in menstruating women and the adrenal glands continue to produce androgens, which are converted to another type of oestrogen in fat tissue.

Other life-style factors, such as alcohol and caffeine abuse, can also contribute to bone loss. Both caffeine and alcohol act as diuretics that can cause loss of calcium and zinc in the urine. Alcohol damages the liver, interfering with vitamin D metabolism. However, one or two cups of coffee or tea, a beer or a glass of wine, or 1½ ounces of spirits daily probably do no harm.

Smoking is a known risk factor in osteoporosis. It is directly toxic to the ovaries. Women who smoke often experience the menopause up to five years earlier than non-smokers, and thus have lower oestrogen levels for a longer period of time. Smoking may also interfere with the body's metabolism of oestrogen, and may affect bone remodelling in other ways.[22] Smoking often accompanies high alcohol or caffeine use. If you smoke, try to stop or at least cut down.

Lack of exercise is another major risk factor that you can control. Part of the geographical and racial differences among women relative to the incidence of osteoporosis may be due to differences in physical activity.[23] In the past, middle-class women didn't exercise vigorously. To sweat was unfeminine, and our society equated femininity with a small frame, low weight, and a passive attitude toward life; certainly there was no approval of a female 'athletic' type. Fortunately it's never too late for us to start exercising. Weight-bearing exercises such as walking, jogging, skipping and dancing all make our bones work harder and strengthen the muscles and ligaments supporting the skeleton. One researcher reported that weight-bearing exercise that excluded upper-body activity resulted in a 3.5 per cent increase in spinal bone during an 18-month period, but a 3.6 per cent decrease in wrist bone.[24] It is important to make our arms work also, by swimming, wearing weights on them as we walk, carrying equally-distributed shopping bags, doing push-ups, or other arm exercises.

Prolonged inactivity, such as bed rest, can speed up the rate of bone-density loss.

ENVIRONMENTAL RISK FACTORS

Fluoridation of drinking water has been successful in the prevention of tooth decay – and it may also prevent bone fragility and osteoporosis.[25] New evidence supports research done twenty years ago (largely ignored at the time) that reported fewer bone fractures in communities with high-fluoride water than those with low-fluoride water.[26] In one study, the number of hip fractures during an eleven-year period was significantly lower in women over the age of seventy in a community with a water fluoride content of 1 mg per litre than in a similar community with only 0–0.1 mg per litre. Levels as low as one part fluoride to one million parts water are reported to reduce osteoporosis by up to 40 per cent.[27] You may wish to check the fluoride level of your public or bottled water supply. Until your water supply is fluoridated you might consider individual fluoride supplementation. In the UK there has been vocal opposition to fluoridation of water supplies, but most medical opinion favours it when natural fluoride content is low. Supplementation by fluoride tablets can lead to medical problems such as inflamed joints and gastric troubles however.[28]

When We Need Professional Help

If you have several of the above risk factors, or just feel you want further information, you can seek out a doctor who is knowledgeable about osteoporosis. Nutritionists can be extremely helpful in planning a preventive diet to your liking; exercise instructors can tailor a regimen that will strengthen the muscles and ligaments supporting your bones;[29] nurses and health visitors can help you establish osteoporosis-prevention habits[30] and understand the politics of the current osteoporosis controversy;[31] doctors can order screening (if available) and medication for osteoporosis.

In the past, most doctors have concentrated on treatment of existing osteoporosis at the expense of early prevention.* They have often prescribed, after a fracture has occurred, the very procedures that might have prevented osteoporosis from developing in the first place – replacement calcium, vitamin D supplements, and weight-bearing exercise. Doctors are presently debating the value of certain drugs, such as hormones and sodium fluoride, in the

*For the first time, a medical organization – the American Society for Bone and Mineral Research – has formally addressed the issue of osteoporosis prevention, announcing guidelines that stress adequate calcium intake, regular weight-bearing exercise, and avoidance of smoking.

prevention and treatment of osteoporosis.[32] Some doctors are very 'pro-medication';[33] others warn of its dangers and encourage exercise and dietary modifications instead.[34]

SCREENING AND DIAGNOSIS

Because the loss of bone cells leading to osteoporosis is so gradual, we need to be very alert to early signs. Screening and diagnosis of this condition can be difficult since low bone density alone does not necessarily indicate osteoporosis. There is substantial similarity in the bone densities of women with and without fractures.[35] Other factors, such as the strength of the muscles and ligaments supporting the bones, also affect susceptibility of bones to fractures.

Loss of teeth during midlife and thinning of the bones supporting the teeth are warning signals. This bone thinning may be detected by dental X-rays. A recent study reports that loss of teeth at midlife occurs more often in women than in men, and in white women much more often than in black women. Women who lost their teeth early and smoked developed osteoporosis three times as frequently as women who did not smoke.[36] However, we women will have to question and convey information between our doctors and dentists, since they so rarely communicate with each other.

Ordinary X-rays don't clearly detect osteoporosis until at least 30 per cent of bone density is lost, and are not suitable for screening purposes. One screening tool is a bone-density scanner, of which there are two types: single- and dual-photon absorptiometry.

Single-photon absorptiometry (SPA) scans are more common and less expensive – they take less than fifteen minutes. Radioactive iodine is directed at the patient's arm, which is submerged in water, and a detector counts how much radiation passes through the bone, thereby gauging bone density. The amount of radiation received from this procedure is less than 1 per cent of that received from an X-ray.[37] This test can detect bone loss as slight as 1 to 3 per cent. However, though SPA is a relatively simple and accurate measure of bone density in the hand and arm, it doesn't measure bone density at the other major fracture sites – the hip and the spine. One researcher found that the test erred an average of 14 per cent of the time when predicting bone mass at the hip or spine based on a scan of the hand and arm, and so cautioned that no single method of bone scanning can definitively predict the risk of fracture before it happens.[38] Other researchers, however, have faith in SPA as a screening technique for detecting osteoporosis. The technique, however, is rarely available in the UK, unless provided privately at high cost.

Dual-photon absorptiometry (DPA) can be used to scan the whole body, including the spine and hip. This method is also low in radiation, but is not generally available due to the high cost of the equipment. The CAT scan, involving even more expensive equipment, is the most accurate method of detecting osteoporosis anywhere in the body. However, it involves exposure to more radiation than the SPA or the DPA.

In order to be certain that osteoporosis is the major problem, and not the result or symptom of another disease, other tests, possibly even a bone biopsy, are needed. A bone biopsy to test for osteoporosis is usually taken from a hip bone.

Most doctors outside of large research centres will probably continue, at least in the near future, to conclude that osteoporosis is the culprit whenever a female patient over fifty fractures a bone. The well-to-do may be able to be monitored and tested early if they wish, but NHS patients generally do not have this option. If screening can predict osteoporosis before a fracture occurs, then it should be available to all middle-aged women.

Such early detection is meaningless, however, unless it is accompanied by incentives for women to make the changes in diet and life-style that will strengthen bone mass or at least slow down its loss. Understanding the risk factors described in this chapter may go a long way toward achieving that end. The screening methods can then be used by those with high risk factors.

The Use of Hormones

As we saw in the Menopause chapter, in recent years American doctors have concentrated on the risk of osteoporosis as the main, or only, reason for prescribing Hormone Replacement Therapy (HRT). In the early seventies in the United States, oestrogen therapy was seen as an answer to all the 'ills' women were supposed to suffer around the time of the menopause. Doctors in Britain were more cautious about prescribing HRT, and despite a certain amount of media propaganda only a small minority of women were treated. Then came the scare – oestrogen administered to menopausal women was linked with an increased risk of endometrial cancer. British women felt that any benefit they might get in the form of improved appearance (unproven) or the relief of depression (also unproven) was outweighed by this cancer risk.

The pharmaceutical companies in the US and the UK then came up with a new formula. Progestogen was added on days sixteen to twenty-five of the menstrual cycle in imitation of the 'natural' production of hormones in a normal cycle in premenopausal women. This combination, it was claimed, would prevent the lining of the uterus from building up to a dangerous, cancer-threatening level.

As we've seen, the thrust of propaganda in the US was switched. Getting away from the earlier 'forever youthful' story, the target was now osteoporosis and its prevention. And in Britain, too, until quite recently, it was being claimed that the only valid reason for prescribing HRT over a longer period than a few months was that hormone replacement did appear to have a slowing-down effect on the thinning of bone that occurs as we age. Few women can have failed to read the media articles that put osteoporosis on the map. Many will have heard on radio of the formation of organizations for sufferers and question-and-answer programmes where experts extolled the virtues of HRT in combating osteoporosis.

What many didn't realize, of course, is the extent to which the pharmaceutical interests were backing these campaigns, directly or indirectly, by funding seminars, publications and groups, briefing journalists and generally changing the climate of opinion in subtle, PR exercises.

Interestingly, some 'experts' were not satisfied with simply treating osteoporosis perhaps because, after all, only 25 per cent of women are badly enough affected to suffer fractures as a result. So by 1988 there were indications that the target had widened again, and some 'experts' were beginning to tell us, through the media, that really *everyone* could benefit from many years of HRT; we'd just be treating the 'deficiency disease' of middle and old age by replacing the natural hormones the menopause had robbed us of. The advantage to the pharmaceutical companies of an acceptance that every woman of forty-five plus ought to have HRT is obvious. Perhaps it is less so for us.

Who Needs HRT?

Research is under way to determine whether the present low-dose HRT – small enough not to cause 'periods' – is effective in the prevention of osteoporosis. And some doctors still won't prescribe HRT as a preventive measure because

- Research on the long-term effects is not yet available;
- Progestogens in the birth-control pill increase the risk of high blood pressure, strokes, and breast cancer;
- This combination of hormones causes menstrual-type bleeding;
- Extra medical examinations – such as regular Pap smears, pelvic and breast exams, blood-pressure monitoring, and endometrial biopsies – are necessary to monitor the effects of these drugs.

There is a fundamental confusion in the medical literature and the popular media between recommending hormone therapy to *treat* osteoporosis and recommending it to *prevent* osteoporosis. In April 1984, a US National Institutes of Health Consensus Development Conference recommended the use of oestrogen for white women to prevent osteoporosis, despite the known risks. Now many doctors are indiscriminately prescribing hormone therapy for prevention.

To recommend widespread use of hormones to prevent osteoporosis without assessing the needs of each individual woman is the same as recommending that everyone take anti-hypertension drugs to prevent high blood pressure. For no other condition is anything as potentially dangerous as hormones recommended for prevention.[39]

One researcher recommends oestrogen therapy both for what he calls Type I osteoporosis – which occurs in women within ten to fifteen years after the menopause, resulting in spinal crush fractures and dowager's hump – and Type II osteoporosis – which affects elderly women and men and is caused by inefficient calcium absorption.[40] Oestrogen therapy does appear to offer some protection against bone loss for three to five years.[41] We must remember, however, that both these types of osteoporosis can be affected by the life-style factors discussed previously, and that if we start hormone therapy and then stop we will lose just as much bone as if we never started.[42] We will just be postponing the bone loss. Many doctors recommend, therefore, that hormone therapy be continued virtually indefinitely if it is to offer any protection.[43] Others limit its use to high-risk women for a short period of time, while helping the women make dietary and exercise changes.

Doctors Disagree

Among doctors, we find a wide range of opinions on hormone therapy as a preventive measure. Some advocate it for all postmenopausal women,[44] some promote it for women 'at high risk of osteoporosis',[45] while others are against mass campaigns that recommend hormones for prevention.[46]

Generally, practising doctors, in contrast to medical researchers, are more likely to use hormone therapy both to prevent and to treat osteoporosis. These doctors have direct contact with women and are thus forced to come to some decision regarding the prescribing of hormones. Women themselves may ask for hormones. The doctor should explain the risks and possible benefits so that an informed decision can be made by the women themselves. Some doctors in the US worry about the possibility of a lawsuit if they do not prescribe hormone therapy for a woman who later develops osteoporosis. A similar situation might develop in the UK. The lawsuit could be based on the contention that the doctor was unaware of 'prevailing use' or 'common medical practice'; after all, there has been a deluge of articles, advertisements, and public-relations campaigns on osteoporosis. But many medical researchers, on the other hand, are concerned with the possible dangers of hormone therapy (especially cancer, cardiovascular problems, and gallbladder conditions).[47]

Lowered oestrogen levels after the menopause are only one of several factors involved in osteoporosis. Almost all studies of bone loss in ageing women show that the process begins before age forty in the bones of the hand, spine, hip, and wrist.[48] Furthermore, researchers have shown that while the age at which the menopause occurs is relatively constant, enormous geographic and racial differences exist in the incidence of fractures related to osteoporosis.[49] Differences in fracture rates may be due to differences in nutrition and physical activity as well as to genetic factors.

Most of us who don't take hormones won't develop osteoporosis severely enough to cause fractures, and many women treated with hormones still experience fractures. There can be a similar amount of bone mass for women with and without osteoporosis, so that selecting appropriate subjects for preventive hormone therapy remains beyond the ability of medicine at this time.[50]

It must also be remembered that the introduction of progestogen in combination with oestrogen is a relatively recent development. Research into long-term results of the combined treatment is therefore not yet completed. Research to date on the results of HRT over a number of years is thus concerned with oestrogen-only therapy. The long-term effects of the current therapy will not be known for some time – they may be good or bad.

One woman with osteoporosis decided reluctantly to take hormones:

I've had a bad back for a long time – I walk stooped over and I can't stand up straight . . . it's got worse, especially the pain. After I was advised by three doctors to take hormones I started on oestrogen and progesterone to prevent further development of osteoporosis. Does it help the pain in my back? No. The disadvantage is that I got my periods again and that feels just awful. It isn't natural for an older woman like me to be having periods. I was really against taking hormones, but when the three doctors told me to I didn't give up on my scepticism, but I did stop resisting. [a seventy-six-year-old woman]

HORMONES AS TREATMENT

Doctors do not agree on the advisability of *treating* osteoporosis with hormones, either. Some believe that since hormones cannot reverse the course of osteoporosis, they only expose women to unnecessary cancer risks without any obvious benefit.[51]

Both doctors I consulted advised me that the history of cancer in my family was so strong – breast cancer particularly – that it was better not to take oestrogen for my osteoporosis. They said it was better to leave it alone, so I did. [a fifty-three-year-old woman]

HORMONE THERAPY: OESTROGEN AND PROGESTERONE

Advantages:

- Possible reduced risk of osteoporosis
- Elimination of hot flushes and sweating associated with the menopause
- Reduction of vaginal dryness

Disadvantages:

- Increased risk of heart disease and stroke
- Increased risk of breast cancer
- Increased risk of gallbladder disease
- Accelerated growth of uterine fibroids
- More medical procedures
- Lifelong dependency on hormones
- Continuation or resumption of periods in women who have not had a hysterectomy

The use of hormones may be appropriate for:

- a woman believed to be at high risk for osteoporosis, such as one who is taking corticosteroids for a life-threatening condition or who has definite multiple-risk factors that she is unable to change
- replacement therapy until the age of natural menopause for a woman who has had her ovaries removed at a young age. This is the only time when the word 'replacement' is appropriate – the use of hormones *after* the menopause is adding, not replacing, hormones.
- a woman who has severe osteoporosis. Osteoporosis is treatable and further bone loss can be prevented.

Another woman decided to participate in an experiment:

I'm short, slim, and light-skinned and worried because my mother developed osteoporosis. I'm willing to be part of a research project in which I'm taking calcium plus oestrogen and progestogen in such low doses that I do not have periods. [a fifty-five-year-old woman]

One physician warns that the questions of whether, when, and how much of what hormone to prescribe should be based on individual evaluations after a diagnosis of osteoporosis has been confirmed.[52] Researchers who claim that hormones are effective commonly fail to have a control group to test for other factors, such as diet, efficiency of calcium absorption, and activity level. **When we have osteoporosis, the most hormones can do is to help prevent further**

THE AMARANT TRUST

The National Osteoporosis Society (see Organizations) publishes booklets on osteoporosis that suggest HRT, but do not discount diet and exercise as preventive measures. Another organization, the Amarant Trust, 'has been set up to promote a better understanding of the menopause, to support and expand research in this field and to make information and treatment available to more women'. Its activities, in part, are supported by drug companies with a vested interest in the treatment on offer and women should be aware of this. Its first clinic is at King's College Hospital, London, where there is a strong medical team involved in HRT treatment and research. Charges are made for consultation, but subsequent prescriptions for HRT supplies are passed on to patients' GPs, most of whom agree to prescribe on the NHS. The Amarant Trust's newsletter, *Feeling Good*, is sponsored by an educational grant from the two drug companies Ciba-Geigy plc, and Novo Laboratories, manufacturers of hormonal products. The Trust disclaims any direct connection with pharmaceutical companies in running its *services*, but these companies frequently fund *research* in this and other medical fields.

bone loss and keep our bones at the level they were when treatment started. Women who should not take oestrogens include those with a history of cancer, breast cysts, high blood pressure, blood clots, atherosclerosis, strokes, kidney, liver, gallbladder, or heart disease, sickle-cell anaemia or trait, asthma, epilepsy, uterine fibroids, endometriosis, adenomyosis, and women who took DES during pregnancy (see below). Though women who smoke are at high risk for osteoporosis, their use of oestrogen increases other risks.

Women who have not had a hysterectomy and who take oestrogens are advised to take progesterones to reduce the risk of endometrial cancer. **Be aware that the effects of long-term use of progesterone are not known.** Progestogen can cause changes similar to those of diabetes, can unfavourably alter blood fats and so may increase the risk of heart disease and strokes, and may stimulate the growth of breast cancer cells, which are more frequent in older women. Some brands of oestrogens also contain tranquillizers or testosterone (see pp. 54 and 403). Some women taking hormone therapy experience nausea, water retention, weight gain, breast enlargement and tenderness, or depression.

If you have been on hormone therapy and decide to stop, consult your doctor on how to taper off. A sudden drop in hormones can cause hot flushes and other discomforts; a gradual drop may be more comfortable.

The Hormone Industry

When a condition has received as much publicity as osteoporosis has recently, as we've seen, there are profit-motives in the drive to prescribe HRT for all women. In the United States there is now an Osteoporosis Awareness Week, during which interested companies go all out to promote their wares.[53] There are signs that something similar might develop in the UK – the drive to bring the condition to public awareness has resulted in the formation of osteoporosis groups and the publication of glossy brochures whose message 'you need HRT' is a good deal more prominent than the small-type acknowledgements to this or that pharmaceutical company which has funded the publication.

The story of DES (diethylstilboestrol) in the United States should act as a warning. This was taken in good faith by American women between 1941 and 1971 for many reasons, notably the prevention of miscarriage. Not only was it proved to be ineffective in this respect, but it was later found to have caused cancerous and non-cancerous tumours in the women who had taken it, and, in some cases, abnormal structural development of the sex organs of the daughters and sons of those mothers who had taken DES in pregnancy, and infertility problems as well.

With this and other stories of 'wonder treatments' that subsequently had to be modified or withdrawn because of ill-effects, it seems that we should look at the HRT propaganda with a healthy degree of scepticism. Of course we should also try, too, to inform ourselves about situations where benefits can outweigh disadvantages. We can always change our nutritional and exercise patterns first, before trying chemical solutions.

The present debate over whether to prescribe hormones to prevent or treat osteoporosis will continue. We believe that it is unethical and medically unsound to prescribe hormones for all menopausal women. Instead, we support a public health campaign to prevent osteoporosis by increasing women's knowledge of the risk factors, by accident prevention strategies, and by encouraging exercise, good nutrition, fluoridation of the water supply, and avoiding or ending the habit of smoking.

SODIUM FLUORIDE

Besides the small amounts of fluoride being added to the water supply, fluoride is also being used in higher doses experimentally to increase bone mass and lessen the chance of new fractures. One study showed that a fluoride-and-calcium regimen was associated with a 10 per cent increase in spinal bone in women with vertebral osteoporosis, compared to a 3 per cent increase in those on a placebo-and-calcium regimen.[54] Another study found that a fluoride-calcium-vitamin D regimen helped hip-fracture patients prevent further fractures.[55] But when fluoride is used therapeutically, the quality of the new bone cells is questionable.

Fluoride in high doses should only be used to treat severe osteoporosis under careful supervision and be accompanied by a good nutrition and exercise programme. Sensitivity to fluoride varies; some people experience nausea and vomiting, inflamed joints, and gastric pain and should not take it.[56]

NEW RESEARCH

Several new drugs are currently being studied for their effectiveness against osteoporosis. These include calcitriol (the body's working form of vitamin D), calcitonin (a thyroid hormone), a synthetic parathyroid hormone, androgenic anabolic steroids (steroids that increase bone mass but cause masculinization), thiazides (diuretics that reduce the amount of calcium lost in the urine), biphosphonates (used to reduce excessively high blood levels of calcium), 'ADFR' (a complex system of several drugs), and various drug combinations.[57] If your doctor offers you these drugs, you should know that their efficacy and safety have not yet been established. We urge an emphasis on natural methods to prevent and treat osteoporosis. We also stress the need for adequate long-term testing for safety and efficacy of any drugs before they are marketed.

Living with Osteoporosis

After I was told that I had osteoporosis I slowly got my act together and began to realize that I, too, must help. I started reading about vitamins and calcium and had long talks with people who had gone the health food route. I changed my diet. This, with walking up to one hour per day, gradually brought my health up to par. [a sixty-seven-year-old woman]

Many of the same steps that help us live with osteoporosis can help us prevent it. An exercise programme as short as six months can reduce the risk of bone fractures.[58] When we have osteoporosis, exercise must be vigorous enough to strengthen but not fracture the bones. Some exercise programmes offer muscle-strengthening regimens and physical therapy in swimming pools.[59]

In addition, look around your home to eliminate hazards likely to cause falls, such as slippery surfaces, loose rugs, and electric wires on the floor. Install rubber mats and handrails in showers and baths, and lights and railings in all stairways. Wear shoes and slippers with low heels and non-slip soles. If you are unsteady on your feet, use a stick or a walking frame. If you need glasses, wear them, but never walk around with glasses that are meant just for reading.

Now the osteoporosis means little to me. My doctor told me not to worry about it. He said, 'You're going to have aches and pains as this thing progresses. Be careful but don't let it ruin your life.' So I didn't. He said, 'Do anything you enjoy, and when it hurts, stop.' I believe that I shouldn't let it interfere with my life-style. [a sixty-year-old woman]

When I was eighty-two I fell down a flight of stairs and injured a vertebra and my hip, and I have pain in one leg. The doctor told me I had osteoporosis, which I had never heard of before. He gave me a lot of information about it. I developed it after being on thyroid medication for ten years. My doctor said there was no cure but we could arrest it. We had a long session about the alternatives. I decided to use exercise and nutrition. I walk at least three to four blocks a day. If the weather is bad I walk up and down the corridors of the apartment building. I use a set of exercises I learned at a course on ageing and I do them every day. I have lost only a little height, am still very flexible and can touch my fingers to the floor. I drink four glasses of skim milk a day. I used to have a lot of salt but now I reduce it. I have red meat only one or two times a week. I like plenty of greens and other vegetables. I'm still very active and belong to many organizations. [an eighty-six-year-old woman]

If the current propaganda that suggests 'HRT for every woman' is successful, the NHS will be faced with massive costs in providing the hormones, and the majority of women who aren't at risk of osteoporosis will be taking medication which *may* lead to breast cancer in later years. Rather than spend vast sums in this way, it would seem both more economical, and safer, for the government to go all-out for accident prevention for everyone and the provision of efficient screening procedures only for those women who are really at risk, and for whom HRT now would outweigh the possible future dangers. If well-informed, these women could then make their individual choice.

Meanwhile, one of the best things you can do if you have osteoporosis is to join a self-help group, or set one up. It is especially important to have a place where we can discuss what we hear about osteoporosis and the pros and cons of HRT – outside the medical arena. Such groups could campaign for more government action, more unbiased information, and at the same time talk together about ways of coping, learn about self-help measures, and help each other to make desirable life-style changes.

NOTES

[1]Morris Notelovitz and Marsha Ware, *Stand Tall! The Informed Woman's Guide to Preventing Osteoporosis*. Gainesville, Fla.: Triad Publishing Co., 1982.

[2]National Institutes of Health, *Osteoporosis Consensus Development Conference Statement*, Vol. 5, No. 3, Washington, DC: US Department of Health and Human Services, Office of Medical Applications of Research, 1984.

[3]Diane M. Raab and Everett L. Smith, 'Exercise and Aging Effects on Bone'. *Topics in Geriatric Rehabilitation*, Vol. 1, No. 1, October 1985, pp. 31–9.

[4]A. Michael Parfit, 'Definition of Osteoporosis: Age-Related Loss of Bone and Its Relationship to Increased Fracture Risk'. Paper presented at the National Institutes of Health Consensus Development Conference on Osteoporosis, 2–4 April 1984. National Institutes of Health, Bethesda, Md.

[5]Betty Kamen and Si Kamen, *Osteoporosis: What It Is, How to Prevent It, How to Stop It*. New York: Pinnacle Books, 1984.

[6]Raab and Smith, op. cit., p. 37.

[7]Notelovitz and Ware, op. cit., p. 32.

[8]Ibid., p. 53.

[9]Mary E. Farmer et al., 'Race and Sex Differences in Hip Fracture Incidence'. *American Journal of Public Health*, Vol. 74, December 1984, pp. 1374–9.

[10]Sadja Greenwood, *Menopause Naturally*. San Francisco: Volcano Press, 1984, p. 55.

[11]Gary M. Chan et al., 'Decreased Bone Mineral Status in Lactating Adolescent Mothers'. *The Journal of Pediatrics*, Vol. 101, November 1982, pp. 767–70.

[12]L. K. Mahan and J. M. Rees, *Nutrition in Adolescence*. St Louis: Times Mirror/Mosby Co., 1984.

[13]Robert Lindsay et al., 'Long-term Prevention of Post-menopausal Osteoporosis by Oestrogen'. *Lancet*, Vol. 1, No. 7968, 15 May 1976, pp. 1038+; and S. Meema et al., 'Preventive Effect of Estrogen on Postmenopausal Bone Loss'. *Annals of Internal Medicine*, Vol. 135, 1976, pp. 1436–40.

[14]Joseph Lane, 'Postmenopausal Osteoporosis: The Orthopedic Approach'. *The Female Patient*, Vol. 6, November 1981, pp. 43–54.

[15]Judy Foreman, 'Study, Anorectic Women May Have Osteoporosis'. *The Boston Globe*, 20 December 1984.

[16]Kamen and Kamen, op. cit.

[17]J. M. Aitken et al., 'Oestrogen Replacement Therapy for Prevention of Osteoporosis After Oophorectomy'. *British Medical Journal*, Vol. 3, 1973, pp. 515+; and Lindsay et al., op. cit.

[18]Notelovitz and Ware, op. cit., pp. 58, 73.

[19]L. G. Raisy and B. E. Kream, 'Regulation of Bone Formation, Part II'. *The New England Journal of Medicine*, Vol. 309, 1983, pp. 83–9.

[20]Kamen and Kamen, op. cit., p. 157.

[21]Jane Porcino, *Growing Older, Getting Better: A Handbook for Women in the Second Half of Life*. Reading, Mass.: Addison-Wesley, 1983, p. 233.

[22]John A. Baron, 'Smoking and Estrogen-Related Disease'. *American Journal of Epidemiology*, Vol. 119, No. 1, 1984, pp. 9–22.

[23]J. Chalmers and K. C. Ho, 'Geographical Variations in Senile Osteoporosis: The Association with Physical Activity'. *Journal of Bone and Joint Surgery*, Vol. 52B, 1970, pp. 667–78.

[24]Fran Pollner, 'Osteoporosis: Looking at the Whole Picture'. *Medical World News*, Vol. 14, January 1985, pp. 38–58.

[25]D. S. Bernstein, N. Sadowsky, D. M. Hegsted et al., 'Prevalence of Osteoporosis in High and Low Fluoride Areas in North Dakota'. *Journal of the American Medical Association*, Vol. 196, 1966, pp. 85–90.

[26]O. Laitinen and O. Simonen, 'Does Fluoridation of Drinking Water Prevent Bone

Fragility and Osteoporosis?' *Lancet*, Vol. II, No. 8452, 24 August 1985, pp. 432–4.

[27]*Fluoridation, Nature's Tooth Protector.* Division of Dental Health, Massachusetts Department of Public Health, January 1986.

[28]B. Lawrence Riggs et al., 'Effect of the Fluoride/Calcium Regimen on Vertebral Occurrence in Postmenopausal Osteoporosis'. *The New England Journal of Medicine*, Vol. 306, No. 8, 25 February 1985, pp. 446–50.

[29]R. A. Yeater and Bruce R. Martin, 'Senile Osteoporosis: The Effects of Exercise'. *Postgraduate Medicine*, Vol. 75, 1 February 1984, pp. 147–58.

[30]Jean Colls, 'Osteoporosis Protocols'. Developed for Inservice Education for the Nurses' Association of the American College of Obstetrics and Gynecology, 1983; Diane Palmason, 'Osteoporosis: Catching the Silent Thief'. *The Canadian Nurse*, Vol. 81, January 1985, pp. 42–4; and A. Mines, 'Osteoporosis: A Detailed Look at the Clinical Manifestations and Goals for Nursing Care'. *The Canadian Nurse*, Vol. 81, January 1985, pp. 45–8.

[31]Kathleen I. MacPherson, 'Osteoporosis and Menopause: A Feminist Analysis of the Social Construction of a Syndrome'. *Advances in Nursing Science*, Vol. 7, July 1985, pp. 11–22.

[32]Lombardo F. Palma, 'Postmenopausal Osteoporosis and Estrogen Therapy: Who Should Be Treated? *The Journal of Family Practice*, Vol. 14, 1982, pp. 355–9; Mack R. Harrell and Marc K. Dreyner, 'Postmenopausal and Senile Osteoporosis: A Therapeutic Dilemma'. *Drug Therapy*, April 1983, pp. 105–15; and Robert W. Cali, 'Estrogen Replacement Therapy – Boon or Bane?' *Postgraduate Medicine*, Vol. 75, 1984, pp. 276–86.

[33]Leon Speroff, 'Menopause'. Paper presented at the District I, American College of Obstetricians and Gynecologists, Copenhagen, Denmark, October 1983; and Robert B. Greenblatt et al., *The Menopausal Syndrome*. New York: Medcom Press, 1984.

[34]Sydney Wolfe, E. Borgmann, C. Lacheen et al., Statement of Public Citizens Health Research Group. Read before the National Institutes of Health Consensus Development Conference on Osteoporosis, Bethesda, Md., 2–4 April 1984.

[35]Pollner, op. cit.

[36]Harry W. Daniel, 'Post-menopausal Tooth Loss: Contributions to Edentulism by Osteoporosis and Cigarette Smoking'. *Archives of Internal Medicine*, Vol. 143, September 1983, pp. 1678–82.

[37]Product Reports, 'Osteoporosis Diagnostic Centers Multiplying Rapidly'. *Hospitals*, Vol. 59, May 1985, p. 126.

[38]Pollner, op. cit.

[39]For a discussion of HRT in relation to endometrial cancer see M. I. Whitehead MRCOG et al., 'The Effects of Estrogens and Progestins on the Biochemistry and Morphology of the Postmenopausal Endomentrium'. *The New England Journal of Medicine*, Vol. 305, 1981, pp. 1599–1605.

[40]Pollner, op. cit.

[41]Cali, op. cit., pp. 276–86; Speroff, op. cit.; Lindsay, op. cit.

[42]Robert Lindsay et al., 'Bone Response to Termination of Oestrogen Treatment'. *Lancet*, Vol. 1, 1978, pp. 1325+.

[43]Speroff, op. cit.

[44]One doctor advises others not to 'get bogged down with fancy tests, most of which aren't sensitive enough anyway', and just to increase the quality of life for midlife women by prescribing hormones. Pollner, op. cit.

[45]C. Christiansen, 'Estrogen/Progestogen as a Prophylactic Treatment of Postmenopausal Osteoporosis'. Paper presented at the National Institutes of Health Consensus Development Conference on Osteoporosis, 2–4 April 1984. National Institutes of Health, Bethesda, Md., pp. 62–5.

[46]Wolfe et al., op. cit.

[47]Patricia Kaufert and Sonja McKinlay, 'Estrogen Replacement Therapy: The Production of Medical Knowledge and the Emergence of Policy'. In Ellen Lewin and Virginia Olesen, eds., *Women, Health and Healing*. New York: Tavistock Publications, 1985, pp. 113–38.

[48]Yeater and Martin, op. cit., pp. 147–58.

[49]Chalmers and Ho, op. cit., pp. 667–75.

[50]Harrell and Dreyner, op. cit., pp. 105–15.

[51]Wolfe et al., op. cit.

[52]Herta Spencer, 'Osteoporosis: Goals of Therapy'. *Hospital Practice*, Vol. 17, No. 3, March 1982, pp. 131–51.

[53]Tacie Dejanikus, 'Major Drug Manufacturer Funds Osteoporosis Public Education Campaign'. *The Network News* (Publication of the National Women's Health Network), May–June 1985, p. 1.

[54]Pollner, op. cit., pp. 38–58.

[55]Lane, op. cit., pp. 43–54.

[56]Riggs, op. cit.

[57]National Institutes of Health, op. cit., section 5 and background working papers.

[58]Yeater and Martin, op. cit., pp. 147–58.

[59]Lane, op. cit., pp. 43–54.

BOOKS AND PUBLICATIONS

National Osteoporosis Society, *Osteoporosis*. (See Organizations.)

Women's Health and Reproductive Rights Information Centre, *Self-Help Approaches to Menopause*. (See Organizations and books on the menopause listed on pp. 203–4.)

A. Smith (ed.), 'Benefits and Risks of Hormone Therapy in the Menopause', *Recent Advances in Community Medicine*. London: Churchill Livingstone, 1984.

20
Dental Health

Dental health is important not only in itself but also for total health and well-being. Yet, although we are among the wealthier nations in the world, 98 per cent of British adults have had caries (dental decay or cavities) and periodontal (gum and bone) disease,[1] and 65 per cent of all British over the age of sixty-five are missing all their natural teeth.[2] Many people believe that tooth loss is a natural part of ageing, but this is not the case.

Prevention of dental disease involves self-care and regular visits to a dentist. Having good dental health can help prevent a whole range of potentially debilitating and isolating conditions among older people. Continual tooth pain saps our energy and can distract us for days and weeks at a time. Tooth loss can prevent us from eating well if we don't learn to substitute nutritious soft foods for those we can no longer chew. If we are embarrassed about our appearance, we may avoid going out. We may avoid smiling and speaking, and we may feel awkward.

FOUR IMPORTANT RULES FOR GOOD ORAL HEALTH ARE:

- Brush your teeth after you eat anything and use dental floss daily.
- Eat well and drink fluoridated water when possible.
- See the dentist regularly for cleaning and checkups (even if you have dentures).

- Keep your natural teeth – avoid dentists who are quick to extract teeth (get a second opinion). A modern dentist **should not** extract teeth needlessly.

Many older people never go to the dentist unless they are in pain. This is partly because they have had bad experiences in the past, but largely because recent changes in legislation have meant that, unless she is on Income Support, a pensioner will have to meet quite high dental charges. The Health Service no longer funds dental checkups, and treatment charges rise almost annually. Private treatment can be astronomically expensive. By writing to our MPs and bringing pressure to bear on our dentists, we can try to reverse the steady erosion of public dental health care on the NHS.

Special Dental Problems of Older Women

The risk of losing teeth increases as we age, and women have higher rates of tooth loss than men.[3] Older white women have a higher rate of tooth loss than white men or black women of the same age. Yet white women practise more careful dental hygiene than white men and have lower rates of periodontal disease than black women. For these reasons, some researchers have begun to suspect that postmenopausal bone loss may be a factor in tooth loss for older white women.[4] Paying attention to prevention of osteoporosis, especially by not smoking and getting enough calcium and fluoride, may have the added benefit of protecting us against losing teeth in our older years.

Home Care for Teeth and Gums

Many of us were not taught as children to take proper care of our teeth and gums. The idea of preventive dental care dates back only to the 1950s. A seventy-eight-year-old woman remembered her father calling tooth brushing a thing 'only sissies do'.

Many dentists believe that an individual's careful attention to diet and self-care will do more to prevent tooth problems than the best professional care.[5] Proper tooth brushing and flossing are essential parts of this. Ideally, brushing and flossing should be done after every meal, but at least once a day. A machine that directs a stream of water to the gumline can be a helpful adjunct but does not replace brushing and flossing.

Tooth brushing guidelines have changed over the years. Now the preferred method is to use a brush with soft, rounded nylon bristles. (Natural bristles act as a bacteria reservoir because they take too long to dry.) Hold the brush alongside the teeth at about a forty-five-degree angle against the gumline, wiggle it in a circular motion and then brush away from the gum.[6] Move the brush back and forth several times using a gentle scrubbing motion. On the biting surfaces of the teeth, again use a back and forth motion. If you can't grasp a toothbrush easily, try wrapping it with adhesive tape or something like a sponge hair curler to enlarge the handle. If you have shoulder problems that make it hard to brush, try an electric toothbrush or extend the length of your toothbrush by gluing a strip of wood or plastic to the handle. Replace your toothbrush when it wears out (after about six months to one year of use) and after each time you have a cold or flu.

A mild, only slightly abrasive commercial toothpaste with fluoride is best for the teeth. Baking soda can be used, but don't brush with salt because salt damages the surface enamel of the teeth. Brush your tongue and the roof of your mouth, too. Bacteria collect on the tongue and then spread to the teeth. Plaque – the sticky, colourless layer of bacteria that forms around the teeth and along the gumline – often forms more quickly and in larger amounts because of reduced saliva flow as we age. (Saliva production is part of the mouth's cleaning process.) After brushing, rinse your mouth with warm water.

Floss between all teeth. Start with an eighteen-inch piece of floss. Wrap the ends of the floss around the third finger of each hand. Use your thumbs and forefingers to guide about one inch of floss at a time between the teeth. Holding the floss tightly, gently insert it to the gumline. Curve the floss against one tooth in a C-shape and gently rub up and down the whole height of the tooth side. Repeat on each adjacent tooth. In case you have trouble holding the floss, you might try cutting a twelve-inch length and tying the ends together to form a circle. You can have someone prepare these for you if you have trouble tying the knots. If you haven't been flossing regularly, your gums will probably bleed when you start but will stop bleeding after a few days.

I hate using floss, but I've had a lot of gum problems and the dentist says I must floss. I've found it's more pleasant to do in the bath. [a fifty-four-year-old woman]

DENTURES

If you have dentures, you should brush them with a soft brush. Soaking dentures, even in a denture cleanser, is never enough. Dentures must be brushed with a commercial denture powder or paste, hand soap, or baking soda. Never use scouring powders, as they damage the denture. Fill a sink about one-third full of water and place a face flannel on the bottom to prevent damage in case you drop the denture. Hold the denture over the water while brushing and brush thoroughly both inside and out. Rinse with cool water (never hot) before putting the dentures back in your mouth. Dentures should never become dry, because they may crack or warp. When they're not in your mouth, immerse them in water. To remove stains from full dentures, soak them overnight in a commercial denture cleanser or a combination of bleach and water (one teaspoon chlorine bleach to eight ounces of warm water). Never use bleach alone, as it can change the colour of the pink base of the denture, and never use bleach at all on a partial denture, as it may harm the metal clasp. To remove stains from partial dentures, soak them in white vinegar or a commercial denture cleanser.

Denture adhesives are not very effective and should be used for a limited time only. The denture will still wiggle, and this cuts the inside of the mouth and interferes with chewing. Overusing adhesive powders can irritate the gums and soft tissue in the roof of the mouth. It is worth the investment to have your false teeth relined when they start to slip. The reason for the slippage can then be determined and the soft tissue checked for damage. You are recommended to have new dentures about every five to six years; impossible for many people, since 1988 legislation has reduced subsidies for appliances as well as treatment.

It is important to wear dentures regularly. If you don't wear them for a few weeks, the shape of your mouth will start to change and the dentures won't fit. The tissues will then have a hard time readjusting to the old set of dentures. And if you don't wear your dentures, you are less likely to eat a nutritionally balanced diet, since you won't be able to chew properly. Make sure you massage and brush your gums and the roof of your mouth daily with a soft toothbrush or flannel.

Denture problems may be caused by poorly made or poorly fitting dentures, not enough mouth tissue to cushion the fit, or even emotional upsets – or a combination of these factors.

I've had false teeth for over twenty years – a full upper plate and a partial on the bottom. I still see my dentist three times a year, since I have periodontal problems with my few remaining teeth and want to keep them at all costs. I have my dentures adjusted almost every time I see my dentist because my mouth tissue keeps changing. No one told me about bone reabsorption when I got my dentures. I've had three dentures made over time and both of the first two relined. Your jawbone just naturally gets narrower and shorter as you get older, though I think having your teeth pulled makes it happen more so. My current dentist is terrific and I can eat raw carrots, apples, and anything I want. But I expect to live another thirty-five years and I worry about whether I'll have enough bone left for my teeth.

My dentist says I should leave my dentures out at night to give my mouth tissue a rest. He may be right, but I don't feel self-confident – and certainly not sexy – without my teeth.

There are times I can't wear my partial for days due to soreness on my gums, not just from cuts but from when I have the flu or am under stress at work. My gums react and are extremely painful. [a fifty-one-year-old woman]

If you leave your dentures in while you sleep, be sure to remove them for some time each day to let the tissues in your mouth repair. Partial dentures increase plaque formation, so remove partial dentures each day and thoroughly clean the remaining teeth.

MOUTHWASHES

Mouthwashes, lozenges, and toothpaste can't cure bad breath. They only cover it up for a brief period of time. Warm, salty water is the best mouthwash. Persistent bad breath may be a sign of a medical or dental problem that needs attention, such as postnasal drip, digestive problems, diabetes, or badly decayed teeth. It may also be caused by medicines or smoking.

DRY MOUTH

If your mouth feels dry, you should discuss the problem with a doctor. A slight decrease in saliva may occur as we grow older, but frequently dry mouth (xerostomia) is caused by prescription or over-the-counter drugs. More than 200 medications, including antihistamines, decongestants, diuretics, and some drugs used to treat Parkinson's disease, ulcers, and cancer, can cause dry mouth. In addition, smoking dries and irritates the mouth. Caffeine and alcohol both have dehydrating effects. Thus, the proper treatment of dry mouth depends on the cause. The treatment may be as simple as rinsing with a salt-water solution several times a day or avoiding very spicy foods. In some cases an artificial saliva may be prescribed. Because saliva is essential for a healthy mouth, not taking care of dry mouth can lead to tissue breakdown, tooth decay, gum disease, and ill-fitting dentures.

NUTRITION

Good nutrition is an important factor in keeping teeth and gums healthy. Here are some pointers to keep in mind:

- Among the many good reasons to eat protein are the facts that it doesn't form plaque and it builds and repairs mouth tissue.
- Eating fibre helps to remove food particles trapped between teeth (chewing gum won't do this).
- Sugar plays a major role in causing cavities, and so keep the use of table sugar low, and watch for hidden sugars in such things as ketchup and lunch meats.
- If you do eat sweets and desserts, eat them with meals rather than in between. Acid produced from the bacteria formed by food particles eats into tooth enamel. The more often you eat decay-promoting foods, the more 'acid attacks' the teeth suffer.
- The longer sugar is in the mouth the more chance the bacteria have to produce destructive acid, so avoid hard toffee or similar sweets, cough drops, or anything else that is high in sugar and is sucked or chewed for a

while. Foods like raisins and honey stick to the teeth and so remain in the mouth a long time.

- As we grow older we need more vitamins C, A and B complex, as well as calcium. Vitamin C helps with healthy gums and tissue repair. Vitamin A keeps tissue soft. Vitamin B complex prevents tissues in the corner of the mouth from breaking down and also prevents sore tongue and other mouth sores.[7] Calcium strengthens the bones that support the structure of the mouth.

Dental Checkups

It's important to have regular dental checkups that include a thorough cleaning. Someone with severe gum disease or diabetes should have a cleaning every three months. For most of us, twice a year is best. Unfortunately research in the UK shows that pensioners who have to pay dental charges are deterred from having treatment. Dental checkups are no longer free. Moreover, according to research carried out in 1985 'at least as far as one vulnerable group is concerned, charges not only deter but tend to deter from checkups and lead to more costly treatment later'.[8] Costlier treatment accounted for 10 per cent of all treatments of pensioners exempt from charges, but only 4.8 per cent of those of fee-paying patients. Emergency treatments were given to 3 per cent of all those of exempt patients, but 12.3 per cent of those of the paying patients.

The dentist does not necessarily carry out cleaning – in many practices this is carried out by a dental hygienist.

It is very important when going to a dentist to make sure that she or he understands that you wish to have treatment under the NHS. This should ensure that any work done on your teeth is charged for at the statutory rate. If the dentist feels that a procedure not allowed for by the NHS is necessary, this should be discussed with you and an estimate of its cost supplied, to enable you to make a decision about private treatment. Don't allow any dental work to be done without getting a full explanation of what it is, the amount of discomfort likely, other possible treatments, the consequences of postponing treatment a few weeks or months, and potential complications. The Age Concern factsheet No. 5, *Dental Care in Retirement* (free with s.a.e. from Age Concern), is full of good suggestions about care of the mouth and teeth, explains what the NHS can and cannot provide, and gives a rundown on costs.

X-RAYS

X-rays are used to detect abscesses or underlying decay, broken tooth roots, bone loss from periodontal disease, and ill-fitting dental restorations. Full-mouth X-rays as part of a regular checkup aren't routine. A clinical examination will not always find cavities between the back teeth and under fillings. X-rays are usually necessary when a problem is suspected. While X-rays are being done, your neck and body should be covered with a lead apron. You may have to pay extra for X-rays.

DENTAL DECAY

Cavities (caries) can form at any age. Drinking fluoridated water reduces cavities in adults by 50 per cent and may contribute to stronger bones, thus reducing the possibility of fractures from osteoporosis.[9] Some evidence is emerging that very small cavities can actually be remineralized – that is, the tooth can rebuild itself – if we drink fluoridated water.[10]

Having work done on a root canal is one way to save a tooth when the nerve of the tooth is infected. In a root canal procedure, the nerve within the tooth is removed, and the nerve canal is cleaned and filled. The tooth can remain healthy and structurally sound. There is an alternative to root canal work, which can be used if decay has reached but not infected the tooth's nerve. In this option, a simple protective sedative is placed over the nerve and covered with a pulp cap.

A crown is a cap or jacket over the stump of a tooth. It is used to support a badly decayed tooth, for cosmetic purposes, or to anchor a fixed bridge. The dentist grinds the natural tooth to a stump, caps it with pure gold or gold mixed with other metals, and sometimes covers it with porcelain. If your dentist suggests crowning a decayed tooth and you can't afford it, ask about having a filling with reinforcing pins, which should cost much less. These procedures may not be available to NHS patients.

PERIODONTAL DISEASE

Periodontal disease is actually a group of diseases involving the gums and the supporting bones under the teeth in an infective process.

More teeth are lost because of untreated periodontal disease than from tooth decay. Studies of the periodontal health of persons fifty-five years old and older show that they have less gingivitis (surface inflammation of the gums caused by irritants) than younger people. However, the proportion of older persons with major periodontal problems has remained unchanged or increased slightly in the past twenty years.[11]

Plaque is the most common cause of periodontal disease. Other causes include grinding or clenching teeth, a bad bite (malocclusion), or bad jaw configuration. In addition, hereditary predisposition, hormonal imbalances, diabetes, and thyroid problems may worsen gum problems, since they impair the body's defence against disease.

The symptoms of periodontal disease include red gums, swollen gums, bleeding, loose teeth, and drifting teeth. It may be painless and often involves no bleeding. Only a dentist or hygienist can detect it in its early stages. Prevention of the disease begins with proper brushing and flossing. If it is caught early enough, treatment involves root planing or smoothing, scraping under the gum, and prescription antibacterial mouthwash. In more advanced cases, where the disease has caused deep pocketing, treatment becomes more complex. In some cases minor surgical procedures are done in a dentist's surgery or, depending on the extent, in a hospital. A local anaesthetic is used and a medical dressing is placed over the wounded area for a week or so while it heals.

Since the late 1970s a non-surgical treatment, the Keyes technique, has been used by some periodontists. This technique combines deep scaling and antibacterial agents applied by the dentist plus a special paste treatment used at home daily. The technique is still controversial and is not available to NHS patients.

SMOKING

Smoking and using snuff or chewing tobacco can damage the tissues in the mouth, increase the risk of oral or nasal cancer, stain the teeth, and cause bad breath. Anyone who uses a tobacco product should see a dentist or hygienist frequently – at the very least once a year. Smoking can also cause dryness in the mouth, resulting in chewing and swallowing problems as well as tissue damage and tooth decay.

DENTAL CARE IN RESIDENTIAL HOMES AND HOSPITALS

Research shows that elderly people in hospital tend to suffer a lot of untreated dental disease. If you are in a residential home you should make sure that you are allowed to go to, or are taken to, the dentist for regular checkups. If you are in hospital, ask to be referred to the hospital dental service.

Age Concern reports that many elderly patients lose their dentures while in hospital. Ask to have them permanently marked for identification. If you can't clean your dentures or teeth yourself, ask the nursing staff to do so.

NOTES

[1]British Dental Association figure.

[2]*Update on Dental Care*, Office of Population Censuses and Surveys, 1983.

[3]Ronald J. Hunt et al., 'Edentulism and Oral Health Problems Among Elderly Rural Iowans: The Iowa 65+ Rural Health Study'. *American Journal of Public Health*, Vol. 75, No. 10, 1985, pp. 1177–82.

[4]Harry W. Daniell, 'Postmenopausal Tooth Loss: Contributions to Edentulism by Osteoporosis and Cigarette Smoking'. *Archives of General Medicine*, Vol. 143, September 1983, pp. 1678–82.

[5]*Health Facts*, p. 4.

[6]Ibid.

[7]Maury Massler, 'Oral Aspects of Aging'. *Postgraduate Medicine*, Vol. 49, January 1971, pp. 179–83.

[8]Health Care UK 1988: *Policy Journals*, the Old Vicarage, Hermitage, Newbury, RG16 9SU.

[9]O. Simonen and O. Laitinen, 'Does Fluoridation of Drinking Water Prevent Bone Fragility and Osteoporosis?' *Lancet*, Vol. II, No. 8452, 24 August 1985, pp. 432–4.

[10]National Institutes of Health, *Challenges for the Eighties*. National Institute of Dental Research Long-Range Research Plan 1985–9, US Department of Health and Human Services, Public Health Service, December 1983, NIH Publication No. 85-860, pp. 2, 19.

[11]Chester W. Douglass, 'The Potential for Increases in the Periodontal Disease of the Aged Population'. *Journal of Periodontology*, Vol. 54, No. 12, December 1983, pp. 721–30.

BOOKS AND PUBLICATIONS

Department of Health, *NHS Dental Treatment: What it Costs and How to Get Free Treatment*. Free leaflet D11 from local offices and Citizens' Advice Bureaux.

Department of Health, *Teeth Need Gums*. Free booklet DH17.

British Dental Health Foundation, booklets and leaflets (see Organizations).

Dental Health Education Initiatives, *Age Well*.

Age Concern, *Age Well* Campaign Unit.

21
Urinary Incontinence

Urinary incontinence, the involuntary loss of urine, is a very common problem among women, and yet we are ashamed to talk about it. The barrier to discussion is only one of the obstacles to finding satisfactory solutions. We also have to deal with how little is known scientifically, poor professional help, and treatments that are of dubious value. Many of us have arrived at adulthood and even old age without ever receiving adequate, accurate information about our bodies and how they work.

Bladder-control problems should not be looked upon either as an inevitable part of ageing or as a disease, but rather as a problem that can be managed and possibly corrected if you are determined to do so. Shame, guilt, anxiety, fear, embarrassment, loss of self-esteem, and depression are common, legitimate accompaniments to this problem. Unfortunately, these feelings are harmful and can only make it worse. Finding the courage to take action is an important step in regaining self-confidence. Realize that you are not alone, and that many other women are finding ways to escape the prison which incontinence problems impose. Be aware that about 30 per cent of incontinence is temporary.

Current figures show that over 50 per cent of all those in long-term care institutions, mainly nursing homes, have urinary incontinence problems.[1] These problems may have contributed to the reasons for their admission or may have developed after they entered the nursing home. Cost estimates for dealing with this problem in hospitals and nursing homes are enormous, accounting for 3 to 8 per cent of the costs of nursing home care in the United States.[2] The cost for the care of the incontinent elderly in all institutions is estimated at over $8 billion per year.[3] British figures are proportionately large. Many of these people might be helped through timely evaluations and care if more staff were hired, through behaviour modification, medication, surgical treatment, or some combination of these techniques. Since women comprise the overwhelming majority of the institution population, bladder-control problems are a major public health issue for women.

Only about 15 per cent of all the incontinent elderly are institutionalized in the US.[4] More elderly incontinent men are cared for outside the institutions, with the direct, unpaid burden of caring for them falling, in the majority of cases, on female carers in the home. In other words, whether we have the problem or whether we care for those who have it, incontinence is overwhelmingly a women's problem. The good news is that increasing attention, more accurate diagnosis, and more appropriate treatment are resulting in complete cure or great improvement in about two-thirds of those with the problem.[5]

Women apparently suffer from bladder-control difficulties far more than men, both in number (approximately two to one) and in degree of severity, and the difficulties increase with each decade of age. These facts tend to reinforce the belief that incontinence is an inevitable accompaniment of female ageing, yet fail to explain why some elderly women have the problem and others don't. Since many doctors believe that nearly 50 per cent[6] of young, normal women have some degree of urinary-control problem, it is easy to conclude that existing figures indicating that 15 per cent of non-institutionalized elderly women are incontinent are too low. It seems as though the problem is underreported. Many women are too embarrassed to speak about this problem, especially to a male doctor; others don't speak about it because they believe nothing can be done. Sadly, many of those who have had the courage to bring it up have found their doctors uninformed, unsympathetic, and often embarrassed themselves.[7]

We women will have to chart our own course to deal with this problem. We hope this chapter will help you know more about how your body functions, what the different types of incontinence are, what you can do about bladder-control problems for yourself or for others, and how to find competent help.

Control of Our Social Lives

One of the very first ways we learn as little girls that we are different from boys is that if we can't 'go' in some places, we can't 'go' at all. Girls may be restricted from certain places or events because there are no toilets. It's usually okay for little boys to simply turn around, discreetly or otherwise, and pee if there isn't a toilet nearby, but it isn't always okay for little girls.

At a festival by the river, the nearest public toilets are several blocks away. I overheard a little girl about five years old say she needed to 'go'. She was then scolded by the man who appeared to be her grandfather. 'Didn't you go before you left the house?' and all that. Because I have incontinence problems, I stepped in and asked whether he would just take a little boy over to the bushes. When he responded, 'Yes, of course,' I suggested he take the little girl there also. He was embarrassed but then the girl's grandmother, who had been sitting nearby, offered to take her. [a woman in her sixties]

Bladder control can be difficult for young girls to learn, and for women to maintain, because while we are being taught to control our bladders and anal sphincters we are also being taught that 'nice' girls do *not* feel or experiment with anything 'down there', especially with the nearby sensations coming from our vaginas and clitorises.

When we are aware of our bladder sensations, we are often required to ignore them. Many of us remember when times to go to the toilet were strictly regulated in schools. Adult women are also restricted in where they can urinate. There are usually no public toilets in shopping malls, grocery stores, and undergrounds, and not enough in sports arenas and theatres, forcing women to brave bars and other places they don't want to enter just to find a toilet. Public toilets are often so filthy and unsafe that women can't use them.

At the Barbican in London there's always a long queue for the ladies' room. When I'm with my husband and we both need to go to the toilet, he's in and out and waiting for me for ages before I reappear. The planners there and in lots of other places seem to assume that fewer women than men need their facilities and forget that a woman takes longer to pee. [a woman in her seventies]

In some workplaces toilet provision for women is inadequate. In fact, one of the excuses some employers use for denying equal work opportunities to women is that there aren't any women's toilets on the site!

Even where toilets are available, women may have to sit hour after hour doing clerical work, with little chance to walk around or get other exercise. When there is a chance to take a break, that, too, is often spent sitting. Sitting is very destructive to the lower abdominal muscles, the pelvic floor, and the entire muscle system of the pelvic girdle. All of these situations can contribute to bladder problems by forcing women to hold urine, which overstretches the bladder, and by weakening muscles. These conditions may in turn lead to chronic infections, cystitis, and bladder-control problems.

Our ability to manage our urine actually controls our social life far more than we realize. Finding a loo is a constant worry for many women, young and old. To lose urine, to wet one's pants visibly, or to smell of urine is simply unacceptable. Not only would we give offence, but we might be thought of as not fully adult – childish, regressed, or even 'senile'. We all try to learn how to 'hold it', often longer than we should, without realizing that doing so may contribute to infections from urine retention. If the anxiety about making it to a toilet in time is too distracting, we may decide not to attempt certain trips, or only do so after we know exactly where the toilet is and are sure we can be near it. We may resort to pads rather than tell anybody. In many cases of incontinence, women feel obliged to withdraw from social life altogether, not going out and often not having people in, either.[8] Use pads and other aids, if necessary, rather than avoiding people and activities, but do not assume that nothing can be done about incontinence.

An older person's inability to control urine is often the last straw for an overstressed carer, and institutionalization often becomes the solution. Pads are often used in place of adequate evaluation and treatment, especially in nursing homes with overworked and untrained staff. What is labelled incontinence is often ignoring a patient's request for a bedpan or toilet until she has no choice except to wet herself.

If you do need advice about pads and other aids, the incontinence advisor at the Disabled Living Foundation can be very helpful (see Organizations). A chronically incontinent older person being cared for at home may be entitled to free protective garments – the GP can arrange a visit from the local incontinence advisor, who will offer specific advice on managing the problem and organize the supply of pads.

How Bladder Control Works

As shocking as it is, even experts know little about the basic anatomy and physiology of the female genitourinary system, as the female genitals and urinary tract together are called. The classic text, *Gray's Anatomy*, devotes several pages to the male genitals and urinary tract but only one sketch to the female urinary system. Most doctors see the female urinary system as an inadequate or defective variation on the male system, rather than as a complex system in its own right. Following is a summary of what experts believe about how the female genitourinary system works.

Urine comes down two tubes called ureters (one from each kidney) to fill the bladder. The bladder and the urethra (the tube opening from the bladder to the outside) constitute a unit for the purpose of storing and emptying urine. Normally, the bladder relaxes while it is filling with urine and the urethra tightens along its whole length from where it joins the bladder neck down to the outside opening, in order to hold urine in. When it is time to pee, the urethra opens along its entire length, and the top of the bladder (the fundus) contracts and drops, expelling the urine. The urethra then closes along its entire length and the whole bladder rises again to its original position to fill with urine again and to expand automatically against the pressure of the closed urethra.

The anus has a true sphincter musculature which is capable of closing off completely in response to a conscious act of will. The vagina never closes off completely. The neck of the bladder and the area near the opening of the urethra have some additional muscle tissue, but we cannot contract it voluntarily the way we contract the anal sphincter. The urinary structure is capable of perfect control, but by the following mechanisms. Normally, the urethra will not open until we decide it should. At a certain point we become aware of the sensation that the bladder needs emptying, but we postpone it rather than wetting ourselves. This is the first stage of control. Though it feels automatic, this postponement until we can get to the right place is a discipline we learned years ago during toilet training.

As the pressure builds up, we deliberately control the muscle surrounding both the urinary and vaginal openings, called the pubococcygeal or levator ani muscle. This muscle is part of a group of muscles woven like a large sling or hammock under the bladder and uterus and around the delicate tubes of the vagina, urethra, and anus. The entire area controlled by this muscle, from the clitoris at the front to the anus at the back, is called the pelvic floor (see diagrams, p. 125 and p. 383). Using this muscle is the second stage of control.

Anxiety about getting in time to a place where they are comfortable urinating plays a role in incontinence for many women, especially if they know from experience that they may not make it. But even for a woman without special anxieties, after postponement has gone beyond a certain point, pain may set in and it will take squeezing her legs together and even holding her hands against her labia to keep urine from escaping before she gets somewhere to pee. This is the third stage of control.

Once at an acceptable place, we have to deliberately decide to release the urine, another act of will, which may be quick or take some time, depending on how distracted we are, how anxious we feel, and how long we have been postponing release. Sometimes sexual arousal may either stimulate or delay the release of urine.

It is also not clear how we know when we are really finished urinating, because we can voluntarily stop and start again. We think we're finished when no more urine comes out and the initial sensation of pressure is gone. Yet some women retain small or large amounts of urine in their bladders even after the sensations cease and the urethra recloses, which makes it clear that it is not just the complete emptying of the bladder that signals the urethra to close.

In fact, bladder functioning is one of the most complicated, sophisticated mechanisms of the female body. As many as thirty different reflexes may be involved in the retention and voiding of urine, and twelve have been shown to play direct, specific roles in incontinence. Incontinence in women involves a complex interaction of anatomical, neurological, social, and psychological factors.[9] Be sure your doctor considers all these factors in your evaluation for treatment.

Types of Incontinence

Experts do not agree on how to describe the various types of incontinence. Since many women have a combination of types, individualized assessment and treatment are needed. We are naming the categories we will discuss as follows:

1. Stress incontinence
2. Urge incontinence
3. Overflow incontinence
4. Irritable bladder

Stress incontinence is a condition in which there is a loss of urine at times when sudden activity increases the pressure in the abdomen and bladder, such as when you cough, sneeze, laugh, or run. This type of incontinence is by far the most common, though experts disagree about whether it is the most common in older women. Often stress incontinence is combined with one or more other types of incontinence. Current theory suggests that urine loss results when the urethra is increasingly unable to maintain control along its entire length against the ever-filling bladder, changing the balance of pressure between the two systems. The bladder neck has probably widened, often in response to relaxation of muscles (against pressure of the bladder); the urethra may be stretched wider and wider at the top, and shortened, much the way a nylon stocking is when you take it off, compared with how it was when you took it out of the package. The only remaining control mechanisms then are a very short area of the urethra near the outlet and the pubococcygeal muscle. Even when weak, the pubococcygeal muscle can usually permit normal functioning, but is unable to handle the 'stress' of the laugh, cough, sneeze, or bearing-down pressure.*

Urge incontinence refers to a sudden, sometimes painful, urge to urinate, which is unexpected and so powerful that it is not always possible to make it to the bathroom. Most gerontologists and urologists believe that urge incontinence is most common among elderly women.

What gets me is that often I'll be fine all day out shopping – no trouble at all. Then just as I get home and start to put the key in the door, I'll suddenly have to go so badly that I can hardly stand it. Sometimes I just make it to the bathroom, but sometimes I lose it right there at the front door.

---

*A few women who have this type of relaxation of the pelvic floor are apparently perfectly continent, and others with stress problems do not seem to have any noticeable relaxation of the pelvic floor, but this is not the general rule.

Overflow incontinence is the problem in a smaller percentage of cases. Usually, it comes on with no warning – no sensation or signal at all – and urine unexpectedly 'overflows' after a woman changes position, such as standing up after sitting, or sitting up after lying down. We may lose a relatively small amount – a few drops – or enough to require a pad. Often there is a desire to urinate again a few minutes later, but very little urine emerges, a sign that the bladder is not emptying completely. The risk of bladder infection is high with this problem, which often happens because we have been sedentary or have learned to hold our urine too long.

'Irritable' or 'spastic' or 'unstable' bladders seem to behave erratically, causing the feeling that we need to urinate even though we may not – often just after the bladder has been emptied.* Irritable bladder may be confused with both urge and stress incontinence, or combined with them, and is often aggravated by anxiety. Because the condition is irregular rather than constant, experts believe it may be more psychological than physical.

Causes of Bladder-Control Problems

AGEING

Ageing does not by itself cause female incontinence, even if the chances of being incontinent do tend to increase as women age. This is probably the single most difficult fact to get across to the medical profession and to the general public.

WEAK MUSCLES

Our whole way of life in this culture has traditionally worked against women maintaining good muscle tone. Many generations of women were brought up to think of exercise as something for men only. In these generations it was poor women who often had adequate muscle tone because of the physical work they did. A general fitness campaign directed at adult women as well as men, and also including the elderly, has only recently been started, and this is too often directed only at the affluent.

After midlife, the muscle tone that we tended to take for granted as younger women slowly decreases. Keeping in shape may take much more effort than previously. This partly depends on how active you have been throughout life. Without a fairly systematic and vigorous programme, already weak muscles

---

*Rarely, a fistula may have occurred as a result of a difficult childbirth, radiation treatments, or surgery, and not be detected. This often results in a more or less continuous drip from a break between the vaginal wall and the bladder or urethra. Most fistulas can be repaired surgically.

may deteriorate more rapidly. Even women who were active previously, however, will lose muscle tone and may gain weight through inactivity. 'Use it or lose it' is as true for the pelvic muscles as it is for any others.

There is solid evidence that weak muscles of the pelvic floor and abdomen contribute to stress incontinence, and perhaps to other incontinence problems. Severe and prolonged immobility can contribute to incontinence problems such as 'overflow'. For incontinent women, exercise such as running, aerobic dancing, even walking may actually aggravate bladder problems because of the

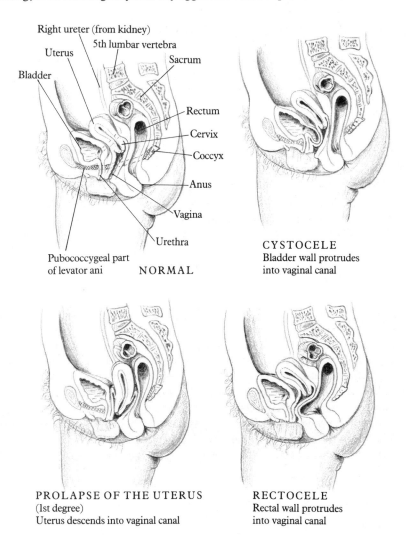

Right ureter (from kidney)
5th lumbar vertebra
Uterus
Sacrum
Bladder
Rectum
Cervix
Coccyx
Anus
Vagina
Urethra
Pubococcygeal part
of levator ani   NORMAL

CYSTOCELE
Bladder wall protrudes
into vaginal canal

PROLAPSE OF THE UTERUS
(1st degree)
Uterus descends into vaginal canal

RECTOCELE
Rectal wall protrudes
into vaginal canal

jarring and gravitational pull on the genital and urinary organs, so exercise is avoided. Breaking the cycle may well begin with pelvic floor exercises for getting control of that key set of muscles in the pelvic floor.

The pelvic floor exercises can be done conveniently and invisibly, whether sitting, standing, lying down, or during sex, and can partly counteract the negative effects of prolonged sitting and passive sex. Women frequently report a noticeable improvement in sexual response as well as urinary control when pelvic floor exercises are practised regularly (see Moving for Health, p. 124).

REPRODUCTIVE EVENTS AND HORMONAL CHANGES

Reproductive events may contribute to a woman's bladder-control problems, or create problems where none existed before. For example, slight bladder-control problems, which may be temporary or permanent, are often associated with childbirth. While childbirth itself is often blamed for these problems, the actual cause may be damage caused by obstetric practices such as the use of forceps, episiotomy, the lying-down position in which most women have been required to labour, and pushing uphill to give birth, often with a partially full bladder.[10]

The reduction of ovarian oestrogen production around the time of the menopause, which may bring some degree of thinning and temporary drying or shrinking of vaginal tissues, often affects the nearby urethra as well. Some women may for the first time experience some type of incontinence, which may be temporary and disappear once the body has adjusted to its different production of oestrogen (less from the ovaries but some from the adrenal glands and fat tissue), or may persist.

INADEQUATE NUTRITION AND WATER

The role of nutrition in incontinence is somewhat controversial, but it is clear that poor diet can contribute to repeated bladder infections and poor muscle tone. Certainly one major factor in certain types of incontinence associated with bladder infections is dehydration due to inadequate water intake.

Magnesium deficiencies have been reported to contribute to bladder instability, but there is no solid evidence for this. However, magnesium (available in fruits and vegetables) is an important mineral for bone strength in elderly women, and should accompany calcium, which is also important for muscle fitness.

INFECTIONS AND INFLAMMATION

One cause of some urinary-control problems is a long-term pattern of chronic bladder and urethral infections. A vicious cycle is often involved in incomplete emptying of the bladder. Infection builds up in the stagnant urine, which may inflame the lining of the bladder and infect the urethra itself. One result may be intermittent, temporary, or permanent urge incontinence. Many women have low-grade infections of this type almost constantly, without even being aware of them until they flare up and overwhelm the system.

Interstitial cystitis also causes frequent urination and pain similar to the symptoms of bladder infection. Urine tests are negative, however, because the symptoms are caused by chronic inflammation and scarring of the bladder lining, which may bleed, rather than by bacterial infection.[11]

MEDICATIONS AND DRUGS

Several specific prescription drugs for hypertension, heart disease, and fluid buildup (diuretics), as well as some sedatives, hypnotics, and tranquillizers, may provoke temporary incontinence. Many types of drugs (including many over-the-counter antihistamines) can cause the bladder to retain urine and lead to overflow incontinence.

TRAUMA AND MEDICAL TREATMENT

Violent sexual penetration, gynaecological surgery – especially hysterectomy and other procedures carried out via the vagina – as well as radiation treatments for cancer all may contribute to problems with urinary control. In the case of hysterectomy, the cause may be physical – the loss of support that the uterus provides for the bladder and urethra,[12] or damage to the urinary structures or nerves during surgery – or it may be hormonal. For many women, hysterectomy causes a drop in oestrogen levels, even when the ovaries have been retained. This drop can, in turn, affect the urinary structures. In some cases, repair of a uterine prolapse or cystocele may remove the blockage which was actually helping to control the urinary flow.[13]

SPECIFIC DISEASES

Other causes of urinary-control problems include diabetes and progressive degenerative diseases involving the brain or spinal cord such as Alzheimer's disease, multiple sclerosis, brain or spinal cord tumours, and Parkinson's disease. Other specific physical causes include spinal cord injuries, stones in the urinary system, obstructive tumours, bladder cancer, strokes, or TIAs (transient ischaemic attacks). Before diagnosing incontinence, a competent doctor should try to rule out each of these conditions, and, if any are present, plan a treatment programme which includes treating the incontinence as well.

EMOTIONAL PROBLEMS

Finally, there are bladder problems which result primarily from stress, anxiety, and depression. Since emotional factors are rarely the sole cause of the problem, it is vital to rule out physical causes first, while recognizing that the state of our emotions may aggravate any bladder-control problem we may have.

I started to wake up at night to urinate – sometimes once or twice, but sometimes every two hours. A gynaecologist put me on oestrogen cream that caused bleeding, so then he wanted to do a D&C. I said goodbye to the cream and to him and also to the leading urologist, who wanted to put me on antidepressants. He had said after observing me – and I was tearful – 'The sorrow that has no tears to cry makes the body weep.' I realized I had this dependency on 'Doctor, doctor, make it better!' The only initiative I was showing was going to doctors. Then I decided to do as much as I could for myself. So I changed my whole pattern of eating to vegetarian (macrobiotic) foods, started swimming and doing pelvic floor exercises regularly. I try to understand what is happening. Now I see that my waking up is related to stress and anxiety. I still expect to wake up once most nights, but when I have had a massage, I usually sleep through the whole night. [a fifty-five-year-old woman]

General Self-Help

Before seeking any type of medical solution to an incontinence problem in the absence of other symptoms, we encourage you to observe and record your problems and take some simple steps to try to help yourself. The first step is to review your diet, hygiene, and exercise habits.

Are you drinking enough water and other liquids? Many women avoid drinking in order to avoid accidents. The result is more likely to be urinary-tract infections and dehydration, which can actually trigger accidents and may even become life-threatening. Try cutting down drastically on caffeine, alcohol, and soft drinks (including 'diet' sodas) and substitute water and clear unsweetened fruit juices such as apple juice. Drink six glasses of water throughout the day, most of them before your last meal.

Toilet hygiene tends to become more important as we age. Some women were never taught that it is important to wipe from front to back to avoid faecal contamination. Some may find that moist wipes do a better job now than conventional dry toilet paper. If you can get access to a bidet or a 'telephone' shower (shower head extension with a flexible hose) for post-toilet cleansing, or switch from baths to showers, you may have fewer urinary infections.

A diet high in whole grains, fruits and vegetables, including some fish, and low in white flour, sugar, fats, and meats, can help keep the acid balanced in the urinary and vaginal systems to discourage infections and also improve overall digestion, muscle tone, and urinary output. Vitamin C, including bioflavenoids, is sometimes helpful. Many women find that unsweetened cranberry juice prevents or fights infections. How do citrus fruit juices affect you? Some women find they irritate the bladder, others that they help control the tendency to infections. Some women find that spicy foods aggravate their problems.

Are you getting enough general exercise, at least walking regularly every day? Decide now that you are not going to stay home or avoid exercise for fear of having an accident, but will find whatever kinds of protective devices and clothing you need in order to have brief walking trips, preferably every day (see Organizations – Disabled Living Foundation). Wear comfortable shoes when walking, and pay attention to posture to correct the alignment of the entire pelvis.

Next, check your overall weight and health. Many women find that losing weight through exercise improves their continence noticeably, though it isn't always clear why. It may be a combination of improved diet and increased exercise, removal of the drag of heavy fat across the abdomen, plus the improvement in self-esteem.

It's estimated that 50 per cent of women suffer from cystitis at least once in their lives. This painful infection can cause us to feel a tremendous urge to urinate when in fact there is very little urine in the bladder – and if a toilet isn't immediately available there can be some leakage. Read the book listed below, or others by Angela Kilmartin, founder of the U and I Club (see Organizations) for self-help measures. Drink plenty of water during an attack – at least one pint an hour; a hot water bottle placed in the groin can ease the pain for some women; and if the problem doesn't clear up within a day, take a urine sample to your GP for analysis. The right antibiotic can clear most infections, but the cystitis attacks can be avoided or at least lessened in frequency by following the suggestions outlined in the book and leaflet we've listed.

If you hold your urine for several hours and then have overflow problems, make an effort to identify earlier the feeling of needing to urinate, which you may be ignoring. Go to the toilet regularly, either at the very earliest sign of fullness, or at scheduled intervals regardless of sensation. If feelings of urgency are *very* frequent, allowing the bladder to fill up more may help.

If you have never done pelvic floor exercises, start today. While exercising

KEEPING RECORDS

While you are taking the initial steps in the self-help process, you may also want to keep a careful watch on your symptoms, both for your own use and to help any professional you decide to consult. A competent doctor will ask you many specific questions as one part of a thorough history and evaluation. Keeping this record will help you to be ready with answers. For example, many doctors ask, 'How many pads do you use in a day?'

Begin by making a note of *every* time you have any type of urine loss or 'accident' – exactly when it happened, what you were doing, where you were, how much urine you lost in ounces (approximately), and what you did about the loss. Try to remember when you first began to have a problem. How did it begin? Does it seem to be getting worse? Did it begin suddenly? Did it start for the first time after an operation or childbirth, after you started taking some new prescription drug, after an accident, after a time of stress, or after some episode of illness? Is it worse during the day or during the night? How long can you hold your urine after you sense a need to go? Do you feel your bladder completely empty? Do you strain to empty? Do you regularly wear pads to catch escaping urine? In some cases, simply keeping a record like this can improve bladder control by helping you pay attention to your patterns.

One of the things you need to establish is whether your condition is temporary or chronic. Try to distinguish between different types of episodes. Do you ever experience pain

this important set of muscles may not prevent or solve all problems of urinary control, it does keep the whole pelvic floor in good condition and almost always brings some improvement in urinary control. Add abdominal toning exercises if you can, slowly, until you can feel the improvement (see Moving for Health chapter, p. 126).

In my early forties I had some stress incontinence which I stopped by doing pelvic floor exercises. In my early fifties I started waking several times a night and, once awake, needed to urinate. When I went on a camping trip I didn't like getting out of the sleeping bag and tent so many times at night. At first I kept a plastic container in the tent to pee in but then I decided to ignore the feeling and go back to sleep. By the end of the trip I was sleeping through the night. For a few years after that I was awakened several times at night because of hot flushes but never had to urinate more than once a night. Now that my hot flushes have subsided I am again sleeping through the night. [a fifty-five-year-old woman] with an accident? What kind of pain (sharp, dull)? Is there itching, burning, or a feeling of pressure? Is it something that happens only when you laugh, sneeze, cough, run, jump, or lift something? Does it happen when you stand up quickly from a sitting position, turn suddenly, or stoop down? All the time or only sometimes? Have you gained weight recently? Do you (or did you) ever wet the bed at night while you are asleep? Do you drink caffeine or alcohol regularly? What does your usual diet consist of (include all liquids and snacks between meals, as well as meals)? Do you sometimes lose urine without any urge or warning? Do you experience sudden, overwhelming urges to urinate that you cannot control? Does the sound of running water cause you to start urinating? Do you have a history of chronic infections of the bladder or urinary tract? What is your menopausal status?

If you answer these questions carefully and keep records for several weeks or a few months, you should be able to get a rough idea of whether or not you fall into one of the major categories of urinary incontinence or whether you seem to have signs of more than one type. Mixed problems will call for several types of treatment, but many women will discover that they fall mainly into one category or another, which clearly calls for a specific set of medical or surgical options, and for which other approaches will probably not be as useful. When you have assembled this information, you will need to learn how doctors use it to make a diagnosis.

Next, review all your prescription and over-the-counter drugs (see pp. 52–5). Your pharmacist can tell you whether any of these drugs or combination of drugs actually aggravate bladder-control problems, as well as whether certain foods or drinks taken at the same time may make a drug's effects even stronger.

As you try all of these approaches, a self-help group can be extremely useful.[14] Composed of other women like you, groups offer an invaluable opportunity to realize that you are not alone, and to hear what others with the same problems have found helpful. Other women are the major source of information on this subject. You may learn from one another who and where the really helpful professional people are and how to avoid inappropriate care. You may find help for these problems in 'menopause' groups because some of the members will also have urinary problems (see Organizations). You may have to start your own group.

Seeking Competent Medical Care

One of the most serious barriers to a better understanding of the connections between the reproductive and the urinary system is their traditional separation into two different areas of specialization: gynaecology and urology. The two physical systems, in fact, are subject to the same hormonal influences and are separated only by a thin layer of tissue. The whole unit is anchored together on the bladder side to the abdominal cavity.

Obstetrician-gynaecologists generally have little training in urology – the study and treatment of the urinary system.[15] Some gynaecologists are so eager to treat any incontinence with standard surgery that they may fail to ask even the most basic questions before proceeding. This often results either in failure to notice an underlying disease or in misdiagnosis of the specific type of incontinence. The urologists, meanwhile, know little more than the basics about female reproductive organs. Few doctors in either specialty are trained to treat middle-aged and older women. Despite repeated attempts to do so, the doctors have yet to get together on a commonly agreed-upon terminology.[16]

Whom should you see? As women, we tend to get referred to gynaecologists for most problems, without always realizing that they are surgeons, trained primarily to offer a surgical solution to many problems that might be better treated in other ways. Sometimes a medical or surgical approach (or combination thereof) is warranted. However, many women continue to suffer from bladder-control problems as a direct *result* of surgical or medical treatment (a phenomenon known as iatrogenesis, or illness caused by medical treatment). In some cases, the doctor did not diagnose the bladder problem correctly, or prescribed treatment such as gynaecological surgery or certain drugs that caused bladder-control problems for the first time. Yet if surgery is appropriate, all of us want to be sure we are in the hands of the most skilled and knowledgeable people. Since so few surgeons have adequate training for successful treatment of female urinary-control problems, you may have to make considerable effort to locate satisfactory care.

A new medical specialty is developing called 'gynaecologic urologist' or 'urologic gynaecologist'. These doctors specialize in female urinary problems. They practise in Europe and even in a few places in the US, but they are rare and very much in demand.

Since you may be unable to afford private consultations or might have to travel very far to find a specialist, your next choice might simply be to rely on your GP. If that doctor refers you to a surgeon (gynaecologist or urologist) after a thorough medical evaluation, request that the doctor continue to work together with you and the surgeon to help define the right approach to treatment. You should decide about surgery in the context of your total health and life situation.

Medical Diagnosis

A diagnosis involves many different processes, and you are an important part of all of them. How you feel and what you experience and remember definitely help the doctor identify the cause of your problem. If you feel you are not being listened to, or are contradicted, or if a detailed history and questionnaire about your bladder functioning are not taken before tests are done, you may want to consult another doctor.[17] The one you choose should make a diagnosis based on an extensive history, your observation of your own symptoms, clinical examination, and, where appropriate, diagnostic tests. A combination of different diagnostic tests and treatment options may be indicated for women who have an overlap between stress and urge incontinence, for example.

DIAGNOSTIC TESTS

Tests alone, as important as they can be, cannot substitute for clinical judgment, and vice versa. **Most experts now agree that a test for stress incontinence performed with the surgeon's fingers alone, while the patient is lying down or standing, is an inadequate basis for planning surgery.**

STANDARD TESTS

A urinalysis and a urine culture should be done first, in order to rule out infection as a temporary or chronic cause of bladder or kidney problems. Some doctors say only a clean specimen taken by catheter is adequate. Part of urinalysis should also include screening for excess sugar, since some bladder problems (like too frequent urination) may actually be an early sign of diabetic or prediabetic conditions. The physical examination should include two pelvic (internal gynaecological) exams, one while the woman is standing and the other while she is lying down, to check that the position of the internal organs is not a problem. Basic neurological testing should rule out damage to the brain, spinal cord, or peripheral nerves. If physical causes are ruled out, a thorough doctor usually looks for depression or other psychological causes of the symptoms.

TRIAL USE OF A PESSARY

One intermediate approach to testing whether or not you are an appropriate candidate for stress-incontinence surgery is the use of a pessary. A pessary is a stiff, doughnut-shaped rubber device varying in size that fits into the top of the vagina, somewhat like a diaphragm, except that it is a little larger and less flexible. Many women used pessaries for uterine prolapse in the days when surgery was not as safe or available (or insured) as it is today. One effect of the pessary is to raise the neck of the bladder to a position more nearly normal, thus reducing the tendency to stress incontinence. Today the pessary is becoming more popular as a non-invasive diagnostic test (in the sense that no body cavity or body system is being 'invaded' as with X-rays or cystograms).

If there is significant reduction of stress incontinence when the pessary is in place, then the chances are improved that surgery (properly performed, of course) will be successful.[18] For some elderly women who are not good candidates for surgery because of other physical problems (heart conditions, etc.) or for any woman who wishes to avoid surgery, the pessary may also prove to be a valuable permanent alternative to surgery, as it sometimes was in the days of our grandmothers. It requires considerable manual dexterity (the kind necessary to use cervical caps, for example) for a woman to remove and clean the pessary herself, but many do. Otherwise, a doctor or nurse will have to do this regularly for you.

I've had the pessary for about a year and a half. Before that everything was sliding down – there was a big 'thing' [the prolapsed uterus] in my body and I had to pee every half hour or so. Once in a while the urine would leak out but mostly I got to the toilet in time. Now I don't leak urine.

I think in the beginning the pessary was too small and it came out. Then they put in a bigger one. It was uncomfortable for about a month but then it was all right. About every two or three months they take it out and wash it and put it back again. It hurts when they are putting it in but once in it stops hurting. [a ninety-one-year-old woman in a nursing home]

NEUROLOGICAL TESTS

Clinicians should test to see whether incontinence could be caused by damage to the nervous system itself. If this type of testing is to be done, however, consider having a separate examination by a neurologist/psychologist team experienced in identifying TIAs (small strokes), Alzheimer's disease, or other neurological problems. Distinguishing among these conditions is difficult but crucial for planning treatment.

URODYNAMIC STUDIES

These tests, also called urodynamic pressure profiles, evaluate how well the bladder, urethra, and anal sphincter hold and release urine. A catheter is inserted in the bladder, filled to capacity, and various measurements are taken while the patient is lying down, standing, and urinating.[19] While they provide a more complete picture than more orthodox methods, they may be stressful and unnecessary for elderly women.[20] Training programmes often bring improvement without such detailed testing.

TESTS IN PREPARATION FOR SURGERY

Today there are multiple diagnostic tests available to surgeons planning specific types of surgery, usually for stress incontinence.

Other common tests include cystoscopy and urethroscopy, a direct look inside to check the condition of the bladder and urethra. Bladder and kidney X-rays, using fluorescent dyes, also help visualize the shape and position of both the urethra and bladder. Some tests have the purpose of determining the precise angle of the urethra, so that the doctor will know how to correct it. Some doctors rely on physical examination for this, while others insert a beaded chain into the urethra, take an X-ray, and then remove the chain.

I went to a urologist who insisted on doing a cystoscopy in his consulting room. He was aware of my great reluctance because an earlier cystoscopy was very painful, even under anaesthesia, but he said he could not determine what he wanted to know when the patient was asleep. He was very reassuring and so was the nurse. He was so gentle and the procedure was so painless that I would not hesitate to recommend having this done in a doctor's room, if done by a doctor of this calibre. After doing the cystoscopy the doctor said he did not find anything wrong except a prolapsed bladder. He said he did not recommend an operation. This doctor said that stretching the urethra, which other doctors recommended, is a very outdated urological technique and he does not do it. [a woman in her sixties]

If your surgeon recommends a test, ask exactly which test it is, how it will be done, what it will show, and how that information will be used in planning the surgery, if necessary. If you do have the test(s) done, ask to see the results yourself and have them explained to you. Together with diagrams of the surgery being proposed, this should enable you to participate more meaningfully in the final treatment decisions.

Medical and Surgical Treatments

Treatments of Mild Stress Incontinence and/or Vaginal Dryness

Many doctors routinely recommend synthetic oestrogen drugs either for complaints of vaginal dryness or urinary-control difficulties around the time of the menopause. A condition mild enough to respond to oestrogen treatment might respond to less risky dietary and exercise changes as well. On the other hand, if these other approaches have been tried and a thorough medical history and evaluation do not reveal any significant anatomical problems with the bladder or urethra (and oestrogen is not contraindicated), oestrogen is an option some women have found helpful. It may be that a low-dose oestrogen cream for a short time is all that is needed for some mild problems (see p. 146). Be sure to check all drugs with your doctor and consult your pharmacist for the availability of newer formulations, and possible undesirable effects.

Treatments for Severe Stress Incontinence

SURGERY

After the less drastic approaches mentioned above have been tried, you and your surgeon may conclude that surgery is the only way to correct the overstretched muscles and/or ligaments in the pelvic area which contribute to stress incontinence.

For example, a woman with fairly severe stress incontinence may feel that the exercise/weight-loss approach, including pelvic floor exercises, is too slow (sometimes it takes several months), or she may have already tried it and found it unsatisfactory. Sometimes she has already had surgery that failed and wants to try again.

The major goal of most surgery for stress incontinence is to restore the bladder neck to its (normal) high position slightly above and behind the major bones that come together at the front of the pelvis (beneath the mons). Ideally, the dynamics of the normal pressure between bladder and urethra will thus be restored. Once raised, the bladder neck is 'tacked' into its new position by attaching it to the bones or ligaments of the pelvis.

We do not have space here to describe all the possible surgical procedures for stress incontinence. Techniques for repositioning the bladder – specifically, the bladder neck – vary from tacks inside the vagina alongside both sides of the urethra (much like creating a short tunnel for a drawstring) to tacking the bladder neck to an abdominal ligament, to more complex sling devices, some made from a woman's own muscle tissue, others made from a synthetic substance like Dacron.

While all of these surgical procedures for stress incontinence *may* result in improvement, all of them do so by permanently altering the relationship of the internal organs to one another – actually cutting the bladder away from its natural attachment to the vagina or anterior abdominal wall. None actually alters the primary cause of the dislocation of the bladder, the stretched or weak levator ani or pubococcygeal muscles of the pelvic floor. Every woman considering surgery should obtain full information on the risks, benefits, complications, and alternatives before giving her consent.

After many years of bladder problems and avoiding a gynaecological examination or evaluation, my mother finally had to submit to a vaginal hysterectomy because of a seriously prolapsed uterus. She was seventy-nine. At the same time, her doctor performed urethrovesical suspension surgery (she called it 'tucking her up'), which has been totally successful. My mother has been liberated from the constant anxiety of having to be near a toilet at all times. She only regrets not having done it much sooner.

SUSPENSION

Many surgeons believe women with stress incontinence need some type of sling that can help support the bladder in a new position. However, this operation may offer only limited benefit if the urethra has become shortened, scarred, and rigid due to repeated infections or surgeries.

DILATION

Some doctors, including respected urologists, still practise a surgical procedure called dilation or dilatation, the insertion of a tube or a scalpel-like coring mechanism into the urethra to break up scar tissue. Today many specialists say this only further damages tissue already scarred from repeated infections, almost never yields permanent results, and frequently makes the condition worse.

Treatments for Urge Incontinence and Irritable Bladder

In prescribing treatment for urge incontinence or irritable bladder, it is vital to distinguish clearly between physical and emotional/psychological factors, but the average doctor is largely unable to do so. Women need to be wary of snap diagnoses offered without thorough evaluations.

Newer approaches to bladder-control problems of either the urge or irritability type are emerging that involve combinations of non-surgical techniques such as biofeedback, exercise, drugs, and even sessions of 'bladder retraining', that is, going to the toilet at timed intervals.[21] These techniques do require competent and committed supervision. Such programmes may use catheters or other devices to measure how much bladder control a woman is able to exert, and how that control is improving over time.

Women who experience irritable bladder syndrome may also be helped by certain antispasmodic drugs. Whenever a doctor recommends drug treatment, however, it is crucial to investigate exactly what is being recommended and why, as well as to make sure that other drugs already prescribed for you are being taken into account. In most cases, all these approaches involve long-term monitoring and follow-up.

Most experts believe that urge incontinence must result from some type of neurological impairment. Unfortunately, the classification 'neurological' means different things to different doctors. Some perceive it as damage or a defect in the central nervous system's ability to transmit messages, perhaps because of a stroke or because of some other disease. Other doctors interpret 'neurological' to mean 'psychiatric', concluding that the problem behind urge incontinence is somehow 'emotional' or 'psychological' in origin, or represents evidence of senility. As a result, they conclude that nothing can be done about it. Most doctors are taught in medical school that complaints without any verifiable anatomical cause are 'functional', implying, in psychiatric language, that, although the symptoms may be real enough, the patient's complaint probably serves some other purpose in the patient's life or relationship with her doctor, such as attracting attention.

However sure a woman is that an anatomical condition is the cause of her urge incontinence, she will usually be met with disbelief. Many older women with urge incontinence have actually suffered unknowingly from some type of neurological problem. Testing for various neurological abnormalities can't hurt and may yield benefits. If, for example, a small stroke is discovered, it is possible to commence both rehabilitation therapy and preventive therapy for future strokes at the same time that the incontinence is being treated.

However, it is entirely possible that no neurological cause will be found, even on the most searching examination. A few practitioners concede that there may be such a thing as an 'unstable bladder' (detrusor dyssynergia), for which no neurological cause can be found – but most doctors secretly or openly doubt it.[22] As a result, the term 'unstable bladder' has become a wastebasket category for many, often unrelated, conditions. The medical imagination is uncomfortable with highly individualized diagnoses and often accepts as one of its primary tasks the assigning of each case to some previously existing diagnostic category.

This prejudice can be devastating for many women. In some cases of incontinence, women are given tranquillizers, which can make the problem worse, or are referred to psychiatrists instead of receiving the neurological examinations they need. Many psychiatrists are also unaware that the complaint of incontinence may require physical and neurological evaluation.

Nevertheless, there may be some psychological aspects to the origin of urge incontinence. Also, the loss of bladder control in and of itself is capable of *causing* depression. This reaction is well within the range of normal, given our culture and given the social loss which this crucial malfunction represents. In fact, most incontinent people report their first reaction to this problem was one of depression. Many women have experienced noticeable improvement when antidepressant drugs are given for incontinence, even in the absence of a diagnosis of depression.[23] It may also be that some forms of depression actually bring on incontinence difficulties.

Drugs are used to help regulate the bladder or urethra during the filling or the emptying phases. Certain drugs reduce the tendency for the 'irritable' bladder to contract. Others may improve the tone of muscles at the bladder opening. However, most drugs to treat incontinence also produce unpleasant effects, such as dry mouth or irritability, and should not be used without consideration of your total health condition and the other medications you take.

Treatments for Overflow Incontinence

In cases of overflow incontinence, specific drugs may help when combined with a programme of regular, frequent, timed trips to the toilet. Such a programme helps re-establish normal signals to prevent overflow and infection. For urine retention, self-administered catheterization or clean intermittent catheterization (CIC) may be desirable. Indwelling catheters are more controversial, and are rejected for overflow incontinence by many doctors because of the high risk of infection, even though they offer improved control. For certain conditions they may be necessary temporarily.

Issues to Consider Regarding Surgery

What factors should you consider in evaluating surgery as an option? First, there is a high failure rate – around 50 per cent. Many surgeons dismiss that figure, saying that of the patients who come to them as 'failures' from previous surgery, a significant percentage show that the original diagnosis was wrong or that the correct procedure was not performed in the first place.[24] However, it is also true that even many successful procedures become failures after several months or a year or two. Most procedures require general anaesthesia, with its known risks. There are also risks of damage to nearby organs. Such damage may not be classified as a failure by the surgeon, but for the woman it most certainly is one.

If something goes wrong after surgery, we need to ask not only 'Was the correct diagnosis made?' but also 'Was the appropriate procedure performed?' The best approach is to take our post-surgery symptoms and complaints seriously and seek a second opinion for verification.

Specialists with a pioneering approach to urinary problems in a few teaching hospitals in the UK are likely to be able to accept referrals from your GP. If you meet difficulties in getting a second opinion, you should press the GP to find out where such facilities are available and ask to be referred there. If you believe that the treatment offered locally has been unsatisfactory, there is no reason, except the GP's reluctance, why you should not be referred to a distant hospital.

A major issue when considering surgery for incontinence problems is whether to have a procedure done 'from below' – that is, entirely through the vagina – or whether to undergo an abdominal, or 'supra-pubic', procedure. As with hysterectomy, there are advantages and disadvantages to both, and disagreement among experts. Many gynaecologists have preferred vaginal techniques in order to avoid two major problems with abdominal surgery: 1) the scar, which even with the so-called 'bikini cut' (near the top line of the pubic hair) may show, especially on older women with less pubic hair; and 2) the invasion of the body cavity, which is always risky and may lead later to adhesions (scar tissue) on the surrounding organs. Nevertheless, the complication/infection rate in the case of hysterectomy, for example, is significantly higher with vaginal surgery than with abdominal surgery. There is also the risk of damage by gynaecologists to the urethra and ureters during vaginal surgery (and during both abdominal and vaginal hysterectomy), which may actually cause incontinence. Many expert urological surgeons do perform corrective procedures through the vagina.[25] A painful bone condition called osteitis pubis, a slow disintegration of the pubic bone, is another complication frequently resulting from surgery that attaches stitches to the bony structure rather than to one of the ligaments. You will have to discuss the choices of techniques, consider your surgeon's experience, and compare your preference with your surgeon's preference.

When we realize how little scientific knowledge is available on this subject, and how poorly prepared most medical professionals are to help us, it is easy to feel depressed about incontinence. On the other hand, the more we learn about prevention and treatment, the more we can break through the barrier of silence surrounding this condition.

NOTES

[1]Neil M. Resnick and Subbarao V. Yalla, 'Current Concepts: Management of Urinary Incontinence in the Elderly'. *The New England Journal of Medicine*, Vol. 313, No. 13, 26 September 1985, pp. 800–5.

[2]Joseph G. Ouslander and Robert L. Kane, 'The Costs of Urinary Incontinence in Nursing Homes'. *Medical Care*, Vol. 22, No. 1, January 1984, pp. 69–79.

[3]Resnick and Yalla, op. cit., p. 800.

[4]Ibid.

[5]Ibid., p. 803.

[6]Estimate from Neil M. Resnick, MD.

[7]Jane E. Brody, 'Personal Health'. *The New York Times*, 5 June 1985; Pamela Jones and Marian Emr, 'Studies Focus on Treatment and Prevention of Urinary Incontinence'. *News and Features from NIH*, Vol. 85, No. 4, 1985, pp. 11–12; and Joseph G. Ouslander et al., 'Urinary Incontinence in Elderly Nursing Home Patients'. *Journal of the American Medical Association*, Vol. 248, 1982, pp. 1194–8.

[8]Jones and Emr, op. cit.

[9]'Structural, Neurological, Psychological Factors in Female Incontinence'. *Ob. Gyn. News*, Vol. 17, No. 12, 15–30 June 1982.

[10]Sally Inch, *Birthrights*. New York: Pantheon Books, 1984.

[11]Betsy A. Lehman, 'Health Sense: Interstitial Cystitis Pain Is Real'. *The Boston Globe*, 22 September 1986, pp. 41–2; and Adriane Fugh-Berman, 'Standard Bladder Infection Treatment May Bring on Interstitial Cystitis'. *The Network News*, Vol. 10, No. 3, May–June 1985, pp. 4–5.

[12]Joanne West, 'Urinary Problems Resulting from Hysterectomy'. *HERS Newsletter*, April 1983, pp. 3–4.

[13]David A. Richardson et al., 'The Effect of Utero-vaginal Prolapse on Urethrovesical Pressure Dynamics'. *American Journal of Obstetrics and Gynecology*, Vol. 146, No. 8, 15 August 1983, pp. 901–5; and Emil A. Tanagho, 'The Effect of Hysterectomy and Periurethral Surgery on Urethrovesical Function'. In Donald R. Ostergard, *Gynecologic Urology and Urodynamics*. Baltimore, Md.: Williams & Wilkins Co., 1980, pp. 293–300.

[14]Ann Landers, 'Incontinence Is Treatable'. *The Boston Globe*, 28 February 1985.

[15]'Women Need Same Services That Urologists Provide for Men'. *Ob. Gyn. News*, Vol. 18, No. 21, 1–15 November 1983, pp. 1–14.

[16]Patrick Bates et al., 'First Report on the Standardization of Terminology of Lower Urinary Tract Function'. *British Journal of Urology*, Vol. 48, 1976, pp. 39–42.

[17]'Chart for Urodynamics and Gynecological Urology History'. In Ostergard, op. cit. (Chart is copyright 1978 by Donald R. Ostergard.)

[18]N. N. Bahtia and A. Gergman, 'Urinary Incontinence: Pessary Test Predicts Surgical Outcome'. *Modern Medicine*, September 1985. Taken from article in *Obstetrics and Gynecology*, Vol. 65, February 1985, pp. 220–6.

[19]Kathleen Poole, 'A Useful Way to Diagnose Bladder Disorders'. *RN*, Vol. 47, No. 8, August 1984, pp. 51–2.

[220]Mark E. Williams, 'A Critical Evaluation of Assessment Technology Regarding Urinary Continence in the Elderly'. Presented at a 1984 conference sponsored by the National Institute of Aging.

[21]William Frewen, 'Role of Bladder Training in the Treatment of Unstable Bladder in the Female'. *Urologic Clinics of North America*, Vol. 6, No. 1, February 1979, pp. 273–7; Evan C. Hadley, 'Bladder Training and Related Therapies for Urinary Incontinence in Older People'. *Journal of the American Medical Association*, Vol. 256, No. 3, 18 July 1986, pp. 372–9; and Kathleen A. McCormick and Kathryn L. Burgio, 'Incontinence: An Update on Nursing Care Measures'. *Journal of Gerontological Nursing*, Vol. 10, No. 10, 1984, pp. 16–23.

[22]'Detrusor Dyssynergia: A Rare Cause of Urinary Incompetence in Women. Questions and Answers'. *Journal of the American Medical Association*, Vol. 241, No. 12, June 1985, pp. 15–30.

[23]Alan J. Wein, 'Pharmacology of the Bladder and Urethra'. In Stuart L. Stanton and Emil A. Tanagho, eds., *Surgery of Female Incontinence*. New York: Springer-Verlag, 1980, pp. 195–6.

[24]Stanton and Tanagho, ibid.

[25]Shlomo Raz, ed., 'Vaginal Surgery'. *Seminars in Urology*, Vol. 4, No. 1, February 1986, pp. 1–61.

BOOKS AND PUBLICATIONS

Dorothy Mandelstam (ed.), *Incontinence and Its Management*. Beckenham: Croom Helm, 1986.

Health Education Authority, *Incontinence: a very common complaint*. Free leaflet from GPs' surgeries, Citizens' Advice Bureaux and local health departments.

Cheryle Gartley (ed.), *Managing Incontinence*. London: Human Horizons/Souvenir Press, 1988.

Angela Kilmartin, *Victims of Thrush and Cystitis*. London: Century/Arrow, 1986.

Health Education Authority, *Cystitis*. Free leaflet from GPs' surgeries.

Aids for the Management of Incontinence: A Critical View. King's Fund Centre. (See Organizations.)

Dorothy Mandelstam, *Incontinence*. Disabled Living Foundation. (See Organizations.)

22
Hysterectomy and Oophorectomy

Our reproductive organs, like most other parts of our bodies, have multiple functions. We are only beginning to identify and do not yet fully understand the many ways these organs affect our health and our sexuality. Therefore, our bodily integrity should never be tampered with unless absolutely necessary. Yet for well over a century in the West, women's uteri and ovaries have been subjected to routine medical abuse. In the United States unnecessary removal of the uterus and ovaries became a scandal. Anyone considering either of these procedures needs to be aware of *all* the possible consequences. Hysterectomy (removal of the uterus) and oophorectomy or ovariectomy (removal of the ovaries) can be life-saving procedures, but before undergoing them every woman must be sure that they are truly necessary.

Unnecessary Hysterectomies and Oophorectomies

Hysterectomy and oophorectomy will always have their place in sound medical practice, mainly as a treatment for confirmed cancer. As women get older the risks of uterine and ovarian cancer increase, so regular gynaecological check-ups including Pap smears are advisable.

In 1985, 670,000 hysterectomies and 525,000 oophorectomies were performed on women in the United States.[1] Only a small proportion of hysterectomies – 8 to 12 per cent – were performed to treat cancer and other life-threatening diseases.[2] Most hysterectomies were elective, that is, not clearly necessary. As a result of this widespread overuse of the operation, almost every American woman began to believe that her hysterectomy was necessary. But studies challenge this. The number of hysterectomies thought to be unnecessary varies between 33 and 72 per cent, depending on the source.[3] Things got to the point where by 1978 the chance that a woman would have a hysterectomy some time in her life was estimated to be greater than 50 per cent.[4]

Fortunately in Britain we have the National Health Service, which, with all its growing deficiencies, has never encouraged doctors to perform unnecessary operations. In the US doctors and surgeons make a great deal of money out of treating, or operating upon, individuals. In Britain, their opposite numbers are, in general, salaried staff or receiving payment per capita (in the case of GPs) for the number of patients registered with them. And so, unless a woman decides to 'go private' she can be sure that her surgeon does not benefit financially from suggesting an operation. In the US there's evidence that poor and minority women are sometimes operated on as 'teaching practice' without being fully informed about what is being done.[5] There is a possibility that in Britain some women are being operated on following childbirth as a form of birth control. The well-known obstetrician and gynaecologist, Wendy Savage, suggests that no woman should succumb to pressure to have a hysterectomy after childbirth until she has had at least six months' reflection.

In countries where there is a national health service, the rate of hysterectomy is half that of the US, and there's no evidence that women's health has suffered as a result.[6] Even in the US the rate of hysterectomy varies from city to city,[7] and is still too high, but there are now signs of a slight decline.[8]

Is Your Hysterectomy Really Necessary?

Although it's unlikely that you will experience pressure to have a hysterectomy or oophorectomy from the medical profession in the UK without sound medical reasons, you may wonder whether, once you've completed your family or have decided that you just don't want children, it might be a good idea to rid yourself of this 'unnecessary' part of your system. If periods are troublesome it would seem an attractive idea to anticipate the menopause.

Then there are those who believe that you'll feel better, enjoy sex more and look younger, although there's no evidence of this.[9] And some psychoanalysts have even suggested that women who experience problems after hysterectomy are affected by emotional problems rather than the surgery – so if you resist having a hysterectomy you may be infantile and 'too attached to the uterus': a sign that you are inappropriately confusing your sexuality with your ability to reproduce! As we shall see, there often *are* problems following a hysterectomy, but studies that document them are often ignored by psychiatrists and some gynaecologists.[10]

A further reason for considering hysterectomy, of course, is the fear of pregnancy in middle age, when menstruation becomes unpredictable and some forms of contraception undesirable. However, removal of uterus and ovaries is an unacceptable form of birth control and anyone without other overriding reasons for having the operation ought to think very carefully about the disadvantages, should she meet with a surgeon willing to operate on birth control grounds alone. (See Birth Control chapter for up-to-date birth control and sterilization techniques.)

Possible After-effects of Hysterectomy and Oophorectomy*

Each woman is different, and it is impossible to tell in advance how a hysterectomy will affect her. Neither age, marital status, work, sexual preference, severity of symptoms before surgery, nor the number of children she has had will indicate how a woman will feel after a hysterectomy. Many women report a variety of adverse physical and emotional effects of hysterectomy, many of which are permanent and irreversible.

Both the ovaries and the uterus have important functions in the body long after the reproductive years are over. A study that tested ovarian function in 2,132 women whose uteri were removed found that many ovaries continued to function for up to twenty-five years after the operation.[11] In fact, hot flushes can appear when a woman's ovaries are removed years after her menopause occurred.[12]

Healthy ovaries should not be removed. Removal of the ovaries from premenopausal women creates an immediate 'surgical menopause' that is often more severe than normal menopause. Today many doctors recommend hormone replacement therapy (oestrogen in combination with progestogen) for premenopausal women who have a surgical menopause. If the uterus has been removed, the major risk associated with oestrogen – cancer of the uterine lining (endometrial cancer) – has also been removed. If the uterus has not been removed, the risk of endometrial cancer is minimized by adding progestogen to the regimen. However, the long-term effects of progestogen are not yet known, and the suspected risks of that hormone include a higher likelihood of heart attack or stroke. Long-term oestrogen replacement may increase the risk of breast cancer, gallbladder disease, and phlebitis. A small percentage of women are allergic to hormones. For some women, such as those who have had endometriosis or breast cancer, oestrogen replacement therapy (ORT) is contraindicated. On the other hand, *not* taking oestrogen after *premature* menopause (whether surgical or natural) can result in premature osteoporosis, bone and joint pain, vaginal dryness or shrinkage, or atherosclerosis.

The relationship between hormones and osteoporosis is discussed in the Osteoporosis chapter. In addition to knowing what is stated there, women should be aware that hormone therapy, either oestrogen or the oestrogen-progestogen combination, does *not* replace the androgens secreted by functioning ovaries. Androgens contribute to the libido (sexual desire).† And the

---

*We wish to be clear throughout this chapter about whether we are discussing hysterectomy, oophorectomy, or both. We will try to avoid the inaccurate, but common, error of referring to the removal of any part of the uterus or ovaries as a hysterectomy.

†Testosterone (one of the androgens) has been used to enhance libido but also results in 'masculinizing' effects such as facial hair, acne, and permanently lowered voice. (See the Boston Women's Health Book Collective, *The New Our Bodies, Ourselves*, Penguin.)

hormonelike substances called *prostacyclins* that circulate in the uterus and help keep arteries open, keep blood platelets from excessive clotting, and help to prevent heart attacks are not replaced through hormone therapy.[13]

Even when the ovaries are left in place, a hysterectomy can cause a significant drop in hormone levels. The uterus is a living, functioning organ that secretes hormones and responds to ovarian hormones for many years after the menopause. It is more than just a 'baby carriage'. When the uterus is amputated, a delicately balanced system (which includes ovaries, fallopian tubes, cervix, vagina, and clitoris and their blood and nerve supplies) is disrupted. Major blood vessels, nerves, and connective tissues are cut, leaving raw edges to heal and scar.

More than a hundred women, who contacted a support group in New York, reported varying degrees of fatigue, memory loss, and loss of sexual feeling following a hysterectomy. **None of the women had been forewarned by their doctors about any possible after-effects.** Those who retained their ovaries had hot flushes for several weeks after surgery, but then the flushes disappeared if the women were premenopausal. Also reported were breast pain, breast enlargement and engorgement, cystic breasts, and feelings of lactation and oily skin. Those who had their ovaries removed reported severe hot flushes, bone and joint pain, and dry skin. Many of the women did not realize that their problems might be linked to their surgery until they talked with other women who had suffered similar problems following hysterectomy.[14]

Other consequences reported by women after hysterectomy with or without oophorectomy are: depression, loss of sexual sensation in the breasts and other parts of the body, lessened sexual desire, weaker orgasms, insomnia, vaginal dryness and shrinkage, loss of firm body tone, hair loss, premature greying, weight gain (despite dieting and exercise), unpleasant vaginal odour, protruding abdomen, bloating, recurrent vaginal yeast infections, urine leakage when coughing or sneezing from loss of the uterus as a support for the bladder, dry eye syndrome, lower resistance to colds, and less intense emotions.

Hysterectomy means the loss of uterine contractions during orgasm, which for many women reduces sexual pleasure. Many women report the loss of pleasure from penetration, fewer sexual fantasies, slower arousal, lack of interest in seeking lovers or a mate, loss of desire to masturbate, and sometimes even an aversion to being touched.

My hysterectomy had a result that I was most unprepared for. With breast stimulation, intercourse, and orgasm, there was a definite loss of a sensation which I can only describe as uterine. Having had a number of losses and having helped others through the losses that seem to come to us throughout life, I felt prepared for anything that life had to offer . . . meaning anything that I could conceive of. This was one thing that I had never conceived of. My greatest need at the time was simply to talk with someone who knew what I was talking about. I received a lot of unhelpful responses. The most insensitive came from female sex therapists. [a forty-one-year-old nurse]

One study reports that 33 to 46 per cent of women experience varying degrees of diminished libido and diminished physical sexual responses after hysterectomy.[15] Oestrogen therapy is of no benefit in this regard.[16]

The worst thing since my hysterectomy is the lack of desire. No more delicious cravings and wonderful radiating feelings of exciting anticipation. I always felt that my desire and enjoyment of sex was a special gift, my own private joy that could never be taken away from me even if I lost material things in life. If something turned me on, whether it was a love scene in a movie, a touch, or a thought, my body would feel all tingly and flushed. Even if I didn't get sex right away, I could luxuriate in thinking about it – how I would do it, where, and when.

Now there is just emptiness inside. I feel I could go one hundred years without sex and I'm aware of the enormous void. To me it is tantamount to death. I was so overcome by the loss that I cried to everyone about it. [a fifty-year-old woman]

For other women, loss of the cervix may prevent orgasm if they were dependent upon cervical stimulation. Some women also report loss of nipple and clitoral sensation; this may be the result of severed nerves and ligaments and loss of blood flow to the pelvic area. Changes in vaginal structure, loss of cervical mucus, and the loss of the copious discharge resulting from monthly ovulation and hormonal changes also contribute to the sexual deficits created by this surgery.

Depression is a common aftermath of hysterectomy. One doctor who had a hysterectomy described her feeling as that of 'chronic sorrow'. One study found that 70 per cent of women suffered depression after hysterectomy, which was double the rate of other postoperative depressions. Depressions usually occur within three to six months after surgery and can be severe. The causes of posthysterectomy depression have not been researched thoroughly enough. One theory is that removal of the uterus lowers the oestrogen level by altering the blood supply to the ovaries, and lowered oestrogen level is associated with a lowered blood level of *tryptophan*, an amino acid that may prevent depression.[18] Other possible reasons for posthysterectomy depression may be the rage resulting from loss of sexual feeling or from concluding that one's surgery was unnecessary.

The removal of the uterus sometimes results in a surprising feeling of devastation over the loss of fertility.

After my hysterectomy, I grieved over the end of my childbearing potential, although I was fifty-five. Before I left the hospital, my concentration on babies became pronounced. I watched a TV programme on adoption and fantasized about a foster child. The woman across the hall told me that she found she could not look at new babies because she was grieving over having had her hysterectomy and never having had children. She was surprised at her grief at being childless because she had, she thought, long ago chosen to be a lesbian and to have no children. Now, she was once again having to reinforce that choice. [a fifty-seven-year-old woman][19]

Some women also regret other changes in their bodies.

I miss my periods so much. I think there's something barbaric about cutting off a woman's periods before her time. Two months after my hysterectomy I developed a raw spot in my internal scar that had to be cauterized. The procedure made me stain for a few days. I tried to pretend that the blood on my pad was a period. But I knew it wasn't and I felt sad. [a fifty-year-old woman]

Not everyone reacts negatively to having a hysterectomy. Some women are pleased with the outcome.

From the moment I woke up from the surgery I was optimistic. The recovery was smooth and swift. About three months later I began having hot flushes. (My ovaries had also been removed, at my wish.) I began a regimen of oestrogen and later a progestogen was added. From the recovery on, I have not had a bad day. It is a joy not to be bleeding either regularly or irregularly and to be interested in sexual activity any day of the month. The sense of security and comfort of not having periods is great. If I knew it would be so easy after the operation I would have had it at thirty-nine, when my heavy bleeding started. My youngest child was then seven and I knew that I wanted no more. [a fifty-three-year-old woman]

The important point is that women should be made aware of all possible reactions to and consequences of hysterectomy before surgery is undertaken.

When the doctor recommended a hysterectomy for a fibroid, I tried desperately to get information from at least ten women who had the operation. Each one willingly told me about her hospital, her doctor, and the anaesthesia she had. Not one of these women told me how she really felt afterwards, or mentioned a single word about after-effects. Some of them encouraged me to have the surgery. From all this I naively concluded that a hysterectomy is not too bad.

When the shock of the sudden, unwelcome changes from my hysterectomy hit me with its full impact, I became overwhelmed with anger and hurt at these women for not telling me anything. I felt betrayed. Why didn't anyone warn me? Could they have all been so satisfied with their results? Could they have been too embarrassed to talk about sexual changes? If I had known more truths I would have tried harder to avoid the surgery!

Could they have simply not wanted to scare me or to assume too much responsibility in case my operation was really necessary? Or is there a baser emotion, a certain reluctance in some people to spare another person from making the same mistake they made – something like 'misery loves company'? When anyone comes to me asking, 'What is a hysterectomy like?' I tell them everything I've experienced and let them take it from there. [a forty-nine-year-old woman]

Perhaps because in Britain relatively few 'unnecessary' hysterectomies are performed, a higher proportion of women who have had the operation seem to be pleased with the outcome. Of seven women I questioned in snap interviews, five said they felt much better, one felt she was still recovering (after eight months) and one attributed her depression to her hysterectomy a year earlier. Obviously such a small sample could be biased – but it may be typical.

JEAN SHAPIRO

When Hysterectomy is Necessary

There are times when a hysterectomy is life-saving; each case must be evaluated individually. Some conditions that may require surgery are:

1. Invasive cancer of the uterus (endometrium), ovaries, cervix, or fallopian tubes. This operation should be planned in consultation with both a gynaecologist and an oncologist (cancer specialist) to review all the treatment options.
2. Haemorrhaging (severe uncontrollable bleeding) combined with anaemia that has not responded to medical treatments – such as a D&C (dilation and curettage, or scraping, of the uterus), hormone therapy, or laser technology – or to non-medical treatments.
3. Fibroid tumours (common, non-cancerous growths) that obstruct bowel or urinary function (a rare occurrence) and that are too large to remove by myomectomy (removal of the tumour alone). Frequent urination is usually not a sufficient reason for a hysterectomy.

4. Advanced pelvic inflammatory disease (PID), in which infection spreads to the peritoneal cavity (membrane that lines the walls of the abdomen). Sometimes a bad infection can be fought successfully with massive combinations of antibiotics (administered intravenously) and complete bed rest.
5. Severe uterine prolapse, in which the uterus descends completely through the vagina.
6. Severe endometriosis (the presence of tissue of the uterine lining elsewhere in the abdominal cavity), if it is untreatable by hormones or other drugs, or if it recurs with severe pain and bleeding after minor surgery.
7. Certain other obstetrical catastrophes and very rare cases of tuberculosis of the uterus.

Some Common Problems and Alternatives to Hysterectomy

The following conditions will often correct themselves with the coming of the menopause. They rarely require hysterectomies and never require oophorectomies.

FIBROID TUMOURS

Fibroid tumours (myomas or leiomyomas) are the most common reason for hysterectomy in women between thirty-five and fifty. Fibroids are knobs of muscle tissue in or attached to the uterus. Do not automatically think of cancer when you hear the word 'tumours'; 99.7 per cent of all fibroids are benign (non-cancerous).[20] Nearly 40 per cent of white women over thirty-five have fibroids, and the incidence is even greater in black women. The growth of fibroids is stimulated by oestrogen, so if you know you have fibroids you should avoid birth control pills and oestrogen therapy. Fibroids may stay the same size or grow in spurts, plateau, and shrink many times during a woman's reproductive years, often peaking just before the menopause. Usually they recede slowly after the menopause as oestrogen levels drop. A uterus can accommodate a surprisingly large number of sizeable fibroids without showing any symptoms. The presence of large fibroids, and even feelings of heaviness and mild pressure, are not necessarily a reason for a hysterectomy.

The three most common types of fibroids, named according to their location in the uterus, are:

Subserous – Located outside the uterus. These usually do not interfere with uterine function, even if they are large (though very large ones may eventually disturb other organs).

Intramural – Located inside the muscle wall of the uterus. May cause pain and bleeding (not true haemorrhaging) at menstruation.
Submucous – Located just under the surface of the uterine lining and jutting out into the uterine cavity, this type of fibroid sometimes causes serious bleeding. Fortunately, this is the least common of the three.

The location of fibroids is determined by uterine X-ray, ultrasound test (sonogram), and D&C. Sometimes a fibroid is attached to the uterus with a *pedicle* or *peduncle*, a narrow-based stalk, which may twist and cause pain. The pedunculated fibroid is the easiest to remove regardless of its size.

We may be alarmed when doctors tell us we have 'large' fibroids. How large is a 'large' fibroid? Hospitals approve surgical removal of a fibroid that grows beyond a twelve-week pregnancy size, or is larger than four to five inches (the size of a grapefruit) when palpable from the abdomen. Some gynaecologists consider a uterus massively enlarged if it is the size of a fourteen- to eighteen-week pregnancy. Unfortunately, some surgeons may perform hysterectomies

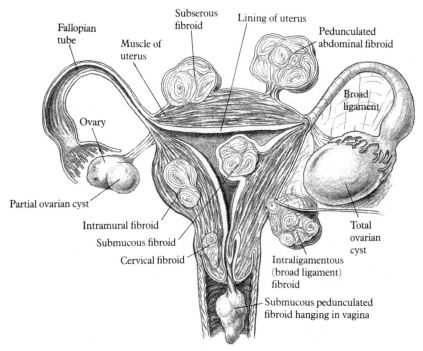

FIBROIDS (MYOMAS) OF THE UTERUS AND OVARIAN CYSTS

for much smaller fibroids. Sometimes nothing more than a surgeon's clinical judgment is used to measure these growths. A slight increase in size can make a fibroid seem enormous to the touch. In the operating room these 'enormous' tumours often turn out to be much smaller than originally perceived.

Some women become alarmed because they think the rapid growth of a fibroid may be a sign of malignancy, although this is extremely rare. How does a woman know how rapid is 'rapid'? Ultrasound tests can be repeated at three-month intervals, in order to compare sizes. A fibroid that increases by one-third its size in three months might be considered rapid growth, although most fibroids that grow rapidly are benign.

Fibroids may have to be removed if they cause extreme bleeding or pain, if they degenerate because they have outgrown their blood supply, or if they become infected. But in such cases the operation of choice is usually a myomectomy, *not* a hysterectomy.

If you are approaching the menopause and have bothersome fibroids, you may choose to wait until the menopause, when fibroids usually recede, before making a decision about surgery. Try the following suggestions in the meantime. Patience is advisable in this situation, because fibroid shrinkage may be very gradual, over a period of months or even years after the last menstrual period.

SELF-HELP FOR FIBROIDS

1. Do not take oestrogen.
2. Do not take steroids, unless needed for a life-threatening illness. (Steroids stimulate the adrenal glands, which also produce oestrogen and so may enlarge fibroids.)
3. Try to keep your percentage of body fat down by exercising. Oestrogen is produced in the fat cells of the body.
4. Reduce the total percentage of fat in the diet. Cut out or cut down on sugar. Increase vegetables and whole grains. Cut out alcohol.
5. Try to manage and reduce stress. Many women recall that their fibroids enlarged after a particularly stressful time. Reactions to stress can stimulate the adrenal glands to produce hormones.
6. Try alternative healing techniques. Some women report help from acupuncture and from visualizing a uterus free of fibroids.

Myomectomy for Fibroids

Myomectomy, or surgical removal of fibroids without removing the uterus, was rarely done in the past and was reserved for younger women who wished to have children. However, with new awareness of the value of retaining organs, an increasing number of skilled surgeons are performing myomectomies on older women who do not intend to have children but who wish to preserve their uteri. In 1985, 35,000 myomectomies were performed in the US.[21]

During a myomectomy the surgeon will make an incision into the abdomen and examine the uterus. Fibroids on the outside of the uterus (subserous) can be removed. If the fibroids are inside the uterus, the surgeon will cut into the uterine cavity and remove the fibroids, which peel out like oranges peel from their skins. She or he will then repair and close the uterus. Uterine tissue heals easily.

I just had my second myomectomy in sixteen years because of extensive fibroids. Before the myomectomy, I had periods that were two weeks long, I looked five or six months pregnant, had to pee frequently because the fibroids were pressing on the bladder, and experienced discomfort during sex because of the fibroid in the cervix. The surgeon compared the sizes of the fibroids to fruits. He said he removed one grapefruit, one orange, several lemons, and a bunch of grapes. [a forty-one-year-old woman]

Though not necessarily more difficult to perform than a hysterectomy, myomectomy does require a surgeon experienced in that technique. Such surgeons are more apt to be found in teaching hospitals: ask your GP to refer you to a consultant with experience of myomectomy, if possible.

Every effort must be made to remove even the smallest fibroid during a myomectomy, since regrowth can occur in 10 to 25 per cent of cases. An older woman is less likely than a younger women to have fibroids regrow to a size that requires a second myomectomy. Fifteen, thirty, and even more fibroids have been successfully removed without damaging the uterus.

New methods of myomectomy with laser beams now exist, which cause less bleeding and require a much shorter recuperation time than conventional surgery.[22] Laser surgery through a hysteroscope (a device that allows the surgeon to see into the cavity of the uterus) can destroy submucous fibroids.[23] Long-term advantages of this technique over a standard myomectomy are being studied.

Unfortunately, gynaecologists who are unfamiliar with or unskilled in performing myomectomies may discourage a woman from having one by telling her that it is dangerous, that it might require a second operation, that it is silly at her age, or that she should accept a hysterectomy instead.

Neither progestogens nor the hormone danazol (Danol) shrink fibroids successfully. Since the growth of fibroids is stimulated by oestrogen (fibroids are never found before puberty and only rarely after the menopause in women who are not taking oestrogens), research on drugs such as buserelin which suppress oestrogen is underway. The drugs (called LHRH agonists) induce a state of pseudomenopause, shrinking fibroids, and also causing hot flushes and vaginal dryness. LHRH agonists may also reduce the beneficial HDL levels and may induce osteoporosis. Though the fibroids will grow back when the medication is stopped, the treatment may be used by itself as a way to 'buy time' until the menopause, or may be used to shrink fibroids before a surgical myomectomy is performed.[24]

Pain During or Between Periods

Do not have a hysterectomy just because you have pain in the lower abdomen during or between periods. Pain can come from many sources. A thorough diagnostic checkup should be done to discover whether the cause of the pain might be from the digestive system, the urinary tract, the bones or the joints. Do not automatically assume that the pain is gynaecological.

Visualization, relaxation training, and hypnosis for pain control are often helpful. Pain can sometimes be caused by *premenstrual syndrome*, which sometimes increases in duration and severity in women nearing the menopause[25] and then subsides after menopause. (See Menopause chapter for an explanation and suggestions.)

If self-help techniques are not effective, prescription drugs may be necessary. An anti-arthritic drug (generic name: ibuprofen; trade name: Brufen) may relieve menstrual cramps and pain from fibroids. This drug contains prostaglandin-blocking substances that often lessen excessive menstrual flow as well.[26] However, anti-inflammatory drugs such as Brufen can also raise blood pressure, trigger asthma attacks in asthmatics, and cause fluid retention and depression. One NSAID (non-steroid anti-inflammatory drug) may work better for one woman than another. (Take these drugs with milk.)

To relieve the pain caused by a fibroid in a tipped-back uterus that is pressing on the rectum, try the knee-chest position several times a day. This position will help straighten the uterus, thus lessening pressure on the rectum.

Heavy or Prolonged Menstrual Bleeding (Menorrhagia)

Even though women are used to menstrual bleeding on a regular basis, unexpected and unpredictable bleeding can be frightening. We need to know that irregular or heavy menstrual flow is very common in women approaching menopause (see chart, pp. 196–7). Discuss prolonged heavy bleeding with your doctor. Also, any bleeding in a woman well past the menopause should be checked.

A hysterectomy should not be done merely to stop heavy bleeding, at least until the reason for the bleeding is determined and all other efforts to control it have failed. Many hysterectomies performed because of bleeding are done without a preliminary D&C, hysteroscopy and suction curettage, or endometrial biopsy. In a letter to a medical journal, an indignant doctor wrote, 'Generally, menorrhagia seems to be diagnosed on the basis of a woman's description of her menstrual loss and is rarely confirmed by the methods available. I am unaware of any other important organ that is electively removed without first assessing its degree of malfunction.'[27]

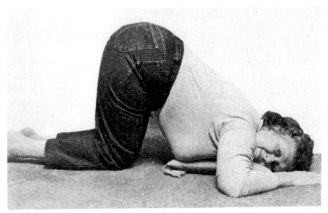

Knee-chest position

Be sure that you do not overestimate the amount of blood lost during a period. We suggest women keep menstrual charts, recording the number of days from the beginning of one period to the beginning of the next period, the number of days bleeding lasts, how many napkins or tampons are used, whether there are clots (red or brown), and any other details that seem relevant. You may be able to establish some pattern to the bleeding to discuss with your doctor.

In addition, heavy loss of blood may lead to anaemia, which causes fatigue, paleness, and heart palpitations. A blood test for anaemia should always be given to a woman who is bleeding heavily. Normal haemoglobin values range from twelve to sixteen grams per 100 millilitres; normal haematocrit values (the ratio of red blood cells to the volume of whole blood) range from 33 to 46 per cent. A mild anaemia can often be improved by eating more iron-rich foods and taking iron supplements after you eat. Foods rich in vitamin C eaten at the same meal as iron-rich foods help increase the absorption of iron.

In my late forties I started to have heavy flooding when I had a period. Some days I just couldn't go to work. My GP referred me to a consultant who suggested a hysterectomy. However, there was the usual waiting list, so the op was delayed. Meanwhile I went on holiday, and when I had my next period it wasn't nearly as bad. Two months later I had a very slight bleed – then no more. By the time a hospital bed was available I'd had no periods for over six months. So I decided to take a chance and cancel the booking. Just as well – that was my menopause. [a fifty-four-year-old woman]

In the absence of any diagnosed pathology, you can try these self-care and alternative treatments for heavy bleeding:

1. Try to remain calm. Anxiety can increase blood flow by raising your blood pressure and making the heart pump faster.
2. Stay off your feet, with your legs elevated, if 'flooding' occurs. An ice pack applied to the abdomen for an hour or two (fifteen minutes on, fifteen minutes off) can stop or reduce bleeding. Also, try applying cold to the lower back with a towel that has been dampened and chilled in the freezer.
3. Avoid heating pads, hot showers, or baths on heavy-flow days. Heat increases blood flow.
4. Avoid aspirin products. They increase bleeding. Garlic and mint may also increase bleeding.
5. Try taking vitamin C with bioflavinoids. In amounts under one to two grams per day, these help to strengthen the walls of blood vessels and may reduce bleeding. Above this amount, vitamin C is sometimes toxic, and may actually increase bleeding.
6. Try taking 10,000 international units (IUs) of vitamin A twice a day (five times the recommended daily allowance for women).[28] Higher doses may be more helpful but should only be taken under the supervision of a doctor or nutritionist familiar with the treatment who will monitor your symptoms and test your blood for toxicity. Amounts in excess of 25,000 IUs per day can be toxic.
7. Calcium, vitamin D, and magnesium encourage blood clotting and blood vessel contractions.
8. Acupuncture and other alternative healing methods have helped some women.

If self-help approaches do not work, some doctors may prescribe progestogens. Use only the smallest effective dosage for the shortest time possible. You and your doctor may have to experiment to find the proper dosage and type for you. Some American doctors are suggesting intrauterine devices (IUDs) containing progestogen for the older woman who has heavy or extended menstrual flow.[29] However, IUDs can cause pelvic inflammatory disease, a major reason for hysterectomies; in addition, IUDs are not recommended at all for women approaching menopause (see Birth Control for Women in Midlife chapter).

A D&C is a diagnostic procedure that can also remove polyps (strawberry-like benign growths) and hyperplasia (the overgrowth of normal uterine tissue) that may be causing bleeding. For routine diagnosis, an aspiration-suction curettage done in the consultant's surgery is safer than a D&C. It involves neither the risk of damaging the delicate lining of the uterus nor the risk of anaesthesia.

Developing from its successful use in eye surgery, an experimental technique, laser surgery, is now used for uterine conditions, especially to treat heavy bleeding. The surgeon needs special training to use a flexible glass rod with a laser beam tip to cauterize the uterine lining. The resulting scar tissue will not bleed. The surgeon is able to view the inside of the uterus through a hysteroscope inserted through the vagina and cervix. Being able to see the lining this way may have advantages over a D&C, which is performed blindly. The newer Nd:YAG laser beam can be focused more precisely than a CO_2 laser. The hormone danazol (Danol) is given for three weeks before the surgery to thin the endometrium. This procedure is not recommended for women with any signs of cancer or active pelvic inflammatory disease. *This procedure causes sterilization* but seems to preserve other uterine functions. It carries risks of anaesthesia and perforation but the heat created and lack of incision minimize infection. Moreover, it can be done with a one- or two-day hospital stay or on an outpatient basis with immediate resumption of normal activities. The procedure has not been in use long enough to evaluate long-term effects.[30] It is unlikely to be widely available in the UK as yet.

Uterine Prolapse (Dropped Womb)

About 35 per cent of hysterectomies are done for uterine prolapse, or dropped womb. In general, prolapse results from stretching of the ligaments that support the uterus and/or weakness of the pubococcygeal muscle, which supports the pelvic floor. There are three stages of uterine prolapse:

First degree – The uterus has descended into the vaginal canal, but not yet into the vaginal opening.

Second degree – The cervix actually appears outside the vaginal opening, in whole or in part.

Third degree (called complete prolapse) – The entire uterus descends to the point that it shows outside the vagina entirely. This type is most common in women over seventy.

To prevent uterine prolapse and to improve your pelvic muscle support system, no matter how slight or severe your prolapse, do pelvic floor exercises regularly (see Moving for Health chapter). Symptoms usually do not occur with first-degree prolapse, except for occasional bearing-down discomfort. **If you cannot tell you have a prolapse, then surgery is not necessary.**

Some women can avoid surgery by use of a pessary, a rubber doughnut-shaped device that helps hold the uterus in place. Pessaries come in various sizes and must be fitted and inserted by a doctor. They must be removed periodically for cleaning. Any woman who is a poor risk for surgery because of age or vulnerability to anaesthesia might find this her best choice.

A less drastic surgery to correct prolapse is uterine suspension surgery. This is abdominal surgery that lifts the uterus into its correct position by shortening the ligaments that hold the uterus in place. Unfortunately, however, some surgeons prefer to remove the uterus rather than repair it, based on their own value judgment that losing her uterus does not matter to a woman beyond a certain age.

Endometriosis

Endometriosis is a condition in which tissue of the uterine lining is found outside the uterus. This tissue thickens and bleeds with the menstrual cycle each month, forming cysts. The main symptoms of endometriosis are pain during menstruation or intercourse and heavy bleeding. The symptoms tend to get worse as the endometriosis spreads and grows. Endometriosis is often a cause of infertility.

Doctors sometimes diagnose endometriosis when they find tender, nodular growths behind the uterus during a manual pelvic exam, but a laparoscopy (examination of the pelvic organs with a lighted, periscope-type instrument through a half-inch incision in the navel) provides the most definite diagnosis.

Endometriosis is often treated with birth control pills or other hormones that bring on a state of pseudopregnancy. This can dry up the growths completely and is effective in about 50 per cent of cases. However, relief is temporary, since the tissue can regrow, and the hormones have certain unpleasant and/or dangerous effects. Birth control pills are very dangerous for women over the age of thirty-five (see p. 164). Danazol (Danol), a derivative of the male hormone testosterone, is reported to be very effective in the treatment of endometriosis, but it is not without its own potential additional effects, namely, depression, liver damage, and masculinizing reactions such as growth of facial hair, weight gain, loss of libido, and deepening of the voice. It is also extremely expensive. Danazol should only be taken under careful medical supervision. Instead of, or in addition to, danazol, you may choose to undergo conservative surgery, in which an abdominal incision is made and the endometrial implants removed, either by laser beams or by electric cauterization.

Hysterectomy is usually a last resort for endometriosis, especially in near-menopausal women whose symptoms will probably recede after the menopause. Since endometriosis, like fibroids, is oestrogen dependent, you can follow some of the same self-help tips for it as you do for fibroids (see p. 410).

Adenomyosis

Adenomyosis is a condition in which endometrial tissue that lines the inside of the uterus (and which is shed each month during the period) is embedded into the walls of the uterus. Previously the condition was called internal endometriosis, since both involved endometrial tissue in unusual places. Adenomyosis, however, is usually found in women in their forties and fifties who have borne children, while endometriosis is most commonly found in younger women who have not borne children. One theory is that the tissue becomes trapped as the uterus shrinks to normal size after pregnancy. Some degree of adenomyosis is so common that it is found in up to 60 per cent of women whose uteri are removed and examined for some other reason. With adenomyosis, the examining doctor may find that the uterus is firm and diffusely enlarged, but only 20 per cent of women may experience heavy or prolonged periods and menstrual pain. A D&C will not help adenomyosis because the tissue is embedded in the wall of the uterus. Since the tissue swells with the increase of oestrogen each month but is trapped in the uterine wall, use of oestrogen or progesterone will only make it worse. See cautions (above) on the use of danazol. Try the self-help suggestions for heavy bleeding, pain, and fibroids. Menopause, with its drop in oestrogen, brings relief.[31]

Precancerous Conditions

Many women have hysterectomies because of supposed 'precancerous' conditions. Always question a doctor's suggestion that an area of tissue is precancerous. It is not clear whether precancerous means the tissue will almost certainly become cancerous or whether it means the condition can revert to normal, become cancerous, or stay the same. Sometimes what is called a precancerous condition may disappear without treatment or can be treated with medication, self-help techniques, or less drastic surgery. If your consultant tells you that you have a precancerous condition, ask your GP to discuss and explain the pathology report and ask for a second, or even third, Pap test several weeks or even a month after the earlier one before agreeing to surgery or any other treatment to destroy questionable cells. If the results of the Pap tests warrant further investigation, the doctor should view the cervix with a colposcope. Areas of the cervix can be removed for study by a *punch biopsy* (removal of a small plug of cells for examination). Suspicious cervical cells have sometimes returned to normal when women had their male sexual partners use condoms to keep sperm from contact with the cervix. Then cauterization (with heat, electricity, or chemicals), cryosurgery (freezing the cells), or laser surgery can destroy small patches of malignant cells. *Cone biopsy*, or *conization* (removal of a ring of the cervix around the opening to the uterus), may also be recommended. These procedures can remove small amounts of tissue, reduce the spread of cervical cancer, and prevent hysterectomies.

The cells of the lining of the uterus (endometrium) can also undergo changes, many of which are not serious enough to justify hysterectomy. One such change, *hyperplasia* (an increase in the number of normal cells), is not cancer, rarely becomes cancer, and can be treated with medication or a D&C. A hysterectomy or even a D&C is not necessary to diagnose uterine or ovarian cancer. An endometrial biopsy performed in a doctor's office can diagnose cancer of the uterus with reasonable accuracy. A laparoscopy (described earlier in this chapter) can provide a view of the ovaries and even take samples of tissue or fluid for examination. This procedure requires general anaesthesia.

Types of Hysterectomy

There are three different types of hysterectomy:

Total hysterectomy, sometimes referred to as **simple hysterectomy** – Removal of the uterus and cervix (mouth of the womb) but not the ovaries and fallopian tubes. A woman continues to produce hormones from her ovaries, but not at her optimum output, and the regular cyclical pattern of ovulation may be interrupted. Sometimes the ovaries are irreparably 'shocked' and never resume functioning after the uterus is cut away.[32]

Total hysterectomy with bilateral salpingo oophorectomy – Removal of the uterus and cervix as well as both tubes and ovaries. Ovarian hormone production ceases abruptly.

Subtotal hysterectomy – Only the body of the uterus is removed. The cervix is left in, with the surrounding stump of uterus. The tubes and ovaries remain.

A subtotal hysterectomy is rarely done today, on the theory that the cervix may develop cancer later. But the rate of cervical cancer is no higher if the

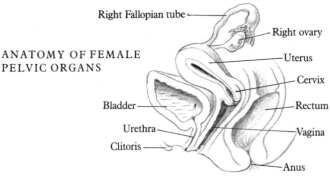

ANATOMY OF FEMALE
PELVIC ORGANS

Right Fallopian tube

Right ovary

Uterus

Cervix

Bladder

Rectum

Urethra

Vagina

Clitoris

Anus

TYPES OF HYSTERECTOMY

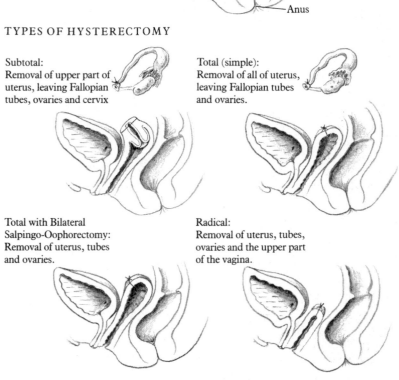

Subtotal:
Removal of upper part of
uterus, leaving Fallopian
tubes, ovaries and cervix

Total (simple):
Removal of all of uterus,
leaving Fallopian tubes
and ovaries.

Total with Bilateral
Salpingo-Oophorectomy:
Removal of uterus, tubes
and ovaries.

Radical:
Removal of uterus, tubes,
ovaries and the upper part
of the vagina.

cervix is left than if all the organs are intact.[33] Researchers do not yet know whether the remaining cervix and piece of uterus will provide the body with beneficial hormones as a piece of ovary will. But leaving the cervix in when a hysterectomy is performed avoids the necessity of cutting the bladder completely away from the uterus, as the surgeon does in a total hysterectomy. The advantage of letting the bladder remain with the cervix is that it may prevent the prolapse of the vault of the vagina, as sometimes occurs after a total hysterectomy.[34] Leaving the cervix in may prevent the loss of sexual response among women who depend on cervical stimulation for orgasm.

If the cervix is left, then be sure to continue to have regular Pap tests.

Hysterectomy: The Operation

As with all surgery, hysterectomy presents hazards. The death rate is one to two per 1,000 women – approximately 800 women in the US die each year from a hysterectomy. Most of these deaths are anaesthesia-related. As many as half of all patients experience some operative complications, including adverse reactions to anaesthesia, haemorrhaging that requires transfusion (one in ten women),[35] abdominal or urinary tract infections, abdominal adhesions, injury to the bladder, bowel, or rectum, and postoperative blood clots.

The surgery commonly involves five to seven days in the hospital and four to six weeks of recovery at home. As with any surgical procedure requiring general anaesthesia and involving opening the abdominal cavity, strenuous activity is usually curtailed for several months. Some women experience prolonged fatigue and loss of energy for six months to a year after surgery.

The operation may be done from inside the vagina (leaving no visible scar) or through an abdominal incision. Vaginal hysterectomy patients show a higher incidence of postoperative fever, bladder and other infections, and urinary tract problems. They also experience greater postoperative blood loss.[36] The number of vaginal hysterectomies has declined since 1975.[37] Since vaginal hysterectomies are performed less frequently and require greater skill, if you do have one it is important to use a surgeon who is experienced in this type of approach. Vaginal hysterectomies seem to involve a shorter recovery period and faster healing. However, many urologists and gynaecologists specializing in the treatment of incontinence believe that the vaginal approach carries too much risk of damage to the urinary system, and that the abdominal approach is preferable for that reason (see Urinary Incontinence chapter).

OVARIES IN OR OUT OVER FORTY?

The threat of ovarian cancer does not justify routine removal of healthy ovaries. Ovarian cancer, while a serious disease, is relatively rare, occurring in less than 1 per cent of all women. While the risk increases in postmenopausal women, it should be noted that the average age of diagnosis of ovarian cancer is sixty-one, and this does not justify routine removal of healthy ovaries from women in their forties or fifties. In the United States a woman has a 1.3 per cent chance of developing ovarian cancer by her seventy-fourth year.[38] One source estimated that 7,500 healthy ovaries would have to be removed to prevent a single cancer death.[39] The risk of ovarian cancer is no higher in hysterectomized women who keep their ovaries than in women who do not undergo a hysterectomy. Furthermore, because ovarian tissue can occur elsewhere in the abdominal cavity, removal of the ovaries does not absolutely guarantee that ovarian cancer will never occur.[40]

Removal of the ovaries in a woman with oestrogen-dependent breast cancer, in order to reduce the amount of oestrogen that stimulates the growth of the cancer, is now virtually obsolete, since hormone treatments achieve the same effect.

During a hysterectomy, the ovaries should be examined for abnormalities. In *advance* of surgery, a woman should discuss with her doctor the conditions under which she consents to the removal of her ovaries. Often a gynaecologist will say, 'If the ovaries are unhealthy we'll take them out,' without specifying what is meant by 'unhealthy'. A cyst, for example, can be cut out from an ovary without removal of the entire ovary. Experts disagree about cysts. Most ovarian cysts in menstruating women are harmless and disappear after several cycles. There is no evidence to date showing that the presence of cysts means an increased risk of ovarian cancer at any age.

If the ovaries are retained after a hysterectomy, regular ovarian checkups are advised. The ovaries are actually easier to examine once the bulky uterus is out of the way, and any question as to their size or consistency can be checked by an ultrasound or laparoscopy.

Do's and Don'ts for Women Contemplating Elective Hysterectomy

A woman who has been advised to have a hysterectomy is often not at her best physically and emotionally. She may feel weak or sick and be under too much stress to be an assertive, active information-seeker. The pressures are often strong to 'get it over with'. But it is important to persist, for a thorough knowledge of your condition is your best assurance of making the right decision.

- *Do* have someone with you when you see your doctor or consultant. Bring a person who will help you ask questions, assess the answers, and support you so you will not feel intimidated into making a quick decision.

- *Do* seek other opinions if surgery is recommended. *Don't* feel it is a *fait accompli* if a second doctor also recommends hysterectomy.

- *Do* talk with other women. *Do* contact the Hysterectomy Support Group (see Organizations). The women there cannot make your decision for you, but they will give you information unavailable elsewhere. Other women's honest assessments are one of your best tools.

- *Do not* have a hysterectomy solely for sterilization purposes (see Birth Control for Women at Midlife chapter).
- *Do not* have a hysterectomy because that was the medical practice popular in your mother's and aunts' era.
- *Do* search out the most current information. Check copyright dates: books written even five or six years ago do not have the newest information about alternatives to and after-effects of hysterectomy. The Women's Health and Reproductive Rights Information Centre (see Organizations) and hospital medical libraries may help you find the newest information. Technical language may be difficult at first, but conquering the jargon is well worth the effort. *Do* check the source of all information read. A pamphlet produced by a drug company, for example, may subtly encourage surgery that would necessitate taking their drug.
- *Do* talk to your GP. She or he is likely to see you as a whole person, not just a set of gynaecological organs. Talk to your GP about non-surgical treatments and ask for a referral to a gynaecologist likely to try other methods before resorting to surgery. Ask friends for names of sympathetic gynaecologists and suggest these to the GP.
- *Do* try to be optimistic. This is very difficult when doctors take a sombre, pessimistic approach to your condition. Some doctors may accentuate the negative.
- *Do* try to reduce stress by every means possible. Stress exacerbates all gynaecological problems.
- *Don't* automatically reject proposed treatments because you do not want to take drugs regularly. Some drugs may be far less risky than a hysterectomy, which involves anaesthesia, prophylactic antibiotics, and possibly long-term hormone replacement therapy, not to mention the potential irreversible after-effects of the surgery.
- *Do* realize that you have a right to refuse or withdraw from any treatment or surgery at any time, even *after* you have entered the hospital.

If You Have Already Had a Hysterectomy

- Make sure you know exactly what was removed during the procedure. Many women do not know that they have had one or both ovaries removed.
- If you want to be sexually active, make extra efforts to promote sexual desire. This may be difficult if your interest in sex is low, but just thinking about sex as well as engaging in it increases hormone production in the ovaries and/or adrenal glands and contributes to health and well-being.
- Pay special attention to your diet. Follow the general suggestions given in Chapter 5. Hysterectomies often produce hormone imbalances that can lead

to low blood sugar (hypoglycaemia). Try to eat small meals high in protein or complex carbohydrates every two to three hours. Vitamin supplements, especially the B complex and vitamin E, may help deficiencies caused by hormone loss.

• Exercise helps to lessen depression and builds stronger bones, helping to prevent osteoporosis. Some women find that yoga, swimming, dancing, and walking are especially helpful after hysterectomy. Exercise helps firm muscles and increase muscle and tendon strength, which is helpful in preventing urinary problems and osteoporosis.

• If you undergo an oophorectomy before the menopause, you may wish to consider oestrogen or oestrogen-progestogen replacement therapy only until the time when the menopause would be expected, tapering down gradually to imitate a natural menopause. If you are undergoing menopausal changes or if you are postmenopausal already, you may prefer not to add hormones when your system has already decreased its production.

NOTES

[1] Estimated figures from the National Center for Health Statistics.

[2] The Boston Women's Health Book Collective, *The New Our Bodies, Ourselves*. London: Penguin, 1989.

[3] The 33 per cent figure is quoted in Niels Lauersen and Eileen Stukane, *Listen to Your Body*. New York: Simon & Schuster, 1982, p. 455. The 72 per cent figure is in Penny Wise Budoff, *No More Menstrual Cramps and Other Good News*. New York: G. P. Putnam & Sons, 1980, p. 1981.

[4] Winnifred Berg Cutler et al., *Menopause, A Guide for Women and the Men Who Love Them*. New York: W. W. Norton & Co., 1983, p. 156.

[5] Claudia Dreifus, ed., *Seizing Our Bodies*. New York: Vintage Books, 1978.

[6] The Boston Women's Health Book Collective, op. cit.

[7] John E. Wennberg, 'Dealing with Medical Practice Variations: A Proposal for Action'. *Health Affairs*, Vol. 3, No. 2, Summer 1984, pp. 6–32.

[8] Richard Sattin and Joyce Hughes, 'Hysterectomy Among Women of Reproductive Age, United States, Update for 1979–1980'. *Urban Health*, Vol. 13, No. 1, January 1984, pp. 44–8.

[9] Nancy Nugent, *Hysterectomy*. New York: Doubleday & Co., 1976, p. 85.

[10] Katherine Dalton, 'Discussion on the Aftermath of Hysterectomy and Oophorectomy'. *Proceedings of the Royal Society of Medicine*, Vol. 50, 1957, pp. 415–18. Surveyed women for ten years after surgery.

[11] Brooks Ranney and S. Abu-Ghazaleh, 'The Future Function and Fortune of Ovarian Tissue Which Is Retained In Vivo During Hysterectomy'. *American Journal of Obstetrics and Gynecology*. Vol. 128, No. 6, 15 July 1977, pp. 626–34.

[12] Sherwin A. Kaufman, *The Ageless Woman*. New York: Prentice-Hall, 1967, p. 127.

[13] James D. Shelton, 'Prostacyclin from the Uterus and Woman's Cardiovascular Advantage'. *Prostaglandins Leukotrienes and Medicine*, Vol. 8, No. 5, May 1982, pp. 459–66.

[14]Personal communication from a member of the group, which has been in existence since 1982.

[15]L. Zussman, Shirley Zussman, R. Sunley and Edith Bjorson, 'Sexual Responses After Hysterectomy/Oophorectomy. Recent Studies and Reconsideration of Psychogenesis'. *American Journal of Obstetrics and Gynecology*, Vol. 140, No. 7, 1 August 1981, pp. 725–9.

[16]Wulf H. Utian, 'Effect of Hysterectomy, Oophorectomy and Estrogen Therapy on Libido'. *International Journal of Gynaecology and Obstetrics*, Vol. 13, No. 3, 1975, pp. 97–100.

[17]J. Anath, 'Hysterectomy and Depression'. *Obstetrics and Gynecology*, Vol. 52, No. 6, December 1978, p. 729.

[18]D. H. Richards, 'A Post-Hysterectomy Syndrome'. *Lancet*, 26 October 1974, pp. 983–5.

[19]From an unpublished manuscript by Carolyn Ruth Swift. The writer has since become a substitute grandmother for a lesbian couple raising a child.

[20]Sandra Beaman Jordan, 'The Facts About Fibroid Tumors'. *McCall's*, July 1985, p. 62.

[21]Estimated figures from the National Center for Health Statistics.

[22]Peggy Eastman, 'Hysterectomy – No Longer the Only Way'. *Self*, September 1984, pp. 183–5.

[23]Robert S. Neuwirth, 'Hysteroscopic Management of Symptomatic Submucous Fibroids'. *Obstetrics and Gynecology*, Vol. 62, No. 4, October 1983, pp. 509–11.

[24]Charles C. Coddington et al., 'Long-Acting Gonadotropin Hormone-Releasing Hormone Analog Used to Treat Uteri'. *Fertility and Sterility*, Vol. 45, No. 5, May 1986, pp. 624–9; and Rodolphe Maheux and André Lemay, 'Uterine Leiomyoma Treatment with LHRH Agonist'. *Progress in Clinical and Biological Research*, Vol. 225, 1986, pp. 297–311.

[25]Niels Lauersen, *PMS: Premenstrual Syndrome and You*. New York: Pinnacle Books, 1984, p. 88.

[26]Lauersen and Stukane, op. cit., p. 61.

[27]M. Greenberg, 'Hysterectomy, Hormones and Behavior: Letter to the Editor'. *Lancet*, Vol. 1, No. 8217, 21 February 1981, p. 449.

[28]'Hysterectomy', in *The Prevention Guide to Surgery and Its Alternatives*. Emmaus, Pa.: Rodale Press, 1980, pp. 287–328.

[29]Jonathan Parmer, 'Long-Term Suppression of Hypermenorrhea by Progesterone Intrauterine Contraception'. *American Journal of Obstetrics and Gynecology*, Vol. 149, No. 5, 1 July 1984, pp. 578–9.

[30]Maryann Napoli, 'Medical Breakthrough. Laser Hysterectomy'. *Ms.*, March 1986, p. 30; and Jane Brody, 'Laser Lessens the Trauma of Surgery in the Uterus'. *The New York Times*, 13 April 1987.

[31]Lynda Madras and Jane Patterson, with Peter Schick, *Womancare: A Gynecological Guide to Your Body*. New York: Avon, 1981, pp. 386–9.

[32]Ranney and Abu-Ghazaleh, op. cit.

[33]Richard Mattingly and John D. Thompson, *Te Linde's Operative Gynecology*. Philadelphia: Lippincott, 1985.

[34]Niles Newton and Enid Baron, 'Reactions to Hysterectomy'. *Primary Care*, Vol. 3, December 1976, p. 793.

[35]The Boston Women's Health Book Collective, op. cit.

[36]Cutler et al., op. cit., pp. 154–76.

[37]Sattin and Hughes, op. cit.

[38]J. L. Young, Jr et al., 'Surveillance, Epidemiology, and End Results: Incidence and Mortality Data 1973–77'. National Cancer Institute Monograph, 1981, p. 57.

[39]Lauersen and Stukane, op. cit.

[40]Joanne Tobachman et al., 'Intra-Abdominal Carcinomatosis After Prophylactic Oophorectomy in Ovarian-Cancer-Prone Families'. *Lancet*, Vol. 3, 9 October 1982, p. 795.

BOOKS AND PUBLICATIONS

Nikki Henriques and Anne Dickson, *Women on Hysterectomy, or How Long Before I Can Hang-glide?* Wellingborough: Thorsons, 1986.

Lorraine Dennerstein, *Hysterectomy: A Book to Help You Deal with the Physical and Emotional Aspects.* Oxford: Oxford Medical Publications, 1982.

Dr David Delvin, *A Patient's Guide to Operations.* London: Penguin, 1981.

Hysterectomy: What's It All About? Thames TV leaflet.

Wendy Savage and Nancy Duin, originally for Thames TV's 'Help' programme, *Hysterectomy.* Women's Health and Reproductive Rights Information Centre, 1988.

23
Hypertension, Heart Disease, and Stroke

Many of us have had someone close to us become ill or suddenly die from cardiovascular disease, the leading cause of death in the United Kingdom. In Scotland the heart disease figures are the worst in Europe. Cardiovascular disease, or disease of the heart and blood vessels, can damage every other part of the body. Some of us have experienced a heart attack or a stroke. Many of us fear being well at one minute and seemingly at death's door the next.

Although healthy habits are no guarantee that we can prevent cardiovascular disease, we do know that high blood pressure, smoking, eating foods rich in saturated fats and cholesterol, and inactivity all increase our chances of developing it. We can decrease the probability of serious illness or premature death by reducing these risk factors, regularly checking our blood pressure, and knowing the early warning signs of heart attack and stroke.

Heart Disease *is* a Woman's Disease

In the past, heart disease was considered a man's disease. Most research until recently did not include women, so much of the information we have about heart disease is based on studies of men, assuming that they are the norm. In fact, heart disease is the leading cause of death in women over sixty today, and women who have heart attacks are more likely to die from them than men. Women are also more likely than men to have strokes. We can no longer afford to ignore the impact of heart disease on women's health – more research is needed on women and heart disease.

Because heart disease is often regarded as a man's disease, many doctors pay less attention to symptoms in women than in men, and don't emphasize preventive steps, such as lowering cholesterol levels. Women often suffer needless discomfort because they or their doctors ignore or minimize early symptoms.

I was lying in bed at about 2.00 in the morning. I felt a pain in my chest, which I thought might be indigestion. Then the pain went into my arm and up to my neck and

*head. That really hurt. I jumped up and it seemed to get better, so I didn't tell my
daughter. The next night it started again. I knew there was a problem, but it went
away again when I jumped up. The next morning I told my daughter but I refused to
go to the doctor. I knew what had happened. But after the pain stopped, I thought
maybe nothing happened. I'm stubborn and we fought for two days. Then I went
and the doctor put me in the hospital for fourteen days.* [a seventy-two-year-old
woman]

HOW THE HEART WORKS

The heart, a four-chambered muscular organ, is divided into a left and right
side. The right side receives blood through the veins that is low in oxygen and
high in carbon dioxide and passes it to the lungs, where oxygen is added and
carbon dioxide eliminated. The oxygen-rich blood from the lungs then goes to
the left side of the heart where it is pumped to all parts of the body through the
arteries of the circulatory system. Valves in each chamber of the heart regulate
this flow of blood. The circulating blood supplies nutrients and oxygen to all
organs and tissues of the body. It picks up waste products from the cells and
carries the waste to the kidneys or lungs to be eliminated. The pumping action
of the heart is controlled by a bundle of nerves that acts as a natural pacemaker.

High Blood Pressure (Hypertension)

Hypertension, or high blood pressure, increases the risk of strokes and often
contributes to heart attacks and other diseases. Most people who have
hypertension experience no signs or symptoms; some may experience headaches, dizziness, fainting spells, ringing in the ears, or nosebleeds.

Blood pressure is the force of blood against the walls of the arteries and
veins. The force is created by the heart as it pumps blood to every part of the
body. Blood pressure is recorded with two numbers, for example, $\frac{120}{70}$, read as
'120 over 70'.

- **Systolic**, the first or upper number, represents the blood pressure in the
  arteries when the heart is pumping blood;
- **Diastolic**, the second or lower number, is the pressure in the arteries when
  the heart is filling with blood for the next beat.

The American Heart Association (AHA) considers any systolic pressure
over 140 to be abnormal. (Other researchers arbitrarily have defined hypertension as blood pressure over $\frac{160}{90}$.)[1] For people over sixty-five, systolic pressures
of 150 to 155 are not uncommon, but the AHA suggests that they be lowered, if
possible. If your diastolic pressure remains above 90 to 95, you are considered
hypertensive.

A painless and simple test measures blood pressure. Taking blood pressure is an easy skill to learn. Since many women are under stress in a doctor's surgery, it may be preferable to check your blood pressure at home or at work. A family or a group could share the cost of the equipment obtainable from a medical supplier. If you are a large woman, be sure that the cuff you use is big enough to fit around your arm, as one that is too small may cause a false reading. Don't rely on coin-operated machines that are available in some pharmacies and supermarkets; they are not always adjusted properly and can give false readings.

A diagnosis of high blood pressure should not be based on only one reading, because blood pressure varies with the time of day, activity, and stress, including the stress of having your blood pressure taken. At least three elevated readings, taken days or weeks apart while both sitting and standing, should be found before hypertension is diagnosed.

Blood pressure tends to rise with age and after the menopause. About 50 per cent of people over sixty-five have hypertension.[2]

More black women than white women develop hypertension, and they develop it earlier in life, more severely, and suffer hypertension-related deaths more frequently. Death rates from strokes, in particular, are much higher among blacks than whites. Some researchers attribute these high hypertension rates to a genetic adaptation useful for survival in the African climate but not needed at colder temperatures. Others criticize this theory and state that these high hypertension rates are related to high-stress lives caused by poverty, and diets high in salt and fats.

I am a sixty-one-year-old black lady who has been diagnosed as having severe hypertension. For thirty-odd years I have tried hard to accept and cope with this problem: no salt, no fat, weight control, etc. It is very hard but if you want to live a fairly normal life, you have to try to do what's best. After having all kinds of tests and medication I have learned one of the best remedies for me is to try and not let things bug me. I try not to get upset over things which I have no control over. Sometimes it doesn't work, but I still keep on trying. My doctor has tried different medications and when something new comes along she will suggest it to me, tell me the side effects, and then leave the decision up to me. Usually I try these medications because maybe something will come along that will help me, or someone else.

WHAT CAN BE DONE FOR HIGH BLOOD PRESSURE?

If you have mild hypertension you may be able to lower your blood pressure without medication, or with less medication, if you adopt the following good health habits.

- Eat well for weight management.
- Exercise. If you are not accustomed to exercise, start by taking a walk each day. If you are not able to get around see the section When Movement is Limited, pages 121–2. Exercising also helps weight management (see Weighty Issues chapter).
- Reduce salt intake.
- Reduce stress and use relaxation exercises (read Ageing and Well-being chapter for a more complete discussion of these suggestions).

MEDICATION/DRUGS FOR HIGH BLOOD PRESSURE

If your hypertension is severe, or if the above suggestions do not lower your blood pressure enough or soon enough, you may need medication to lower it. However, good health habits will contribute to your well-being and should be continued even if you take medication.

If medication is necessary, the first type of drug tried is usually a diuretic (often called a 'water pill', because it reduces the amount of fluid in the body). Possible effects include a low potassium level and elevated uric acid and blood glucose levels, which can cause fatigue, muscle weakness, leg cramps, and other problems. Do not take over-the-counter diuretics without consulting a doctor. Anyone taking diuretics should be carefully monitored for signs of dehydration and urinary problems. If you are taking a potassium-depleting diuretic, you should eat four servings a day of potassium-rich foods.* If you cannot eat enough of these foods, you may have to take a prescribed potassium preparation.

If diuretic therapy alone is not effective, you may be given additional medications. *Beta-blockers*, such as propranolol (Inderal), metoprolol (Lopressor, Betaloc), nadolol (Corgard), and atenolol (Tenormin), lower the heart's demand for blood. Beta-blockers are not considered a good choice for treating hypertension in black people, some older people, or people with asthma or heart failure. For others, in low doses, beta-blockers effectively treat heart pain (angina pectoris) and irregular heartbeats (arrhythmias). Some women may experience other effects from beta-blockers, such as nausea, cold feet, insomnia, tiredness, depression, a slow heartbeat, or wheezing asthma. Sometimes, though not often, these medications may cause lower sexual desire. Too high a dose can cause dizziness and fainting spells. If you are taking insulin for diabetes, you should carefully review any possible reactions with your doctor. **Never stop taking beta-blockers abruptly; you must taper off gradually.**

---

*Apricots, avocados, bananas, broccoli, cabbage, cantaloupe, dates, figs, raisins, grapefruit, molasses, mushrooms, oranges, peanuts, pineapple, plums, potatoes, prunes, pumpkin, radishes, rhubarb, tomatoes, water melon, wheat germ, whole grains, cooked dried beans.

Calcium-channel blockers are still being tested but are increasingly used as the second step, rather than beta-blockers, in medically treating hypertension. Because calcium-channel blockers prevent spasms of the coronary arteries, they keep the supply of blood flowing into the heart and are useful when spasms play a role in causing angina pain. They also slow a racing heart rate.

Vasodilators are another kind of drug commonly taken for high blood pressure. These relax the blood vessel wall, allowing more blood to flow through. Some women who take them complain of headaches, swelling around the eyes, heart palpitations, shortness of breath, dizziness, or aches and pains in the joints. If these symptoms continue after the first few weeks, talk to your doctor about changing medications.

A combination of small doses of various hypertensive drugs is often more effective for older persons than a single form of medication. Attempting to lower blood pressure over a period of weeks or months, rather than suddenly, produces better results with fewer side effects.

SOME GENERAL SUGGESTIONS FOR REDUCING HIGH BLOOD PRESSURE WITH DRUGS

- Your pharmacist is a valuable resource. Ask her or him about the medicines you have been prescribed; food and drinks to avoid; and best times to take medication.
- Don't mix drugs. Tell your doctor and pharmacist about all drugs (prescription and over-the-counter), including vitamins and birth control pills, you are taking and any drug reaction you have had in the past.
- Keep to your schedule for taking drugs. Your blood pressure is only lowered while the drugs are working, so you must keep a continuous supply in your body. Some people need medication for the rest of their lives; others may be able to reduce or stop medication if changes in life-style lower their pressure sufficiently over a significant period of time.
- Do not stop medication because your blood pressure is normal or because you feel okay. Remember, you have to *keep* your blood pressure normal.
- Drink little or no alcohol.
- Know your blood pressure. Keep a record of it. You can only know your blood pressure by measuring it, not by how you feel.

Atherosclerosis

Atherosclerosis, often called 'hardening of the arteries', is a condition that underlies cardiovascular diseases. With this condition, over time the walls of the arteries become thickened with deposits of a combination of fat (cholesterol) and calcium, called plaque, which can narrow or block the arteries leading to any part of the body, including the heart and brain. The deposits are likely to form where damage has occurred because of high blood pressure. The deposits can cause intense pain in the heart (angina pectoris) if there is partial blockage; heart attack, if total blockage occurs in a coronary artery; or a stroke, if the blockage occurs in arteries in the brain.

Angina can occur whenever less oxygen reaches the heart than is needed. Exercise, extremes of temperature, reactions to stress or strong emotions, or other causes, such as anaemia, may cause angina. Some of us experience pain but can live full lives with it for many years, even when the cause is not clear.

Cholesterol is one of several blood fats (lipids) in the blood. Lipids must be combined with proteins, forming lipoproteins, to transport fat in the blood. High-density lipoprotein (HDL) contains the highest proportion of protein and is important in transporting fat away from body cells, preventing the accumulation of cholesterol and other fats within the artery walls. Women tend to have higher levels of HDL than men. Athletes also have high levels, especially long-distance runners. Smokers have lower levels of HDL.

Low-density lipoprotein (LDL) contains the largest proportion of cholesterol of any of the lipoproteins. LDL is a factor in the accumulation of fatty materials in the artery walls and is significantly related to risk of heart attack and stroke.

Lowering the cholesterol level in the bloodstream reduces heart attacks and heart attack deaths. Every 1 per cent drop in the cholesterol level means a 2 per cent decrease in the likelihood of a heart attack.[3] Although women have not been included in most past studies, a recent study shows that women benefit more than men from low-cholesterol diets.[4]

In addition to food sources, the body also produces cholesterol. Blood cholesterol levels generally increase with age. An estimated 15 million American women have blood cholesterol levels of 260 milligrams per 100 millilitres (250 mg/100 ml) or above, placing them at high risk of developing heart disease. Recommended levels of blood cholesterol vary among medical professionals – some set the desirable level under 200 mg/100 ml for adults,[5] while others suggest 100-plus-your-age (up to a maximum of 160) mg/100 ml.[6] The average American adult consumes between 400 and 700 milligrams of cholesterol each day.[7] The British diet is generally just as full of cholesterol and in Scotland (where heart disease is so prevalent) it is particularly so. The American Heart Association recommends that Americans limit cholesterol intake from food to no more than 300 milligrams a day (a medium-sized egg yolk contains about 275).

Preventing Cardiovascular Diseases

We can do a lot to reduce the factors that affect our chances of having a heart attack or stroke. The first step is understanding the role of hypertension and other risk factors. Then we can make changes to improve our health and reduce the risks. Understanding these factors is the first step.

SMOKING AND HEART DISEASE

Cigarette smoking definitely increases the risk of heart disease.[8] Women who give up smoking can lower that risk. Studies show that smokers who stop return to non-smoker risk levels for heart disease within approximately ten years.[9] Some studies suggest that after age sixty-five the influence of cigarette smoking on heart disease declines,[10] though all the other negative effects of smoking continue.

Smoking affects the circulatory system in a number of ways. It damages the linings of the arteries, making it easier for plaque to build up in them. Nicotine from cigarettes overstimulates the heart. Smoking causes the oxygen in the blood to be displaced by carbon monoxide, causing the heart to work harder to remove the carbon monoxide. Finally, smoking harms the respiratory system (see pp. 41–4 for help in stopping smoking).

EXERCISE AND WEIGHT

Regular aerobic exercise helps regulate weight, raises beneficial HDL levels, and increases overall cardiovascular fitness by improving blood circulation throughout your body. Exercise is especially important for those whose bodies produce high levels of cholesterol. If you have cardiovascular disease, check with your doctor before starting an exercise programme, to make sure you know the level of exercise suitable for you (see the exercise cautions on p. 122).

Research shows that those of us who are very overweight are at greater risk for developing hypertension. Some studies show that increasing exercise to lose weight can be as effective as diet and drugs in controlling hypertension; others suggest that regular exercise is more important than weight loss.[11]

As we age, the eating patterns of our younger years tend to stay with us, but we often exercise less, causing an increase in fat in our bodies. Women who accumulate fat around the waist and abdomen are at higher risk of heart attack, stroke, hypertension, and diabetes than others who accumulate fat around the hips and lower extremities.[12]

DIET

Diet influences HDL and LDL levels in the blood and therefore influences the likelihood of developing heart disease. We can reduce this risk by: (1) replacing saturated fats with polyunsaturated fats, (2) eating less food high in cholesterol, (3) eliminating 'empty calorie' foods with little nutritive value, and (4) increasing exercise to reduce the ratio of fat on the body.

Salt contributes to fluid retention, increasing the amount of energy the heart must exert. It also counters the effect of diuretics, which are often prescribed for hypertension. Take the salt cellar off the table and avoid most canned foods, baking soda, ketchup, relishes, and delicatessen meats, all of which contain high amounts of salt.

Eat poultry and fish rather than meat. Limit meat to lean cuts, trimming all visible fat. Replace butter and shortening with oils such as corn, canola, sunflower, and safflower oils. Eliminate coffee.[13] Try reducing egg yolks to no more than three a week. Eat more garlic, onions, whole grains, fruits, and vegetables. Choose low-fat milk and cheeses, but take care not to eliminate calcium (which is found in dairy products) from your diet, since calcium is a factor in the prevention of both hypertension and osteoporosis.

Reports indicate that eating fish two or three times per week reduces risk of atherosclerosis. Not only does eating fish reduce the number of high-cholesterol, red-meat meals you consume, but fish oil contains omega-3 polyunsaturated fats, which appear to have beneficial effects on blood cholesterol.[14] Some people take daily doses of cod-liver oil, in liquid or capsule form, and some doctors recommend this.

STRESS FACTORS

Although reactions to stress vary, most doctors agree that reducing emotional stress benefits general health and particularly heart disease. The Framingham Study, a long-term project in the US that looked at various aspects of heart disease, found that women who work outside of the home have fewer heart attacks than women who do not. However, women who have children, work in stressful clerical jobs, and have unsupportive bosses and husbands, are the most frequent victims of heart disease.[15] A few employers offer employees stress reduction programmes to reduce lost time on the job and prevent stress-related disease: this is more often offered to executives than to 'lower level' workers. Relaxation and yoga classes are run at many Adult Education Centres (see Disarming Stress, p. 21). Many of us, as we get older, need to balance rest and activity. Take a rest in the afternoon if you feel tired and can fit it into your routine.

HEREDITY

Some medical researchers believe there is a link between family history and likelihood of developing cardiovascular diseases. Others think this link reflects family behaviour more than inherited traits. We not only pass on genetic traits to our children but often also eating, smoking, and exercising habits, which may have greater effects than hereditary factors. Nonetheless, if several members of your family have died of heart attacks or strokes at a young age, you should pay particular attention to preventive measures.

AGE AND GENDER

Although heart disease is not directly related to ageing, it does occur with greater frequency after the age of forty. On the average, it occurs in women ten years later than in men. Up to age fifty-five, men have higher death rates from heart attacks and stroke. After that, women catch up.

HORMONES AND HEART DISEASE

The relationship between hormones and heart disease is not fully understood. Oral contraceptives, which contain hormones, cause a twofold or greater increase in risk of heart attacks and strokes – an increase well beyond their blood-pressure-raising effect.[16] Smoking has an additional harmful interaction with hormone use. Women who use oral contraceptives and smoke are ten times as likely to suffer from coronary heart disease as non-smoking women who take oral contraceptives.[17] Among a group of heavy smokers (twenty-five or more cigarettes per day), aged forty to forty-nine and currently using oral contraceptives, the risk of a heart attack was thirty-nine times greater than that of women who neither smoked nor used oral contraceptives.[18]

Because heart disease among women increases at about the same age that the menopause occurs, the assumption was made that the hormone oestrogen offers some protection. The menopause, especially when caused by the early surgical removal of the ovaries, reduces oestrogen and seems to remove some of our protection from heart disease. Oestrogen use in women seems to reduce LDL cholesterol and increase HDL cholesterol, both effects which should protect against cardiovascular disease. However, the research results in women have been mixed and have not shown a significant association, either positive or negative. In fact, oestrogen use among men increased heart disease.[19] The hormone progesterone (progestogens or progestin) may increase LDL cholesterol and lower HDL cholesterol, and it has been linked to an increased risk of heart attack and stroke.[20]

While one study that took cigarette smoking into consideration supported the hypothesis that the postmenopausal use of oestrogen therapy reduces the risk of coronary heart disease,[21] another study published at the same time found no benefits from oestrogen use but rather an increased stroke rate among non-smoking oestrogen users and an increased heart attack rate among smoking oestrogen users.[22]

More research is needed on the effects of postmenopausal hormones (both oestrogens and progestogens) on cardiovascular diseases. Unfortunately, the 2 million to 3 million women in the United States and the increasing numbers in the UK, who are taking these hormones before all the long-term effects are known, are themselves the unwitting subjects of this research. See pages 355–61 for further discussion of HRT.

Heart Attack

When the supply of blood to the heart is interrupted, because of narrowed arteries or a blood clot, part of the heart muscle dies from lack of oxygen and nutrients. This is called a heart attack, or myocardial infarction (MI).

How to Know You Are Having a Heart Attack

You will be the first one to suspect you are having a heart attack. Look for these signals:

- Uncomfortable pressure, fullness, tightness, squeezing, or pain in the centre of your chest, lasting two minutes or more. The pain may fade away and then return. Unlike the pain of angina, the pain of a heart attack does not go away after physical or emotional stress ceases.
- Pain that spreads to your arms, shoulders, neck, jaw or stomach.
- Severe pain, dizziness, fainting, sweating, nausea, or shortness of breath.

Everyone does not experience all these symptoms. If you experience any of these conditions, try to stay calm. Do not panic, but do not wait. Get help immediately. The sooner you begin treatment, the greater your chances of surviving. Dial 999 or go to the emergency department at a nearby hospital. There, a doctor will take your history, give you a complete physical exam, take an electrocardiogram (ECG), and draw blood for lab tests.

DIAGNOSIS OF HEART DISEASE

A wide variety of tests exists to determine whether someone has heart disease or has had a heart attack. All tests are not necessary for everyone who suspects heart disease – some are expensive and will only be performed when necessary. Ask your doctor why a particular test is being ordered and what you will learn from it.

An *electrocardiogram* (ECG) to identify abnormal heart rhythms is usually the first test performed when heart disease is suspected. This is normally done in the outpatients department of a hospital.

Exercise testing, or *stress testing*, primarily determines the nature and cause of any chest pain and is useful in the early detection of coronary heart disease. Through graded exercise, the stress test determines whether the coronary circulation is capable of increasing the oxygen supply to the heart muscle. Unfortunately, the results for women often show damage when none exists (called a false positive result). Some doctors, therefore, always order thallium scanning (radionuclear imaging) along with stress testing for women. Others, to avoid unnecessary testing and save expense, order thallium scanning only if the stress test is positive.

Radionuclear imaging, sometimes called a *thallium test* or *thallium scanning*, is a technique in which a small amount of thallium, a short-lived radioactive substance, is injected into an arm vein. The thallium circulates with the blood and concentrates in the heart. There it gives off gamma rays that are translated by computer into a picture. The doctor can tell if any areas of heart muscle have been damaged by heart attack, or if any part of the heart is not getting enough blood and oxygen, the cause of angina. This test may also be done while exercising.

Echocardiography uses sound waves to study the heart's structure and function. It is non-invasive (does not penetrate the body and therefore does not cause pain or discomfort). It can be helpful in identifying patients with disease of the heart valves, an often overlooked problem with the elderly.

A *Holter monitor exam* is a twenty-four-hour ECG. You wear a portable ECG machine for twenty-four hours. This gives the doctor a longer record of your heart's activity than she or he can get in the examining room.

Coronary arteriography, sometimes called *cardiac catheterization*, is a procedure in which a long tube, or catheter, is inserted in an artery and dye is passed through it. The dye allows X-rays to show whether any arteries to the brain or heart are blocked. Catheterization is not recommended for everyone, especially not for the elderly. If your heart disease can be managed with medication, or if you are considered a high-risk candidate for bypass surgery, little useful information will be gained from performing a catheterization.[23]

Treatment for Heart Attack

Most people who have suffered a heart attack are admitted to a hospital coronary care unit (CCU) or intensive care unit (ICU). Here their heart is monitored, and life-saving services are available in case they are needed. For some people, however, the atmosphere in the ICU or CCU is itself tension-producing and may slow recovery.

Two kinds of drugs are prescribed for people who have suffered a heart attack: those that increase the flow of blood, bringing extra oxygen to the heart; and those that reduce the need for oxygen.

After a heart attack, the blocked artery that was responsible for the heart attack may need to be opened, allowing the heart to get adequate oxygen. New treatments to open blocked arteries have been developed. These use the same process as cardiac catheterization. One method involves injecting streptokinase, a clot-dissolving drug, through a catheter or directly into the artery. If used within a few hours after a heart attack, streptokinase will dissolve the clot within twenty minutes. It is not recommended for anyone who has a bleeding disorder or who has recently had surgery. Although streptokinase is no longer considered experimental by most doctors, it is not widely used, especially not in small hospitals. Tissue plasminogen activator (TPA) is a newer drug with fewer adverse effects that is beginning to replace streptokinase. The sooner you get treatment after you suspect you have had a heart attack, the more likely it will be effective.

Another method used to clear a blocked artery is balloon angioplasty. In this treatment, a small balloon is inserted and is inflated at the site of the obstruction to clear a partially blocked artery. For some patients, this procedure is a less expensive alternative to coronary bypass surgery. It does not require the chest to be opened and involves shorter hospitalization, and shorter recovery time. This procedure is increasingly available in the UK – generally in large or teaching hospitals. Laser procedures combined with angioplasty are more effective than angioplasty alone.[24]

Cardiac bypass surgery is sometimes performed when an artery is blocked and cannot be cleared with medication or balloon angioplasty. Surgeons use a vein, usually taken from the leg, or an artery from the chest[25] and construct a detour, or bypass, around the blocked artery. In bypass surgery, the chest is opened and a heart/lung machine keeps blood circulating while the new segment is attached to the heart.

If you saw me at my Over-Sixties Keep Fit Class you wouldn't know I'd had a coronary bypass operation. It was after two heart attacks and two years of anxiety and depression about my condition that I agreed to the op. It's been a huge success –

and it's changed my life-style. Now I walk instead of taking the bus, go swimming and have become a near-vegetarian. (I eat fish but no red meat.) My GP says there's every reason I should survive to my nineties. [a seventy-three-year-old woman]

Some women who have bypass surgery experience dramatic relief from pain and lead physically active lives again. However, bypass surgery primarily relieves pain; there is no proof that surgery increases life expectancy for most people. For only one group, those with obstruction of the left main coronary artery, does surgery improve chances of survival. Yet in the US over 100,000 operations are performed each year at a total cost of over $1.5 billion.

Several studies have shown that a more conservative approach is as effective as bypass surgery for most people.[26] These studies suggest that bypass surgery could be avoided through the use of medication, exercise, diet, stress reduction, and smoking cessation. These changes must be made even with surgery or the bypass may clog.

Before having bypass surgery, you may want to ask for a referral to a cardiologist who specializes in the *medical* rather than surgical treatment of heart disease. This will ensure that you get opinions from two different perspectives. Finally, death rates for bypass surgery vary from hospital to hospital. Generally, medical centres with specialized surgical teams have the best records. The more often a team operates, the better their record. **Never consider undergoing bypass surgery at a hospital where fewer than 200 procedures a year are performed.**

Many women are concerned about how their scars will look after surgery, and they should ask.

My scar starts above my ankle and goes almost up to my throat. I love to swim, but the scar turns blue when I get it wet. This summer I didn't swim or wear shorts. I don't care too much about my chest scar. They sewed it on the inside and it doesn't show as much as the scar on my leg. Some women only wear turtlenecks or high-neck blouses, because they don't want anyone to see their scar. [a sixty-eight-year-old woman]

Some Other Surgical Procedures

Modern heart surgery may extend life and improve its quality. Unfortunately, it can also hold out false promises and be performed unnecessarily, at great cost to the individual and to society.

PACEMAKERS

A bundle of nerves in the upper-right chamber of the heart – our natural pacemaker – transmits electrical impulses that control our heartbeat. When these impulses slow down or become irregular or blocked, we may not experience any symptoms or we may experience weakness, breathlessness, slow pulse beat, lack of increased pulse beat when exercising, or even loss of consciousness.

No treatment is needed in many instances. In some instances, a battery-powered artificial pacemaker is used externally for a time or implanted permanently under the skin of the chest wall. The artificial pacemaker controls the heart rate by sending out rhythmic electrical impulses to activate the contractions of the heart. The implantation carries a risk, as does any surgery. The Food and Drug Administration in the United States reviews the safety and effectiveness of new models of pacemakers developed since 1976, but does not review so thoroughly those pacemakers which are similar to models developed before passage of the 1976 medical-device amendments to the US Food, Drug and Cosmetic Act.[27] Controversy continues about whether unnecessary or no-longer-necessary pacemakers should be removed.[28]

An artificial pacemaker's batteries usually last an average of four years, despite claims made by some manufacturers that theirs will last longer. Make sure to keep the regular checking appointments, so that problems can be detected before they are serious. A recent study of pacemakers led to the suggestion that they be checked more often and earlier than some manufacturers recommend.[29]

VALVE REPLACEMENT

Some procedures, such as replacement of the valves in the heart, can affect positively both the length of life and its quality.

For at least two years I had progressively less strength and was feeling more and more tired. I couldn't do physical activity like gardening, which I loved. I also felt psychologically under a cloud, that my life was draining out. I wasn't feeling pain in my chest but I was feeling spasms, quivering, palpitations, and butterflies that I thought would go away. I kept attributing these symptoms to getting older, but when I had headaches, which I never had before, and couldn't do a lot of walking, I knew something was the matter.

My doctor referred me to a cardiology department where they did all the tests and said that I needed a valve replacement within a month. I read up on it a bit first and then went into the hospital for twelve days, five of them in intensive care. After I came home the stairs were difficult for a while and there were some days when I couldn't walk very far. I gradually went back to work. I started feeling really great after about six months. [a fifty-four-year-old woman]

TRANSPLANTS AND ARTIFICIAL HEARTS

Research in cardiology today often emphasizes sophisticated treatment of existing disease conditions at the expense of prevention and early intervention. Newspapers are filled with stories about some patients receiving procedures costing huge sums, while funds for health education and specifically for heart disease prevention programmes are minimal. The few heart transplant operations performed each year in the UK get a lot of publicity. There is very little for courses on cardiopulmonary resuscitation, which could help to save lives. Ask your local branch of the British Red Cross about classes on mouth-to-mouth resuscitation and heart massage.

Stroke

A stroke occurs when the blood vessels that supply oxygen to the brain are blocked. One of the most common forms of stroke, cerebral thrombosis, occurs when a clot develops in an artery damaged by atherosclerosis. In cerebral embolism, a wandering clot, or embolism, lodges in one of the arteries, blocking blood to the brain. In a cerebral haemorrhage, a burst artery floods the brain tissue with blood, causing blood loss to the brain and pressure on the brain tissue. This bleeding can be caused by a head injury or an aneurysm – a blood-filled pouch that balloons out from a weak spot in the artery wall.

Long-standing hypertension is a major cause of strokes. Diabetic women, especially those with hypertension, are at greater-than-average risk of stroke and should especially take action to keep their blood pressure normal.

How to Know You Are Having a Stroke

The following symptoms may be warnings that you are about to have a stroke or are having little strokes already. Even if they are temporary, you should not ignore them.

- Temporary weakness or numbness in the face, arm, or leg on one side of the body.
- A severe, persistent headache.
- Temporary loss of speech or difficulty speaking or understanding speech.

- Temporary dimness or loss of vision.
- Dizziness or unsteadiness, possibly causing you to fall.
- Memory loss.

I was frightened to realize that there were parts of three days I couldn't reconstruct. I usually have a fabulous memory; people call me for details from a meeting held seven years ago. And now I couldn't recall last week's appointments, phone calls, or letters. I was in a real panic by the time I got to the doctor.

A thorough examination turned up things I hadn't even noticed – a generalized weakness on my left side, the inability to make a fist, a little problem with my speech, and bruises on my left leg that suggested I'd been bumping into things. My blood pressure was very high. The doctor referred me to a neurologist as an emergency. After many tests the final diagnosis was made – I'd had several strokes. [a sixty-year-old woman]

Little strokes, or transient ischaemic attacks (TIAs), sometimes precede a major stroke by days, weeks, or months. These are generally warning signs of a major stroke to come. If you experience any of the symptoms listed above, **see your doctor right away.**

TREATMENT FOR STROKES

Treatment for strokes starts with treatment of those very conditions that are also risk factors for strokes: hypertension, cardiac disease, TIAs, high haematocrit (percentage of red cells in the blood), and diabetes. TIAs are treated with aspirin or other anticlotting medication to reduce the possibility of forming new clots.

None of what followed my stroke was easy. Getting my hypertension under control proved to be difficult. I found it hard to let my children and my friends do things for me. Most of all, I had to face my own feelings. I felt older. I was depressed and scared. Would I have another, more crippling, stroke? Just how much would my life have to change?

I continued to work and now, three years later, I'm about to take a new job. I don't forget anything important. I walk and use a stationary bike and have cut down on fats and sugar, so I feel great and thinner. My blood pressure was 130 over 70 yesterday. The amount of medication has been reduced over time. Taking it has become just one more thing I do regularly each day – like brushing my teeth. [the same sixty-year-old woman]

Recovery and Rehabilitation

After heart attacks and surgery, people often re-evaluate their lives and find new directions.

I now celebrate two birthdays – the day I was born and the day I had the surgery! [a sixty-nine-year-old woman after bypass surgery]

After surgery I took a trip abroad. I felt well physically and I was beginning to think of alternative things I might do. Seeing people dress and think differently had an effect on me. New possibilities presented themselves. I felt a physical and emotional connection between my heart and my experience I hadn't completely grasped before.

When I came home I started seeing a therapist. She said, 'Now you have a new life and want to figure out what to do with it.' One of my goals is to make more connections and to get involved in organizational and political work. I'd like to change my job to one where I can meet more people. I realize I'd be better off if I had more friends and more associations with other women. [a fifty-four-year-old woman]

Formerly, a person who had a heart attack was told to rest in bed for three weeks. Recent evidence shows that this can be harmful. Rehabilitation programmes help people who have had a heart attack or cardiac surgery return to health. Many programmes begin in the ICU or CCU, where you can begin doing ankle circles and limited-range exercises while your heart is monitored. By the time you leave the hospital, you will be walking and climbing stairs. In a good programme you will learn exercises to continue at home and diet changes to follow. You should be fully informed about any medications you will be taking.

WHAT ABOUT SEX?

A common myth about heart disease is that having sex will cause heart attack or even death. This is not true. Nor does a heart attack or heart surgery or stroke mean an end to a satisfying sex life. Most women find that after their initial recovery, lovemaking is as pleasurable as before. (See Sexuality chapter.)

The second phase of rehabilitation should be an outpatient programme lasting about twelve sessions. This would combine monitored exercise, discussion groups, and education. Here you have a chance to increase your physical capacity and talk about your concerns with people who have experienced a similar trauma. Such programmes are seldom offered in the UK. Contact the Chest, Heart and Stroke Association for advice.

Physical, speech, and occupational therapy help people who have had strokes regain all the skills possible. A stroke can affect speech, behaviour, thought patterns, memory, and ability to understand, and sometimes can cause paralysis.

In the past, rehabilitation stressed compensation for the disabled parts of the body, so the stroke victim depended more on the unaffected side of the body. Today's approach to rehabilitation emphasizes relearning control over the affected side.

She heard the doctor say as he left her hospital room, 'There can be no hope of recovery from this.' She could see everything; words were exploding in her mind but none escaped into sound. She couldn't believe the doctor's words. Would she be helpless for years to come? She was a photographer. Would she never take another picture?

'It isn't so!' The voice of the nurse reached her. She was leaning over the bed, her face very angry. 'He shouldn't have said that!' The nurse was whispering furiously. Recovery was possible. She had seen it often in people who put their will into it. A tremendous sense of confidence welled up in her. Of course, she knew the nurse was right. Relief flooded her, and she became possessed of a single thought: recovery. The nurse stayed with her for an hour, talked with her, encouraged her.

That night, she slept soundly, dreamlessly. The next morning she glanced down at her hand on the white sheet. Two fingers on her right hand flickered. Watching her hand, she willed it to happen again. Slowly her forefinger lifted, then her second finger. The little movements occurred slowly, bit by bit.

On the third day her speech returned. By the tenth day she was able to lift her right hand up to her chest. The next day she lifted both hands, a few inches below her heart. A deep sigh went through her. It would be all right, just a matter of time and effort. She wanted to tell her family, the nurse, everyone, just what it meant to her to lift her hands in that gesture with just enough space to hold her camera. That was how she knew she wasn't finished. She could go back to work again. [a seventy-year-old woman]*

---

*Adapted with permission from the section about Eleanor Milder Lawrence in *Gifts of Age: Portraits and Essays of 32 Remarkable Women* by Charlotte Painter and Pamela Valois. San Francisco: Chronicle Books, 1985, pp. 126–9.

Families and friends should be included in the rehabilitation of persons who have had strokes. Not only must they be kept up-to-date about expectations for the patient, but they can help in the process by encouraging her or him to reach the highest level of independence possible.

A massive stroke impaired my ability to function independently and seriously damaged my physical and emotional stability. Facing life was difficult. Learning to swim was one of my most effective coping techniques. Two swimming sessions weekly (forty-five minutes each) increased my strength and endurance. The constant verbal encouragement by the therapist and members of the group for even a tiny accomplishment provided enormous support and was a tremendous morale booster. We adopted the motto 'Press on regardless.' I discovered that working in a group was the most effective technique for helping me and my family cope with a long-term disability. [a thirty-eight-year-old woman]

NOTES

[1]Franz H. Messerli, ed., *Cardiovascular Diseases in the Elderly*. Boston: Martinus Nijhoff, 1984, p. 65.

[2]Ibid., p. 77.

[3]John Langone, 'Heart Attack and Cholesterol'. *Discover*, Vol. 5, March 1984, pp. 20–3.

[4]"Study Says a Low Cholesterol Diet Does Little to Increase Longevity'. *The Boston Globe*, 1 April 1987, p. 11. Note that the headline states the finding for men at low risk for heart disease, not the different finding for women.

[5]National Institutes of Health, *Lowering Blood Cholesterol to Prevent Heart Disease*. Consensus Development Conference Statement, Vol. 5, No. 7, 10–12 December 1984, p. 5.

[6]Nathan Pritikin with Patrick McGrady, Jr, *The Pritikin Program for Diet and Exercise*. New York: Grosset & Dunlap, 1979, p. 16.

[7]American Heart Association, *An Older Person's Guide to Cardiovascular Health*. National Center of the AHA, 7320 Greenville Ave., Dallas, TX 75231, 1983.

[8]Walter C. Willett, 'Cigarette Smoking and Nonfatal Myocardial Infarction in Women'. *American Journal of Epidemiology*, Vol. 113, No. 5, May 1981, pp. 575–82.

[9]R. Paffenburger, 'Physical Activity and Fatal Attack'. In E. Amsterdam, ed., *Exercise in Cardiovascular Health and Disease*. New York: York Medical Books, 1977.

[10]Francis D. Dunn, 'Coronary Heart Disease and Acute Myocardial Infarction'. In Messerli, op. cit., p. 156.

[11]Ulf Smith, Report at the American Heart Association Seminar, Monterey, Cal., 1985. Cited by Richard A. Knox, *The Boston Globe*, 18 January 1985, p. 8.

[12]Per Bjorntorp, 'Regional Patterns of Fat Distribution: Health Implications', in *Health Implications of Obesity*, programme and abstracts. National Institutes of Health Consensus Development Conference, 11–13 February 1985, p. 35.

[13]Dag S. Thelle et al., 'The Troms Heart Study: Does Coffee Raise Serum Cholesterol?' *The New England Journal of Medicine*, Vol. 308, No. 24, 16 June 1983, pp. 1454–7.

[14]Daan Kromhout et al., 'The Inverse Relation Between Fish Consumption and 20-Year Mortality from Coronary Heart Disease'. *The*

New England Journal of Medicine, Vol. 312, No. 19, 9 May 1985, pp. 1205–9; and Beverly E. Phillipson et al., 'Reduction of Plasma Lipids, Lipoproteins, and Apoproteins by Dietary Fish Oils in Patients with Hypertriglyceridemia'. *The New England Journal of Medicine*, Vol. 312, No. 9, 9 May 1985, pp. 1210–16.

[15]Suzanne Haynes and Manning Feinleib, 'Women, Work, and Coronary Heart Disease: Prospective Finding from the Framingham Heart Study'. *American Journal of Public Health*, Vol. 70, No. 2, February 1980, pp. 113–41.

[16]Nancy R. Cook et al., 'Regression Analysis of Changes in Blood Pressure with Oral Contraceptive Use'. *American Journal of Epidemiology*, Vol. 121, No. 4, April 1985, pp. 530–40.

[17]Boston Women's Health Book Collective, *The New Our Bodies, Ourselves*, London: Penguin, 1989.

[18]Charles H. Hennekens et al., 'Oral Contraceptive Use, Cigarette Smoking and Myocardial Infarction'. *British Journal of Family Planning*, Vol. 5, 1979, pp. 66–7.

[19]Patricia A. Kaufert and Sonja M. McKinlay, 'Estrogen-Replacement Therapy: The Production of Medical Knowledge and the Emergence of Policy'. In Ellen Lewin and Virginia Oleson, eds., *Women, Health, & Healing: Toward a New Perspective*. New York: Tavistock Publications, 1985, p. 116.

[20]Erkki Hirvonen et al., 'Effects of Different Progestogens on Lipoproteins During Postmenopausal Replacement Therapy'. *The New England Journal of Medicine*, Vol. 304, No. 10, 5 March 1981, pp. 560–3.

[21]Meir J. Stampfer et al., 'A Prospective Study of Postmenopausal Estrogen Therapy and Coronary Heart Disease'. The Nurses' Health Study. *The New England Journal of Medicine*, Vol. 313, No. 17, 24 October 1985, pp. 1044–9. See also Graham A. Colditz et al., 'Menopause and the Risk of Coronary Heart Disease in Women'. *The New England Journal*

of Medicine*, Vol. 316, No. 18, 30 April 1987, pp. 1105–10.

[22]Peter W. F. Wilson et al., 'Postmenopausal Estrogen Use, Cigarette Smoking, and Cardiovascular Morbidity in Women over 50'. The Framingham Study. *The New England Journal of Medicine*, Vol. 313, No. 17, 24 October 1985, pp. 1038–43.

[23]Messerli, op. cit., p. 155.

[24]Larry Tye, 'Lasers Show Promise for Heart Patients'. *The Boston Globe*, 20 January 1987, p. 6. Report of the American Heart Association held in Monterey, California, 19 January 1987.

[25]Floyd D. Loop et al., 'Influence of the Internal-Mammary-Artery Graft on 10-Year Survival and Other Cardiac Events'. *The New England Journal of Medicine*, Vol. 314, No. 1, 2 January 1986, pp. 1–6.

[26]Marcia Millman, *The Unkindest Cut: Life in the Backrooms of Medicine*. New York: William Morrow & Co., 1978; and Office of Technology Assessment, US Congress, *Assessing the Efficacy and Safety of Medical Technologies*, GPO Stock No. 052-003-00593-0, 1978; and Kenneth M. Kent, 'Coronary Angioplasty: A Decade of Experience'. *The New England Journal of Medicine*, Vol. 316, No. 18, 30 April 1987, pp. 1148–50.

[27]Esther R. Rome and Jill Wolhandler, 'F.D.A. Is Lax in Enforcing Medical Regulations'. Letter to the Editor, *The New York Times*, 30 November 1985, p. 22.

[28]'Correspondence: Complications of Permanent Cardiac Pacemakers'. *The New England Journal of Medicine*, Vol. 313, No. 17, 24 October 1985, pp. 1085–8, in response to B. Phibbs and H. J. L. Marriott, 'Complications of Permanent Transvenous Pacing'. *The New England Journal of Medicine*, Vol. 312, No. 22, 30 May 1985, pp. 1428–32.

[29]Leonard Dreifus and Douglas Zipes, report at the American College of Cardiology Meeting, March 1985. Associated Press report in *The Boston Globe*, 12 March 1985, p. 3.

BOOKS AND PUBLICATIONS

Women's Health and Reproductive Rights Information Centre, *Women's Health and Heart Disease*. Broadsheet. (See Organizations.)

Mary Ann Haw, 'Women, Work and Stress: a Review and Agenda for the Future'. *Journal of Health and Social Behaviour*, Vol. 23, June 1982, p. 132.

Health Education Authority, *Exercise. Why Bother?* Free booklet. (See Organizations.)

Health Education Authority, *Look After Your Heart*. Free booklet.

Dr Caroline Shreeve, *A Healthy Heart for Life:*

The Secret from the Sea. Wellingborough: Thorsons, 1988.

Dr D. J. Thomas, *Strokes and Their Prevention*. Wellingborough: Thorsons/British Medical Association, 1988.

Health Education Authority, *Beating Heart Disease*. Free from HEA and local health education departments.

'How Well Can We Predict Coronary Heart Disease?' *British Medical Journal*, 12 May 1984, p. 1407. Findings of the UK Heart Disease Prevention Project.

24
Cancer

Forty-nine years ago when I had my first surgery and radiation for ovarian cancer, people were so afraid of cancer that they couldn't use the word. They would say, 'She has C.' They lied to me but I knew they were lying when they gave me radiation. I'd read enough to know I had cancer. Today things are better, more open, people talk more. Now I visit other cancer patients and they mostly know. They can talk about it more now. [a seventy-five-year-old woman]

The diagnosis of cancer is not a death sentence; many live long lives with the disease and eventually die of other causes at a ripe age. Most of us know at least one person who has lived many productive years after a diagnosis of cancer. The same woman continues:

Eight years ago, at age sixty-seven, I developed colorectal cancer and had a colostomy. I went back to work afterwards and I wear a bag all the time. I do everything I did before. I'm in a relationship with a man and it doesn't make any difference to him. I walk a lot. I like to keep my shape. I tell my doctors, 'I feel good, I just get cancer once in a while.'

While it is true that most of us will never get cancer, three out of ten of us will; so we need to know more about it for ourselves and for those close to us. We have heard stories of painful, lingering death and of treatments that sound more miserable than the disease itself. We may worry that we will lose a breast or go bald and be less attractive, less womanly. Cancer is still one of the most feared diseases, even though women's risk of death from heart and circulatory diseases is much higher.

What is Cancer?

We call it by one name, but cancer takes many forms, alike only on a basic biological level. The cancerous patch of skin removed from a forehead bears little resemblance to breast cancer or to leukaemia until we understand how cancerous cells develop, grow, and spread through a living body.

Most cells in our bodies reproduce themselves and grow in order to repair or replace damaged organs and tissues. But sometimes the cells change so that they lose their ability to function properly, and they begin an abnormal process of uncontrolled growth. Cancerous lung cells, for example, lose the ability of normal lung cells to transfer oxygen into blood cells. Scientists think this change begins as a result of contact with carcinogens (cancer-causing agents). While the process of normal cells evolving into cancer cells is not fully understood, it appears that the abnormal change happens in steps. Some carcinogens *initiate* the change and others *promote* the process. Some carcinogens may be both initiators and promoters. Others work as a destructive team, as when alcohol promotes mouth and throat cancers started by tobacco.[1]

Some inborn genetic factors may predispose a woman to developing a cancer, making her more vulnerable to carcinogens. Many experts now believe it is likely that everyone has some cancerous cells at one time or another, but our immune systems eliminate them before they develop sufficiently to cause problems. Virtually all experts agree that 85 to 95 per cent of all cancers are *environmentally* caused, that is, from substances in cigarettes, air, water, food, cosmetics, or from workplace hazards or medical treatment. Increasing concern about the links between environmental factors and cancer has led to public pressure on government and industry to control pollutants and dangerous substances.

How Cancer Grows

At its earliest stage, a cancer is limited to one location, one organ, perhaps one cell. The number of cancer cells may increase rapidly or very slowly. (Some cancers are not discovered until up to twenty years after the first cells change.) A cancer may totally destroy the ability of that one organ to function without ever spreading to other parts of the body – or it may spread.

One kind of spread occurs when the mass of cancerous cells in one organ (a 'primary' cancer) touches another organ and begins to grow in it, also. This regional growth (sometimes called a 'secondary' cancer) should not be confused with a new cancer (called a second 'primary') that grows in another place.

Another kind of growth occurs when cancer cells are carried to other parts of the body from the primary site by the blood or lymph system and begin to replace normal cells in other organs; the cancer has then become 'systemic' or 'metastatic'. This may never occur, or may not occur until many years after cancer is first discovered. It also may happen simultaneously with the first growth of cells in the primary site. Many cancers are slow-growing, produce no symptoms, and are not discovered until many years after the cancer begins. Both regional spread and systemic distribution of cancer may be referred to as metastasis (plural, metastases).

A number system (I–IV, from localized to metastasized) is used to describe the stages of cancer according to where it appears to have spread. When evaluating research and other people's experiences with various treatments, always take the type and stage of the cancer into consideration.

Risk and Prevention

Lists of cancer risk factors are based on statistics and on scientific studies. Many risk factors are identified by the fact that, since so many people with a particular cancer have them, it seems unlikely to be mere coincidence. Some risks, such as exposure to asbestos, have also been studied in laboratory tests on cultured cells in dishes (in vitro) or in animals, where scientists have been able to observe the cancer-causing process.

If you know about some risk factors, you may decide to change your habits to reduce the risk. Those risks you cannot control – things that happened at work years ago, your family health record, where you live – may alert you to watch for symptoms and to be conscientious about regular checkups. Even though early cancer detection does not guarantee cure, it does help in many cases.

Some risk factors may involve things you do not want to give up. If you are eighty years old and love pickles and bacon, giving them up is not likely to make much difference in whether you will ever have cancer (though there are other reasons to avoid the salt and the fat they contain). On the other hand, research has shown that giving up smoking, even for people who have smoked for fifty years, very quickly improves health.[2] **Smoking is the number one controllable cause of cancer.**

Anyone who has a history of cancer is at risk of developing another one. Reducing the risk factors, especially stopping smoking, may help prevent further cancers. Regular checkups with a doctor can help discover new cancers early.

Sometimes we make important choices for our bodies in spite of known future risks. For example, the immune system has to be suppressed in anyone receiving an organ transplant so that the organ from the donor will not be rejected. People who have had a kidney transplant have a higher risk of cancer years after the transplant than people who did not undergo such treatment.

Things You Can Do to Reduce Your Risk of Cancer[3]

(In the list below, factors which minimize the risk of breast cancer specifically as well as other cancers in general are marked with an asterisk.)

*1. Don't smoke. Avoid smoke-filled places. Smoking also markedly increases the risks from other carcinogens such as alcohol, asbestos, and industrial agents. Don't use any other tobacco products.

  2. Know the risks and follow the health and safety rules of your workplace. Where needed, wear protective clothing and use safety equipment. If your employer does not enforce safety rules, ask for help from your trade union or the Health and Safety Executive.

*3. Avoid unnecessary X-rays whenever possible. Don't hesitate to ask your doctor if an X-ray is necessary, but do not refuse an X-ray needed for a diagnosis because you fear cancer. If you need an X-ray, be sure shields are used to protect other parts of your body, especially the trunk.

*4. Avoid taking oestrogen except for severe symptoms that have not responded to other treatments. If you do take oestrogen, ask about combining it with progestogen, which reduces the risk of endometrial cancer. (Progestogen does not reduce the other risks of using oestrogens, such as gallbladder disease, and progestogen may even increase the risk of breast cancer and heart disease. See Osteoporosis chapter.)

  5. Eat a well-balanced diet with a variety of foods (see Eating Well chapter).

- Eat a variety of whole grains, vegetables and fruits rich in bran and fibre – grown without pesticides (if available and affordable).
- Eat foods high in beta carotene and vitamin A: carrots, pumpkin, sweet potatoes, cantaloupe, spinach, winter squash, greens, apricots, broccoli. Eat cruciferous vegetables such as kale, broccoli, cauliflower, cabbage, Brussels sprouts, greens, kohlrabi, and turnips. Vitamin A pills are *not* a substitute for beta carotene, and high doses can be toxic.
- Eat foods high in vitamin C: citrus fruits, sweet peppers, leafy greens, broccoli, cauliflower, tomatoes, fresh potatoes, berries, melons, bean sprouts. Eating the whole fruit gives you more nutrients than just drinking the juice.
- Eat foods high in selenium: brewer's yeast, garlic, onions, asparagus, tuna, shrimp, mushrooms, whole grains, brown rice. Eggs, liver, and kidneys contain selenium but are also high in saturated fat. Selenium can be toxic in high doses, so it is best to get it in foods instead of pills.

*6. Reduce the fat in your diet (see Eating Well chapter). Adding fish may be beneficial.

  7. Minimize consumption of smoked, salted, or pickled foods, and avoid chemical additives, including food colouring.

*8. Limit or eliminate alcohol.

*9. If you are substantially overweight, try to take off weight by increasing exercise and by reducing fat and sugar in your food. There is evidence that people who weigh more than 40 per cent over recent recommendations have higher rates of cancer.

10. Maintain frequent and regular bowel movements by exercising, drinking water, and including fibre in your diet.
11. Avoid sunburn and excessive tanning, especially if you have light skin. You do need some sun for vitamin D, or foods or supplements with vitamin D such as cod liver oil, if you live in Britain.
*12. Avoid hair dyes made from petroleum bases.

Most of the above are really basic cancer preventive care measures that also promote general good health. Doing as many of them as your willpower, interest, and life-style will allow should make your body all the stronger to prevent cancer or to help you fight it. While stopping smoking, eating better, or making other changes will not guarantee you a cancer-free life, they will influence your statistical chances and should make you generally healthier. Some choices seem to be contradictory. Cancer experts may warn you against alcohol, while heart experts may advise that a couple of ounces a day is good for you. Fat women have higher cancer risk but lower risk of osteoporosis. Given the incomplete knowledge of these diseases today, the best you can do is emphasize moderation in life-style and understand your own body and health history.

Environmental and Occupational Risk Factors

It can be worrying to read cancer statistics for your area if you happen to live where there seem to be higher than average rates of specific cancers. TV and radio coverage, research published by bodies such as Friends of the Earth, and reports from some scientists are quickly countered by official denials from government departments and industry, but in Britain many of us have become extremely sceptical about what we see as whitewashes. We haven't forgotten the delays in banning the sale of lamb raised in districts affected by fall-out from the Chernobyl disaster; we note with wry amusement the statements of scientists who say that it's perfectly safe to live near an atomic power station but who, when pushed, admit that they themselves wouldn't actually choose to bring up children there. For many of us the point has been reached when we know that there's real and urgent cause for concern; when the evidence of our own eyes tells us that the North Sea is full of sewage and chemical waste; when seals and fish in estuaries are dying or diseased; when we learn that for some 'unexplained' reason it just happens that cancer rates are higher in people living near estuaries; when, tardily, industry has to take note of pressure for banning certain kinds of propellants used in aerosols; and when as a result of public concern the government itself is forced to turn its attention, at last, to the damage being done to our environment. As Friends of the Earth, the Chemical Cancer Hazard Information Service (see Organizations), and other environmental groups point out in numerous well-researched reports and publications, a very large proportion of these substances are directly or indirectly linked with forms of cancer. A reading of some of the publications listed below makes plain just how dangerous to our health and that of our children and grandchildren further uncontrolled pollution with atomic and industrial waste will be. As in Europe, it's likely that these issues will become major political factors and will colour the attitudes of all of us in the future, regardless of the party politics of the past.

Of course, some higher rates of cancer may be caused by natural environmental factors such as the radioactivity levels associated with the underlying granite-type rock in some parts of the country, and the fierce sun some of us court when holidaying in countries nearer to the Equator. We're becoming increasingly aware of the risk of skin cancer, but sadly many of us still take that risk rather than return untanned from a Mediterranean fortnight.

There are clear links between certain occupational hazards and diseases. Many common household products contain carcinogens, and some studies show that housewives have higher than average rates of cancer. Artists, craftswomen, laboratory and medical workers, and others should seek information about the proper handling and ventilation of the materials they use. There is increasing evidence that chemicals used in the microchip industry can cause immune system problems.[4] Always investigate the risks of any chemicals or equipment used at your work site.

OTHER RISK FACTORS YOU CANNOT CONTROL

Age. The longer you live, the greater your chances of discovering some kind of cancer. Half of all cancers are diagnosed in people over sixty-five. The cancer incidence begins to rise at about age thirty-five for women (and a little later for men). In the US cancer is the leading cause of death of women thirty-five to fifty-four, second for ages fifty-five to seventy-four, and third for ages seventy-five and older.[5] In the UK lung cancer is diagnosed in 40,000 new patients a year, increasing numbers of older women among them.

Gender and Race. A higher percentage of men than women, and blacks than whites, die from cancer. Controllable factors such as variations in smoking rates, access to health care, eating habits, and exposure to occupational hazards can account for some of the differences in these cancer statistics.

One in four people in the United Kingdom will die of cancer. Estimates of the main causes are:

- Diet 35%
- Tobacco 30%
- Sexually transmitted disease (wart virus) infection 10%
- Reproductive and sexual behaviour (e.g. multiple partners) 7%
- Occupation 4%
- Geographical factors 3%
- Alcohol 3%
- Pollution 2%
- Medicines and medical procedures 1%
- Industrial products less than 1%
- Food additives less than 1%
- Unknown 3%

Figures from Dr Tony Smith, 'Self Health'. *Cancer*, 20 September 1988.

Family. Some cancers are found more often in people whose parents or close family members have had them. Be sure to inform your GP if anyone in your family has had or has died from cancer. Some cancers can be stopped early when family members are alert to a familial disposition or a common environmental hazard.

Let's Not Blame the Victim

Cancer patients face stigmas that have yet to be obliterated. Some people still think cancer is 'catching', despite research that proves otherwise. Others believe that all cancers are inevitably fatal. These stigmas can lead to personal isolation and to discrimination in employment. We should fight for definitions of 'disabled' to include people with cancer who require regular treatments over an extended period or who are unable to carry out major activities.

People with cancer often feel shame or guilt, wondering what they have done to be so punished. Sometimes they blame themselves, and others blame them also, for exposure to the risk factors that might have predisposed them to the disease. Many people still try to hide the fact that they have cancer – even from close family and friends. But the stigma will never go away until we all learn as much as possible, as well as talk much more to each other, about our cancer experiences. We should not accept isolation when we most need support.

After my operation, a lot of my friends came to cheer me up. But I had to put them at ease first. They didn't know what to say. The cancer was like a wall between us. So I just took a deep breath and started talking about it. Then it was all right. [a forty-year-old woman with breast cancer]

Much of what has been written about cancer ends up 'blaming the victim'.

Particular personality traits have been attributed to persons with cancer, just as they were attributed in the last century to persons with tuberculosis.[6] Some years ago there was a lot of publicity surrounding a 'finding' that depressed women were likely to contract cancer – another way of telling people to 'pull themselves together, or else . . .' Doctors themselves tend to hold patients responsible for their progress, giving great credit to 'gallantry and grace in the face of hardship', and therefore by extension blaming those who do not get well for 'not trying hard enough'.[7]

There are two dangers in believing that your state of mind is the major influence on the course of your cancer: (1) You may suffer guilt and feelings of failure if your cancer advances to more destructive stages in spite of your own efforts. (2) You might abandon medical therapies that might actually help you. It is very important to get the best treatment you possibly can. Periods of anger, fear, grumpiness, depression, hopelessness, and passivity are common, as you can discover by talking with others who have experiences with cancer. The success or failure of any treatment is not caused by the strength or weakness of your faith in it, by living right, or being a happy person. One study found no relationship between 'psychosocial' factors such as marital status, other companionship, work and life satisfaction, and hopefulness and how people with advanced cancers responded to treatment or how long they lived.[8] People who are at all times full of courage, grace, faith, and endless, cheerful endurance are rare. On the other hand, we should not abandon all sense of control. We have many decisions to make about how we will live and what treatments we will choose. Sometimes both the person with cancer (or other chronic disease) and those in relationships with her or him take more control over their lives and are stronger than before. It is this possibility that lies behind the claims of places like the Bristol Cancer Help Centre (see below).

Cancer Research

Money and institutional support for cancer research come from private organizations, individuals, and government agencies. Scientists as individuals and in groups ask for more funding than is given out each year. Decisions may speed up one researcher's project while forcing another to delay or abandon research. Many factors go into deciding who gets how much money for which kind of research: assessments of how many people could be helped; how close the investigator is to a breakthrough or to being able to put a discovery to a practical use; what other experts think of the excellence of the project; the applicant's past record; the reputation of the research institution (university, hospital, etc.); and a number of even more subjective criteria including the potential profitability of any new drug.

The special interests of politically powerful groups also influence funding of cancer research. Some trade unions, for example, have demanded answers when their members have occupation-related cancers. The anti-smoking movement has spurred research on links between smoking and various kinds of cancer. At the same time business and industry have used their economic and political power to block legislative action on substances and practices that seem to cause cancer, or to limit the funding of relevant research.

PHYSICIAN, DO NO HARM!

Too often drugs or other methods for treating medical conditions are adopted without sufficient research; and too often they prove useless, and even harmful, only after many people have been exposed to them. Examples include radiation to pregnant women, resulting in leukaemia in the child; radiation to the neck in childhood that leads to an increase in thyroid cancer in adulthood; DES (diethylstilboestrol) prescribed during pregnancy, leading to a rare cancer in some female offspring, abnormalities in some male offspring, and an increased risk of breast cancer in the mother many years later. Inform your doctor if you had radiation to the upper body as a child to increase the chance that any possible cancers can be diagnosed and treated early.

Although by 1953 it was known that DES (a synthetic form of oestrogen) was ineffective in preventing miscarriage, its use in pregnancy in the US was permitted up until 1971, when its link with cancer was finally admitted.[9] American women, and any others whose mothers or who themselves were taking DES, should get a breast examination annually, in addition to doing their own regular breast examinations.

Diagnosis

Why find out early? With some cancers, early detection offers the possibility of cure or substantial remission with years – even decades – of symptom-free life. Many cancers are more easily treated and controlled when discovered early. Certain skin cancers, cervical, and colorectal cancer are common and can be detected early and cured:

- Basal- and squamous-cell skin cancers are visible, grow very slowly, and cure rates approach 100 per cent following removal.
- Cervical cancer, which grows unnoticed, can be stopped before it leaves the cervix. A Pap smear every one to three years will catch cervical cancer at its earliest stages. The NHS has provided smear tests at five-year intervals for women over thirty-five, but there is pressure to include all adult women,

and at shorter intervals. (Canadian research suggests every three years.) Heterosexual women who are sexually active and whose partners do not use condoms should have regular tests. Not all abnormal Pap smears mean that cervical cancer will develop, however, and it is crucial to try to reverse changes in the cervical cells (dysplasia) before agreeing to surgery (see Hysterectomy and Oophorectomy chapter).

Other, less common cancers may also be treated effectively if discovered early. Sometimes, however, early detection does not prolong life. It only bolsters statistics on survival rates because, while the person survives only as long as most others who have the same disease, the counting starts sooner. Improved survival rates for lung cancer and breast cancer, for example, seem to be a direct result of earlier diagnosis and better record-keeping rather than of improvement in actual survival rates. Many cancers cannot be detected earlier than the time when they produce symptoms.

Some women would rather not know they have cancer at all, especially if the symptoms are not likely to disturb their lives until a late stage shortly before death.

By the time my mother had cancer in her early forties, she had already had two close women friends about ten years older than her die of cancer. She was terrified of the disease and of the idea of death itself. So when her lung cancer was diagnosed, we didn't want anyone to tell her. But an X-ray therapist did anyway. She died about two months later, and it was as awful for all of us in the family as it was for her to die so young. [a forty-year-old woman]

Others take steps immediately:

My second husband had cancer, but I remember so many good times in our all-too-short marriage when his treatments led to remission. So when my mammogram showed a suspicious shadow, I was very motivated to do something about it. Yes, I was scared, but I knew I could get some help. As it turned out, my doctor urged me to wait a couple of months before having a surgical biopsy, and the second mammogram was clear. [a sixty-year-old woman]

If you have one of the following warning signals publicized by the American Cancer Society, tell your doctor:

- Change in bowel or bladder habits
- A sore that does not heal
- Unusual bleeding or discharge
- Thickening or lump in breast or elsewhere

- *I*ndigestion or difficulty in swallowing
- *O*bvious change in a wart or mole
- *N*agging cough or hoarseness

None of these is a sure sign of any disease, and all have other possible causes besides cancer. But you should at least talk it over with a doctor you can trust.

Diagnostic Methods

You may want to make choices about diagnostic methods in cases where several approaches are possible. Breast cancer is the most widely publicized disease where you can make these choices (see p. 471). Ask your doctor to explain exactly the methods she or he uses, whether there are others, and why those others are not suggested for your specific condition.

X-rays, including mammograms, can suggest but not definitively diagnose cancer. Often cells are taken from a suspicious mass (the procedure is called a biopsy) to make a more certain diagnosis. A few cells can be removed and sent to a pathologist for examination. Needle biopsies can be done for breast, lung, or pancreatic tumours. A corkscrew-shaped needle (trucut needle biopsy) may be used to draw tissue out of a solid lump. A D&C (dilation and curettage) or an endometrial biopsy of the inside of the uterus yields cells to examine for endometrial cancer. Biopsies can be done through a small incision using an endoscope (a device consisting of a tube and an optical system) to reach polyps in the colon and stomach, and lung tumours.

Depending on the size and location of a lump, and whether there is more than one, the surgeon will recommend *incisional* or *excisional* biopsy. Incisional means taking a small slice, usually of a larger mass. Excisional means removing the entire lump (lumpectomy). The tissue removed is divided and prepared into permanent sections and sometimes frozen sections on glass slides for the pathologist to examine. Results from the frozen section are known quickly, while the permanent section, which is more accurate, takes at least twenty-four hours. Sometimes, as in abdominal surgery, the decision for additional surgery during the operation is made on the basis of the frozen section in order to avoid another operation. In other sites, such as breast cancer, there are good reasons to wait for the results of a permanent section before deciding on further treatment, so a frozen section is not needed.[10]

The slides prepared from the sections become part of your medical record. Slides and X-rays should be available if you want the opinion of another pathologist or radiologist.

Some women report complications of the diagnostic surgery itself; so, when asking for a referral, try to make sure your surgeon is experienced in dealing with your specific condition and preferably has a reputation for conservative, but adequate, surgery.

Living with Cancer

'How long will I live?' is a frequently asked question. We fear death, and the statistics, showing little improvement in survival rates for many cancers, only compound the fear.

Every time a friend of mine dies of cancer, it's not necessarily the same kind of cancer as mine. It's not the same stage or in the same place, etc. But knowing that doesn't keep me from getting frightened. I wonder if I will keel over this afternoon or tomorrow. It's not intellectually sound, but I do feel that way. [a fifty-seven-year-old woman now being treated for cancer]

How many stories have you heard about people who were only supposed to live two years . . . or one year . . . or six months . . . five years ago? We marvel to see them 'still going strong at seventy-five'. Stories like these, mostly true, are one reason why doctors hesitate to set time limits for survival with cancer diagnoses, even for very advanced cases. You might want to know how long you will remain active or will live because you have things to get done, relationships to mend or a book to finish, but what will you do as you approach that time limit?

Time limits for living with cancer come from two basic sources: statistics that count hundreds of thousands of people, and the individual physician's own experience with the specific disease. Remember that half the people live longer than the often quoted 'median' figure for survival of any given cancer. Those who live longer can live anywhere from just a little longer to very much longer – maybe even decades longer.[11]

Doctors often use the word 'cure' for what should be more correctly five- to ten-year survival rates. Statistics for remission (a temporary stopping of growth and of related symptoms, and shrinkage of the cancer) and for cure (disappearance of all detectable signs of cancer) should never rule the outlook of an individual with cancer. Hope is essential, and many of us find that knowledge makes the reality of cancer easier to live with.

I feel very positive about recovery – wrong word – how about remission? My playful platelets are good and high, blood tests terrific and blood pressure down. I feel better than ever. [an active seventy-year-old woman with breast cancer]

TAKE ALONG A FRIEND

Whether you suspect that you have cancer or a diagnosis of cancer has been confirmed, you should consider taking someone with you whenever you go for diagnostic work, checkups or treatment, particularly when decisions have to be made. You can probably use the moral support of someone who cares about you, and you may need help getting home after some procedures. It is useful to have a second person to ask questions and to listen to the answers, even to take notes, and to talk things over with afterward. The person you take could be your partner, your sister, a friend, or a volunteer from a women's group, the local cancer society (e.g. CancerLink), or other helping organization.

Everyone asks if you have any questions, but you just don't know what to ask when it's your first consultation. My doctor kept asking if I had any more questions and I really didn't just then. [a fifty-seven-year-old woman with cancer]

I had been to enough meetings on women's health issues to know I should take someone with me when I went to hear the results of my mammogram. I took my cleaning lady and she turned out to be just the support I needed. [a sixty-year-old woman]

SUPPORT AND MUTUAL-HELP GROUPS

It has taken many years to break down the barriers keeping people with cancer from talking to each other. Now there are groups such as CancerLink (see Organizations) and other bodies set up locally, as well as BACUP (see Organizations) which can provide telephone counselling and a great deal of information about cancer. Often those close to us need help and support just as much as we do. If there isn't a group in your area, start one, perhaps by contacting local women's organizations for names of members likely to be interested.

Treatments

Each of us must be able to trust the decisions we make when cancer is found in our bodies or in our loved ones, in spite of the contradictory recommendations in the media and even within conventional medical circles. Gather all the information, advice, and support you feel you can use – but ultimately you will have to make the choices about which treatments to accept or reject.

I am their pet patient at the moment though they learned to treat me rather gingerly

QUESTIONS TO WHICH YOU NEED ANSWERS*

Select from this list the questions that pertain to you. *Similar questions will apply to other diseases.* Ask your doctor to give, or help you find, the answers. Use the organizations listed at the end of this book and any others you hear of to give you this vital information for making decisions.

1. Exactly what kind of cancer do I have? Can you tell if it is slow- or fast-growing?
2. What therapies are available? Where?
3. How effective is each therapy? What is the probability of cure? What definition of 'cure' is being used?
4. What benefits can I expect? Prolonged life by months? Years? Reduced symptoms? Reduced pain?
5. What percentage of people treated benefit from the therapy? How is that benefit measured?
6. Will I be able to continue my regular activities during therapy? What about sex? Working? Exercise?
7. Will the therapy require overnight stays in the hospital or can it be done on an outpatient basis?
8. What are the potential negative effects of the treatment? How serious are they? What percentage of people get them? Are they permanent? Are there any drugs that will help alleviate these effects? Do these drugs themselves cause any negative effects? How soon after treatment are symptoms likely to begin and how long do they usually last? (For example, does nausea generally start

after I refused to start chemotherapy until my incision stopped draining. Blew the young oncologist out of his chair when I remained firm, especially after he said he'd talk it over with my surgeon. To which I replied, 'You can talk to her till hell freezes over – this is not a medical decision; it is my personal decision since it is my personal body.' The surgeon, a great woman, agreed. [a seventy-year-old woman]

It is particularly important for an NHS patient whose GP has made a preliminary diagnosis of possible cancer to talk to her or him about the consultant or hospital to which she is to be referred. Once you have seen a hospital consultant, you will be expected to undergo any surgery or other treatment at that hospital. You should try to ensure that the consultant to whom you are referred is not only a recognized specialist in the treatment of

*Adapted from the Boston Women's Health Book Collective, *The New Our Bodies, Ourselves*. London: Penguin, 1989.

immediately, within twenty minutes, or several hours later? How long does it last?)

9. How long will the therapy last? Each session? How many sessions?

10. How many people get recurrences after this treatment? How soon?

11. Are there statistics on survival, cure, mortality, and remission rates for this therapy for my type of cancer, considering such factors as stage of cancer, age, sex, race, socio-economic status, occupation, geographical location?

12. Who is my doctor while I am undergoing therapy? Whom do I contact, and how, if I have new symptoms while I am in therapy? After I finish the therapy?

13. May I speak to some of your other patients? Do you know of any local groups for people with cancer? Any groups for family members and friends?

14. Whom do I call, and when, if I have further questions?

You should take a written list of these questions with you to your doctor's consulting room and make notes, take a tape recorder, and have someone with you. This is a lot of information to assimilate at one time; it may take more than one question-asking session. But having these answers will make you a well-informed patient, and your consultant will know it. Most doctors will respect you for asking such questions and try to keep you informed of your progress.

cancer (an oncologist) but that she or he has a reputation for considering the patient's wishes when it comes to accepting or rejecting any particular kind of treatment, and explaining possible or probable outcomes.

Treatments for cancer range from high-technology radiation and chemical therapies to home remedies found in family herb gardens. All treatments for any disease are experimental to the extent that no one knows for sure exactly how *you* will respond to any given treatment or combination of treatments.

The three most common orthodox treatments for cancer are surgery, radiation, and chemotherapy (including hormone therapy and immunotherapy). These may cure the disease, slow it down, or relieve symptoms and make your life easier.

Surgery removes cancerous tumours, tissues, or areas where cancer cells have invaded normal tissue; or it can open up a blocked system or ease painful pressure on other body parts.

Ask how the surgery will help your specific condition. Get second or third opinions, especially if a doctor suggests removing some healthy part of your body to prevent it from becoming cancerous. Breasts, ovaries, and uteri have too often been removed just in case they might develop cancer someday; medical literature has no accounts of men having anything removed 'just in case'.

While your surgeon may urge you to decide immediately whether to have surgery and tell you a delay will allow the disease to spread, you always have time to get those additional opinions unless you have an emergency condition such as intestinal or bladder blockage. A cancer will rarely cause sudden life-threatening symptoms, but even if it does, you can get a second opinion.

Radiation therapy uses X-rays or radioactive substances to destroy cancerous cells instead of cutting them out. Sometimes the radiation is used instead of surgery; often it is used before surgery to shrink a mass, or after surgery to destroy remaining traces of the cancer.

Radiation is also used for palliative reasons without curing, for example, to ease bone pain.

Radiation may cause nausea, diarrhoea, fatigue, and burns, depending on the part of the body treated. But radiation therapy may also prolong active, meaningful life when used for some cancers, especially for Hodgkin's disease and some stages and forms of cervical, lung, nose, and throat cancers.

I just had modest side effects. I had a rash that developed after about the second or third week, a very itchy rash. I couldn't put anything on it because cream affects the way the beams go through. And I had a rash on the front that went all the way through so I had a sunburn on my back as well as on my front. The rash went away in a relatively short time. [a woman in her fifties]

In general, the more radiation, whether larger doses (more units of radiation – rads) or over a larger area, the more complications arise. Some of these do not show up for many years. Complications are minimized by dividing the therapy into several treatments.[12] You might be willing to put up with more adverse effects if the radiation holds the possibility of cure than if it is only intended to make you more comfortable.

Radiation therapy often causes nitrogen and other nutrient deficiencies. You can prepare yourself by eating a high-protein diet with a good balance of vitamins and minerals before you start radiation therapy; and you can try to put on a little weight in case you become nauseous and can't eat.

Both radiation and chemotherapy aim to destroy the abnormal, cancerous cells. The aim is to do so without harming too many normal cells nearby or elsewhere in the body. Techniques are being refined to make cancer cells more vulnerable than normal cells to treatment or to restore damaged normal cells more quickly. One technique is to apply heat, especially to tumours near the body surface, as an adjunct to both chemo- and radiation therapy. Implanted heat sources may work on deeper tumours. A number of drugs are being investigated either to make the cancer cells more vulnerable or to reinforce normal cells, protecting them against radiation. Techniques to salvage and restore bone marrow are being tried.

Cancer cells tend to have less oxygen than normal cells (to be hypoxic) and tend to block the effects of radiation. So researchers are trying to find ways to oxygenate cancer tumours before irradiating them.[13]

Large university (teaching) hospitals are likely to have the most modern equipment and technology, plus well-trained personnel. You should always ask about the age of radiation equipment, when it was last inspected, and how often the therapists' training is updated. If the equipment is more than ten years old or you have doubts about the staff, ask BACUP for the name and number of the nearest teaching hospital with radiation therapy and oncology departments.

Chemotherapy – treating cancer with chemicals or drugs – is the only method which has the potential to reach cancer cells in every part of the body. It is called a systemic therapy. It is the basic treatment in cancers such as leukaemia (cancer of the white blood cells) and a supplemental (or adjuvant) therapy to destroy cancer cells that are beyond the reach of primary surgical or radiation therapy. Chemotherapy sometimes has other effects, because anything strong enough to kill cancer cells damages other cells as well. Possible temporary adverse effects of chemotherapy are hair loss, nausea, diarrhoea, and cessation of menstrual periods. Possible long-term and serious effects include perma- nent cessation of periods in premenopausal women over forty, kidney damage, heart disease, a weakened immune system, and leukaemia. But many drugs and many combinations of drugs are used. Not everyone gets sick from them, and many people have been helped.

Have had two and about to have a third chemo treatment (injection of combined drugs) and NO side effects! Absolutely none. [a seventy-year-old woman]

When my hair grew back, it was all grey, and soft like a baby's hair. And curly! I had straight dark hair before. [a sixty-eight-year-old woman]

When a woman in my cancer support group said she was going to have chemotherapy, I told her I had had the same exact thing. No problems at all. But she turned out to be as sick as a dog. Now we both laugh about it, and we both know how different each person is. [a fifty-seven-year-old woman]

Your doctors should have enough experience with the chemicals they propose for your treatment to be able to explain exactly how they work, what could go wrong, and how well the treatment works on your specific cancer at the stage you are in. You should not have to carry a pharmacy textbook to the hospital to understand what they tell you. If they cannot be clear about the therapy, talk to another doctor; get another opinion or two. You should also be aware that some therapies can actually *shorten* your life if given inappropriately.

Hormone therapy is slower-acting and generally less toxic than most chemotherapy. Hormones are substances which originate in one gland or organ of the body and are carried through the blood to stimulate another part of the body. Hormone therapy changes the hormonal environment in which the cancer is growing by removing the source of the hormone (surgically or medically), adding hormones, or using substances which block the action of hormones (antihormones), such as tamoxifen. Hormone therapy is used to treat breast, uterine, ovarian, and thyroid cancers as well as leukaemia (cancer of the white blood cells), lymphomas (cancers of the lymph system), and other cancers. Corticosteroids (hormones from the adrenal glands) are also used to control nausea and vomiting caused by some chemotherapy and for treatment of tumours in the central nervous system.

Immunotherapy is an attempt to stimulate the body's immune defences to recognize and attack cancer cells. Many substances are under study for their possible effectiveness.

Experimental/Investigational Therapies. New drugs or combinations of drugs are constantly being studied. You may choose to take part in an experimental or investigational cancer treatment programme. Before you give your consent, you should understand all the potential risks as well as benefits, and the investigators should take all the time needed to answer your questions. They should explain how you were selected for the study, who is funding it, what outcomes they expect, what risks are known, and how the study could benefit you as well as others. They should tell you how the experimental treatments differ from the standard protocol (treatment plan) for someone with your diagnosis. In addition, they should tell you what any doctor should tell you about any treatment recommendation: how it works, what effects to expect, what your possibilities are for relief, remission, and/or cure.

Alternative Treatments

The things you can do to reduce your risk of cancer can also help the body fight existing cancer. Most alternative treatments have little or no statistical data to help you decide how well they have worked for large numbers of people like you with your specific cancer. You will have to judge them according to the kind of cancer you have, the experiences of people who have tried them, what you know about the practitioners who offer them, and by your own feelings about trying something outside the mainstream of current medical practice.

Some alternative treatments may be combined with conventional treatments. But promoters of many alternative methods claim their treatments will not work if you have had radiation or chemotherapy because of the damage these therapies may have done to the body. If so, you might have to choose between an established therapy with only fair outcomes and a treatment that is severely questioned or totally rejected by your doctor. However, some hospitals now offer alternative treatments along with radiation or chemotherapy.

Many alternative approaches were originally developed by doctors, but are either ignored or considered invalid by the medical establishment. Often these alternatives seem logical in their approach, and a great many people credit them with curing or controlling their cancers. The preventive diets now being tested by several medical research centres are based on the same principles as some alternative cancer therapies.

Remember that no alternative practitioner is allowed to claim that she or he can treat or cure cancer. This does not mean that such practitioners have not helped some people either to prolong their lives or even to secure a significant remission. It is understandable that someone whose orthodox treatment has proved unsuccessful, or whose experience leads her to believe that the surgery or other treatment offered by doctors will be so painful or undermining as to destroy the quality of her life, should look for other ways of handling her situation. One centre which has claimed success in enabling cancer sufferers to lead happier lives and develop a positive approach to their illness is the Bristol Cancer Help Centre (see Organizations). Patients attending the centre don't have to follow a strict, pre-determined regime but are helped to adopt a way of life which takes the whole person into account, using diet, relaxation, music, drama, meditation, and any other therapy, in a calm and hopeful atmosphere. There are some residential places, but the centre draws most patients from the Bristol area who attend regularly on a day-time basis. Fees are charged, and these can be quite high, but in cases of real hardship they may be waived.

I don't know whether the Bristol Centre actually gave me a longer lease of life – I can't prove anything. But it has helped me to accept better what is happening to me and to take positive action over things that may be beneficial. That in itself – the feeling that I am more in control of the illness, that something is actually being done about it, may be the reason why, although I certainly do still have cancer, I don't feel so helpless and despairing. [a fifty-five-year-old woman]

Some books about the Bristol Cancer Help Centre and the diet it recommends are listed below. *New Approaches to Cancer* supplies relaxation and meditation tapes, and lists 'alternative' people willing to help cancer patients.

Some alternative therapies receive so much publicity that public demand forces the medical establishment to evaluate the treatment's safety and efficacy. One such case is that of Laetrile. Laetrile was finally tested in the US and considered useless after thousands of people with potentially controllable cancers spent their energy and considerable money travelling to foreign countries where the unapproved drug was available. Yet some people still place their faith in it.

Many alternative therapies are simply another kind of chemotherapy, using natural or synthetic substances in different forms or amounts than in ordinary use. *Consumer Reports* recounts its investigation of 'Drugs in Disguise' – mostly disguised as 'nutritional supplements'.[14] American marketers of these supplements claim they cure ills ranging from herpes virus to many forms of cancer. The contents of these food/drugs range from herbs and citrus extracts to ground-up animal glands to industrial solvent. In the US, Congress has been making some attempts to reduce, or at least regulate, this 'quackery', as Consumers Union labels it, and in the UK it is illegal to claim that such substances can 'cure'. The safety of herbal medicines is not, in general, tested by the Committee on Safety of Medicines, however.

We do not know yet how to mobilize fully the body's self-healing capabilities and the mind's ability to influence the body's recovery. Many methods, such as the Simonton technique, whereby the body's strength and the treatments chosen are imagined (or visualized) to fight the cancer, are used both to treat symptoms of cancer and to enhance the effectiveness of the treatment. They have reportedly induced remission. Prayer, meditation, and religious rituals are especially useful as supplements to other treatment choices; sometimes they are credited with cure, and sometimes not with cure but an enriched life.

The risk of relying solely on faith healers and psychics is that a person whose cancer has a chance of responding to medical treatment may forgo that treatment and rely only on this method until her cancer has progressed to a stage that is much more difficult to treat.

SCIENTIFIC BREAKTHROUGHS

The media frequently report new wonders of science that may help cure cancer. The sad reality for most people with cancer is that these reported discoveries are in the laboratory stage, at most being tested on animals. Even those that have had successful human trials are usually many years away from being available outside a few teaching and research institutions.

When you read or hear about something new that you think may help you or a friend, you can call your doctor, your local hospital, the closest medical school, BACUP or even the university or hospital mentioned in the report. You might also write to your MP urging his or her support of the research if it sounds worthwhile to you.

As we move into the 1990s some of our most respected cancer scientists are coming to a different conclusion. Because cures for most cancers are not likely in the near future, focusing so much money and energy on treatment research may be actually robbing us of the motivation and resources to try to prevent cancer.[15] Also, by focusing more on the quality of life than the quantity of life, we could better help those people who already have cancer to live with the disease constructively.

Lung Cancer

There are several types of lung cancer, caused by different environmental conditions or carcinogens, but the most common one is bronchial carcinoma, caused by smoking. It is possible to get lung cancer if you never smoked or lived with a smoker, but more women now die of lung cancer caused by smoking than from breast or any other cancer. The chances of getting bronchial carcinoma depend directly on how much you have smoked and for how long. Stopping pays off – after only ten years your chances of bronchial cancer are the same as a non-smoker's, though passive smoking (breathing the smoke from other people's cigarettes) probably continues your risks.

Lung cancer is the best example of how prevention is superior to cure, because the disease is so difficult to detect until its advanced stages. A persistent cough is usually the only warning. Lung cancer is usually treated with a combination of surgery, radiation therapy, and chemotherapy. Only 13 per cent of people with lung cancer live five or more years after diagnosis.[16]

I didn't feel well for a long time but a year ago nothing showed up on a checkup. Six months ago I was down to 101 pounds and didn't care about eating. It was a blow to find out I had lung cancer. I had smoked since I started college – everyone did. Have you noticed how much smoking there was in the old movies? Katharine Hepburn, all the stars I admired, smoked in the movies. After the diagnosis I just stopped smoking even though I still have the urge. I got a lot of lectures from everyone. I get chemotherapy every three weeks. I lost my hair but I'm feeling better. My appetite has returned and I'm up to 115 pounds. I'm doing pretty well now but I wish no one else had to go through this. I've been to two funerals for women who have died of lung cancer in less than a month, and now my dental hygienist has lung cancer also. My faith and my friends are helping me. [a seventy-five-year-old woman]

What is diagnosed as lung cancer may also be a metastasis from a malignancy elsewhere in your body, even one which was apparently cured years ago. Many of these have a better prognosis if detected early.

Cancer of the Ovary

Ovarian cancer is rare, and while it did increase for a brief period, it now appears to be declining again. Because this disease has been so difficult to detect until considerably advanced, it is often fatal, with five-year survival rates of 38 per cent for all stages combined.[17] Newer diagnostic technology may improve earlier detection but it remains to be seen whether earlier treatment will actually improve survival. Early warning signs are usually intestinal upsets of different kinds and often pain in the shoulder. Ovaries feel swollen to the examining doctor.

For a long time a lot of things I ate would make me gassy, but I thought, 'I'm just getting old, I can't eat the things I used to.' I went to the doctor and he gave me fluid pills [diuretics] for the swelling I had, but he never examined me 'down there'. It wasn't until I started bleeding down there that I found out what I had. I nearly died in surgery, they couldn't get it all, and though the radiation made me sick, I'm a little better now. [an eighty-four-year-old woman, during remission, who later died of ovarian cancer]

Even though the risks of removing healthy ovaries clearly outweigh any benefit, some doctors believe the poor prognosis for ovarian cancer justifies the removal of healthy ovaries during other abdominal surgery. But ovarian cancer tissue can and does grow in the abdomens of some women after the ovaries are removed (see Hysterectomy and Oophorectomy chapter).

While researchers don't completely understand the causes of this cancer, some factors are becoming clearer. The fewer children you have, the greater the risk, childless women being at greatest risk. Women who already have cancer of the breast, intestines, or rectum appear to be at increased risk, as are women whose jobs involve electrical, rubber, or textile manufacture. The use of talcum powder, especially in the genital area, may increase the risk as much as three times. Cornflour is a safe substitute for bath powders containing talc.

Most recent studies are beginning to suggest that some of the same preventive changes in diet which could reduce breast cancer may also reduce ovarian cancer, specifically fat in the diet. This may help to explain why women who are significantly fat, who have taken menopausal oestrogens (see Osteoporosis chapter), or who have a family history of ovarian cancer also appear to be at increased risk. Oestrogen overproduction is the central factor here. Treatment of ovarian cancer usually involves surgery, radiation, and chemotherapy, with surgery and chemotherapy currently showing the most favourable results.

Colorectal Cancer

Colorectal cancer (cancer of the large intestine) is the third most common cancer among women in the US. Almost half of all people with this disease are cured, usually by surgery. Many experts say survival rates could be improved if the cancer were discovered earlier. Early detection not only improves the chance of survival but often makes it possible to save greater portions of the large bowel because the cancer has not yet spread so far.

Women should be examined for colorectal cancer, particularly if they are, for one reason or another, considered to be at higher than usual risk of developing this kind of cancer. Colorectal cancer grows slowly; it may take months or years before it causes symptoms. Bleeding or changes in bowel habits such as constipation, more frequent movements, or diarrhoea may be the first symptoms.

You should see a doctor as soon as possible if you notice that any of the symptoms described above persist or if you have abdominal pain that doesn't go away. In doing an evaluation, the doctor will take a complete personal and family history, give you a physical examination (including a rectal exam) and perform laboratory tests; special attention will be paid to your large bowel, including tests for blood in the stool and looking into the bowel with an instrument (colonoscope or sigmoidoscope). X-rays of the bowel are often taken; they require a barium retention enema.

Since at this time we know very little about the prevention of colorectal cancer (a well-balanced diet rich in fibre and low in fat is the only recommendation available),[18] the only other thing that can be done is to promote early detection.

WHO IS AT HIGHER THAN USUAL RISK?

1. *All people when they get older.* Up to age forty, this risk is very low unless special circumstances are present (see 2 and 3 below). From then on, the

risk doubles every ten years. Thus, a person at age seventy-five has an eight times higher risk of developing colorectal cancer than one at age forty-five. This is why the American Cancer Society recommends that people, *even if they feel completely healthy*, should routinely have certain tests beginning at age forty or fifty. Such tests are not available on the NHS, unless the GP suspects trouble. These tests are: an examination of the rectum with a gloved finger (digital rectal); a test for blood in the stool (guaiac test); a 'procto', which means inspection of the inside of the bowel with an instrument called a proctosigmoidoscope or with a flexible colonoscope (which allows examination of more of your bowel). New flexible instruments cause less discomfort than the rigid instruments used in the past.

2. *People with a personal or family history of colorectal cancer, breast cancer, or cancer of the endometrium* (lining of the uterus). Since such individuals have colorectal cancer more often than others – sometimes also at a younger age – doctors should take careful family histories and should do periodic examination for colorectal cancer regardless of age. Again, this is unlikely to be NHS routine. It is only recently that researchers have noticed this family tendency. They also recommend such examinations for blood relatives of these patients, beginning at age twenty or thirty. In this situation, the whole bowel may be inspected by colonoscopy.

3. *People with bowel diseases which are not cancer in themselves but often lead to cancer.*
   (a) Inflammatory bowel disease (ulcerative colitis or Crohn's disease – sometimes called regional ileitis or enteritis). If one of these conditions exists for eight or ten years, the chance of developing colorectal cancer is greatly increased.
   (b) Familial polyposis. In this condition, the bowel is studded with polyps and examinations should begin much earlier, even in adolescence. The disease is inherited and leads to cancer in 50 per cent of the cases. Close blood relatives of anyone who has this condition should be examined early and periodically, for they might develop the same life-threatening disease.
   (c) Single polyps, especially of the cell type called 'adenomatous', are also associated with cancer of the bowel. These should be removed surgically (not a major operation), and the surgery followed by regular examinations.

LIVING WITH AN OSTOMY

When a part of the intestine must be removed, the two cut ends are sewn together to maintain a passageway for food. When this is not feasible, an opening (a 'stoma') is made in the abdominal wall, through which the undigested matter can pass into a pouch (appliance). The operation is called a colostomy when the stoma is made in the colon, and an ileostomy when the stoma is made in the portion of the small intestine called the ileum. People with colostomies may or may not return to a predictable time of bowel evacuation, depending on the location of the colostomy in the large intestine, on prior bowel habits, on the presence of other medical conditions, on use of medicines, or other cancer treatments. Some people with a colostomy flush or irrigate the stoma with water to promote a bowel movement at a certain time of day, others prefer to wear an appliance most of the time. Those with ileostomies must keep the bag in place all the time.

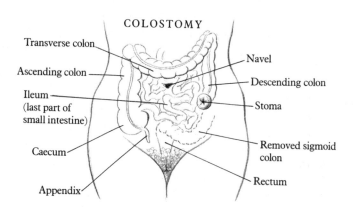

People often fear that a diagnosis of colorectal cancer leads automatically to a colostomy. This was never the case, and is even less true today because of new surgical techniques that reconnect parts of the large intestine after removing the cancerous section. Furthermore, living with an ostomy today is signifi-cantly easier than it was in the past. Women who have an ostomy can lead completely normal lives that include sexual relations (see publications of the Colostomy Welfare Group. See also the Sexuality chapter).

Very many women, including some much in the public eye, have col-ostomies – and can wear most normal clothes without any difficulty. The Colostomy Welfare Group can put you in touch with women who have lived for years with a colostomy and can help you develop a positive attitude to your future.

Breast Cancer

To women, breast cancer is perhaps the most familiar and the most frightening of all cancers. The older we get, the more we hear of friends and relatives who have the disease, and the more likely it is that we ourselves have experienced it.

Statistics on the disease cause us concern. Breast cancer was long the foremost cause of cancer deaths in women, and is now second only to lung cancer. Overall, one out of every ten women develops it, but the risk of developing it before age seventy is much less – one in seventeen. Breast-cancer incidence rises rapidly in women between thirty and fifty, then continues to rise, but more slowly, after age fifty.[19] Approximately 80 per cent of all breast cancers occur in postmenopausal women.[20] It is more common in white women than in black women, but this seems to be changing; among younger black women, the incidence is now similar to that in younger white women.[21]

But these statistics mask other facts about breast cancer, facts that are both reassuring and complex. Breast cancer is actually many different diseases, some aggressive and rapidly fatal, some so indolent and slow that they may not kill, and many between these two extremes. The rate at which breast tumours grow varies enormously, as does our immune systems' ability to fight them. Although many women with breast cancer die within a few years of diagnosis, others live as long as thirty or forty years before dying either of breast cancer or of other causes in old age.[22] **Sixty per cent of women with breast cancer live as long as their peers without the disease.**[23]

Nonetheless, some researchers think that some or all breast cancers spread immediately, and as cancerous cells leave the breast through the lymph nodes or bloodstream, others remain in the breast to form a lump. But when breast cancer spreads, it does not necessarily kill. Whether or not a spreading breast cancer is fatal seems to depend on the same vital factors: How fast or slow is the cancer? Can the immune system keep it under control?

As with other forms of cancer, smoking has been shown to make us more vulnerable.

DETECTION

The Breast Self-Exam
Although most breast lumps are benign (non-cancerous), a lump is the most frequent first sign of breast cancer, far more frequent than pain or nipple discharge. Unlike cancerous lumps in other parts of the body, a sizeable lump in the breast is relatively easy to feel. For this reason, doctors usually encourage us to examine our breasts regularly for lumps in order to detect cancer 'early' if it is there. But is the breast self-exam actually beneficial?

Researchers now know that breast cancer is in the body not months, but years, before it is detected through a lump in the breast. In most cases, by the time a lump is large enough to be felt, it has been in the body at least three to five years, more likely five to fifteen years, depending on its rate of growth.[24] If it is going to spread at all, it has probably spread long before we can feel its presence.

But even if breast cancer has already spread, there are arguments for early detection: (1) removing the lump as early as possible leaves the immune system free to fight cancer cells that have spread rather than having to fight the cells in the lump as well; (2) the longer a cancerous lump remains in the body, the more time it has to populate the body with additional cancer cells, making it harder for the immune system or cancer treatments to fight them.

However, many women question the emphasis on breast self-exam and feel blamed if a cancerous lump is found and they didn't find it 'early enough'. In the US a Federal panel recently supported women's doubts by deciding that there is not enough evidence in favour of the breast self-exam to advocate it as a detection test.[25] It is unlikely, but still not definitely known, whether the practice of monthly breast self-exams can lengthen a woman's life. Statistics show that in fact most women do not examine their breasts regularly, partly out of fear of finding a lump and partly because, as healthy women, they don't want to look for disease. Other women like the idea of becoming familiar with their bodies by monitoring normal, cyclic changes in their breasts. They see regular or occasional breast exams as a way of taking care of themselves, and they examine their breasts when the time feels right for them.

Mammogram Screening

A mammogram, an X-ray picture of the breast, is now the most widely publicized method of regularly checking or screening healthy women for breast changes. Its purpose is to locate a suspicious lump in the breast so it can be removed and examined under a microscope to see if it is cancerous. A mammogram itself cannot diagnose cancer and it is not a treatment.

Theoretically, the arguments in favour of breast self-exam hold true for the mammogram, with the advantage that, in some women, a mammogram can indicate the possibility of a small cancerous lump years before it is large enough to be felt. Large-scale studies in Sweden and in the United States show that women over fifty benefit from regular mammogram screening with 30 per cent lower breast-cancer death rates.[26] The same advantage has not been shown for younger women. Some researchers believe that mammograms are equally effective for women in their forties. However, there are no reliable statistics yet to prove or disprove the value of this practice. In the meantime, these studies contradict the American Cancer Society's recommendation that women in their forties be screened every one or two years.

Mammogram screening has its dangers. One is that radiation from an X-ray can cause breast cancer. Radiation is cumulative: many small doses over time equal one large dose. No one knows how large a radiation dose has to be to

cause breast cancer, and the amount probably varies from woman to woman.*
But the breast seems to become less vulnerable with age, the adolescent breast
possibly being the most vulnerable to radiation. Since it takes ten to twenty
years or more for radiation-induced cancer to appear, the older you are, the less
risk.

If you decide to have a mammogram screen at a Well Woman or private
clinic make sure that the radiologist uses the lowest feasible dose of radiation.
If possible as low as 0.1 or 0.2 rads per examination. Also, it appears that
screening only every two or three years, using a single X-ray exposure for each
breast, may be just as beneficial as yearly screening with double exposure.[27]
The practice in this country is to take at least two views of each breast, and
some radiologists argue that this provides better accuracy. Check to assure that
the mammograms are kept on file for future comparisons.

Mammograms do not distinguish a cancerous lump from a benign one. Since
some breast lumpiness is normal in women, many mammograms interpreted
as 'suspicious' lead to needless worry and to countless unnecessary breast
biopsies. The breast biopsy rate is increased by doctors who are afraid of
malpractice accusations and who protect themselves by recommending biopsies 'just to make sure'.

Perhaps the most disturbing aspect of mammogram screening is that of over-
treatment. A mammogram can find lumps so small they are difficult to
diagnose correctly under a microscope. Some of these lumps are cancers that
may not spread, called *in situ* cancers. Women with such cancers may be
misdiagnosed and treated as though they have rapidly spreading disease. Also,
these women will be called 'cured', thus distorting figures on the supposed
benefits of the mammograms and the treatment.

Mammograms also find fields of what are called microcalcifications, tiny
spots of calcium deposits that show up almost like grains of sand in the
mammogram. While it is true that calcium deposits are often present in cancer
cells and are one of the signs radiologists look for in the screening process, it is
also true that 75 per cent of microcalcifications are normal and do not indicate
cancer.[28]

To date, mammography is the only imaging method of screening which can
show benefit to women. Other forms of breast pictures, such as thermography,

*Estimates for mammograms indicate that one rad (radiation absorbed dose) to the breast per examination can
result in six cancers per one million women beginning ten years after exposure. Another estimate shows that
approximately 788 cases of breast cancer per year are caused by X-rays. However, this figure includes all X-rays
in which the breast was exposed to the rays, such as X-rays of the chest and back, and CAT scans, as well as
mammograms. I. Craig Henderson, 'Breast Cancer', in John A. Spittell, Jr, ed., *Clinical Medicine*. Philadelphia:
Harper & Row, 1986, p. 4; and John S. Evans, John E. Wennberg and Barbara J. McNeil, 'The Influence of
Diagnostic Radiography on the Incidence of Breast Cancer and Leukemia'. *The New England Journal of
Medicine*, Vol. 315, No. 13, 25 September 1986, pp. 810–15.

diaphanography, and ultrasound, are not yet reliable enough to be beneficial. Further study of effective screening methods that do not involve radiation is needed.

THE 'HIGH RISK' CONTROVERSY

You may have read or heard a long list of factors that supposedly make a woman a high risk for breast cancer. The list includes having fibrocystic disease (see below), early menarche and late menopause, Jewish ancestry and many more. More recent studies show that most of those factors do not actually increase a woman's risk.

Women who are more likely than others to develop breast cancer are those who:

• Have already had breast cancer;
• Have a mother or sister who had breast cancer before age forty, especially if she had it in both breasts;
• Have taken oestrogens after the age of fifty,* or the synthetic oestrogen diethylstilboestrol (DES) during pregnancy.†

• Have had frequent high-dose X-rays that exposed the breast.

No risk factor warrants removal of the breast to *prevent* breast cancer, a procedure called a prophylactic mastectomy. Some American doctors actually urge women to undergo this operation. These doctors overrate the significance of risk factors and of microcalcifications and do not know that *removal of a healthy breast is no guarantee against breast cancer*. A cancerous lump can grow in any remaining breast tissue or on the chest wall, and there is always a chance that breast cancer is already somewhere in the body. Breast reconstruction after a mastectomy makes detection of a later cancer even more difficult.

IF YOU HAVE A HIGH RISK OF BREAST CANCER

If you have already had breast cancer it is worth having regular mammogram checkups no matter what your age, since cancerous lumps often recur in the same or the other breast. Also, the benefits of mammogram screening probably

*Women without ovaries who took 1.25 mg of oestrogen for three years after the age of fifty had double the risk of breast cancer compared with women who did not take oestrogens. The risk of breast cancer was 2.5 times higher among women whose ovaries were intact. Ronald K. Ross et al., 'A Case-Control Study of Menopausal Estrogen Therapy and Breast Cancer'. *Journal of the American Medical Association*, Vol. 243, No. 16, 20 April 1980, pp. 1635–9; and P. A. Wingo et al., 'The Risk of Breast Cancer in Menopausal Women Who Have Used Estrogen Replacement Therapy'. *Journal of the American Medical Association*, Vol. 257, No. 2, 9 January 1987, pp. 209–15.

†E. R. Greenberg et al., cited in note 9.

outweigh the risks if you are over fifty and have a higher than average risk of breast cancer. If you are at high risk for breast cancer, but under fifty, have a mammogram every one or two years if it helps put your mind at ease, but remember that benefits for women your age are not yet proven.

IF YOU FIND A LUMP

If you or your partner or doctor find a lump in your breast, keep in mind that 80 to 90 per cent of lumps are benign (non-cancerous). Breast lumps are common and normal in women, and most conditions causing change, lumps, or pain in the breast are not cancer. Probably the majority of older women have found one or more isolated lumps in their breasts through the years, and a general lumpiness of the breasts is common in half of all women. Many doctors call lumpiness or even one isolated lump 'fibrocystic disease'. But lumpy breasts are not a disease and do not increase our risk of breast cancer. For this reason, some doctors more appropriately refer to breast lumpiness as a fibrocystic condition.[29] Most benign lumps are related to the hormonal fluctuations of menstruation, however, so a new lump after the menopause should be checked. There is no sure way of reducing non-cancerous breast lumps, but some women find that reducing fat, salt, caffeine, chocolate, and cigarettes, while adding dietary supplements of vitamin E and evening primrose oil (available in health-food stores), has helped.

There is no harm in monitoring a lump yourself for a few weeks. If a lump fluctuates with your period, this is an indication that it is a harmless cyst, or fluid-filled sac. If you are past the menopause, check the lump on the same date each month, since women continue to have cyclical changes in their breasts even after periods cease.

If your lump does not fluctuate and/or worries you, have an experienced doctor or nurse examine your breast. Many women find that their own general practitioners do not know how to examine the breast properly, nor are they knowledgeable about how to distinguish a benign lump from a cancerous one. If you or your GP are worried, ask for a referral to a Breast Clinic. You can see a surgeon simply for a diagnosis of your lump. You do not have to plan on surgery or agree to it. The doctor should give you a thorough breast exam in both seated and supine (lying down) positions, palpate your underarms for swelling and your abdomen for suspicious masses, listen to your lungs, and take a complete blood count. These examinations are a precaution to check for cancer in the body. If your lump is large and feels like a cyst, the doctor may omit these examinations and try an immediate needle aspiration.

Diagnosis. If both you and your doctor think your lump is harmless, you may choose to forgo any further procedures. However, even if the lump feels harmless, you should consider a biopsy if you are considered in a higher-risk category of breast cancer or if there are other symptoms of possible cancer present, such as hard, swollen glands in the armpit, a skin rash on the breast, nipple discharge, or dimpling or puckering of skin around the nipple. There are two basic diagnostic procedures to determine whether a lump is cancerous, both of them office procedures.

1. *Needle aspiration*: your doctor inserts a needle into the lump. If the lump is a cyst, fluid is withdrawn and the lump collapses. If the lump proves solid, or if it is too small to insert the needle accurately into it, the next step would be a surgical biopsy.

2. *Surgical biopsy*: the removal of the lump in order to examine it under a microscope. The surgery can usually be done under local anaesthesia – unless you prefer general anaesthesia, which entails risks and requires longer recovery time. **Do *not* agree to a biopsy under general anaesthesia so that the surgeon can remove the entire breast immediately should your lump prove cancerous.** This 'one-step' procedure is unnecessary and detrimental.

It is best to remove an entire solid lump (excisional biopsy), since some lumps are made up of both benign and cancerous cells. If only part of the lump is removed and proves benign, the part left in the breast could still be cancerous. The excised lump should be analysed by permanent section, which may take a few days, but is more reliable than the quick frozen section. There is no need of a bone scan or any further tests unless your lump is diagnosed as cancerous.

If you have a biopsy make sure your doctor plans to order an immediate oestrogen-receptor test on the lump if it turns out to be malignant. This test will show whether or not your tumour cells contain a certain protein called an oestrogen receptor. This test is vital to planning future treatment and must be done upon the diagnosis of cancer, without delay.

Fine needle aspiration of a solid lump and *trucut needle biopsy* are less common and are not definitive. If the needle shows only non-cancerous cells, the cells remaining in the lump could still be cancerous. But if your lump is so large that removing it would greatly distort the breast, these procedures can help you decide whether or not to have surgery.

Wire localization biopsy may be used if a mammogram shows a suspicious area such as microcalcifications which can't be felt but which your doctor thinks should be removed. While an X-ray shows a picture of your breast, the radiologist inserts a fine wire into the breast under local anaesthesia, and points the wire to the area in question. The surgeon then follows the wire and removes the tissue at the end. Further examination is done to confirm that the correct area was removed.

A mammogram is not appropriate for diagnosing a lump which can be felt. However, some doctors recommend a mammogram before a biopsy to see if there are other suspicious masses in the same or the other breast.

IF YOUR LUMP IS CANCEROUS

If your lump proves cancerous, there is no need to rush into action. Give yourself time to adjust to the powerful feelings you will have and to find out which treatment, if any, might be most beneficial for your special case. There is no harm in taking up to six weeks before making any decisions.

Making a Decision About Treatments

Since breast-cancer treatments are so controversial among doctors, and new studies are constantly clarifying treatment options, it is especially important to get second or even third opinions about the right treatment for you. Be sure to find out the results or trends of current studies, especially larger 'randomized clinical trials'.

You and your doctor need to know as much as possible about your cancer in order to make a sound judgment on possible treatments. The first step is the oestrogen-receptor test. Your tumour cells may contain an oestrogen and/or progesterone receptor (called an oestrogen/progesterone-positive cancer, or OR+ and PgR+). This indicates a hormone-sensitive cancer, which is often a slower-growing one. It is most prevalent in postmenopausal women. The absence of this receptor is called an oestrogen/progesterone-negative cancer, or OR− and PgR−. Oestrogen/progesterone-negative cancers tend to be more aggressive than oestrogen/progesterone-positive cancers.

As a second step, your doctor may suggest removing a few lymph nodes from your armpit. The presence of cancerous cells in the nodes (called 'positive nodes') is a sign that cancer may be elsewhere in the body and that your immune system, in which lymph nodes play an active role, is not successfully fighting the spreading disease. Conversely, cancer-free lymph nodes (called 'negative nodes') indicate that your immune system is more successful in fighting the disease elsewhere in your body than if the nodes are positive.[30] Lymph-node sampling is for diagnosis only, to help decide which treatment might be beneficial. Removing them does not help eliminate cancer from the body. Removing more than about ten nodes may cause arm problems later.

Your doctor should also do an abdominal exam and order blood tests, a chest X-ray, and possibly a bone scan. If any of these tests show that cancer has already reached a detectable stage in a distant part of your body such as the bone or liver, available treatments can only relieve uncomfortable or painful symptoms. They are not likely to lengthen life more than a few months, and this small advantage must be weighed against the negative effects of the treatments.

Treatment Options

1. LOCAL THERAPIES

The purpose of local therapies is to remove (surgery) and/or kill (radiation) cancerous cells at the site of the lump and in the surrounding area.

Lumpectomy. Lumpectomy is the surgical removal of the lump with varying amounts of surrounding tissue. If your biopsy included the entire lump and some surrounding tissue, this is considered a lumpectomy and you probably need no further surgery.

A recent study shows that women with tumours up to one and a half inches in diameter live as long with lumpectomy alone as with lumpectomy and radiation, or with mastectomy.[31] Although this US study is relatively new, it is supported by Canadian and European research with up to twenty-five-year results. This study included women with positive and negative nodes but with no evidence of distant spread. However, it probably also applies to women with obvious distant spread. It is what happens in the rest of the body that counts.

The possible adverse effects of a lumpectomy are some scarring and disfiguring of the breast.

Lumpectomy with Radiation. In this procedure, after the lump and surrounding tissue have been removed, the area surrounding the site of the lump is irradiated by X-ray beams and sometimes by temporary implants of radioactive materials (radiation implants). Radiation can evidently help prevent a cancerous lump from growing back again in the same breast, but it does not prolong life. Although radiation can have adverse effects, some women choose it to reduce the risk of a repeated lump and surgery in the same breast. However, this is a matter of choice. If you have a lumpectomy you do not have to agree to radiation also.

Adverse effects can include fatigue, dry, red, itchy skin, extreme sun sensitivity, muscle pain, and occasional cracked ribs or a temporary lung ailment similar to bronchitis. Theoretically, radiation therapy can also cause breast cancer, but this appears to be rare.

2. SYSTEMIC THERAPIES

Chemotherapy. Drugs in the form of pills or injections attempt to kill cancer cells nesting or circulating in distant parts of the body. Two major studies showed that 14 to 24 per cent of premenopausal women with positive nodes live longer as a result of chemotherapy.[32] Women in this category who have one to three positive nodes or whose tumours contain poorly differentiated cells (cells in an undeveloped, embryonic state) seem more likely to be helped by chemotherapy than women who have four or more positive nodes or whose tumours have well-differentiated cells.[33]

A combination of drugs called CMF (cyclophosphamide, methotrexate, and 5-fluorouracil) may work better than single drugs used separately, and a six-month regimen seems just as beneficial as longer use. But the optimal drug dosage, timing, combination and duration of treatment are still being debated. Studies are underway to see if chemotherapy can help premenopausal women with aggressive cancers but no node involvement, but there are no clear answers yet.

Doctors now tend to overuse chemotherapy for breast cancer, routinely giving it to women with no sign of cancer in the lymph nodes and regardless of their menopausal status. This is a dangerous trend, since the drugs used can take a serious emotional and physical toll. Further research is needed to pinpoint which women are most likely to benefit from chemotherapy.

Hormone Therapy. Some hormones, in the form of pills or injections, aim to repress or eliminate oestrogen in the body, thus curbing the spread of cancer. The hormones most commonly used are tamoxifen and male hormones.

There are no definite answers yet on the effectiveness of hormone therapy, but current estimates indicate that tamoxifen can prolong life in some postmenopausal women, especially those whose lumps have been diagnosed as oestrogen-positive and whose nodes show signs of cancer.[34] Long-term use (two years or perhaps longer) seems to be more effective than shorter use. The drug evidently has few adverse effects on women past the menopause except hot flushes and vaginal dryness. Therefore, many feel it is worth trying without awaiting more definite study results, although it is fairly expensive and may not be offered on the NHS.

Doctors sometimes include tamoxifen in chemotherapy regimens. Premenopausal women should not take tamoxifen until test results of such mixed treatments are more conclusive. Ask your doctor which drug will be included in your regimen and why.

Current studies show that postmenopausal women with oestrogen-receptor-negative cancers and those with no node involvement may also benefit from hormone therapy. Further studies on tamoxifen are underway for these women. For a discussion on HRT and breast cancer see Osteoporosis chapter.

3. OUTMODED OR RARELY NECESSARY TREATMENTS

Surgical Techniques to Limit Oestrogen Production. These techniques include adrenalectomy (removal of the adrenals) and hypophysectomy (removal of the pituitary gland). The drugs discussed under hormone therapy can generally produce the same effects with fewer problems. There are still open questions about oophorectomy (removal of the ovaries), and studies are underway.

Mastectomy. Mastectomy is surgical removal of the entire breast. This procedure, long thought the only way to treat breast cancer, is often no more effective than removal of the lump alone. A mastectomy is probably only necessary if:

a. Your breast is small and the lump so large that a lumpectomy would be more disfiguring than removing the entire breast, or

b. The cancerous cells have not formed a lump but are diffuse in tiny clusters throughout the breast. In this case, many women and doctors want to 'get it all out' by removing the entire breast, although there is no proof, even then, that a mastectomy prolongs life. The decision about opting for a lumpectomy or a mastectomy should be yours.

Writing in *Good Housekeeping* (November 1988) Jay Trett, a forty-two-year-old woman, described her reasons for preferring a lumpectomy. Her tumour was small, and she gathered all possible information from her surgeon and the Bristol Cancer Help Centre about the probable outcome of lumpectomy or mastectomy in her case. She opted for lumpectomy and a course of radiotherapy. Subsequent checkups showed that the cancer hadn't spread and that there was only a 10 per cent chance of recurrence. Eighteen months later she was able to write that she had made the right decision: left with no permanent reminder of the disease, she intended to put it all behind her. But another woman says:

Although I used to believe that mastectomy was a brutal anti-woman treatment for breast cancer, when it came to the point I decided against a lumpectomy. My reasons? I feared how exhausting, debilitating and even mutilating [because of possible skin burns] the radiation therapy I would have had after lumpectomy might be. And I did feel that somehow I'd rather have the whole growth removed and the surrounding breast with it rather than risk the odd cell remaining in my breast ready to develop another tumour. It wasn't any easy decision, but I'm glad I made it. [a forty-nine-year-old woman]

It is our right to have all the facts and it is our right to make our own decisions. A radical mastectomy, also called the Halsted radical (removal of the breast, underlying muscles of the chest wall, and lymph nodes), is *never* necessary. However, some surgeons still recommend and perform it.

If You Have Had a Mastectomy

The mastectomy has been standard practice for over one hundred years. Between 1970 and 1985 over one and a half million American women had mastectomies of some kind, including the Halsted radical.[35] In the belief that time was essential, surgeons often performed the operation while the patient was under general anaesthesia given for the biopsy. A woman awoke to find that she had cancer and had lost one or both breasts. This can still happen in the UK and that is why it is so important to state in writing that you do not want the surgeon to do this when performing a biopsy.

Most one-breasted women wear a prosthesis, a breast form made of foam rubber or silicone. Some have had surgical reconstruction to take the place of the amputated breast. If, on a warm summer day when light clothing would normally be worn, all women who had mastectomies decided not to wear a prosthesis, or could temporarily discard their reconstructed breasts, we would see in the streets, the shops, and beaches many one-breasted women.

Women who have lost one or both breasts face the emotional trauma of losing a part of their body so strongly associated with sexuality and a sense of womanhood.

It's been a long process coming to terms with the loss of my breast. The mastectomy seemed unreal for a long time. I would look in the mirror and not believe it! I think it takes a lot of courage to say goodbye to a part of your body no matter what your age. But I was very young, and it seemed especially sad to lose my breast before I had lived with it and enjoyed it fully. I hadn't seen it get full of milk and breastfed with it; hadn't watched it age. Only long after the operation was I able to really say goodbye to my breast. [a thirty-nine-year-old woman]

For some women, the physical discomfort and pain resulting from a radical mastectomy are also a lasting concern. When the lymph nodes have been removed and the lymph and blood vessels cut during surgery, the lymph fluid in the arm cannot drain off and sometimes accumulates, causing swelling in the arm and even pain. At times, women who have had less extensive mastectomies or only a lymph-node sampling experience a similar, but milder, discomfort. There is no cure for this condition, called *lymphedema,** but there are ways of

---

*Lymphedema can occur in the leg after lymph nodes are removed from the groin. Try the same methods mentioned below for the arm to alleviate discomfort in the leg.

making it easier to live with. Wearing an elastic custom-fitted sleeve, and treatment with an inflatable sleeve (pneumo-massage) can alleviate discomfort. Some women find that exercise, especially under the instruction of a physiotherapist, reduces the discomfort of lymphedema as well as any stiffness and numbness in the shoulder and arm.

Counselling after a mastectomy should be provided by the hospital in which the operation has been performed, and in some places this is always offered. However, many women find that there is no one available to offer them support either at the time or afterwards, and some GPs don't know about the valuable service provided by the Breast Care and Mastectomy Association (see Organizations). Counsellors from the Association (themselves women who have had mastectomies) will visit breast surgery patients in hospital and at home, offer advice on the selection of prostheses and, most important, give support as long as it is needed.

NOTES

[1]National Cancer Institute, *Cancer Prevention*. National Institutes of Health Publication No. 84-2671, February 1984.

[2]Robert L. Rogers et al., 'Abstention from Smoking Improves Cerebral Perfusion Among Elderly Smokers'. *Journal of the American Medical Association*, Vol. 253, No. 20, 24–31 May 1985, pp. 2970–4.

[3]Adapted from the Boston Women's Health Book Collective, *The New Our Bodies, Ourselves*. London: Penguin, 1989.

[4]Amanda Spake, 'A New American Nightmare'. *Ms.*, March 1986, pp. 35–42ff.

[5]William Mann, 'Reproductive Cancer'. *Women and Health*, Vol. 10, No. 2/3, Summer/Fall 1985, p. 63.

[6]Susan Sontag, *Illness as Metaphor*. New York: Random House, 1979.

[7]Marcia Angell, 'Disease as a Reflection of the Psyche?' *The New England Journal of Medicine*, Vol. 312, No. 24, 13 June 1985, pp. 1570–2.

[8]Barrie R. Cassileth et al., 'Psychosocial Correlates of Survival in Advanced Malignant Disease'. *The New England Journal of Medicine*, Vol. 312, No. 24, 13 June 1985, pp. 1551–5.

[9]E. R. Greenberg et al., 'Breast Cancer in Mothers Given Diethylstilbestrol in Pregnancy'. *The New England Journal of Medicine*, Vol. 311, No. 22, 29 November 1984, pp. 1393–8.

[10]Office of Cancer Communications, National Cancer Institute, *The Breast Cancer Digest*. US Department of Health and Human Services, Public Health Service, NIH Publication No. 84-1691, 2nd edition, April 1984.

[11]Stephen Jay Gould, 'The Median Isn't the Message'. *Discover*, Vol. 6, No. 6, June 1985, pp. 40–2.

[12]Martin B. Levene, 'Radiation Therapy'. In Blake Cady, ed., *Cancer: A Manual for Practitioners*. Boston: American Cancer Society, Massachusetts Division, 6th edition, 1982, pp. 49–51.

[13]'Overcoming Tumour Resistance in Therapy. Dr Coleman Cites Efforts to Enhance Response to Cancer Treatment'. *Focus*, Harvard Medical Area News Office, 19 October 1985.

[14]'Drugs in Disguise'. *Consumer Reports*, May 1985, pp. 275–83.

[15]John C. Bailar III and Elaine M. Smith,

'Progress Against Cancer'. *The New England Journal of Medicine*, Vol. 314, No. 19, 8 May 1986, pp. 1226–32.

[16]American Cancer Society, *1985 Cancer Facts & Figures*, p. 9.

[17]Ibid., p. 14.

[18]Peter Greenwald and Elaine Lanza, 'Dietary Fiber and Colon Cancer'. *Contemporary Nutrition*, Vol. XI, No. 1, 1986.

[19]John L. Young, Jr, Constance L. Percy and Ardyce J. Cesire, eds., *Surveillance, Epidemiology, and End Results: Incidence and Mortality Data, 1973–77*. US Department of Health and Human Services, June 1981, pp. 2081–2330.

[20]*Health Facts*, April 1985. Center for Medical Consumers, Inc., 237 Thompson Street, New York, NY 10012.

[21]H. Austin, Philip Cole and Ernest Wynder, 'Breast Cancer in Black American Women'. *International Journal of Cancer*, Vol. 24, 1979, pp. 541–4.

[22]I. Craig Henderson, *Breast Cancer Management: Progress and Prospects*. Wayne, NJ: Lederle Laboratories, 1982, p. 5.

[23]M. S. Fox, 'On the Diagnosis and Treatment of Breast Cancer'. *Journal of the American Medical Association*, Vol. 241, 1979, pp. 489–94. The National Cancer Institute reported a rise of 7 per cent in the breast-cancer death rate among white women under fifty between 1983 and 1984. It is not yet known whether this figure will hold or drop again.

[24]P. M. Gullino, 'Natural History of Breast Cancer'. *Cancer*, Vol. 39, 1977, pp. 2697–2703.

[25]Michael S. O'Malley and Suzanne W. Fletcher, 'Screening for Breast Cancer with Breast Self-Examination'. *Journal of the American Medical Association*, Vol. 257, No. 16, 24 April 1987, pp. 2197–2203.

[26]S. Shapiro et al., 'Periodic Breast Cancer Screening in Reducing Mortality from Breast Cancer'. *Journal of the American Medical Association*, Vol. 215, No. 11, 15 March 1971, pp. 1777–85; and L. Tabar et al., 'Reduction in Mortality from Breast Cancer After Mass Screening with Mammography'. *Lancet*, 13 April 1985, pp. 829–32.

[27]Tabar et al., op. cit.

[28]'Differentiating Benign Breast Conditions, Breast Ca[ncer]'. *Ob. Gyn. News*, Vol. 20, No. 20, 15–31 October 1985, p. 41.

[29]Susan Love et al., 'Fibrocystic "Disease" of the Breast – A Non-disease'. *The New England Journal of Medicine*, Vol. 307, No. 16, 14 October 1982, pp. 1010–14.

[30]Loren J. Humphrey et al., 'Immunologic Responsiveness of the Breast Cancer Patient'. *Cancer*, Vol. 46, 1980, pp. 893–989.

[31]Bernard Fisher et al., 'Five-Year Results of a Randomized Clinical Trial Comparing Total Mastectomy and Segmental Mastectomy With or Without Radiation in the Treatment of Breast Cancer'. *The New England Journal of Medicine*, Vol. 312, No. 11, 14 March 1985, pp. 665–73.

[32]Gianni Bonadonna, 'Results of the Milan Adjuvant Chemotherapy Trials'. In *Adjuvant Chemotherapy for Breast Cancer*. National Institutes of Health Consensus Development Conference, 1985, pp. 31–4; and I. Craig Henderson, ' "Adjuvant Systemic" Therapy of Early Breast Cancer'. In J. R. Harris et al., *Breast Diseases*. Philadelphia: J. B. Lippincott Co., 1987, pp. 324–53.

[33]Edwin R. Fisher, 'Pathologic Features as Prognostic Variables'. *Adjuvant Chemotherapy for Breast Cancer*. National Institutes of Health Consensus Development Conference, 1985, pp. 26–7; and I. Craig Henderson, 'Adjuvant Chemotherapy of Breast Cancer'. *Journal of Clinical Oncology*, Vol. 3, No. 2, February 1985, pp. 140–3.

[34]'Consensus Report: Adjuvant Chemotherapy for Breast Cancer'. National Institutes of Health Consensus Development Conference, September 1985. In *Clinical Insights*. Meniscus Ltd, Health Care Communications, Philadelphia.

[35]Figures from the National Center for Health Statistics.

BOOKS AND PUBLICATIONS

Marion Stroud, *Face to Face With Cancer*. Tring: Lion, 1988.

Dr Trish Reynolds, *Your Cancer: Your Life*. London: Macdonald Optima, 1988. Discusses causes, treatments, options (including right to refuse life-prolonging treatment) from a radical viewpoint.

Judith Arvey, Sue Mack and Julian Woolfson, *Cervical Cancer*. London: Faber & Faber, 1988. Practical information in question and answer style.

Michael Baum, *Breast Cancer: The Facts*. Oxford: Oxford University Press, 1981. The orthodox medical viewpoint from a cancer specialist.

Sir Ronald Bodley Scott, *Cancer: The Facts*. Oxford: Oxford University Press, 1981. Medical overview.

Sir Douglas Black, Chairman, *Investigation of the Possible Increased Incidence of Cancer in West Cumbria*. London: HMSO, 1986. The Black Report which sought to allay fears surrounding Sellafield. Friends of the Earth publishes *Critiques of the Black Report*. (See Organizations.)

John Urquart, *Leukaemia and Nuclear Power in Britain: The Evidence So Far*. London: Friends of the Earth, 1986.

Friends of the Earth Press Release, 'Pesticide Residues in Food', 1 August 1988.

Simon Best, 'The Electropollution Effect'. *Journal of Alternative and Complementary Medicine*, May 1988, p. 17.

F. Clifford Rose and M. Gawel, *Lung Cancer: The Facts*. Oxford: Oxford University Press, 1988.

Lesley Doyal et al., *Cancer in Britain: The Politics of Prevention*. London: Pluto Press Ltd, 1983.

Shirley Harrison, *New Approaches to Cancer*. London: Rider & Co., 1987.

Penny Brohn, *The Bristol Programme*. London: Century, 1987. Describes the Bristol Help Centre's methods. (See Organizations.)

Brenda Kidman, *Gentle Way with Cancer*. Revised edition of *Cancer: A Gentle Way*. London: Century/Arrow, 1986. This was the first book to describe the Bristol Approach.

Sadhya Rippon, *The Bristol Recipe Book*. London: Century, 1987.

John Elkington and Julia Hailes, *The Green Consumer Guide*. London: Gollancz, 1988. Sources of organically grown food, non-carcinogenic garden chemicals and household products, etc.

25
Diabetes

Diabetes is a major health challenge today. Statistics show it to be the third leading cause of death in the US because it is the underlying cause of much heart and kidney disease.[1] In recent years, however, we have learned measures to prevent some diabetes and to allow those who have it to live fairly healthy lives. These measures include the same practices that also keep all of us active and healthy during and after midlife.

Diabetes is of special concern to women over forty. Women are more likely to develop diabetes than men.[2] Black and Hispanic women are even more at risk.[3] The disease is not only dangerous in and of itself, but also because people with diabetes often develop complications that result in severe disability and even death.[4] Because it involves our eating habits, those of us with diabetes may suffer from guilt as well as anxiety in connection with the disease.

For a long time I felt really guilty about being diabetic because doctors told me that what I ate was causing some difficulty in my body and that if I would take care of myself I would be in better shape. I think a lot of diabetics stay in the closet about their diabetes because of the guilt. [a fifty-three-year-old woman]

Anything to do with food and eating touches issues of 'ideal body weight', dieting and body image, and our own needs in relation to our role as nurturer in our homes and in society.

What is Diabetes?

In diabetes the pancreas does not produce enough insulin. The pancreas is the part of the communication system in the body that directs the use and storage of energy from foods. This system is an awesome network of biochemical signals that maintains the body's energy balance whether we are at rest or running, hot or cold, old or young, sick or well. Appreciating this balance (called homeostasis) helps us to collaborate with our bodies, even when we are not healthy, instead of viewing our bodies as enemies.

Insulin is a vital link in this communication system. A slow trickle of insulin is normally produced in the body at all times, with larger amounts secreted when eating. Insulin facilitates the movement of fuels from the food we eat into our cells so that these fuels can be used for energy, growth, and healing. The main such fuels are glucose from carbohydrates, amino acids from proteins, and fats from the fat in our diet. When insulin is lacking, glucose builds up in the bloodstream because it is unable to enter cells, and we are short of energy. Some proteins then combine with the abnormally high level of glucose in the blood, blood fats are increased, and blood-vessel walls are damaged. This sequence of events causes further injury throughout the body's tissues and nervous system.

Insulin performs another important task. When we eat more than we can use right away, it promotes the storage of those extra calories for future use. The extra calories are stored in the liver and muscles as glycogen, and in fat cells as fat. That trait helped prehistoric people survive times when food was not available. However, today in our country, where most of us are able to eat every day, this trait is no longer so useful.

Two Types of Diabetes

Diabetes really should be thought of as a plural noun. There are at least two types and possibly more. The two main types differ in cause, inheritability, and treatment. They are now called Type I, insulin-dependent, and Type II, non-insulin-dependent. Type I usually occurs in young people and used to be called 'juvenile-onset'. People who have Type I are usually thin, no matter what age they are when it develops. Type II usually appears after the age of forty and used to be called 'adult-onset'; 80 to 90 per cent of people with Type II diabetes are fat.[5] It is now known that each type can occur at any age.

Diabetes, especially Type II, is on the increase in industrialized countries like ours, where the natural balance between physical work and eating has been disturbed.[6] Our society is food-oriented and sedentary.

More than 6 million people in the United States have diabetes. It is estimated that there are another 6 million who have it and don't know it yet.[7] In the UK about one person in thirty in the age-group sixty plus has diagnosed diabetes. Most of those who are undiagnosed have Type II diabetes. Unlike those with Type I, they still have some of their own insulin available and so may not have any dramatic symptoms. The warning signs for *both* types of diabetes include fatigue, thirst, frequent urination, slow healing of cuts and bruises, vaginal infection and itching, steady weight gain or recent weight loss, dental disease, and difficulty with eyesight. In Type II, these come on gradually and can easily be mistaken for 'just getting older'. Some people have undiagnosed Type II diabetes for many years.

In both types of diabetes, not enough insulin is secreted by the pancreas to regulate the blood sugar within the narrow range (60–140 milligrams per decilitre) needed for normal health. However, there the similarity between the two types stops. In Type I diabetes, the cells in the pancreas that produce insulin have been destroyed. The pancreas fails to produce any insulin and the body is quickly starved. The person becomes rapidly and acutely ill and diabetes is easily diagnosed. Recovery is also rapid when insulin is given. Type I has been the most publicized kind of diabetes, but only 10 per cent of the people with diabetes in this country have Type I.

Though some people do develop Type I diabetes as they grow older, middle-aged and older women are at more risk for Type II diabetes. The most important thing to keep in mind about Type II diabetes is that people who have it still produce generous amounts of their own insulin. However, their bodies have become resistant to insulin, and they are not able to make enough insulin to compensate for this resistance. Though why this happens is not yet completely understood, it is clear that becoming overweight and relatively inactive has a lot to do with insulin resistance.[8] So our sedentary and food habits have a lot to do with the increase in Type II diabetes.

Type II diabetes is inherited much more often than is Type I. Knowing your family history is useful. People who are overweight often feel guilty because they have long been indirectly and unfairly blamed for their condition. Now science tells us that some people have genetic traits that give them a tendency to store excess calories as fat. They may also have another genetic factor in the way insulin influences the energy balance inside the cells of their body.

There's been so much stuff in the media about 'too much sugar' in the average diet, and I knew that somehow sugar was associated with diabetes. So when I developed some symptoms I felt very guilty about the sweet tooth I'd always had. I felt that the diabetes was chickens coming home to roost. But at the Diabetic Clinic when I told the doctor this, he said that there is a lot more to diabetes than eating too much sugar. He told me that there's a strong hereditary factor – and of course I remembered my uncle who'd died quite young, and all that had seemed wrong with him was that he was very fat. It was only later the family realized he must have been a diabetic. [a fifty-year-old woman]

Those who have inherited the likelihood of getting diabetes if they get fat are at an unfair disadvantage in our overfed society, especially if they were brought up in families where heavy eating was encouraged. In addition, people often use food as a comforting substitute when they are scared, lonely, or angry, and this can make it hard to change eating habits. Understanding how these environmental and cultural elements interact with inherited tendencies can relieve feelings of guilt and helplessness about diabetes. We should not be blamed for genetic defects, but we don't have to remain at their mercy. We should offer the same respect and support to those struggling to change eating habits as we do to those who have to inject insulin every day.

TYPE II IS *NOT* A 'MILD' FORM OF DIABETES

Because people with Type II don't usually need to take insulin, it has been called a 'mild' form of diabetes. However, it is now known that this is not the case. Type II diabetes can cause such long-term complications as large-blood-vessel disease and loss of vision and kidney function, just as Type I can.[9]

When my doctor discovered I had diabetes, he said, 'But it is only mild.' So I assumed it was not necessary to be careful and ate sweets anyway. Then I remembered my brother who had recently died of kidney and liver failure and was totally blind. His urine never showed any sugar. The first symptom he had was when he awakened one morning, blind. The eye doctor said he had had diabetes for fifteen years to have such severe haemorrhage in his eyes. I hope these types of accidents can be prevented more now with the new light on Type II diabetes. [a sixty-eight-year-old woman from a family of ten, five of whom have diabetes]

There is a brighter side to this picture. When people with Type II diabetes lose weight and increase their physical activity to maintain a steady weight, their own insulin often comes back into healthy play. If so, they may be able to avoid the inconvenience and possible reactions of taking insulin or pills.

I have had Type II diabetes for several years. When I was fifty-six years old, I was on 34 units of insulin, my blood sugar was 180 and I weighed 210 pounds. Then I cut down on my calories but kept the healthy foods such as plenty of vegetables. In three weeks I had to stop taking insulin because of reactions. My doctor knew I was doing this and has records on it. I had lost 20 pounds. I did some bike riding. I had had a heart attack a year before, but now my heart seems okay. One year later, my weight is 148, my blood sugar 125, and I'm walking five to ten miles a day, am insulin-free and feeling wonderful! [a fifty-seven-year-old woman]

People with Type II diabetes who have a great deal of difficulty in keeping to a treatment plan of diet and exercise may need insulin injections or the pills for diabetes called oral agents, either separately or in combination. However, neither of these interventions works without the diet and exercise aspects too. Diet and exercise are necessary to restore the body cells' sensitivity to insulin. Insulin cannot be taken by mouth because it is a protein and would be digested in the stomach. In addition, there are some disadvantages to taking insulin without implementing a diet and exercise programme as well. Insulin makes you hungry, so it's harder to keep calories down. This may lead to a cycle of weight gain which, in turn, increases insulin resistance and calls for higher doses of insulin. Oral agents can be used in Type II diabetes, in which people still produce their own insulin. The oral agents help to increase the release of the body's insulin. Although the oral agents are now considered to be very useful for many people, they must be prescribed and utilized appropriately for each individual and be very carefully monitored.

My diabetes was diagnosed when I had to have a medical checkup when applying for a job. I was told to see my GP. He confirmed that I had Type II diabetes, and told me that I could control it with diet and exercise. Now I watch what I eat, walk to work rather than take the bus, and go for long walks at weekends and on holiday. I've lost weight, feel fine, and have been discharged from the diabetic clinic because the blood and urine tests are negative. I think that as long as I look after my health like this and get regular checkups, I should have no more need of the label 'diabetic'. [a forty-seven-year-old woman]

HEED EARLY WARNING SIGNS

If you have a strong family history of obesity, gave birth to a baby with a high birth weight, or developed temporary diabetes during pregnancy, you may be able to prevent Type II diabetes both for yourself and your children by following the life-style recommendations in this chapter. You will have a good influence on your family's diet and exercise habits at the same time.

Gestational diabetes is the 'temporary diabetes' which sometimes surfaces during pregnancy. Even if we don't plan to have more children, or are past the menopause, we can alert our daughters, granddaughters, and other younger women to the dangers of developing sugar in their urine during pregnancy. Sixty-five per cent of women who have gestational diabetes and who *also* are overweight during pregnancy eventually develop full-blown diabetes.[10] If they can be persuaded to change their habits while they are still young, to keep their weight down, and to increase their activity, they may improve their chances of avoiding diabetes.

When I had my second baby ten years ago I was told I had diabetes, but that once the pregnancy was over there would be no more problem. So I went on as I had before, eating lots of sweet things and always gaining a little weight every year. I got fat, and lazy with it. I think it's terrible the way doctors can let you go away from the situation that caused the diagnosis in the first place and not tell you you've got to be careful from then on, because it can happen later when you aren't pregnant. Anyway, I did start having trouble again and I'm now on tablets plus much more exercise and a careful diet. [a forty-two-year-old woman]

Many people with Type II diabetes don't need to take oral agents or insulin unless their supply of insulin is so reduced that there isn't enough to overcome insulin resistance. However, those with Type II may need to take insulin temporarily during times of physical or emotional stress, such as before, during or after surgery, or during a personal crisis. They are faced with the demanding task of losing weight and becoming physically active, sometimes after having been sedentary for years, and the lifelong task of remaining active and keeping their weight down.

Conquering these challenges is well worth the effort. People with either type of diabetes who succeed in effective self-care feel well most of the time and lead productive lives of normal length.

COMPLICATIONS OF DIABETES

The worst aspect of diabetes is that people who have undiagnosed or poorly managed diabetes are more likely to develop complications than those who keep control of their blood glucose. The most common of these are heart disease, stroke, kidney failure, visual impairment, sexual problems, and amputation of legs and feet. All of these problems are caused by inadequate circulation of the blood in both the large and small blood vessels. For example, diabetes causes one-half of the 80,000 leg and foot amputations performed annually in the US because the blood flow in the arteries has been damaged.[11]

I didn't take care of myself when I was told I had diabetes at age eighty. My husband was sick and I had to pay more attention to him. I didn't go on a diet, I would drink too much sweetened orange juice and have no exercise at all. After my husband passed away my diabetes came right down on me. It was then that I went to the hospital and was told I had no circulation in my leg at all so that's why I had to have my leg taken off. [an eighty-four-year-old black woman]

Women with diabetes and hypertension should take special care to keep their blood pressure normal (see p. 440) as well as their blood-glucose level. When blood glucose is normal the quality of all aspects of life improves. If your blood glucose is high, so is your urine glucose. Sugary urine turns the vaginal area into a perfect environment for infections and breakdown of the tissues. The resulting discomfort is a major barrier to sexual satisfaction for women with diabetes. However, there is now evidence that working hard at keeping your blood-glucose level as close to normal as possible may minimize, postpone, or prevent these complications.

Diabetes is the leading cause of blindness in adults. Too many GPs supervising diabetic patients not attending diabetic clinics forget to remind them to have annual eye checks (sadly, no longer free under the NHS). **Be sure to arrange annual eye tests. Since they are not part of a diabetic clinic's work, you will have to go to an optician or to an eye clinic.**

Self-Care

Diabetes is the supreme example of the value of self-care. Since it is a disorder of the body's use of the fuel we get from food, we always have to think about energy-in (eating) and energy-out (work and exercise) in relation to each other. Recently there has been a real revolution in the treatment of diabetes, with new tools for self-care and some techniques for treating complications if they do develop.

One of these tools is a blood test that can be self-administered at any time of day or night to find out how well your treatment plan is working. A drop of blood is obtained with an automatic spring-loaded finger lancet and the blood-glucose level is read from a test strip. The finger prick is practically painless with good equipment, and if the sides of the fingertips (rather than the central pads) are used. This self-blood-glucose-monitoring (SBGM) allows you to read your body signals with regard to food and exercise. It rewards you with immediate feedback. Self-blood-testing takes the mystery out of the daily chores of living with diabetes and puts the power of management of diabetes squarely in your hands. You can share your record with your supervising health professionals, who will help you stay up to date on new advances and make suggestions that fit your particular needs.

The British Diabetic Association can advise on the most suitable kit. Unfortunately you will have to pay for it yourself – it isn't provided by the NHS.

What are other daily tasks of self-care for the person with diabetes? They differ according to the type of diabetes. People with Type I have to take insulin injections two to four times a day, and they have to learn to match their food intake with their energy output and the dosage of insulin. There are many alternatives to choose from in accomplishing this difficult routine, including the use of insulin pumps, which are worn outside the body and can be programmed to give insulin automatically. The greatest daily hazard faced by people taking insulin is an unpredictable lowering of blood sugar (hypoglycaemia) called 'insulin reaction', which requires immediate ingestion of sugar.

People who have diabetes should carry medical identification at all times. Again, the BDA can provide information about bracelets, medallions etc., as well as cards to be carried in wallets or pockets.

Support Groups

The British Diabetic Association (see Organizations) is a very active body with branches all over the country which support and educate people with diabetes and their relatives. The Association runs holidays for children with diabetes and publishes up-to-date information on treatment and self-help. The Association's magazine (included in the annual subscription) is a model for other voluntary groups – readable, informative and attractively designed. It plays a part in educating diabetics about so-called diabetic foods, showing that they are unnecessary and expensive when there are plenty of alternatives.

Exercise

Exercise plays an important part in the self-care of people with diabetes. We are all familiar with the many reasons for remaining as active as possible throughout life (see Moving for Health chapter). In addition, persons with diabetes are at high risk for osteoporosis and must exercise in order to utilize the calcium in food to strengthen bones (see Osteoporosis chapter). For those of us with diabetes, exercise brings the added benefit of increased sensitivity of the body's cells to the actions of insulin.[12]

The management of exercise as a vital part of self-care differs for the two types of diabetes. For Type I diabetes, this means that in order to avoid having too much insulin when exercising, each individual has to learn how much to reduce insulin dosage and increase food intake in order to exercise safely. For Type II diabetes, exercise not only burns unwanted calories but also helps to overcome the inherited resistance to insulin. In fact, there are many people with Type II diabetes who have normalized their blood sugar by exercise, even though they do not lose all the weight they had gained over the years.

If I forget my exercise for two weeks, I am depressed and tired. When I exercise, I feel fine because my blood glucose is within normal range. So it's worth it to keep at it, though I've had to accept the fact that my body will never be really slim again. [a fifty-two-year-old woman]

In addition, those who make the switch to a more active life find it has lasting psychological benefits, although the routine may not be easy to establish.

I'd got really sluggish. When the doctor told me I must take more, regular exercise, I balked at the idea. I had to force myself to walk, then jog, then run round the park four or five times a week. But I did begin to feel better – buying some snazzy running gear probably helped! Then I began to realize that I wasn't feeling just physically better, but mentally more alert, too. As my blood sugar level dropped my spirits rose! [a forty-three-year-old woman]

Diet

Everyone says that diet restrictions are the most irritating part of living with diabetes. Today, however, dieticians are taking a new and more flexible approach to food for people with diabetes.[13] Most dieticians now recognize that social, cultural, and emotional habits of eating have to be taken into consideration, and that when people eat food, they are not necessarily thinking about nutrients. You can adjust your diet to include your preferences as well as your caloric needs, but you will need to know about the components of foods to do so. Your diet will vary depending on your age and general level of activity as well as general health and type of diabetes. For this reason, the services of a dietician can be of great value.

Most people who monitor their blood carefully and are willing and able to exercise vigorously can eat at least a little of almost everything.

There has been a move away from the severely restricted diet of the past, when carbohydrates were top of the hit list. The good news now is that the sort of diet we are *all* advised to follow – lower fat, more fruit and vegetables, wholemeal bread, beans and pulses, drastic reduction of sugar and salt – is the ideal diet for most people with diabetes, making family meals easier. It is really now only a small minority whose diet has to be so restricted as to constitute a hardship.

No Smoking

As well as adopting new diet and exercise habits, there is another vital self-care decision to be made. That is the decision not to smoke. Smoking does a great deal of damage to the body's circulatory system. Nicotine acts to constrict the smaller blood vessels and thus increases the risk of hypertension. Combining that hazard with the risk of damage to blood vessels from the high blood glucose and blood fats of diabetes is virtually inviting heart attacks, strokes, and other serious complications.[14] Therefore, although it may be difficult to quit smoking, doing so is a crucial investment in a longer, healthier life for those of us with diabetes.

USING THE HEALTH SERVICE

As with any illness or disorder, it's your GP who will refer you to a diabetic specialist if she thinks you may have diabetes – a suspicion she will probably have confirmed by having a test done on your urine or blood. At the Diabetic Clinic or department you will be given further tests and the type of diabetes and its severity will be assessed. You will then be given a prescription for insulin or suitable drugs, if necessary, and given advice about diet and life-style. Thereafter you should keep regular appointments with the clinic so that your progress can be monitored and treatment adjusted if necessary. If a consultation with the dietician is not suggested, ask for it, and make sure that you are given a diet sheet to take away with you. If you develop any unexpected problem between appointments, contact the clinic or your GP.

Diabetes and Stress Management

The way our bodies respond to stress goes back to prehistoric times when the threats were to life and limb, calling for quick energy for flight or fight. Chemical signals mobilize fuels stored in the liver and muscle and raise the heartbeat and breathing rates for rapid circulation of energy. This outpouring of glucose was fine when we had to run away from a lion, but it is not useful or healthy for a person who is caught in a traffic jam or angry with her boss. The rise in blood sugar, with no way to compensate for it through physical action, is not good for those of us who have diabetes. We need the support of people who are coping successfully in order to learn how to avoid stress and to minimize it when it develops.

Diabetes causes stress both for those of us who have it and for our families and friends. Maintaining the balance of food, activity, and insulin takes time and money and requires planning that limits freedom of choice and spon-taneity. Diabetes is yet another challenge to test our native adaptability and lifelong experience. Others may not understand why we have to eat right on time or why we have to avoid certain foods. We need to let them know what we need and why. We must respect our personal needs and learn to meet them even when they differ from the needs of those who share our lives.

NOTES

[1] National Diabetes Data Group, *Diabetes in America 1985*. NIH Publication 85-1468, National Institutes of Health, Rockville Pike, Bethesda, MD 20014, Chapter 1, pp. 3–4; and J. K. Davidson, *Clinical Diabetes*. New York: Thieme-Stratton, Inc., 1986.

[2] P. H. Bennett, 'The Epidemiology of Diabetes Mellitus', in *Diabetes Mellitus*, Vol. 5, H. Rifkin and P. Raskin, eds. A Diabetes Association Publication. Bowie, Md.: R. J. Brady Co., 1981, p. 87.

[3] National Diabetes Data Group, op. cit., Chapter 8, p. 1, and Chapter 9, p. 1; and American Diabetes Association, *1985 Fact Sheet on Diabetes*.

[4] National Diabetes Data Group, op. cit., Chapter 1, pp. 1–4.

[5]Bennett, op. cit., p. 92.

[6]E. A. H. Sims, 'Effects of Overnutrition and Underexertion on the Development of Diabetes and Hypertension: A Growing Epidemic?' in *Malnutrition: Determinants and Consequences*. New York: Alan R. Liss, Inc., 1984, pp. 151–63; and E. S. Horton, 'Role of Environmental Factors in the Development of Non-Insulin-Dependent Diabetes Mellitus'. *American Journal of Medicine*, Vol. 75, 1983, pp. 32–40.

[7]National Diabetes Data Group, op. cit., Chapter 1, p. 1.

[8]M. Rosenthal et al., 'Demonstration of a Relationship Between Level of Physical Training and Insulin-Stimulated Glucose Utilization in Normal Humans'. *Diabetes*, Vol. 32, 1983, pp. 408–11.

[9]National Diabetes Data Group, op. cit., Chapter 1, pp. 1–4.

[10]J. B. O'Sullivan, 'Body Weight and Subsequent Diabetes Mellitus'. *Journal of the American Medical Association*, Vol. 248, 1982, p. 979; and J. B. O'Sullivan, 'Gestational Diabetes: Factors Influencing the Rates of Subsequent Diabetes'. In Sutherland and Stowers, eds., *Carbohydrate Metabolism in Pregnancy and the Newborn*. New York: Springer-Verlag, 1979, pp. 425–535.

[11]American Diabetes Association, *1985 Diabetes Facts*.

[12]C. Bogardus et al., 'Effects of Physical Training and Diet Therapy on Carbohydrate Metabolism in Patients with Glucose Intolerance and Non-Insulin-Dependent Diabetes Mellitus'. *Diabetes*, Vol. 33, 1984, pp. 311–18.

[13]F. Q. Nuthall, 'Diet and the Diabetic Patient'. *Diabetes Care*, Vol. 6, 1983, pp. 197–207.

[14]US Office of the Assistant Secretary for Health and Surgeon General, *The Health Consequences of Smoking for Women*. Rockville, Md.: US Department of Health and Human Services, Public Health Service, 1983. US Government Printing Office, No. 410-889/1284.

BOOKS AND PUBLICATIONS

British Diabetic Association, *Balance*. Magazine included in annual subscription to BDA. (See Organizations.)

Jim Anderson, *Diabetes: A Practical New Guide to Healthy Living*. London: Macdonald Optima, 1981.

Dr Rowan Hillson, *Diabetes: A Beyond Basics Guide*. London: Macdonald Optima, 1987.

Dr Jim Mann and the Oxford Group, *The Diabetics' Diet Book: New High Fibre Eating Programme*. London: Macdonald Optima, 1982.

Sue Hall, *Cooking for Your Diabetic Child: From Lunch Box Snacks to Birthday Treats – Recipes for Children That All the Family Will Enjoy*. Wellingborough: Thorsons, 1988.

26
Gallstones and Gallbladder Disease

Gallstones are a common problem faced by many women in midlife. Women have a higher incidence of gallbladder disease than men. In the UK about one in five women and one in twenty men of sixty plus may have gallstones present. Certain ethnic groups appear to be more susceptible than others. In one study, 35 per cent of Mexican–American women had symptoms of gallstones by age sixty-five.[1] Such high rates in certain groups warrant special study and care.

Gallstones have been disparagingly labelled by some specialists as an affliction of women who are 'fat, forty, and flatulent'.[2] Some add 'fertile' to the list. This label discloses a bias against ageing women in general and fat women in particular. Because of these prejudiced attitudes, we must be certain that any recommendations for treatment are carefully considered and truly helpful, and not made just on the basis of stereotypes. We must be able to recognize this bias when it surfaces so that we can look for more enlightened care.

Symptoms of Gallbladder Disease

The gallbladder is a small sac located on the right side of the abdomen under the liver. It serves as a reservoir for bile, which is produced in the liver. Following a meal, the gallbladder contracts to release bile into the duodenum (the beginning of the small intestine), where it assists in the digestion of food.

Bile is made up of cholesterol, lecithin, bile salts, and bilirubin (yellowish pigment). When this balance is disturbed and there is too much cholesterol in the bile, the excess separates out in the form of hardened matter called stones, or very fine material called sludge or sand. One type of stone contains mostly cholesterol; another type contains mostly bilirubin (often called pigment stones). Some stones are a mixture of these two types.

Many common signs of indigestion (dyspepsia), such as belching, bloating, and heartburn, are rarely symptoms of gallbladder disease as well. But such signs should be investigated early on, especially if accompanied by nausea, acute pain, fever, chills, vomiting, or jaundice, which are the most common indicators of gallstones, and possible infection.

Once formed, if a gallstone stays in your gallbladder, you usually suffer no pain or only mild pain, belching, bloating, or nausea. Any pain would probably be caused by the stone rubbing against the lining of the gallbladder, producing irritation and inflammation. However, if the stone lodges in the cystic duct, the bile duct, or the pancreatic duct (see illustration), you will suffer severe pain in the upper abdomen (often more pronounced on the right side) which travels through to the back and under the right shoulder blade. This pain, known as biliary colic, comes on suddenly, frequently, after a meal, and usually remains very intense for several hours.

THE BILIARY DUCTS

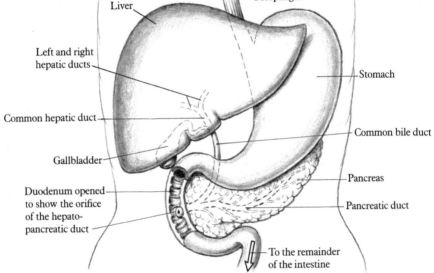

In addition, when a stone is lodged in the cystic duct, the gallbladder becomes inflamed (a condition known as cholecystitis), and fever, nausea, and vomiting may develop. When the stone lodges in the common bile duct, jaundice and infection of the liver may develop. In either duct, the stone can block the draining of bile from the gallbladder into the small intestine. If a stone obstructs the pancreatic duct, it may cause severe inflammation and the destruction of the pancreas. Pancreatitis, as this complication is known, is a potentially fatal condition.

If the gallstone can enter the duodenum, it passes out in the faeces and causes no further problem. If an attack of biliary colic subsides spontaneously, a stone that was temporarily lodged in a duct may have passed into the duodenum or passed back into the gallbladder.

What Causes Gallbladder Disease?

Dietary Factors. While many gallstones are caused by an overabundance of cholesterol in the bile, there is no direct relationship between the amount of cholesterol in the diet or blood and the cholesterol content of the bile. Cholesterol not only comes from the food we eat, but also is manufactured within the body. Some studies claim that a high-cholesterol diet has not been firmly linked to gallstone formation – but a correlation has been found between gallstones and a diet high in calories and sweets. Yet high-calorie diets are high-calorie often because they contain high amounts of fat, which in turn contains high amounts of cholesterol. Still, cutting down on cholesterol (though that kind of modification is recommended for prevention of coronary artery disease) does not seem to prevent gallstones altogether.[3]

There is conflicting evidence as to the connection between a diet high in *saturated* fat and gallstone formation.[4] Some studies find a significant correlation and others do not. However, saturated fats do bring about gallbladder attacks, as follows: fats stimulate the pancreas to produce certain hormones, which in turn cause the gallbladder to contract. The contracting gallbladder may force stones out into the ducts, where they create the symptoms of a gallbladder attack. *Thus, a low-fat diet is crucial for the treatment of an already diseased gallbladder.* It should be noted here that the most common symptoms of fatty food upsets, such as indigestion, belching, and bloating, are seldom caused by gallbladder disease. Indeed, the simultaneous presence of gallstones and indigestion is usually a matter of chance. For example, in one study, only twenty-four of 142 women who complained of 'chronic indigestion' had gallbladder disease.[5] It is therefore critical to establish that gallstones are indeed the culprit before surgery is considered.

Many fat women are warned to follow a strict weight-reduction programme once they suffer a gallbladder attack in order to prevent further attacks. The amount of cholesterol in the bile is greater in fat people than in thin people. The cholesterol level in the bile may increase further during weight loss and then stabilize at a lower concentration when a lower weight level is maintained. Therefore, alternately losing and gaining weight increases the risk of gallstone formation.[6]

In addition, it is likely that the high fat and sugar content of a high-calorie diet sets off gallbladder attacks in fat women, rather than excess weight itself.[7] Thin or average-weight people who ingest a lot of fat are also vulnerable to gallbladder attacks. It is cruel and unfortunate that in our 'thin society' the fat woman with gallbladder disease is made to feel that her weight caused her medical problem, and that therefore she is her own worst enemy.

Studies show contradictory results regarding the effect of wheat fibre on cholesterol metabolism. Oat bran has been shown to have some effect on lowering cholesterol. Foods high in sulphur, such as cabbage, asparagus, Brussels sprouts, celery, cauliflower, onions, and radishes, stimulate the flow of bile and may be included in both prevention and management programmes. Some experts recommend adding supplements of lecithin, taurine and methionine (amino acids), copper, vitamin B_{12}, folic acid, vitamin C, and magnesium to a low-fat diet to increase the solubility of bile.

Some holistic nutritionists believe that gallbladder disease may be related to food allergies, especially to eggs. Some suggest that the gallbladder can be stimulated to flush and clean out sludge, although this is not effective with large stones. Others say they will not supervise such a programme because of the danger that a piece of stone will get lodged in a duct and require emergency surgery.

Unfortunately, an improved diet, though promoting health in many ways, does not seem to dissolve gallstones that have already formed. Thus, changing your diet does not reduce the risk that a stone will block a duct and cause serious complications. However, avoiding fatty foods does help *prevent symptoms* when stones are present.

Hormonal Factors. Oestrogen appears to raise the fat content of bile, which in turn contributes to the formation of gallstones. A 1974 study showed that women taking oestrogen after menopause were *two and a half times* more likely to develop gallstones than women not taking oestrogens.[8] This study was virtually ignored in the wake of controversy over oestrogen as a carcinogen and in the promotion of oestrogen as a prevention for osteoporosis. The 1979 US National Institutes of Health Consensus Conference on Oestrogen Replacement Therapy did list gallbladder disease as a risk of taking oestrogen, but said more study was needed.

The incidence of gallbladder disease is high in women who use oral contraceptives, in pregnant women and in women who have had several pregnancies, because oestrogen level is high during pregnancy. The incidence of gallbladder disease in the US among women was even higher between 1961 and 1971, before the amounts of oestrogen in the oral contraceptives were reduced.[9] Oral contraceptives and oestrogen are not recommended for anyone with gallstones, gallbladder disease, or liver disease, or for anyone who drinks a lot of alcohol.

Diagnosis

Many people who have not reported symptoms of gallbladder disease are often discovered to have gallstones when they undergo tests or an X-ray for other, unrelated reasons. Currently the most widespread diagnostic test is an abdominal ultrasound. A machine emitting sound waves is moved over the abdomen, and the rebounded echoes are recorded on a machine that shows an outline of the gallbladder and any gallstones that may be present. This test involves no pain, no exposure to ionizing radiation, or known danger. Until recently, the most popular diagnostic test was an oral cholecystogram, which is still used in questionable situations after an ultrasound shows no stones or structural irregularities. Sometimes a cholecystogram shows poor gallbladder functioning when the dosage of dye given for the test is too low. If the test is repeated with more dye, and the gallbladder is still not clearly outlined, then poor functioning of the gallbladder is assumed.

Treatment Methods

In many cases, gallstones may never cause any problems at all – or any severe enough to warrant removal of the gallbladder. Studies of autopsies in the US show that 20 per cent of women who never had their gallbladder removed had gallstones at the time of death.[10] This raises several questions: will 'silent' gallstones that are not producing symptoms cause problems later? What, if anything, should be done about them and when?

In 1985, of 475,000 people in the US who had their gallbladders surgically removed, 69 per cent of them were women.[11] Removal of the gallbladder (cholecystectomy) and hysterectomy are the most frequently performed unnecessary operations. While the removal of the gallbladder is sometimes necessary, in other instances the decision of whether and when to operate is not so clear. Is removal of the gallbladder, like hysterectomy and oophorectomy, recommended frequently because it is a good learning experience for surgeons-in-training? Do some doctors recommend the operation as a good way to silence the complaints of a woman who is 'just a menopausal whiner'? Are doctors assuming that every complaint by a middle-aged woman is related to the menopause and ignoring signs of gallbladder disease until the last minute, when surgery is necessary?

What is clear in any case is that when a gallstone is lodged in a duct, immediate hospitalization and (usually) prompt surgery are required. This condition is potentially life-threatening. But when you have a 'silent' gallstone – one that is causing no symptoms, or only mild, painless symptoms – the gallstone does not necessarily have to be treated with medication or removed surgically. Many women with a silent or painless gallstone simply follow a prudent low-fat diet and undergo no further treatment.

Many surgeons advise the removal of a gallbladder with silent gallstones because they may cause life-threatening complications in the future by lodging in a duct. Every individual must weigh the risk and pain of surgery against the risk of developing these complications.

Two and a half years ago, an X-ray for a slipped disc showed a number of stones the size of chick peas. An ultrasound confirmed the stones and a lot of sludge, and I was strongly advised to have surgery right away. In retrospect, I had been having symptoms of fatty food intolerance for a long time. I did not want to have major surgery since I would be moving across the country to start a new job in a month. When I moved I found a good woman GP and told her that I knew I might face an emergency if a stone lodged in the duct and became infected. She encouraged me to wait until the balance of problems outweighed my not wanting to have surgery, and encouraged diet changes. So I waited. At the end of the second year, I became sick with a fever and weakness and pain. That was the signal that the time had come. I had the surgery six weeks ago. I believe the surgery was then necessary and I am also glad I waited. [a forty-year-old woman]

Some experts consider cancer of the gallbladder a threat if gallstones are left untreated, though others do not.[12] A study was done at the University of Michigan on 123 faculty members with silent gallstones. It was found that over fifteen years none of them died of gallstone complications or developed cancer of the gallbladder. Only sixteen of the 123 developed symptoms of biliary colic. The researchers concluded that very few people with untreated silent gallstones will die from gallbladder disease and that an elective cholecystectomy need not be considered unless attacks of biliary colic occur.[13]

A person with gallstones who also experiences abdominal discomfort or mild pain, especially after a fatty meal, should be considered in the category of people with 'symptomatic' gallstones. Someone who has had one or more attacks of biliary colic that have subsided spontaneously (which means that a gallstone was temporarily lodged in a duct and then either passed back into the gallbladder or passed out to the duodenum) also faces a dilemma about whether or not to have surgery.

I had two attacks while away on holiday. The symptoms were excruciating. Pain in the upper abdomen and across the back made me wonder if I was having a heart attack. During the second attack I went to the hospital. They called my symptoms biliary colic and said they were due to fine sand [a form of stones] in my gallbladder, which I should have surgically removed. They described the complications that could occur if I didn't do so, that is, that sand could slip out of my gallbladder into the ducts and cause infection, requiring emergency surgery. This presented me with a terrible dilemma. Since my condition was not life-threatening at the moment I decided to go back home for further opinions there. The second opinion I received concurred with the need for surgery. The third opinion argued that the presence of sand did not require immediate surgery. This consultant did not want to operate on me, since I was very fat, and recommended weight loss and a fat-restricted diet. I went along with the third opinion and have been well now for five years. [a fifty-five-year-old woman]

For two years I suffered with flatulence, belching, and stomach aches that were mild but annoying. Tests did not reveal gallstones, but the registrar suspected them from my symptoms. He wanted them surgically removed. The surgeon refused to operate on stones that weren't visible on the tests. I initially decided that a low-fat diet was preferable to the pain of surgery and the time I would need for recuperation. However, I found that maintaining such a strict diet was enormously stressful and ultimately decided in favour of surgery. Was I ever glad I did! The surgery revealed multiple stones that might have caused me complications. [a forty-nine-year-old woman]

For years I was uncomfortable after eating the least amount of fat and had to watch myself like a hawk. Gallstones were never diagnosed. Finally, after a severe attack of biliary colic, my doctor suggested gallbladder surgery, though no stones could be seen at all in my tests. The surgery revealed that sludge [fine sand] had lodged in the common duct and that the pancreas duct and gallbladder were also infected. I was furious that the diagnosis of gallbladder disease hadn't been made earlier, for if surgery had been done earlier I might have been spared all this infection and post-operative discomfort. [a fifty-six-year-old woman]

I could not face the possibility of ever again having an attack like this one. I dreaded the presence of little demons inside me threatening to strike again at the least expected moment. So I insisted on surgery, and do you know, I sailed through it with no complications, despite my age? They found thirty-two small stones in my gallbladder! Now I guess it took me longer to recuperate than a younger person with this same surgery, but that's to be expected at my age and with my medical problems. [an eighty-two-year-old woman]

Alternative Holistic Treatments

Some people who have gallstones find that alternative holistic treatments, such as acupuncture and imagery, have helped them (though not in emergency situations, when a stone is lodged in a duct).

An acupuncturist stimulates specific points on the body by inserting needles, applying heat, pressure massage (acupressure), or a combination of these methods.

During my acute gallbladder attacks my friend massaged my back to give me some relief from the agony I was experiencing. As she touched a certain point in my back I asked her to dig in deeply to reach the pain inside. She did so and the pain suddenly disappeared, totally and completely, in these few seconds of deep pressure. I embarked on a series of acupuncture sessions. This felt similar to the experience when pressure relieved my pain. The acupuncturist I chose said that acupuncture was unlikely to dissolve the stones, but could possibly rectify the bile imbalance and other physical dynamics that were forming them. I haven't been troubled by any gallbladder attacks since that series and I attribute it, in part, to this treatment, along with careful diet and imagery work. [a fifty-five-year-old woman]

Imagery is a technique that encourages the body to fight disease by visualizing the body as a strong heroine overpowering the disease. The same woman continues:

I was familiar with the use of imagery to fight cancer, and use imagery regularly myself to relax or envision how a design project will look when completed. It comes easily to me and I believe in it. So I imagined my bile salts armed with spikes shattering the stones that were plaguing me and excreting them effortlessly out of my body. I did this imagery work daily during the six weeks I was undergoing acupuncture. It made me feel less anxious about my condition because I felt I was doing something that could potentially cure me.

Surgery

A cholecystectomy is considered by doctors to be a simple operation. An incision is made below the right rib cage; the gallbladder is removed, and the abdomen is explored for any problems not related to the gallbladder. Your surgeon should not remove your appendix unless you give your consent in advance. If the presence of a stone in the common bile duct is suspected, or if there has been an infection, a small plastic drain that protrudes through the surgical wound to the outside of the body is left in place for several days. As with any abdominal surgery, you may have several days of pain and discomfort.

Most people are able to return to work and normal activity two to four weeks after the operation. Some people complain of difficulties with digestion after a cholecystectomy, because bile will be entering directly into the duodenum without the gallbladder to time its entry. On rare occasions, a stone may form in the common bile duct, necessitating another operation.

The likelihood of complications from gallbladder surgery depends on your age, your general physical health before surgery, your surgeon's skill, and the length of time it takes to perform the operation. The older you are, the more likely you are to experience complications. If you are jaundiced and infected at the time of surgery, the likelihood of complications also increases. The most common among these are infection (which can usually be controlled with antibiotics), pneumonia and other lung problems, phlebitis, clots in the lung, and operative errors. A hernia may develop at the site of the incision.

Several new experimental methods of treatment are currently being studied. Percutaneous ultrasonic lithotripsy (PUL) involves inserting a catheter through the skin, which traverses the liver into the cystic duct and from there into the gallbladder. A collapsible basket attached to the catheter snags the gallstone and removes it. The gallbladder is left intact. The advantage of this procedure is that only local anaesthesia is required, and you can return home the same day and get back to work and normal activity immediately. It thus costs considerably less than surgery, does not require hospitalization, and inflicts minimal discomfort.

Drugs to Dissolve Stones

No drug has been found yet that dissolves all gallstones without other injurious effects, though many are being tried singly or in combination. Synthetic bile acids include chenodeoxycholic acid (chenodiol or CDCA or Chendol) and ursodeoxycholic acid (UDCA). In one study of CDCA,[14] gallstones were completely dissolved in only 13.5 per cent of those who received 750 milligrams daily and in 5.2 per cent of those who received 375 milligrams daily. When the drug worked, it usually did so within nine months. Drug-induced diarrhoea was common but responded to treatment. A more serious problem was that the drug altered liver function and caused liver inflammation in many patients, more severely in those on the higher dose of CDCA.

UDCA is more effective but is expensive, since large daily doses are required for six to twelve months. In 85 per cent of patients taking 600 milligrams per day, cholesterol stones smaller than 15 millimetres in diameter were completely or partially dissolved.[15] The drug caused very little diarrhoea and appeared to carry no risk of liver damage.

The currently preferred drug, mono-octanoin, usually requires three to twenty-one days to dissolve cholesterol duct stones but is successful only one-third of the time, irritates the gastrointestinal and biliary tracts, and may cause pain, nausea, and vomiting.[16]

Another experimental procedure involves placing a catheter through which methyl tertbutyl ether (MTBE) is infused into the gallbladder to dissolve the stones in place, without removing the gallbladder.[17] Careful studies are needed to confirm the safety over time of the use of this toxic substance.

Another experimental method for treating gallstones uses a combination of bile-acid drugs and very loud shock waves from a machine called a lithotriptor already used to smash kidney stones. The procedure is administered under anaesthesia because it is potentially painful. This method was not successful for everyone in the first small study, but only for those with cholesterol stones no larger than 25 mm and a functioning gallbladder. Damage to nearby organs is possible, but did not occur in this study.[18]

To date, drugs are not being seen as a general panacea for dissolving gallstones, but as an alternative for the sufferers who cannot or will not undergo cholecystectomy.[19] If you are taking any of these drugs, it is imperative that you have blood tests of the liver at regular intervals to detect any possible damage. You should also bear in mind that even if gallstones are completely dissolved, they may recur once you've stopped taking the medication. Having to take the drugs for a long time may be a serious drawback since they are expensive and their long-term effects are not known.

NOTES

[1]Kenneth M. Weiss and Craig L. Hanis, 'All "Silent" Gallstones Are Not Silent'. *The New England Journal of Medicine*, Vol. 310, No. 10, 8 March 1986, pp. 657–8.

[2]Quoted in 'The Gold Bladder (Gallbladder)', Chapter 1 in Siegfried Krat and Robert Boltax, *Is Surgery Necessary?* New York: Macmillan, 1981. Now available in paperback from New American Library.

[3]'The Gallbladder and Gallstones, Part 1'. *Harvard Medical School Health Letter*, Vol. II, No. 9, July 1977.

[4]L. J. Bennion and S. M. Grundy, 'Risk Factors for the Development of Cholelithiasis in Man, Part 2'. *The New England Journal of Medicine*, Vol. 299, 1978, pp. 1221–7; R. K. R. Scragg, L. J. McMichael and P. A. Baghurst, 'Diet, Alcohol, and Relative Weight in Gall Stone Disease: A Case Control Study'. *British Medical Journal*, Vol. 288, 1984, pp. 1112–19.

[5]'The Gallbladder and Gallstones, Part 1', op. cit.

[6]L. J. Bennion and S. M. Grundy, 'Effects of Obesity and Calorie Intake on Biliary Lipid Metabolism in Man'. *Journal of Clinical Investigation*, Vol. 59, 1975, pp. 996–1001.

[7]Bennion and Grundy, op. cit; Scragg, McMichael and Baghurst, op. cit.

[8]Boston Collaborative Drug Surveillance Program, 'Surgically Confirmed Gallbladder Disease, Venous Thromboembolism, and Breast Tumors in Relation to Postmenopausal Estrogen Therapy'. *The New England Journal of Medicine*, Vol. 290, 1974, pp. 15–19.

[9]Ann Jarnfelt-Samsioe et al., 'Gallbladder Disease Related to Use of Oral Contraceptives and Nausea in Pregnancy'. *Southern Medical Journal*, Vol. 78, No. 9, September 1985, pp. 1040–3.

[10]American Medical Association, *Family Medical Guide*. New York: Random House, 1982, p. 489.

[11]Statistics from the National Center for Health Statistics.

[12]P. Goulin and L. M. Preshow, 'Silent Gallstones'. *Medicine North America*, Vol. 20, 1985, pp. 2676–80.

[13]W. A. Garcie and D. F. Ransonhoff, 'The Natural History of Silent Gallstones'. *The New England Journal of Medicine*, Vol. 307, 1982, pp. 798–800.

[14]L. J. Schoenfield et al., 'Chenodiol (Chenodeoxycholic Acid) for Dissolution of Gallstones. The National Cooperative Gallstone Study. A Controlled Trial of Efficacy and Safety'. *Annals of Internal Medicine*, Vol. 95, 1981, pp. 257–82.

[15]Tokyo Cooperative Gallstone Study Group, 'Efficacy and Indications of Ursodeoxycholic Acid Treatment for Dissolving Gallstones'. *Gastroenterology*, Vol. 78, 1980, pp. 542–8.

[16]Erwin K. Kastrup et al., eds., *Facts and Comparisons*. St Louis: J. B. Lippincott Co., 1986, p. 315e.

[17]M. J. Allen et al., 'Rapid Dissolution of Gallstones by Methyl Tert-Butyl Ether'. *The New England Journal of Medicine*, Vol. 312, No. 4, 24 January 1985, pp. 217–20.

[18]Tilman Sauerbruch et al., 'Fragmentation of Gallstones by Extracorporeal Shock Waves'. *The New England Journal of Medicine*, Vol. 314, No. 13, 27 March 1986, pp. 818–22.

[19]M. C. Bateson, 'Dissolving Gallstones'. *British Medical Journal*, Vol. 284, 1982, pp. 1–2.

BOOKS AND PUBLICATIONS

G. C. L. Lachelin, *Liver Disease and Gallstones: The Facts*. Oxford: Oxford University Press, 1988.

Dr Malcolm Bateson, *Gallstones and Liver Problems*. Wellingborough: Thorsons/British Medical Association, 1988.

27
Vision, Hearing, and Other Sensory Loss Associated with Ageing

Our senses – sight, hearing, smell, taste, and touch – connect us to the world outside ourselves. There are substantial differences from one person to the next, but most of us can expect the acuity of our senses to dim somewhat as the years pass. Usually changes occur so slowly that we adapt without being aware of the differences in perception.

Someone else may be the first to point out to us that we don't seem to be hearing or seeing as well as we once did. We might lose our appetite before we notice that our sense of taste or smell has diminished. Our sense of touch may become less dependable for such formerly rote tasks as fixing the clasp on a necklace, separating notes in a wallet, or turning pages.

While all of the above may seriously interfere with our efficiency and enjoyment, the most serious effects of sensory losses have to do with health and safety. Changes in our sense of touch may result in burns due to failure to withdraw from a hot surface in time. Older persons are actually less sensitive to changes in temperature. As a result their body temperature may drop to a dangerous level (hypothermia) before they are aware of it. Changes in the sense of balance increase the risk of falling and injury.[1]

Some changes are genetically determined; some are influenced by injuries or environmental factors, such as exposure to noise; some are caused by illness or disease. Some change is inevitable with ageing, but no one should settle for a medical dismissal of her concerns as 'simply ageing' without a careful diagnosis of the cause of any changes in vision, hearing, or other senses. There *are* things we can do when we recognize changes in our senses.

Vision Changes

At this very moment, your eyes and your brain together are producing the images you are now perceiving on this page. The eye has the ability to adjust to see near and far objects, shading and colours, and variations in lighting from almost complete darkness to sudden emergence into light.

Most people retain good vision into their older years and don't need to worry about losing their sight. For some of us, though, changes in vision, whether minor or quite serious, can bring troubling changes in our lives. Age-related changes in vision occur in two primary areas of the eye: the lens and the retina.

Presbyopia is the term used to describe slowness in changing the focus from far to near, stemming partly from the loss of elasticity in the lens.[2] The eye's ability to accommodate for near distances starts diminishing at age ten, but not enough for us to take notice of it until about age forty or so. According to medical textbooks, the loss in flexibility of focus is usually fixed by age fifty-five to sixty, though there are ways to promote flexibility. With proper correction (reading glasses, bifocals, contact lenses) and/or self-help eye exercises, sight can be restored to normal.

I now wear bifocals – originally an embarrassment – and find reading increasingly tiring, a big problem for someone who has been a compulsive reader since childhood. [a fifty-year-old woman]

I really thought they had changed the size of newsprint. I complained that they were making the type size of phone books and the eyes of needles smaller to save money. I'd never had any problems with vision before, so it was a slow realization that it was really me that was changing. [a woman in her seventies]

If you need simple magnification in both eyes and have no other conditions that require correction, it is tempting to try over-the-counter reading glasses, which may now be available in some shops. Always begin with the weakest glasses with which you can read. These glasses do not correct for any other visual problems, nor do they allow for differences in each eye. If you don't have regular checks, you are at risk of having a serious eye disease overlooked. It is for this reason, as well as the obvious commercial ones, that opticians do not recommend over-the-counter glasses. Unfortunately NHS eye tests are no longer free for most of us.

But do not neglect regular eye exams: a complete eye examination is important to check for glaucoma and other serious eye diseases and may detect other undiagnosed systemic conditions such as diabetes and hypertension. Everyone over forty should have her eyes checked every year by an ophthalmologist or optician and a test for glaucoma should be performed at every eye examination of persons over twenty-five, though this is not always offered. The intra-ocular-pressure reading test takes only a few seconds, but good diagnostic procedure requires, in addition, taking a family history, checking for structural abnormalities, and viewing the optic nerve with an ophthalmoscope, a flashlight-like instrument that allows the eye-care practitioner to see the optic nerve at the back of the eye. If you have a family history of glaucoma, or have had test results which are borderline or glaucoma-suspect, you should have your eyes tested at more frequent intervals.

Minor problems, such as excess tearing and dry eye, can become annoying as we age. Eyelid skin becomes thinner with age. Because the lid skin does not hug the eyeball as tightly as it once did, drainage function may be affected. Increased sensitivity to wind, light, and/or temperature can cause over-production of tears. If you tear easily, you can help yourself by more frequent blinking and other exercises to relax your eyes (some women wear large-lensed sun glasses in cold or wind),[3] and for dry eyes, by using artificial tear or lubricating drops. Do not use drops that 'get the red out' (called vasoconstrictors). These are not helpful for dry eyes and can even lead to some types of glaucoma in predisposed individuals.

Self-Help Alternative for Healthy Eyes

THE BATES METHOD

This system of eyesight training, sometimes called Vision Therapy, claims that defects in vision are not irreversible: many are due to tension and poor function of the muscles that control the accommodation of the eye to different distances. Accordingly, exercises aimed at retaining flexibility of these muscles, plus relaxation techniques, are suggested by advocates of the method.[4]

To rest and focus your eyes, try:

Blinking: Blink about once per line when reading, and always when a change of focus is needed, as when looking up from reading or if you experience any momentary blur.

When reading or doing close work: Look off and focus on something at a distance for about five seconds, at least every five minutes to keep your eye muscles from stiffening.

Palming: Lean your elbows on something to support them, then close your eyes and cover them with your palms. Breathe and relax. With your mind, either observe your breath, counting in-out cycles of ten, or visualize as clearly as possible pleasant memories and/or fantasies. Include as many of your senses as you can. Do this whenever your eyes feel tired, including once before you sleep.[5]

NUTRITION FOR HEALTHY EYES

Growing interest in the role of nutrition as a factor in preventing eye disease has prompted some new research which is still in a fairly preliminary stage. For example, one study found a lower incidence of cataracts in people who ate a diet high in antioxidants, that is, vitamin E, vitamin C, and beta-carotene.[6]

Eye Care Practitioners

There is some confusion about the role and function of the various practitioners concerned with our eyes.

Most people's first contact with various branches of this profession is the optician – but here, too, there can be confusion. An *ophthalmic optician* is qualified to examine eyes, without the use of drugs, for abnormal vision problems not due to disease. She can prescribe, fit and supply glasses or contact lenses. She is permitted to test for glaucoma. If she suspects this or any kind of eye disease she should refer the person to her GP or an ophthalmologist. An *optician* is a skilled technician who can dispense and fit glasses prescribed by an ophthalmologist.

An *ophthalmologist* (known in the past as an oculist) is a doctor who has specialized in the examination of the eye, and in the prevention, diagnosis and treatment of its defects and diseases. She is also qualified to perform eye surgery.

Eye tests are no longer free, but pensioners on Income Support may be exempt from charges. If you think you have eye problems, you can be tested by an ophthalmic optician, and if she finds no sign of eye disease she will prescribe suitable glasses. This is as far as most of us need to go. The prescription she supplies can be dispensed either at the same firm, or, if you prefer, you can take her prescription to another optician. National Health Service glasses are now not available for most adults (see Chapter 16) so many are faced with the need for spectacles but are unable to pay for the now quite expensive frames. The cost of lenses is more or less standard from optician to optician, but the price of frames can vary, so it is worth shopping around.

If on test, signs of disease are found, you will be referred to the ophthalmology department of a local hospital.

Diseases of the Eye

Four diseases are the principal causes of visual impairment and blindness in older persons: cataracts, glaucoma, macular degeneration, and diabetic retinopathy.[7]

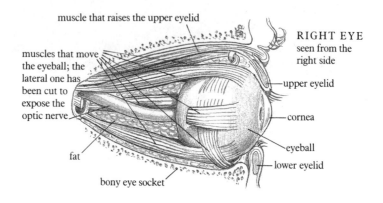

muscle that raises the upper eyelid

muscles that move the eyeball; the lateral one has been cut to expose the optic nerve

fat

bony eye socket

RIGHT EYE
seen from the
right side

upper eyelid

cornea

eyeball

lower eyelid

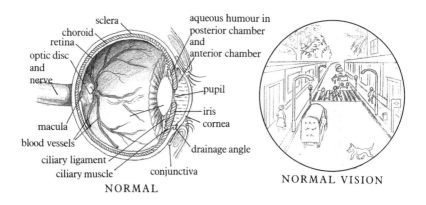

sclera

choroid

retina

optic disc and nerve

macula

blood vessels

ciliary ligament

ciliary muscle

aqueous humour in posterior chamber and anterior chamber

pupil

iris

cornea

drainage angle

conjunctiva

NORMAL

NORMAL VISION

Cataracts involve no pain or discomfort, just less clarity. Gradually the lens of the eye becomes cloudy until there is no longer enough light passing through to the retina to focus a clear image. Vision becomes hazy or blurred and sensitivity to light and glare increases. Sometimes cataracts are caused by injury, radiation exposure, infections, or inflammation within the eye, but by far the most common type is associated with ageing. Around 90 per cent of people over sixty-five have some evidence of cataracts.

Not all cataracts develop to the point where removal is necessary. Some people can live with considerable loss of vision; others may have their livelihood or hobbies threatened by even mild vision loss. There is no need to have surgery unless you experience vision loss that seriously limits your activities.[8] Before agreeing to cataract surgery, be sure to ask whether other eye problems exist which could seriously interfere with vision. Cataract surgery

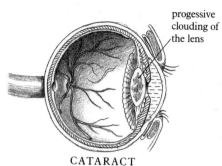

progessive
clouding of
the lens

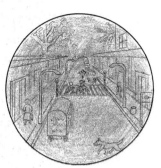

CATARACT

BLURRED VISION

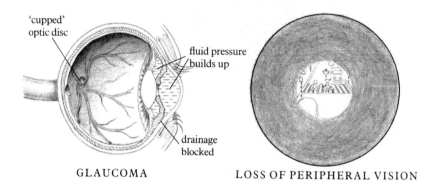

'cupped'
optic disc

fluid pressure
builds up

drainage
blocked

GLAUCOMA

LOSS OF PERIPHERAL VISION

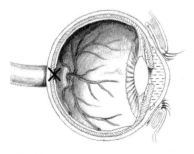

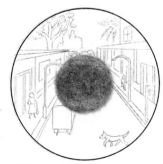

MACULAR DEGENERATION

LOSS OF CENTRAL VISION

should not be performed unless vision will be significantly improved.[9] Given a long life span, a person is more likely to undergo a cataract operation than almost any other surgery. And according to one report, no other operation in medical practice is as dramatically successful so much of the time.[10] Sight is restored after removal of the lens by implantation of an artificial plastic lens (during the same surgical procedure as the removal), or by wearing eyeglasses or extended-wear contact lenses. The contacts or implanted lenses restore a full field of vision; there may be some distortion with glasses.

Glaucoma is one of the more common and potentially severe eye disorders in people over forty.[11] Glaucoma occurs when there is too much fluid pressure in the eye, causing internal eye damage and gradually destroying vision. It is a myth that glaucoma inevitably leads to blindness. With *early detection* and *prompt treatment*, it can usually be controlled and blindness prevented.

Chronic Wide-Angle or Open-Angle Glaucoma (75 per cent of glaucoma cases) seldom produces early signs, and usually there is no pain from increased pressure. Symptoms can include blurred vision that comes and goes, difficulty in adjusting to dark rooms, and reduced side vision. Testing for glaucoma should be part of every routine eye examination but not all ophthalmic opticians provide it. Try to find one who does.

Chronic glaucoma is more common among blacks.

I first noticed a spot six years ago. I thought it was a spot on my glasses but it was still there after I cleaned my glasses several times. I believe that eyes are precious and have always taken care of mine so I went to my GP who referred me to an ophthalmologist. He said I had glaucoma in one eye and started me on medication, but it did not bring the pressure down enough. Laser therapy was new then but I was willing to try it. Then two years later the pressure started in the other eye so I had laser therapy in that eye also. The pressure is down now but I will have to stay on medication for the rest of my life. [a seventy-one-year-old black woman]

Treatment for chronic glaucoma involves bringing down the pressure in the eyeball as quickly as possible with eyedrops and oral medication. This treatment continues throughout life and, with regular checkups to monitor progress, usually ensures that no further loss of vision will take place. If the drugs fail to reduce the pressure, the eye-care practitioner may recommend surgery (usually done with a laser beam) to create an artificial drainage channel.[12]

In **Acute Glaucoma** (about 25 per cent of glaucoma cases), a sudden blockage occurs in the network of tissue between the iris and the cornea that is called the drainage angle. In far-sighted people, the distance between the cornea and the iris is shorter than normal and the drainage angle narrower, thus making it more likely for pressure to build up.

Sometimes preliminary (subacute) attacks occur, but usually with no permanent damage to vision. Early symptoms of acute or subacute glaucoma are foggy vision, coloured rainbows around lights, sudden pain in the eyes, headache, nausea, and vomiting. In an acute attack, permanent loss of vision can occur, especially if treatment is neglected. Early treatment is essential. If you experience such symptoms, go **immediately** to your doctor or to the Emergency Department of your hospital. Emergency treatment consists of eyedrops to bring the pressure down, followed within a day or two by a surgical procedure called an iridectomy, in which a small piece of the iris is removed to relieve the pressure. This is usually done with a laser beam.[13] Laser therapy is sometimes done preventively in persons who may be predisposed to acute glaucoma because of an especially narrow drainage angle in the eye.

Retinal Disorders. The retina is a thin lining on the back of the eye made up of receptors that receive visual images and pass them on to the brain. Retinal disorders include macular degeneration, diabetic retinopathy, and retinal detachment. These are the major causes of blindness.

Age-Related Macular Degeneration. The deterioration of the macula, a centre spot in the retina responsible for sharp colour and fine-detail vision, is more common in women than in men. It is the most common cause of vision loss in adults over fifty-five years of age. Side vision is usually retained. Macular degeneration is thought to be caused by a breakdown in the supply of blood to the retina. An early sign of macular degeneration is wavy distortion of horizontal or vertical lines. Check yourself periodically by looking for a few seconds at a line of print, a door, or a stairway to see if this occurs. Use an object with strong contrast such as light colour against black. Sometimes laser therapy can help with one form of macular degeneration, but it must be done promptly. A variety of low-vision aids (magnifying glasses, telescopic glasses, light-filtering lenses, and electronic devices) can in many cases compensate for visual difficulties.

Diabetic Retinopathy was uncommon a few decades ago. Improved survival rates for diabetes mean that many diabetics live to suffer complications of the disease. Diabetic retinopathy is at present the leading cause of new blindness in the United States for adults ages forty-one to sixty. Early diagnosis increases the chances of controlling this disease of the retina's blood vessels and eye fluid (see Chapter 25).

It never occurred to me that I would ever become blind. Even knowing I had diabetes and knowing it was a possibility, I still never believed that it would happen to me. [a fifty-three-year-old woman]

Detached Retina. Frequent eye complaints include spots that seem to swim in front of the eye; these so-called 'floaters' are common and usually insignificant, caused by changes in the eye's vitreous fluid. **Warning:** Sudden, new, or unusual floaters that do not move or flashes of light or loss of side vision may indicate a torn or detached retina. Get emergency medical attention at once: go to the Accident and Emergency Department at your local hospital, where you should get sent on to a consultant immediately.

I developed floaters in my eyes and was told I'm at high risk for detached retina. My father lost his sight in one eye. I'm a visual person, I love colour and nature and beauty, and blindness terrifies me. I don't want to go crazy if it happens, so to compensate I'm learning touch typing, flute, and drums. [a fifty-four-year-old woman]

Degrees of Vision Loss

Very few people actually lose all their vision to the point of not seeing light or dark. Three primary degrees of vision loss are:

Low Vision: Imperfect vision that cannot be improved with conventional eyeglasses or other medical or surgical means. Low-vision aids, such as telescopic lenses, can help the wearer use her remaining vision, but do not restore vision to near 20/20. About half the people with low vision are over sixty-five.

Severe Visual Impairment: Inability to read ordinary newspaper print, even using glasses; 4 per cent of older people in the community and 26 per cent of those in nursing homes have severe visual impairment.

Legal Blindness: Defined as 20/200 vision (or less) in the better eye as corrected by glasses, or as having peripheral field (side vision) of no more than 20 degrees diameter or 10 degrees radius.[14] Of the 1 to 2 million legally blind Americans, 70 per cent are over the age of sixty.[15] Many British people resist being labelled 'registered blind', yet it is a status that makes one eligible for a number of concessions and allowances.

GETTING HELP

There are many skills in getting around and managing on one's own with a loss of vision. These can be learned with help from others. The ability of eyes to adjust to changing amounts of light diminishes somewhat with age. Dark glasses reduce visibility; yellow shades cut glare without reducing visibility. Night driving can be a problem, but glancing at the left side of the road instead of at oncoming headlights, installing halogen headlamps, wearing yellow shades and keeping the windscreen clean can help. Having to give up night driving can be isolating if our community doesn't have public transportation or if we are reluctant to ask for help.

I had to learn patience. I used to wait until the last minute to jump into the car to do an errand or to meet someone. Now I have to make a lot of time for whatever I am

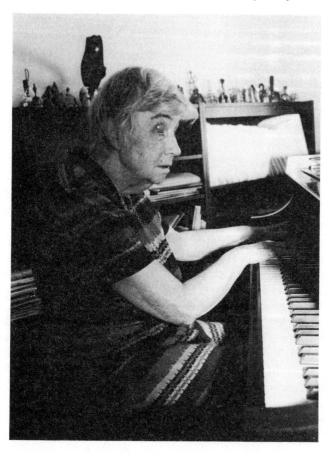

doing because I either go on a bus or by cab or I have to ask someone to pick me up. These all take some time and waiting. [a fifty-three-year-old woman whose vision loss started at age fifty]

Local Social Services Departments or local societies for blind people acting as agents for the local authority are responsible for compiling registers of blind or partially-sighted people in their area. A consultant ophthalmologist completes a certificate of examination and the health authority forwards the necessary information to the local authority.

Once registered, a blind or partially-sighted person is entitled to: a portable VHF radio from the British Wireless for the Blind Fund, distributed by the Social Services Department; a reduced-price TV licence; Braille and Moon type books sold by the Royal National Institute for the Blind; free loan of such books from the National Library for the Blind; the British Talking Book Service (recorded books on tape cassettes); special equipment and aids (through RNIB); a guide dog if suitable, through the Guide Dogs for the Blind Association; holidays organized through Social Services or the RNIB; travel concessions; voting concessions; and some other services. It is therefore essential to be in contact with the Royal National Institute for the Blind, either directly or through the Social Services Department.

For information on benefits, etc. see Chapters 14 and 16.

Hearing Impairment in the Older Years

As we reach our fifties and sixties it is increasingly likely that we will experience some degree of hearing loss: 25 per cent of people over sixty-five and 40 per cent of those over seventy-five have some degree of hearing impairment.[16] Severity of loss tends to be greater for men than for women.

Hearing loss is invisible; thus it is often overlooked by others, who would be more helpful if they were aware of the problem. Because hearing loss begins so gradually, we ourselves may not be aware of it for some time. We may gradually begin avoiding situations with groups and/or with a lot of background conversation or noise. We may appear to go on with our lives as usual but become progressively more isolated. Even a mild-to-moderate hearing loss can be isolating. We may go through a grieving process in stages similar to mourning a death before we can accept ourselves as having a hearing impairment.[17]

I have hearing loss and cannot hear speech when there is competing loud noise. That means I cannot talk to anyone in the clubs, a primary social gathering place for gay women. It has become an impossibility for me to carry on conversation in any public place (restaurant or club) where there is competing music in the background. The louder sounds mask or distort the voices of my companions. I am reluctant to go to these social gathering places and am becoming more of a stay-at-home. I feel increasing stress in wanting and needing social contact with other women and at the same time having consciously to avoid the very places where I am most likely to meet people. [a fifty-year-old woman]

For those of us who have not experienced any hearing loss, it is difficult to comprehend the isolation and frustration experienced by someone who is losing one of her major sensory connections to society, and along with it, access to information and social cues.

My two hearing aids help in communication, at least sometimes they do. Often the light, particularly enjoyable part of the conversation doesn't get through. The punch line of the jokes gets lost. The resulting smile, if I produce one, is artificial. I may use the occasion to educate my hearing friends. Other times I don't. At least my judgment

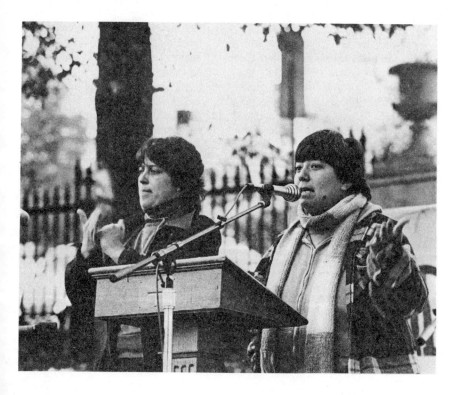

of others is tempered as I remember how often I was thoughtless about hearing problems before I had one of my own.

And I think of various ways by which I can experience lightness, relaxation. Since my sight is adequate, foreign movies in the cinema or on TV with English subtitles are a godsend for me. There we are, all of us, whether we can hear well or not, using those subtitles together. It makes me feel more part of the group. [an eighty-two-year-old woman]

TIPS FOR TALKING WITH A PERSON WITH A HEARING DIFFICULTY[18]

1. Don't talk from another room or from behind her.
2. Reduce background noise. Turn off radio or TV if possible.
3. See that the light falls on your face, so she can use visual clues.
4. Get her attention before speaking. To help her focus attention, address her by name and state the subject before beginning, as, 'Marge, we are discussing plans for the picnic. Will you bring salad?'
5. Face her directly, and on the same level if possible.
6. Keep your hands away from your face. Avoid speaking while you are smoking or eating.
7. Don't shout. Speak naturally but slowly and distinctly – and continue that way without dropping your voice.
8. She may not hear or understand something you say. If so, try saying it in a different way rather than repeating.
9. Recognize that she will hear less well if tired or ill.
10. Be patient. Even hints of irritation or impatience hurt.
11. Be an attentive listener. It's probably easier for her to talk than to listen.

Sensitivity on the part of others is crucial. Those of us who have hearing loss, and others of us who have close friends or family members with hearing loss, have learned a variety of skills to improve communication. It should be accepted practice for all cultural and political events to be signed for the hearing-impaired. Regrettably, this is still the exception and still requires strong advocacy on the part of every one of us.

The Structure of the Ear and How It Works

The ear is an intricate structure that can process and distinguish over 350,000 different sounds. Sound is funnelled into the ear canal and transmitted by vibrations to the eardrum where it is pushed along through the middle ear by bones known, because of their shapes, as the hammer (malleus), anvil (incus), and stirrup (stapes). It is the stirrup that starts the fluid in the cochlea of the inner ear vibrating. The hair cells then convert sound energy to electrical impulses which telegraph sound interpretations through the nervous system to the brain.

The cochlea looks like a spiral seashell and has approximately 25,000 sensitive hair cells lined up on its membrane. The mechanism by which pitch is discriminated can only be theorized at this time, but it seems to depe '

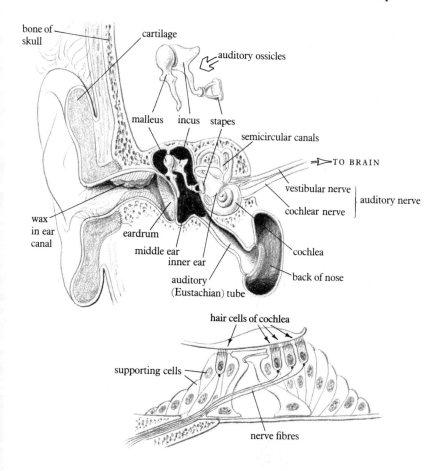

which hair cells are stimulated. Those cells near the base of the cochlea are the high-note cells and those farther along are the lower-frequency ones. Changes in the inner ear, particularly the loss of hair cells associated with high-frequency hearing, have been shown to accompany the ageing process. Loss of hair cells is irreversible and occurs throughout our lives from exposure to jet takeoffs, loud music, machinery, and a myriad of other recreational and occupational noises we encounter.

The loud sound systems at rock concerts and in clubs really impair hearing, and should be a health concern for everyone. Tests of hearing in the population at large show that the hearing of people in their twenties and thirties has already begun to deteriorate, and is often as impaired as that of older people. Unless young people take steps to protect their hearing, hearing impairment in old age will increase even more in the decades to come.

RECOGNIZING AND ACKNOWLEDGING THE SIGNS OF HEARING LOSS

As a slight hearing loss progresses to the point where we become aware of missing much of what is going on, we may react to the first signs of hearing loss with disbelief and denial. Before we can act to help ourselves we must come to terms with our feelings of loss and the consequent change in our image of ourselves.

I can't say exactly when it started. Hearing and understanding telephone conversations is the first difficulty I recall. I found myself asking people to speak up: 'This is a poor connection.' Sometimes an abrupt silence followed my comment, indicating it had not been entirely appropriate. 'I must be more attentive. It's not considerate to the other person for me to let my mind wander while talking.' The next clue was that I could hear when someone spoke to me from another room but I could not understand what was said, and it made no difference how loud the person was speaking. A year or two or three passed and these two problems became worse before I took action. [a woman in her fifties]

Signs of hearing problems to look out for in ourselves and others:

- Consistent difficulty in hearing over the telephone or hearing the telephone ring:
- Saying 'What?' or 'Please repeat' frequently;
- Leaning forward or tilting head to hear better;
- Preferring the television louder than others do;
- Complaining that others are mumbling;
- A ringing in the ears or feeling a blockage.

If our hearing loss develops slowly, we may be the last to become aware of it. Family members and close friends are usually the first to notice the problem because they find themselves raising their voices when speaking. The advance of the loss is almost imperceptible to the one experiencing it. But even a mild loss is well worth checking out. There are hearing aids geared to all kinds of losses, and hearing specialists who can instruct us on ways to improve overall communication.

The degrees of hearing loss are:

Mild	Difficulty hearing faint speech
Moderate	Frequent difficulty hearing normal speech
Severe	Can understand only very loud or amplified speech
Profound	Cannot hear very loud or amplified speech

A common misperception is that hearing loss is a simple reduction in the volume level of sound. This is true for a conductive loss – but not for the type of loss caused by very gradual but irreversible changes in the inner ear.

The main types of hearing loss are:

Conductive Hearing Loss, which involves blockage or impairment of the structures of the outer or middle ear so that sound waves are not able to travel properly. Packed ear wax, extra fluid, abnormal bone growth, or infection can cause this condition. The symptom: your own voice sounds abnormally loud and other voices sound muffled. Flushing the ear, medication, or surgery may correct the condition.

I started going deaf at about age thirty-six. I was examined by an ear, nose, and throat specialist and by an audiologist and both thought it was nerve deafness, which my mother also had. I didn't know to question the diagnosis at that age. I tried several kinds of hearing aids, which helped only a little. I had four or five really tough years until another audiologist told me she didn't think it was nerve deafness and suggested that I go to another doctor. What I had was otosclerosis – a tiny growth which prevents the stirrup from vibrating and so causes conductive deafness. I had an operation called a stapedectomy in one ear when I was forty-two. At that time they used an artificial material to replace the stirrup. When they did my other ear last year they actually used a bit of my own ear lobe. I had a little dizziness for a week or two each time and then it went away. I can hear normally now. [a fifty-eight-year-old woman]

Sensorineural Hearing Loss, caused by damage to the inner ear and/or the nerve pathways to the brain. A high fever or severe infection, head injury, use of certain drugs, vascular problems, and lengthy exposure to loud noises are among the causes. This condition cannot usually be treated medically or surgically. A hearing aid can improve hearing of those with sensorineural loss but won't restore hearing to normal. For some, speech reading and aural rehabilitation can be beneficial.[19] Aural rehabilitation classes teach how to use one's remaining hearing to best advantage by positioning oneself with the better ear toward the speaker, using light and vision effectively, etc. This can be done with or without a hearing aid.

Some hearing loss is temporary and may just go away. Aspirin in large doses (20 to 30 per day), sometimes prescribed for arthritis, may cause a temporary hearing loss. Switching to a non-aspirin product will often remedy the problem. Discuss this with your doctor.

Age-Related Hearing Loss (Presbycusis), a sensorineural hearing loss, and the most common type among older persons. As we grow older, many of the hair cells of the inner ear disappear or wither, causing words to sound mumbled. In most cases there is an increasing loss of sensitivity to high-pitched sounds.

I went to a violin and piano concert and I only heard the piano! [a woman in her eighties]

The symptoms vary, but often people with presbycusis have a problem with 'speech discrimination', or the ability to understand words when spoken loud enough to be easily heard. For example, the words 'sail', 'fail' and 'tail' all begin with high-pitched consonants; with this type of hearing loss, it would be difficult to tell them apart.

Manipulating the Environment

Once we get used to the idea of having a hearing loss, we can learn to help ourselves by arranging the environment to enhance the hearing we still have.

For many of us hearing is not a problem in an ideal quiet environment with well-articulated face-to-face conversation. At home we can sit facing others and can use sound-proofing materials such as carpets and soft furnishings to improve the acoustics. Also, there are many sound-amplifying devices that can be attached to the telephone, television, radio, alarms, doorbell, etc. In addition, visual signalling can be used when you can't depend on hearing. Devices such as a 'moonbeam alarm clock' or smoke alarms that light up your bedroom are available. Ask your hearing-aid dispenser how to order such devices or contact the Disabled Living Foundation (see Organizations).

Manipulating the outside environment is more difficult. What we can do is physically to position ourselves to maximize lighting and acoustics.

At home or away, we can ask people we are conversing with to repeat sentences more clearly and slowly, and to emphasize consonants. We can learn to deal with impatient people, be persistent in our requests for clear speech, and learn to listen better ourselves.

I began confronting the reality that my hearing acuity was less than normal. I quietly but firmly informed friends, relatives, peers, supervisors, and clients that I had a partial hearing loss and needed them to face me, to speak more slowly and distinctly and in lower tone ranges.

Prevention

Unfortunately, GPs working in the NHS are seldom able to offer complete checkups, and therefore it is only when you go to your GP because you are experiencing hearing impairment that you will be referred for specialist assessment. (Private screening services such as that offered by BUPA do include hearing tests.) If screening for pure-tone sensitivity is not done routinely,[20] make sure to report your difficulty to the GP as soon as you notice it – if you wait too long the condition could develop too far for medical help.

How to Seek Help

When your doctor refers you for examination at the Ear, Nose and Throat (ENT) department of a local hospital, tests will be performed to establish what your difficulty is and what remedy – medicine, surgery or a hearing aid – is appropriate. You may be tested by an audiometer which emits carefully calibrated pure tones as well as recorded or live voice speech. It precisely measures and records a patient's hearing threshold, the quietest level at which a person can hear a specific sound stimulus 50 per cent of the time. Doctors may use audiological test results to diagnose specific hearing problems. This testing is particularly significant because it can be repeated over time to detect changes in hearing.

The audiologist may help the doctor evaluate test data to determine whether you would benefit from a hearing aid and in some cases may recommend a particular type. For example, some hearing devices amplify only those frequencies which you need to have amplified. If you tried a hearing aid in the past and were not able to use it, you may want to try again, as they have been improved a great deal in recent years, especially in their capacity to screen out background noise.

Marketing of hearing aids without proper professional testing has resulted in some useless and distressing 'aids', many very costly, being bought by people dissatisfied with NHS aids. If you are dissatisfied with your NHS aid, go back to the department that provided it, in case replacement or adjustment can be made. Some older people have found that they can only get a really satisfactory aid by 'going private' – if you are tempted to do this make sure that you go to a firm recommended by an audiologist or ENT specialist. Sadly, since many of these aids are imported and ear moulds and suitable adjustments are difficult to make, the cost is far beyond the means of many older people.

Adapting to a hearing aid can be trying because, in most cases, all sounds are amplified – not just the sounds you want to hear. It takes time and practice to learn when and where and how to use your hearing aid.

The first few weeks almost convinced me that I wanted only to retreat into 'my silent world' and manage as best I could. It was like living in a noisy factory. It was a constant bombardment of sound, and all of it too loud! Finally all the fine adjustments were made and now I can enjoy films and concerts and theatre again. I can hear my grandchildren as they learn to make sounds and form words and conversation.

All is not as before though. Large gatherings of people are simply noisy confusion. Driving my car with the window down is very tiring emotionally because of the assault of noise, and I must regularly visit the dispenser to adjust the aid. [a fifty-eight-year-old woman]

If you do buy a 'private' aid, the firm should offer a trial thirty-day period during which you may reject the aid, and you should be covered by the firm for any adjustments and further tests necessary during the first twelve months. After that you should return for annual checks, for which you will have to pay.

Services for the Deaf

Some Social Services Departments employ special workers with skills in working with deaf people. All Social Services Departments provide services for those handicapped by hearing loss, providing information about local and national organizations, and aids such as flashing doorbells and telephone light signals, and can arrange special audio equipment through British Telecom. They can usually provide an interpreting service for important situations. There are three categories of deafness recognized for administrative purposes – the deaf without speech who need to use British Sign Language, signs supporting English, finger spelling, mime, gesture or writing; the deaf with little or no speech even with hearing aids and who lip-read; the hard-of-hearing who have some useful hearing with or without aids, and who can communicate by speech, listening and lip-reading. The majority in this third category are people in middle or old age. Social Services Departments liaise with voluntary groups such as the Royal National Institute for the Deaf (RNID) and the British Deaf Association. The former can provide residential care for elderly, profoundly deaf people, and help with holidays for this group. The RNID is a valuable source of general information for deaf people and has a technical department offering advice on hearing aids and other technical devices. The British Deaf Association has over 170 local branches, and an information and library service (for addresses see Organizations).

NOTES

[1]Jeffrey R. M. Kunz, *The American Medical Association Family Medical Guide*. New York: Random House, 1982, pp. 720–1.

[2]Gay Becker et al., *Vision Impairment in Older Persons*, Policy Paper No. 9, 1984. Aging Health Policy Center, University of California, San Francisco.

[3]Personal communication, R. G. Gordon, DBO (Diploma of British Orthoptists), vision therapist.

[4]Ibid.

[5]Ibid.

[6]Personal communication, Allen Taylor, Ph.D. Laboratory for Nutrition and Cataract Research at the USDA Human Nutrition Research Center on Aging. Tufts University, Boston, MA 02111.

[7]Becker, op. cit., p. 10.

[8]'Cataracts'. *Health Letter*. The Public Citizen Health Research Group, Vol. 3, No. 3, March 1987, pp. 1–6.

[9]Ibid.

[10]T. J. Liesegang, 'Cataracts: What They Are, What to Do About Them'. *Mayo Clinic Proceedings*, Vol. 59, August 1984, pp. 556–622.

[11]Kunz, op. cit.

[12]Ibid., p. 322.

[13]Ibid., pp. 320–1.

[14]Fran A. Weisse and Mimi Winer, *Coping with Sight Loss. The VISION Resource Book*. Watertown, Mass.: Vision Foundation, p. 3; and Jane Porcino, 'Vision Capacity of Women Over Forty', in *Growing Older, Growing Better*. Reading, Mass.: Addison-Wesley, 1983, pp. 301–2.

[15]Personal communication, Annette Maleson, Massachusetts Commission for the Blind.

[16]Gay Becker et al., *Management of Hearing Impairment in Older Adults*, Policy Paper No. 13, 1984. Aging Health Policy Center, Room N631, University of California, San Francisco, CA 94143.

[17]Beatrice A. Wright, *Physical Disability: A Psychological Approach*. New York: Harper, 1960. Quoted in Maurice H. Miller, 'Restoring Hearing to the Older Patient: The Physician's Role'. *Geriatrics*, Vol. 41, No. 12, December 1986.

[18]Reprinted with permission from the Boston Women's Health Book Collective, *The New Our Bodies, Ourselves*. London: Penguin, 1989.

[19]*Aging Notes*, US Senate Special Committee on Aging, 8 January 1985, p. 2.

[20]Maurice H. Miller, 'Restoring Hearing to the Older Patient: The Physician's Role'. *Geriatrics*, Vol. 41, No. 12, December 1986.

BOOKS AND PUBLICATIONS

John Dobree, *Blindness and Visual Handicap: The Facts*. Oxford: Oxford University Press, 1982.

Eyecare for the Elderly. Free leaflet. Optical Information Council, Temple Chambers, Temple Ave., London EC4Y 0DT.

Royal National Institute for the Blind, *Information for People Losing Their Sight*. Free leaflet. (See Organizations.)

RNIB, *Running Your Own Home*. (See Organizations.)

Glaucoma. Free leaflet – send s.a.e. International Glaucoma Association, Kings College Hospital, Denmark Hill, London SE5 9RS.

Visual Handicap Advisory Service, Disabled Living Foundation: pamphlets, publications, bibliography. (See Organizations.)

Margaret Ford, *In Touch with Cataracts*. London: Age Concern.

Robert Slater and Mark Terry, *Tinnitus: A Guide for Sufferers and Professionals*. Beckenham: Croom Helm, 1987.

Susan Natrass, *Sound Sense: How Local Groups Can Help Hard of Hearing People*. London: Age Concern.

Age Concern, *Why Do People Mumble So Much?* Free leaflet.

28
Memory Lapse and
Memory Loss

As we grow older, some of us find ourselves becoming more forgetful. We notice that we cannot remember names as easily, forget errands, or often misplace keys or household items. Frequently what we notice is not a memory loss but a memory lapse. It simply takes us longer to retrieve names, addresses, and dates from our memories than it used to. When this happens in our older years we may see it as a sign of age and become flustered, frustrated, embarrassed, or angry with ourselves. We may even think this forgetfulness could be a sign of senility.

When I'm with friends of my age and I forget a name of something – we laugh. That makes it easy. Not so when I'm with younger people. For example, when I'm giving information to a salesperson – I know where I live but occasionally I have to think a minute to remember my address. And I always feel as though they're looking at me thinking, 'Oh, this senile old thing.' I'm not senile! Now I just say to myself, someday they'll be my age and they'll know what this is like. [a seventy-three-year-old woman]

The dictionary definition of *senility* is 'a loss, associated with old age, of mental faculties'. But the word has no real meaning, because it has become a catch-all term for any forgetfulness or mental disorder experienced by an older person. Until recently doctors assumed that senility was an inevitable part of old age. This assumption kept them from identifying and treating true memory disorders.

Alzheimer's disease is gradually replacing senility as a specific focus of our concerns. Media coverage of Alzheimer's can lead to unnecessary fears over signs of forgetfulness. This emphasis on the negative – on potential losses as we get older – can make us feel that forgetting names or misplacing objects is more significant than our interests, our knowledge, and our wisdom gained over the years. It also obscures research that shows that some intellectual abilities often increase with age.[1] It is important to put memory changes into perspective and to understand the differences between normal forgetfulness and memory disorders. We want to stop feeling uneasy about forgetfulness – but we also want to know when to seek help.

There are three categories of memory lapse or memory loss associated with age.

1. Normal forgetfulness, *benign senescent forgetfulness*, is part of the normal ageing process. But it does not necessarily worsen with the years and does not interfere with our lives in any significant way or endanger our health.

2. Memory loss related to disorders or conditions such as depression or malnutrition. These conditions and the resulting memory loss are reversible and can and should be diagnosed and treated.

3. A disease of the brain, *late-life dementia*, or *senile dementia*, not normally part of the ageing process. It is irreversible and progressive, preventing the individual from carrying out even simple responsibilities. Late-life dementia needs medical diagnosis and special care. The most common form of late-life dementia is Alzheimer's disease.

The difference between normal forgetfulness and the early stage of Alzheimer's disease is not always clear-cut. But in Alzheimer's disease memory loss becomes progressively worse and is accompanied by a general decline in intellectual abilities and changes in behaviour.

Benign Senescent Forgetfulness

Throughout our entire lives, beginning at birth, the brain loses nerve cells that are not replaced through regeneration. From around age fifty, parts of the brain can show other signs of change, such as cell tangles (abnormal protein substances in nerve cells, also known as neurofibrillary tangles) and senile plaques (degenerated nerve cells that form scars). These changes can be accompanied by a decline in memory, but for many of us such a decline never occurs, and we can continue to live well into our eighties and beyond experiencing little or no change in our mental vigour.[2]

It is not known why some of us experience a decline in memory and others do not. But our brains, like other parts of our bodies, differ from person to person because of genetic factors and in response to emotions and to physical and environmental changes.

Throughout our lives, including our older years, fatigue, anxiety, inattention, stress, and depression can cause moments of memory lapse or periods of memory decline. As we grow older we also become particularly vulnerable to changes in our social situations. Deaths of loved ones, relocation to an unfamiliar place, or increased social isolation can bring about emotional changes that trigger forgetfulness, confusion, and disorientation. Diseases and physical disorders can be accompanied by emotional distress that can lead to increased forgetfulness, especially when treatment in an unfamiliar place, such as a hospital or nursing home, is required. A loss of sight or hearing contributes to mental confusion by restricting a person's knowledge of the world around her and by putting additional stress on already weakened learning abilities and memory. Eye and ear impairments can also worsen a sense of social isolation or actually cause us to avoid social contact, possibly bringing about depression and a decline in mental functioning. These causes of forgetfulness, confusion, and disorientation are reversible, and mental capacities can return to normal after an adjustment period with proper medical treatment or sometimes with the help of friends and family.

HELPING OURSELVES REMEMBER

Often we notice ourselves being forgetful for no apparent reason. Our memory changes can become bothersome to the point that some of us develop strategies for remembering. We avoid interruptions when concentrating on a task, knowing that distracted attention can be detrimental to our work. We write lists and notes to ourselves instead of relying on our memories. We adjust our surroundings to help us find objects (including our lists) more easily.

In the morning when I wake up I go through what I call a name exercise. I have various friends whose faces come before me, and then I go through that exercise of recalling the names I need for the day, up to ten or twelve at a session. I find that very useful. Sundays before going to church, I try to recall many names of church members who may be present so that they're fresh in the front of my memory. I do this same exercise before I go to meetings or social gatherings. In my bedroom I have my cupboards organized so I can find things. I even organize my refrigerator! [an eighty-six-year-old woman]

An orientation area can also be helpful: a room or corner with a calendar and bulletin board for written reminders, and a place to keep essential items such as glasses, keys, umbrella, and writing accessories. Such a special area can save energy we would otherwise waste in being upset over forgetting, losing, or misplacing something.

Disorders and Drugs that Can Lead to Memory Loss

A number of specific disorders and drugs can lead to memory loss and mental confusion. These effects are not limited to the elderly, but the older brain is more vulnerable to them. *Most of them are reversible and should be identified and treated.* Correct diagnosis is extremely important, since the mental symptoms of these disorders often resemble those of Alzheimer's disease and can be misdiagnosed as Alzheimer's or as 'senility' and left untreated.

Sometimes a person hospitalized because of some apparently medical condition is found to be suffering from the effects of a huge variety of medicines, each of which has been prescribed without relation to the others she is taking. Once off the medication, she recovers mental function.

ORGANIZE, DON'T MEMORIZE³

What to buy and tasks:
Make a list rather than relying on your memory. Keep a pad available to jot down items as needed.

Taking medication:
Place medication in a special receptacle each night for the following day. When you see the receptacle is empty, you know the medication you have taken.
or
Use containers (paper cups, saucers, an empty egg carton, or boxes sold for this purpose), each marked for the day of the week. This is especially helpful if you take different medications on different days. (Caution: Do not leave medications within the reach of children.)

Turning off the cooker, removing the laundry, leaving on time for an appointment:
Use a timer with a bell, or wear a watch with a timer. Set it for the appropriate time, and take it with you around the flat or house so you will be sure to hear it.

Names and ages of grandchildren, names of friends and acquaintances:
Write the grandchild's name and date of birth under each photo in a photo album or frame. Write names under pictures of friends. Periodically look through your address book to refresh your memory or to recognize a name you are trying to think of.

Paying bills:
Place all bills to be paid in one place. Mark on your calendar the date on which to pay the bills. Cross off the reminder after you pay the bills.

Ask your local librarian for books on techniques for remembering. And remember: *You don't have to remember everything.*

Depression. Some of the symptoms of depression include a slowing of movement and speech, slowing of thought, changes in sleep and eating habits, decreased pleasure in activities, underestimation of one's true capacities, and low self-esteem. Depression is probably the disorder most commonly misdiagnosed as Alzheimer's disease, particularly when low self-esteem causes poor results in tests for brain damage, depression and other conditions. The profound changes in thinking and memory sometimes associated with depression have been called *pseudodementia*. However, thorough neurological and neuropsychological examinations usually differentiate depression from dementia. The two are different in both onset and behaviour. The onset, or beginning, of depression is usually more sudden than the slow and gradual process of Alzheimer's disease. And a depressed person is more likely to

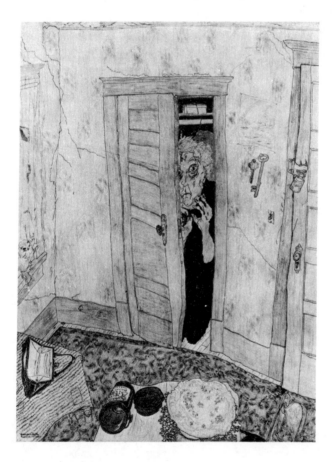

exaggerate her or his difficulties, while a demented person will try to hide, deny, or minimize them and usually will not be aware of her declining mental abilities. In many cases of pseudodementia there is a previous history of depression. There are currently a number of very effective treatments for depression, and a hospital department with experience in treating older persons should be consulted if this is suspected.

Drugs and Alcohol. As we grow older our tolerance for drugs (including prescription medicines and over-the-counter preparations) and alcohol decreases and our reactions to drugs may differ greatly from those of younger people. Certain drugs alone, as well as alcohol alone, can affect mood, memory, and speed of reactions. Alcohol can worsen depression, and drugs or alcohol can worsen the symptoms of Alzheimer's disease. Chronic, long-term alcohol abuse may lead to serious decline in memory and other cognitive functions. Recent studies have also shown that drugs that diminish or inhibit acetylcholine, a chemical in the brain, can produce significant memory loss in the elderly.[4] Such anticholinergic drugs include several prescription medications and over-the-counter remedies for diarrhoea, nausea, and coughs. The older we get the more likely we are to be taking numerous drugs simultaneously to treat medical conditions or chronic diseases.[5] The brain is very vulnerable to drug interactions that can produce symptoms similar to those of dementia. Drugs are often necessary and valuable, but we need to be aware of the possible negative effects of any drug, *including over-the-counter remedies*, and of what the effect may be when we take two or more drugs at the same time, or combine a drug with alcohol.

Nutritional Deficiency and Anaemia. As we age we may develop health problems that can cause malnutrition and anaemia. Also, some of us develop poor nutritional habits because of physical infirmity or loneliness. A restricted budget can limit our choice of fresh and wholesome food, and weakness, frailty, or infirmity can make us reliant on others for transportation, food shopping, and food preparation. One or a combination of these factors can lead to malnutrition. Malnutrition (especially a vitamin B_{12} and folic acid deficiency) or anaemia (a shortage of red blood cells and/or low haemoglobin content of these cells) can cause a person to appear disoriented and confused, to have severe memory lapses, and even to appear delusional. These deficiencies can be ruled out by blood tests and corrected by an adequate diet and supplements and by treating any underlying health problem.

Diseases and Other Health Problems. Some diseases and physical conditions can cause memory loss and mental confusion. These include thyroid disease, diabetes, kidney or liver problems, lung disease, gallstones, and syphilis. Other health problems such as heart and lung ailments, feverish conditions, and even constipation can cause mental confusion. Generally speaking, as we grow older we are less likely than before to develop specific symptoms when we become ill. We may become confused or withdrawn instead.

Brain Disorders. Disorders of the brain or central nervous system that can lead to memory loss include Parkinson's disease, a single stroke, brain tumour, trauma to the brain, subdural haematoma (bleeding in the brain because of trauma), and hydrocephalus (abnormal increase in the fluid surrounding the brain). Often these disorders can be treated, and timely treatment can prevent further damage.

Late-Life Dementia

Late-life dementia refers to a group of diseases of the brain that most frequently afflict those over sixty-five. The dementia influences all aspects of behaviour, not only memory but also judgment, temperament, and social interaction. Late-life dementia is a neurological disorder (a disorder of the nervous system), not a psychological disorder, and it has nothing to do with a person's previous intelligence, education, or mental health. An estimated 90 per cent of all late-life dementias are primarily caused by two irreversible conditions: multi-infarct dementia and Alzheimer's disease.[6]

Multi-infarct Dementia

Multi-infarct dementia is a condition of the brain caused by many small strokes. A stroke is a rupture or blockage of a blood vessel in the brain, which stops the flow of blood and destroys an area of brain tissue by depriving that area of oxygen and other necessary nutrients. The accumulated damage of many small strokes leads to an inability to function in various ways, depending on which parts of the brain are damaged. The mental and behavioural symptoms of multi-infarct dementia can be identical to those of Alzheimer's disease. However, multi-infarct dementia may also involve early signs of physical dysfunction, such as impairment of vision or sensation and muscle weakness or paralysis. The condition may begin abruptly and can be episodic, with short-term improvements and exacerbations. (This contrasts with Alzheimer's disease, which is hardly noticeable at first and progresses gradually.) Risk factors for multi-infarct dementia include atherosclerosis, previous strokes, heart attacks, severe chest pains (angina pectoris), high blood pressure, and diabetes. High blood pressure should be treated in order to prevent further small strokes (see Hypertension chapter).

Multi-infarct dementia is preventable to the extent that we can prevent heart disease, strokes, and diabetes by not smoking and by drinking alcohol only in moderation, exercising regularly, eating well, and getting early treatment for high blood pressure.

Multi-infarct dementia alone makes up an estimated 15 to 20 per cent of late-life dementias. It can also occur in conjunction with Alzheimer's disease.[7]

Alzheimer's Disease

I'm going to fight it. Now what I do is write down everything I want to do. As I get them done I mark them off. Also I read a lot. This is the way I'm fighting it. It makes me so mad that every day I pound the table with my fist, because I don't want to be like this. I'm going to fight it every way I can. I'm stubborn. [a seventy-two-year-old woman in an early stage of Alzheimer's disease]

Since Alzheimer's disease, alone or in conjunction with multi-infarct dementia, makes up an estimated 75 per cent of cases of late-life dementia, the term *Alzheimer's disease* has come to be the term most frequently used for late-life dementia. It is often abbreviated as SDAT (Senile Dementia of the Alzheimer Type). It afflicts an estimated 5 per cent of those over sixty-five, rising with age to approximately 20 per cent of those over eighty.[8] The incidence is expected to triple as the number of elderly people increases within the next three generations. It is more common in women than in men (two to one), although this seems to be a result of women's longer life span. Alzheimer's disease ranks as the fourth or fifth leading cause of death in the United States.[9] Currently dementia, of which Alzheimer's is the major cause, afflicts an estimated 4 million Americans.[10]

Abnormalities in the chemistry of the brain and changes in the structure of brain cells prevent nerve cells from functioning. The cell tangles and senile plaques that occur in normal ageing (see p. 540) are more frequent and widespread in Alzheimer's disease. As more and more cells degenerate and parts of the brain die, the person's functioning deteriorates.

STAGES OF ALZHEIMER'S DISEASE

At the beginning of the disease relatively few brain cells are affected, and the symptoms of memory loss may be noticed only by the victim herself* or, more typically, by a partner or employer. The victim may begin to forget once-familiar names or where she has put things, have difficulty finding words, become withdrawn, lose energy, anger easily, or avoid the unfamiliar. These can be signs of the first stage of Alzheimer's disease. But since an increase in forgetfulness can also be a part of the normal ageing process, it should not cause concern unless it grows progressively worse and is accompanied by other symptoms which noticeably reduce the person's ability to carry out everyday activities.

---

*Since more women than men have Alzheimer's disease, the afflicted person is referred to as 'she' throughout the text although the information applies to men also.

I first began to suspect my mum might have Alzheimer's when I noticed a marked change in her personality. I was getting all kinds of nasty notes and telephone calls from her. She would call me thirteen times a day asking the same question. She couldn't remember what day it was and couldn't remember to take her medication. She was getting angry, frustrated, and more and more forgetful. [a thirty-eight-year-old woman]

When forgetfulness *is* a sign of Alzheimer's it will eventually be accompanied by rambling and repetition in conversation, lack of concentration, difficulty with orientation and travel, and spatial disorientation. These symptoms signal a more advanced stage of the disease. At this stage most people will no longer consciously recognize the symptoms and may deny them, since their reasoning and judgment become impaired. However, some people may have periodic insight into their deficiencies and become depressed or frustrated by them. The depression, frustration, or anxiety can, in turn, complicate the symptoms.

As the disease progresses the person may forget the names and faces of intimate family members; become disoriented in the home, or wander off and get lost; become unable to drive a car; become emotionally unstable and irritable; become incontinent; and eventually forget how to speak, eat, dress, and use a toilet. Some become agitated and occasionally abusive and assaultive while others may become increasingly withdrawn and apathetic. At this stage the person is completely dependent on others for basic human needs and can no longer survive without full-time care.

For unknown reasons, during the later stages of the disease the patient often loses weight. Muscle control diminishes, making any form of exercise difficult or impossible. The person may eventually become confined to a wheelchair or bedridden. The immobile or inactive person becomes more vulnerable to disease, infection, or heart attack. Pneumonia, viral infections, and heart attack are the most frequent secondary causes of death, the primary cause being Alzheimer's disease itself. The disease shortens life expectancy, but many people live for years in the final stages. Survival after the earliest symptoms varies anywhere from four to twenty years. The average survival is seven to ten years. In most cases the person will eventually require twenty-four-hour nursing home care unless the carer(s) can provide or hire private assistants around the clock.

DIAGNOSIS

As larger numbers of the population become sixty-five and older, incidence of Alzheimer's disease will increase. Research on the disease has become more urgent and extensive, but to date there is no cure for Alzheimer's disease, nor any treatment to reduce its intensity or halt its progression. Nonetheless, careful diagnosis is extremely important in order to rule out treatable disorders that can cause mental confusion as well as other forms of dementia such as multi-infarct dementia, viral dementia (such as Creutzfeldt-Jakob disease or sometimes AIDS), and hereditary dementia (such as Huntington's disease). Diagnosis is also important in order to help the person who has the disease and to help future carers understand what they are dealing with and obtain the necessary social, psychological, and medical support. When the afflicted person and her family finally know she has Alzheimer's, the disease is recognized as the reason for bizarre behaviour. This may alleviate the anger family members feel toward the afflicted relative and soften the blame they sometimes place on her for inappropriate behaviour. It may also help to alleviate the victim's own embarrassment and self-blame.

My mother has Alzheimer's disease, but she was first diagnosed as having 'geriatric depression'. We went through years of her behaviour getting worse and worse and driving me up the wall. If only we had had an earlier correct diagnosis, it would have saved us so much emotional pain and strain and turmoil. Now that the disease has been diagnosed it makes it easier for me to at least put a reason to her behaviour. When you know what Alzheimer's disease is all about, the diagnosis is a relief – and not a relief. [a thirty-eight-year-old woman]

To date, the only definite diagnosis of Alzheimer's disease is a postmortem examination of the brain. The only direct means of diagnosing the disease during the person's lifetime is the surgical removal and examination of brain tissue, a procedure too dangerous to perform routinely. Therefore, diagnosis takes place through the careful elimination of all other possible causes of a person's mental confusion. Diagnostic tests should include a complete health history and physical examination, a neurological and a psychiatric examination, neuropsychological and neurodiagnostic tests, and a functional evaluation to discover how much the person can do for herself. The physical exam should include diagnostic tests for endocrine, hormonal, liver, kidney, and heart problems. The doctor should also ask about family history and any history of mental disturbances, as well as the patient's social and occupational background, including education and exposure to toxic chemicals. The possibility of a fall or accident within the last six months should be explored. The neuropsychological examination tests functions such as a person's ability to remember, to concentrate, to do abstract reasoning, to do calculations, and to copy designs.

Neurodiagnostic tests are procedures to evaluate brain function and include a brain wave recording (electroencephalogram, or EEG) and a CAT or CT scan (computer-assisted tomography), which forms a picture of the brain from X-ray images. The CAT scan can also locate possible brain cell loss, and can rule out the possibility of a stroke or brain tumour. Nuclear magnetic resonance (NMR) may be used to assess structural changes in the brain, and the PET scan (positron emission tomography) is sometimes used to evaluate the metabolic activity of the brain. NMR and PET scans are valuable in research on Alzheimer's disease but are as yet too experimental to be useful in routine diagnosis.

Extensive diagnostic testing can be an exhausting trial. It is important to find a team who understand the condition, and who will not upset or exhaust the person by forcing too much testing at one stretch.

Treatment of Alzheimer's Disease

There is currently no treatment that cures, halts the progress of, or has a predictably and reliably helpful effect on Alzheimer's disease. However, many studies are underway. There is much false information in the media concerning possible cures. This misinformation takes advantage of our understandable need for encouraging, hopeful news. It is important to get reliable information on the results of new research. Your doctor, nurse, social worker, and the Alzheimer's Disease Society can be of help. Some large hospitals and research centres are conducting studies of drugs that may help treat Alzheimer's disease and related disorders. You may want to consider entering the affected person in such a study if one is being conducted near you.

Some symptoms of Alzheimer's disease such as uncontrollable agitation, sleeplessness, night-wandering, and hallucinations, are extremely hard on the carer; drugs to control these behaviours without harming the stricken person are urgently needed. Sometimes sedatives will make the stricken person's behaviour more tolerable. However, all drugs, especially those that alter mental function, can have negative effects. It is important that drugs be administered under the care of a knowledgeable doctor. In general, it is advisable to be cautious with all tranquillizers and to begin with the lowest possible doses, advancing slowly. Carer and doctor should closely watch the stricken person for positive as well as adverse effects of all prescribed drugs, and they should frequently re-evaluate the need for continued doses.

Cause and Prevention

There is probably no single cause of Alzheimer's disease but instead many contributing factors that work together to lead to the development of the disease. Since the cause or causes are not known, prevention is also a matter of speculation. The ageing of the brain may in itself be a main contributing factor, accelerated and augmented by other factors such as smoking, environmental toxins, hormonal changes, nutritional deficiencies, stress, a slow virus, hereditary and familial predisposition, or malfunction of the immune system. Research showing concentrated forms of aluminium in the brains of Alzheimer's victims has led to speculation that exposure to aluminium contributes to Alzheimer's disease. However, there is no higher incidence among aluminium workers than among the general population; and exposure to aluminium in daily life, for example through ovenware, does not lead to higher aluminium concentration in the body.[11] It is equally likely that higher brain levels of aluminium are a consequence rather than a cause of the disease.

A small group of people develop Alzheimer's disease earlier – between the ages of thirty-five and sixty-five – and experience a more rapid progression of the disease and an early death. For this subgroup, hereditary factors seem to be stronger, and their children, brothers, and sisters have a higher risk of getting the disease than the rest of the population. Researchers have found a defective gene which may be a cause of this familial form of the disease. However, it appears that the relatives of those with late-life Alzheimer's (onset after age sixty-five) have no higher risk of the disease.[12] People with Down's syndrome develop Alzheimer's disease if they live long enough. A gene that produces the amyloid protein found in the plaques in the brains of people with both early and late-life forms of Alzheimer's disease has been located in the same chromosome that is involved in Down's syndrome and in the familial form of Alzheimer's. However, it is not yet known whether this will prove to link the diseases genetically.[13]

Counselling for Carers and Persons with Alzheimer's

In some areas, departments of geriatric medicine or special geriatric units attached to psychiatric hospitals can provide continuous support for people with Alzheimer's disease, offering memory-training sessions to those in the early stages. Although there is little evidence that such training improves the condition, it serves a useful purpose in maintaining interest and social interaction. Carers, too, can be given specific information about the disease and advice in handling the condition. However, for most carers, local groups of people caring for a wide variety of disabling conditions may provide the best source of help. More information is to be found in Chapter 15.

The carers' support group certainly has been one thing that has kept my sanity together. Some group members are up to date on all of the resources for care and support agencies and are tremendously helpful. Also, I think just the feeling that you're not the only one in the circumstances is helpful. We're there to support each other with whatever knowledge and information we have or to hand out tissues to those who are in tears. [a fifty-seven-year-old woman]

Personal Impact of Alzheimer's Disease

Alzheimer's disease and other progressive dementias perhaps cause more stress and change in the stricken person and within the home than any other conditions. This is because of the devastating personality change and loss of control that the stricken person experiences.

IMPACT ON THE STRICKEN PERSON

I feel like half a person. Where's the rest of me? I really hate this and I'm frightened. Maybe listening to me will open a world that's closed to a lot of people. Nobody knows what it's like. They just don't understand. [a seventy-two-year-old woman in the early stage of Alzheimer's disease]

With the disease, both recent and remote memory are eventually lost. Losing recent memory means forgetting what happened an hour or even a minute ago and being unable to learn new information or lay down new memories. For the person with Alzheimer's, life is like continually walking into the middle of a movie, with no idea of what happened before, and no understanding of what is happening now.[14] She may forget the names and faces of recently met friends and acquaintances, forget recent births and deaths in the family, and forget that she has just eaten and ask when dinner will be ready.

Losing remote memory means forgetting the past, including what we learned as children. This includes activities we take for granted – brushing our teeth, taking a bath, getting dressed, holding a conversation, using the toilet. As the disease progresses the victim regresses. She may forget how to use eating utensils, forget how to dress, forget the sensations of hot and cold, forget how to control bowel and urine, forget what food is, and how to chew and swallow. She may forget inhibitions learned in childhood and may expose or touch her sexual parts in public. The person with Alzheimer's loses a sense of time and can no longer look forward or back, or turn to the collected knowledge of her life for help. With such helplessness, partnerships between adults slowly change to parent/child-type relationships, or an adult child may have to become responsible for a stricken mother or father.

I miss having a partner. Max used to go to the office and stay all day five days a week. Now he doesn't go anywhere at all without me, and that makes a difference in my home life, because I'm very conscious of this individual who is solely dependent on me. And going to parties – well, anywhere – Max used to go to church with me sometimes, and he always did the driving – he was an excellent driver. I find that I've lost the independent mind and gained a dependent one. [a seventy-six-year-old woman]

The stricken person's response to dementia is complex, changes as the disease progresses, and varies greatly from person to person. During the early stages the person may notice the changes within herself and be frightened and depressed by them. She may lose her job because she is progressively incompetent or because of personality changes unacceptable to those around her. She may be aware of her changed role within the household, as more and more responsibilities are taken from her.

It's like being in a ship by yourself. I can't function as I did before and I feel as if I'm odd. I'm so different from everybody else and I wonder if they like me. I'm so forgetful that I'm afraid when I'm with other people I'm going to sound stupid. But when friends ask me out, I go. And I find I'm much more relaxed once I'm with them. They're very kind to me. [a seventy-two-year-old woman in the early stage of Alzheimer's disease]

Throughout the course of the disease, but especially in the early stages, the stricken person may notice changes in the way others treat her and react with anxiety and embarrassment at her own behaviour. But usually she is unaware of her declining capacities and may blame the carer for hiding things she cannot find or for keeping dates and names a secret. She may become angry with the carer who prevents her from driving or managing her bank account.

IMPACT ON THE CARER

I think Alzheimer's disease is probably harder on the carer than it is on the victim. But I wouldn't change places for anything. [a seventy-eight-year-old carer]

Mourning to Do

The new year and a fresh fall of snow,
The new year and mourning to do
Alone in the lovely silent house,
Alone as the inner eye opens at last –
Not as the shutter of a camera with a click,

But like a gentle-waking in a dark room
Before dawn when familiar objects take on
Substances out of their shadowy corners
And come to life. So with my lost love,
For years lost in the darkness of her mind,
Tied to a wheelchair, not knowing where she was
Or who she had been when we lived together
In amity, peaceful as turtledoves.

Judy is dead. Judy is gone forever.

I cannot fathom that darkness, nor know
Whether the true spirit is alive again.
But what I do know is the peace of it,
And in the darkened room before dawn, I lie
Awake and let the good tears flow at last,
And as light touches the chest of drawers
And the windows grow transparent, rest,
Happy to be mourning what was singular
And comforting as the paintings on the wall,
All that can now come to life in my mind,
Good memories fresh and sweet as the dawn –
Judy drinking her tea with a cat on her lap,
And our many little walks before suppertime.
So it is now the gentle waking to what was,
And what is and will be as long as I am alive.
'Happy grieving', someone said who knew –
Happy the dawn of memory and the sunrise.

MAY SARTON*

Caring for someone with Alzheimer's disease takes a tremendous physical and emotional toll on the carer. In addition to the usual strains of caring for anyone with a long-term illness, unlimited patience and self-control are needed to cope with repetitive or unintelligible conversation, with complete silence, with extreme agitation, sudden aggression, or assault, or with any other of the possible changes in a stricken person's character. Along with this comes anger at the stricken person and inevitable feelings of guilt for becoming impatient, angry and resentful, and showing it.

If I'm a little tired and Bob pursues a subject until – you have no idea how people like that can pursue a subject – I can feel myself getting tense and angry. Occasionally, only when I get really angry, does he stop. But I don't like to get angry like that. It's hard on me, and I feel that I've got to work something out to help. I've thought about biofeedback that lets you know how tense you are so I can learn to relax. That might help me, relieve me. [a seventy-seven-year-old woman]

We literally had to watch Mother minute by minute because she was active enough then to put an empty pot on the stove and turn it on. She wasn't sleeping at night so at midnight she thought it was morning, would dress herself in several layers of clothing, and walk down the stairs and out the door. We were chasing her all night long. I didn't have the emotional energy to think out some of the solutions like having a bell on the door which would buzz when she went out. All those things you figure out when you have enough leisure to think them through, but when you're in the middle of it you're so exhausted, so overwhelmed, that you're just sort of getting through the next second. We were all just grimly going step by step, putting one foot in front of the other. [a woman in her forties]

The carer may feel deserted as she takes on more and more responsibilities in the home and perhaps becomes the sole means of financial support. Unlike people with diseases that mainly affect the body, a person with Alzheimer's disease often gives little or no thanks or recognition. The carer may feel resentful at the lack of reward for constant care. This resentment can be fed by a feeling that she is caring for a stranger – for someone whose behaviour has become odd and embarrassing and who no longer knows or loves her. Added to this may come further feelings of guilt, as the carer feels love dying under the strain, and perhaps wishes for the death of the stricken person.

Carers of sexual partners experience a loss of companionship and intimacy and often turn to others for close friendship. They have to decide whether such relationships will include sex. Painful conflicts between loyalty to an ailing partner and one's own needs often result.

The strain of caring for a demented person leads to a high rate of stress-related disorders. Over 50 per cent of carers show symptoms of anxiety and depression including insomnia, headaches, irritability, and increased blood pressure.[15] The carer can become increasingly forgetful under stress, and fear that she or he too is developing the disease. In addition, when whole families are involved in the caregiving process, family life may virtually cease under the burden.

When we took my stricken dad in to live with us, supper table conversation became nonexistent. When you've got relationships within a family, you've got to have time to get together as a family, go away together – just have a meal together and talk together. I have two college-age daughters. One is saying, 'I can't wait to get away from this place.' The other is saying, 'Home's the most awful place in the world.' I feel terribly guilty and also frightened that they will never want to come home; that they won't remember home with enough pleasure to want to spend time with me. [a woman in her forties]

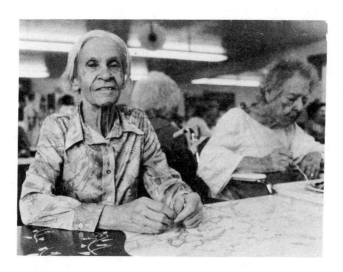

The financial burden of caring for a family member with Alzheimer's often far exceeds the social security allowances payable to carers, particularly when loss of the carer's earnings is taken into account. It's important to give such support as you can offer to organizations that continue to campaign for a better deal for carers and patients – the Alzheimer's Disease Society and the National Association of Carers. See Chapters 14 and 15 for further information on benefits and social services.

THE SPECIAL ROLE OF FAMILY AND FRIENDS

In such a difficult time, the support of friends and relatives becomes more important than ever. With Alzheimer's disease such support is difficult to sustain, since the stricken person loses the social traits that drew others to her: a sense of humour, kindness, special interests and talents. She also loses control over language as a means of communication. The stricken person becomes a stranger to relatives and friends, who may react with withdrawal and avoidance, appalled at the loved one's condition. In addition, visits can be

CARING FOR THE CARER

Public discussion of the need for care, information, and financial aid is increasing. Many of us who are carers have become vocal in demanding more help and are working with others through local associations.

We need:

- Health professionals who are trained in the diagnosis and care of Alzheimer's disease and related disorders, and who will take the time to listen and talk to us.
- Current, reliable information about research on the cause, prevention, and cure of Alzheimer's disease.
- A supportive community of persons sharing their caring experiences.
- Regular periods of relief from daily caregiving – relief in the form of adult day care or aides in the home.
- Regular one- to two-week periods of respite from looking after the afflicted person in order to maintain our own physical and mental health.

Government-funded respite centres and home nursing are needed to make this possible.

- Nurse practitioners who can make home visits to prevent unnecessary disease complications.
- Hospital and nursing home staff trained in caring for the demented who will treat our loved ones with dignity and with respect for their humanity.
- Help of lawyers trained to advise us when a victim becomes legally incompetent.
- Financial guidelines to protect assets from being completely depleted by the cost of full-time care.
- Police and Fire Brigade personnel who are informed about Alzheimer's disease and related disorders to help lost and wandering afflicted persons and to intervene in serious crises.
- Support of family and friends.

difficult to manage since the victim is often confused by any changes in the daily routine and embarrassed by her inability to remember who the visitors are. The resulting isolation of the victim may also lead to isolation of the carer.

As relatives or friends of Alzheimer's disease victims, it is important for us to remind ourselves that the stricken person still needs and recognizes affection even if she may neither remember nor return it. Often just quietly holding the stricken person's hand will help. We should also keep in mind the carer's needs for social contact, a change of scene, and an understanding ear. However, our instinct to withdraw is understandable, since many of us fear becoming demented more than we fear any other illness or infirmity that may come with age. Understanding as much as we can about the disease may help alleviate our anxiety, especially when we know that in most cases the increased forgetfulness that many of us experience is not a sign of disease. For those of us who do not have friends or relatives with Alzheimer's, understanding the disease will help us give support to those who do. It will keep us from isolating stricken people and their carers out of fear.

NOTES

[1] K. Warner Schaie and James Geiwitz, *Adult Development and Aging*. Boston: Little, Brown, 1982, pp. 217–39.

[2] Some studies show that approximately 33 per cent of those between eighty and eighty-five show no decline on neuropsychological tests, including tests of memory, compared with younger age groups. A. L. Benton et al., 'Normative Observations on Neuropsychological Test Performances in Old Age'. *Journal of Clinical Neuropsychology*, Vol. 3, No. 1, May 1981, pp. 33–42.

[3] Adapted from Florence Garfunkel and Gertrude Landau, *A Memory Retention Course for the Aged: Guide for Leaders*. Washington, DC: National Council on the Aging, December 1981.

[4] 'Memory Loss May Follow Use of Anticholinergics'. *Medical World News*, 12 August 1985, p. 51.

[5] Robert N. Butler, 'Clinical Needs Assessment Studies Can Benefit Research on Aging'. *Hospitals*, Vol. 55, No. 8, 16 April 1981, pp. 94–8.

[6] Barry Reisberg, *A Guide to Alzheimer's Disease: For Families, Spouses, and Friends*. New York: The Free Press, 1981, p. 14.

[7] Incidence of concurrent multi-infarct dementia and Alzheimer's disease is unknown. One estimate is 25 per cent of late-life dementia. See ibid.

[8] This estimate is from the *Report of the Secretary's Task Force on Alzheimer's Disease*, US Department of Health and Human Services, September 1984. However, accurate statistics on Alzheimer's are relatively new and in the process of revision. Some researchers consider 20 per cent a conservative estimate, and say

that prevalence may rise to 30 to 40 per cent in those over eighty and 50 per cent in those over eighty-five years of age.

[9] US Department of Health and Human Services, *Alzheimer's Disease Handbook, Vol. I*. San Francisco: Aging Health Policy Center, University of California, April 1984, p. 2.

[10] Donald B. Tower, 'Alzheimer's Disease – Senile Dementia and Related Disorders: Neurobiological Status'. In Robert Katzman, R. D. Terry and K. L. Bick, eds., *Alzheimer's Disease: Senile Dementia and Related Disorders*, Vol. 7, *Aging*. New York: Raven Press, 1978, p. 1.

[11] Conversation with Dr Lon White, Chief, Epidemiology Office, National Institute on Aging; and 'Smokers Risk Alzheimer's Disease'. *ASH Review*, August 1986, p. 10.

[12] L. L. Heston and J. A. White, *Dementia: A Practical Guide to Alzheimer's Disease and Related Illnesses*. New York: W. H. Freeman & Co., 1983, p. 57.

[13] Harold M. Schmeck, Jr, 'A Form of Alzheimer's Is Linked to Defective Gene'. *The New York Times*, 20 February 1987, p. 1. This article mentions four recent research reports.

[14] Nancy L. Mace and Peter V. Rabins, *The 36-Hour Day: A Family Guide to Caring for Persons with Alzheimer's Disease, Related Dementing Illnesses, and Memory Loss in Later Life*. Baltimore: Johns Hopkins University Press, 1981, p. 24.

[15] J. R. A. Sanford, 'Tolerance of Debility in Elderly Dependents by Supporters at Home: Its Significance for Hospital Practice'. *British Medical Journal*, Vol. 3, No. 5981, 23 August 1975, pp. 471–3.

BOOKS AND PUBLICATIONS

Barbara Gray and Bernard Isaacs, *Care of the Elderly Mentally Infirm*. London: Tavistock Publications, 1979.

Alan Baddeley, *Your Memory: A User's Guide*. London: Penguin, 1983.

King's Fund Project, *Living Well into Old Age: Applying Principles of Good Practice to Services for People with Dementia*. (See Organizations.)

Tim Dowdell, *Forgetfulness in Elderly Persons: Advice for Carers*. London: Age Concern. (See Organizations.)

Alzheimer's Disease Society, *Caring for the Person with Dementia*. (See Organizations.)

In a World of Their Own: Home Care of the Confused Elderly. A Publication for Relatives. Free booklet – send s.a.e. Hambro Life Charitable Trust, Allied Hambro Centre, Swindon SN1 1EL.

Nicholas Coni, David Williamson and Stephen Webster, *Ageing: The Facts*. Oxford: Oxford University Press, 1984.

Dr J. P. Watts, *Confusion in Old Age*. Wellingborough: Thorsons/British Medical Association, 1988.

29
Dying and Death

In many cultures, preparing for and making sense of death is the work of women, especially of old women. Whether or not it's fair or best, women in most societies, including our own, still act as the nurturers, carers, and custodians of those near death. Even with the removal of death to the institutional sphere, dying remains the province of women who work in those institutions.

The last person most of us see on earth is a woman – the nurse or student nurse (significantly one of the least paid and least valued workers in our society). . . . These are, in a sense, the midwives of death.[1]

Thus, it is most often women who meet the emotional and pragmatic needs surrounding death.

By the age of fifty-seven I had nursed my husband through terminal cancer, lived through widowhood, and been close to two dear friends who died. I assisted one friend and supported her family through the process of her committing suicide. I feel that my middle years have been significant in bringing me into close and familiar contact with dying and death.

Bereavement and Grief

On a rational level, we know that any fully lived life inevitably contains the experience of death. But observers like psychiatrist Elisabeth Kübler-Ross have remarked that almost everyone who goes through the process of mourning her own impending death or that of a loved one does it in stages: first, denial ('This can't be happening'), then anger ('It's not fair'), followed by bargaining ('Maybe if I do exactly as the doctor says, I'll beat this'), depression ('I can't bear this sadness'), and finally, often with great sorrow and regret, a time of acceptance.[2] Although these different facets of the process of mourning are sometimes referred to as stages – implying that each one is fully experienced and comes to an end before the next begins – it is more likely that these different emotions and thoughts come and go, mingling with each other over a period of years.

The following is excerpted from a woman's journal recording her feelings about her lover's death over a period of years:

In what later seemed to be extraordinary word usage, the doctor called me to say the operation on Karen was 'successful'. They resectioned her colon and took out the tumor; she would not need a colostomy. But the tumor has metastasized and she will die; six months to two years is all they give her. No real hope.

It is 2:30 A.M. and I can't sleep because of rage at God, and then because of guilt. And because of fear for myself. How will I live without Karen to tell me I am brilliant and beautiful?

Images run through my head. Her hand warming my asthma-congested chest. Her step – quick, strong, fast up the stairs. As I remember that sound, I smile; the pain recedes. But if I shut my journal, the pain will return.

Does everyone who is dying look bewildered? Her head in my lap; her body spooned in pain. Dying means dependency. Pain. Listlessness. Fever. Exhaustion. Dying is frightening.

Death is final, but dying can drag on and on and on, destroying everyone. It saps the strength of the healthy and makes them sick.

My first birthday without her. Our anniversary. Her first birthday dead. My first Christmas and first New Year without her. One year it was the greatest New Year of my life, and the next year the woman who gave it to me was dead.

Each marker brings Karen to me and takes her. Soon my first spring without her. My first summer. Then a year since I last saw her will pass. A year since her death; a year since her funeral. And I will put a headstone in my heart: Karen, my dearest.[3]

Any one loss can remind us of all the other losses we have known – especially the earliest ones, which might not have been fully understood or explored.

When my lover died I was fifty-six. Over the next two years I relived, in a way, all of the other great sadnesses of my life – when my father left us when I was little, my mother's death, the endings of other love affairs. I don't think I had realized how much there was for me to mourn. [a sixty-two-year-old woman]

Acceptance of death can come only after a full experience of mourning that may last many months or even years.

My daughter died almost forty years ago, when she was ten. I'm still angry, and I still miss her. But for years after she died I couldn't quite believe that it had really happened – I kept thinking I heard her in the house. Now I can accept what happened, even if I don't like it. [a seventy-eight-year-old woman]

My husband died eighteen years ago and even though today I have a happy, full life, I still miss him. I am often reminded of what he is missing, especially at happy moments, such as the children's college graduations, which are tinged with the wish that he was alive to share the joy. [a fifty-four-year-old woman]

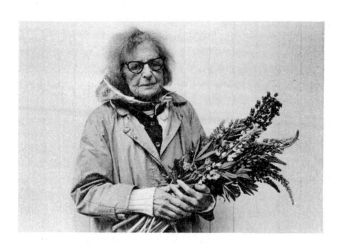

Mental health experts have observed that 'troubled mourning' can be a principal reason for unhappiness and problems later in life. Mourning can go wrong in a variety of ways. We may be unable to grieve at the time of loss, feeling too numb to cry or to express our feelings in any way at all. We may begin to grieve but cut the process short, because of pressure to appear self-possessed for a job or family or friends. Or we may suppress our grief, drive it underground, in which case it is likely to erupt again, perhaps with surprising intensity, at the time of some later loss.

In these cases, we may try to protect ourselves from the pain of grief by adopting a self-protecting mask of composure which allows us to carry on with life as usual. Sometimes a physical illness may appear, or self-destructive behaviour such as drug or alcohol addiction, an eating disorder, or repeated involvements in unsatisfactory relationships. One or more aspects of mourning can become exaggerated. We may dwell on guilt, self-blame, anger, anxiety, or sadness until we become completely incapacitated and such feelings take the place of grieving.

In each of the above cases, the underlying problem is that the person who mourns has in some way not completed the mourning process. Sometimes, friends or relatives, in a misguided desire to be helpful, urge us to 'get on with it', when in fact what we need is to honour the urgency and depth of our feelings for as long as we need to do so. Paying attention to our feelings and talking about them with friends or relatives is extremely important.

When my husband was dying people helped us so much. They came to visit and brought food so that I could spend more time with him. They gave flowers and hugs, gave the children extra attention. Some people were too frightened to visit and I understood. But the friend who came fifteen hundred miles to see him before he died, the friend who came five hundred miles to hold my hand during the funeral, and the friend who stayed at the cemetery to cover his grave after the service will forever have my gratitude.

I was comforted by the notes and cards people sent me. I read them over and over again for many months, nurtured by the care, sympathy, and support they provided. Best of all were the handwritten notes that included something about the writer's relationship with my husband or memories of times together – sometimes things that were new to me. I received notes from people I had not known and was strengthened by their consideration. Even the printed cards and the simplest notes indicating that someone was thinking of me comforted me. Nineteen years later, I still have all the messages in a box so our now-grown children can share with their children how the grandfather they will never know touched the lives of so many others. [a fifty-four-year-old woman]

When my husband died it was like I was paralysed socially for months after. My two good friends did me a great service just by sitting with me. Sometimes I would cry and sometimes I'd just be angry. Sometimes I was so sad I could hardly talk. They'd come over to visit me at least twice a week, and they stayed with it for more than a year. When I felt better I could be a good friend to them again. [a sixty-four-year-old woman]

I learned a lot about anger after my mother died. Somehow, when I was mourning, lots of anger came out that I didn't know was in me. My daughter suggested beating a pillow with a stick to get the anger out, and finally I got so I could talk with my husband and also with my daughter about some of the reasons why I felt so much anger at my poor mother. [a forty-three-year-old woman]

Observing religious and/or cultural traditions, writing about our feelings in a journal, talking to family and friends, meditating, reading poetry, watching emotion-evoking movies or plays and singing or listening to familiar songs can all help us feel our grief as deeply and fully as we need. Joining a self-help group of people who are grieving, such as Cruse or the National Association of Widows (see Organizations), or a hospice group, can be a great comfort. Such groups help us realize that what we are feeling is 'normal' and is shared by others.

HOW TO HELP A DYING OR RECENTLY BEREAVED PERSON

- Give them the time and quiet listening to express their feelings. Express your own sadness and regret, but do not presume to tell a bereaved or dying person that a death is 'for the best', even if after a long illness. We don't really know how someone feels unless they tell us.
- Offer distractions, other topics of mutual interest, but be comfortable with silence and resist the need to fill every minute with words. Your very presence will help.

- Offer help, and be specific in your suggestions. Say, 'I have two hours free on Saturday. Do you want me to shop for you, or is there something else I can do that would be helpful?'
- Take care of a dying or bereaved person: do not expect her or him to take care of you. Bring food if you visit someone's home.
- Do send cards or notes if you can't visit.

For some of us it is useful to get professional help – from a clergyman, for example, or perhaps from a bereavement counsellor – to deal with the process of mourning.

I functioned extremely well most of the time (everyone always said how well), but I felt like I was just going through the motions, waiting for my husband to come home. Three times in the past four years I've arrived at the point where I felt a need for counselling. Each time I've learned more about myself. The counselling has helped me grow and find new meaning in my life. [a woman in her fifties]

The loss of a child or grandchild can be particularly painful. If death is caused by a sudden, unexpected accident that allows little or no time beforehand for preparation, as is often the case when someone we love dies young, the loss may be even more difficult to come to terms with. We cannot comfort ourselves by saying, 'Well, she's lived a long and full life and it was her time to die.' Even if we lose a child in her or his middle or late years, we may feel a sense of unfairness, as if the natural order of things has been violated. This was not a loss we expected to sustain.

When my husband died at age thirty-nine, his mother cried out how against nature his death was. She said, 'I was supposed to die first.'

When death is expected, not only the person who is dying but also those who expect to be survivors have time to make some preparations, get relationships and business affairs in order, and to reminisce and say goodbye.

My father died of a heart attack and my mother died of cancer. My father's death was a surprise and a shock, and my mother's death was a long ordeal. I know that people sometimes think that a sudden and quick death is easier, but for me it was important to talk with my mother and even just to sit and hold her hand, and though those last weeks and months were hard I'm grateful we had them. With my father there was no time to say goodbye. I wish there had been. [a forty-nine-year-old woman]

When we are faced with the shock of a sudden, unexpected death, we often console ourselves with the knowledge that the person we loved did not suffer. While having time to prepare for a death may be easier on our survivors, many of us would choose an unanticipated and painless death for ourselves.

For myself, I want my death to be sudden, quick and easy for me, even if it is harder on those who survive me. [a woman in her fifties]

When death comes at the end of a prolonged and chronic illness, our feelings may take longer to sort out. We may have already grieved, years ago, for the loss of the whole, well person we used to know.

My sister developed the first symptoms of Alzheimer's when she was sixty-two. I took care of her, moved into her flat for five years so she could stay in familiar surroundings. Then I had to put her into a nursing home, where I visited her twice a week. I never missed a week for nine more years until she died. There was very little that anybody could do for her. It was very hard to see her become just a thin little curled-up ball in her bed. For the last seven years she didn't recognize me or even talk at all. She was my only sister, and it was terribly sad for me. [a sixty-two-year-old woman]

We may feel a sense of release for ourselves and for the person who died after prolonged suffering. But later, intense, renewed feelings of loss may surface.

Even though I thought I had prepared myself mentally for the inevitable, I found I was terribly shocked, even surprised, when my mother finally did die. I understand now that shock after a death is common among those close to a person, even when the death was expected.[4]

Coming to Terms with Our Own Deaths

One of the important developmental tasks of the second half of life is coming to a personal understanding, perhaps even an acceptance, of death. Some of us continue to feel ambivalent and scared about acknowledging death.

A few of my friends have died young. We all knew each other for so long. (We had a card-playing group.) Three of them were my age. One of them I met recently and recognized her name from primary school, and so we were the same age. Another one was a few months older, so we were all in the same age bracket. Now my sister-in-law just died and she was only sixty-three. This has been on my mind so much lately, you know, reaching this point that people my age are starting to go. I never used to think of these things before. Like if an aunt or an uncle died that's one thing, but now it's cousins! One cousin my age died this summer, so I start to think 'It's our turn' and in what order are we going! [a sixty-seven-year-old woman]

Intellectually, I'm very glib about it, but in my gut I can't accept that one day I won't be here. [a seventy-four-year-old woman]

Maybe no one can ever be fully 'ready' for death in the sense of knowing about and fully accepting the experience in advance. But we can prepare ourselves in a variety of ways.[5]

I feel a greater awareness of a mystery and beauty in life since I have accepted death as a personal eventuality for me. I don't remember exactly when that awareness came. Before then, I had thought of death 'out there', and now I know that one day it will be a reality for me. Eventually I am going to die. In a way, that has released me for more vivid living. [a seventy-eight-year-old woman]

I've dealt with losing loved ones many times in my life, and after seventy years of repetition of that experience of grief I find the thing that's so hard to deal with is that some person who has been a reality in your life no longer exists. When you're a kid, you learn how to separate fantasy from reality. But then, when you get older, you have to learn how to let go of a reality – that person no longer exists. I've got a handle on that from years of experience with it. So I no longer worry about my own personal death. [a seventy-three-year-old woman]

Some of us are comforted by religious, spiritual, or humanistic beliefs about life and death.

I believe that I am not just a body which is perishable but I am a spirit which is eternal. I believe that death is only an exit from this temporary life of unreality into a glorious new life of reality. I hope, therefore, that there will be only rejoicing, not grief, at the time of my release. I am trying to avoid being 'earthbound' by releasing my attachments to material objects and persons before I enter this transition. [a ninety-two-year-old woman]

What I've been aware of lately because of a number of instances of my being thrown up against death is that I have a different perception of relationships. Death is not a termination of my life because my influence will continue until the last person who knew me has died. [a woman in her fifties]

I do not look to the future with dread. It has to be shorter than my past but it does not have to be less rich. I'm more relaxed. I don't try to do everything.
That means I can take time for quiet, for meditation, alternate this with activity, and see how I can keep a moving, living balance between the two. [a seventy-eight-year-old woman]

Death, I am learning through my own experience, need not be frightening. After all, we are all born terminal cases, because we will all die, at one time or another. Death is part of life. I have lived life fully and enjoyed it greatly, which makes it easier to consider bowing out than if you feel that you have missed out on a lot.★

Providing support to others can also help us come to terms with death. We can serve as resources for one another and create supportive networks that give us the strength and companionship we need to get through hard times.

On the day before her fifty-eighth birthday, my friend Maggy Krebs died in a Boston hospital. Maggy was a feminist artist.† Her humor, her drawings and paintings, and her music had filled many lives with joy. Because I believe that the final months of

---

★Tish Sommers, age seventy, in a letter to members of the Older Women's League in the United States about her expected death. Tish founded and led the 23,000-member organization after her cancer was diagnosed.
†See p. 268 for cartoon by Maggy Krebs.

her life and her death were models for all independent women, I want to tell you part of the story.

For months, Maggy gathered around her a group of her friends, who tended to her at her home and at the hospital. In addition to caring for Maggy, we met each other regularly, often weekly, to share our grief and anger at the anticipated loss of a friend, to find ways to share the responsibility of taking care of her and to support one another. We became a family for Maggy and for each other.

One of Maggy's legacies to us is the pride we feel that we were able to give her the comfort and love she needed. But Maggy also left a legacy of hope to all women who feel themselves to be alone by teaching us that we can support each other through the depths of illness, exhaustion, fear and loss.[6]

Sharing the responsibility as this women's group did avoids the guilt women sometimes feel when they can't do everything by themselves. An illness support group allows each woman to participate to the extent she is able to do so.

In the last four years I have come from the depths of despair to feeling that life is good and that there still is a reason and a need for me to be in this world. Helping to train hospice volunteers continues to be therapeutic for me. With the death of my husband, things which I'd only read about in books or heard others talk about became very real and personal to me. Much of my own grief work was done with the volunteer training classes, where the volunteers gave me the opportunity to talk about my experiences and my life, and the aloneness I felt at the loss of my best friend and life's companion. [a woman in her fifties]

Most of my friends are gone. You just have to say to yourself that it's something that's going to happen. But it's not easy. It helps to do all you can for your friends while they're living. I do a lot of calling on the telephone. I have a friend I call every day. He's been in the hospital a long time. I have another friend who lives down in another town who's quite ill that I call at least once a week. Death used to be scary to me. Four or five years ago, if I thought of dying, I'd push it out of my mind. But now, I think, after all, I've lived out my days and I know I've got to go. [a woman in her eighties]

Another way to prepare ourselves for dying is to take care of any unfinished business in our lives. Most of us have unresolved relationships – some that go back quite far – that we may want to work out or perhaps just make a final statement on. We can seek out people with whom we have unfinished business and see to it that some old unforgiven hurts are healed – and recognize that some can't ever be healed. Those who have made the effort to do this say it is very important.

Before her death my sister asked to see each of her five brothers and sisters. We talked about the ways we had been close and trusting with each other, and we also talked about some of our long-standing fights and grudges. I know that the hour that she and I spent going over our times together was very important to me. It was one way to say goodbye. And I think it was important and healing for her, as well. [a forty-seven-year-old woman]

The Medicalization of Death

Understanding death has become more difficult and complicated because, in our culture, death is often a medical event. Most people in the last stages of life are in hospitals and nursing homes, and are thus 'out of sight'. Life-threatening situations at any age often take place in a hospital. Institutional methods of caring for the sick and dying make it difficult for us to experience and understand death as a natural end to life.

I can remember the day my grandfather died, in a tractor accident on the farm. The men brought him in from the field to the house, and my grandmother, my mother, and my aunt bathed and dressed him. It was a loving act, and a ritual, and I was terribly impressed. I was eight at the time. My own father went from the hospital bed where he died to a funeral home, and I know my mother doesn't feel like she was a part of his dying. I'm trying to understand that difference, and what I myself want to do in that regard. [a sixty-seven-year-old woman]

In some cultures, death is understood to be a natural transition at the end of life. Among some Native American tribes, for instance, each life is seen as a road that is expected to come to an end. The healers in those societies see themselves as 'keepers of the road', guardians of health for as long as the journey goes on – not as persons who work to prevent the journey from ending in its expected transition.

But in our contemporary culture, we invest heavily in science and want to believe that through it we can control all the events of our lives. We have hope that the discoveries of science will allow us to prolong life and prevent death. These attitudes make it hard to look on death as the natural, expected end of life, and make it harder to accept the inevitability of death.

Doctors often use every possible means to prolong life without regard for its quality. The result can be feelings of anguish and helplessness on the part of the dying person, relatives and friends.

When my husband had his heart attack I thought I should rush him to the hospital. The ambulance came right away but by the time they resuscitated him he already had a lot of brain damage. He never recovered consciousness. Everyone in the ICU [Intensive Care Unit] worked very hard to save his life, and he did live for another two weeks, but as far as I'm concerned he wasn't really alive – just a body attached to a lot of tubes and machinery. I wish now that I had just held him, cradled his head, when he first fell. I could have said goodbye that way. [a sixty-five-year-old woman]

As some medical professionals are beginning to recognize, focus on the inappropriate pursuit of a cure when the situation is clearly beyond hope can lead medical personnel to make a person's last days more painful and difficult than necessary. Of course, there are situations of acute emergency in which one cannot be sure whether recovery is possible; it is very hard to know the right thing to do in such a case. But some medical treatments designed to cure, such as chemotherapy and radiotherapy, may increase the dying person's discomfort.

Many of us may feel more secure in a hospital when we are very ill. Or we may feel we want to try, or should continue to try, medical remedies on the chance that one may heal us.

My daughter died of breast cancer at age forty-two. We thought she wanted to die at home and we were ready to take care of her there. But in the end the doctors urged her to try one more round of treatment with chemotherapy and she went back into the hospital. She never came home again, and for the last week she was so sick and in such pain that she didn't even want her teenage children to visit her. [a sixty-eight-year-old woman]

Discomforts such as pain, shortness of breath, weakness, nausea, and vomiting often precede death. The last days of living can be eased by concentrating on comfort rather than cure. (See 'Dealing with Pain' in the chapter Habits Worth Changing, p. 58.) Occasionally, treatments such as radiotherapy or even surgery may be used to bring relief of pain and discomfort, though it is more common to use high doses of pain-relieving drugs.

We were lucky enough to find a doctor who was willing to come to the house and could prescribe drugs for Grandma's pain and also for the nausea. We heard about the doctor because she had performed the same service for a neighbour down the street, and she made a hard time much easier than it might have been. [a thirty-six-year-old woman]

Taking Control of Our Own Deaths

Many of us would prefer not to be subjected to machines and tubes and complex technological procedures that may extend life a few extra days, weeks, or months at the expense of whatever quality it may be possible to achieve. Some of us who have such thoughts, however, will surely die in the very circumstances we deplore. How does this happen?

We tend to forget experiences that most of us have had as patients, like being moved from one treatment to another with little explanation of what is really thought to be wrong, how the treatment is supposed to work, and what to expect next, as if once we become patients we have given over the right or desire to make choices. The doctor often doesn't present alternatives from which we can choose; the alternatives of *no* treatment or of treatments such as acupuncture or herbal remedies are rarely discussed. This failure to present alternatives makes it difficult for the ill person to make informed decisions. Being a patient can feel like being on a slippery slide you can't easily get off.

My daughter spent the last months of her life going to the hospital for outpatient treatments, and feeling terrible. I won't ever do that. I'm not saying it's any better to be sick from the cancer, but at least you'd feel like it's your body and your life. I'd want to have some time to myself to live a little if I thought I was going to die soon. [a fifty-nine-year-old woman]

Here are some things to remember about doctors and dying:

- Doctors cannot actually predict recovery, death, or future disability for any single patient; they can only make broad, educated guesses based on statistics for large populations. They deal in group probabilities.[7]
- Many people whose death was predicted with firm certainty by medical experts have recovered; this happens with sufficient regularity to remind us that illness is not fully understood by science.
- Each individual has a right to say how she or he will live out the last days of a soon-to-be-ended life. If living outside a hospital or without the discomfort of medical treatment is what you want, your right to do so ought to be honoured.

Ten years ago, when I was forty-five, I was told I had breast cancer. For the next year I had chemotherapy and radiation – I was sick and worried the whole year. But now I feel that when the cancer comes back I just want to live with it, except for painkillers when I need them. I feel that if I'm going to live on, or die, I want to be able to experience each day as my day. I've written letters to each of my children to let them know how important this is to me.

Even when we try to stay in control, an illness can become overwhelming and may deplete our energy reserves, especially if we do not have a dependable support system. Though we may aspire to a serene death for ourselves or a loved one, surrounded by familiar faces, we must recognize that humans have never been able to control or predict death.

I felt like I was in a dream. I had promised my husband I wouldn't send him back to the hospital, but I was up for twenty hours each day taking care of him and I just couldn't go on. He agreed to go back because I promised him that I would stay in the hospital with him. The last ten days he didn't talk but he seemed to be comfortable. They were giving him morphine intravenously. The doctor woke me at 3 a.m. to tell me he had died while I was sleeping. It bothered me that I was sleeping when he died because I had promised him that I would be with him. I don't know if he would have said anything if I had been awake. No matter how hard you try, it doesn't always work out the way you want. [a woman in her sixties]

The Living Will

If you decide that you want to die at home, or that in some circumstances you would prefer to have no treatment, or treatment for comfort only, you have a right to make that decision and to refuse treatment. For a discussion on this option see *Your Cancer: Your Life* (listed below). It is a good idea to put your wishes in writing, in the event that you are unable to participate in decision-making yourself. In order to do so, you will have to think now about the possibility of your death. For some of us this can be very difficult. The pressure for the ill and dying to become and remain 'patients' is often so great that your spoken word alone may not be enough to give your family and friends the strength to carry out your wishes.

My mother at age ninety-seven was in a nursing home. By then she was hard of hearing and blind, so we communicated by touch. She had often told me that she wanted to die in the nursing home, not in an unfamiliar hospital. However, she became ill and was sent to the hospital, where she lapsed into a coma for three weeks. Then they wanted to put a feeding tube in. I threatened to sue unless they sent her back to the nursing home. The doctor and I stood over her bed arguing. He said, 'You are murdering your mother.' I said, 'No, I want it to be her choice.' My mother opened her eyes and looked at me and said, 'Thank you.' I got her back to the nursing home that night. Next day she was up, all over the home, and talking with everybody. Then the nurse called, telling me that my mother wanted roast duckling. I baked it and pureed it in a blender. She ate the whole thing. That night she threw her false teeth down the toilet and she died three days later. [a sixty-five-year-old woman]

My mother always said that she didn't want to die in a hospital and didn't want lengthy, complicated, and expensive care at the end of her life. But when she got weaker and weaker because of her failing heart, she was treated with one drug after another. When she got pneumonia, again she was treated and hospitalized because she seemed to be having trouble breathing. I said to my Dad, 'Of course she's having trouble breathing, she's old and she's weak and she's dying.' But he was too scared to let her stay at home. If she had made a legal record of her wishes we could have done as she asked. Weak as she was, I felt that I had betrayed her by letting her go into the hospital and die there. [a fifty-six-year-old woman]

In the United States a 'living will' is accepted in many states – the person can write in advance that she wishes to refuse treatment that could prolong life in circumstances like the above.[8,9] In the United Kingdom it is theoretically possible to refuse treatment, but doctors exert great pressure on the dying person and her relatives to accept it. In the UK only financial restraints imposed on the Health Service (e.g. the inadequate provision of kidney machines) are likely to prevent a patient receiving all reasonable treatments which might prolong life. The Hospice movement (see below) and the organization The Voluntary Euthanasia Society (see Organizations) may be able to offer advice.

Dying at Home

At one time, almost everybody could have expected to die in their own homes – even in their own beds. Now, death more often occurs in a hospital or nursing home. Recently, however, more people are insisting that they be allowed to die outside of these institutions.

I don't want anyone to tell me what to do. I lived all these years with my eight children and made decisions, right or wrong, about how we'd live. I want to decide for myself now. I've no need for medicine, drugs, or hospitals, never have, and I don't want to start now. I want to die with dignity. I'm comfortable in my home among my own things and with my family around me. They'll care for me. They'll respect my wishes. I can see who I want in my own home. I can eat what I want to eat. I know my own body and what it needs or can handle. I'm a private person. There's no privacy in the hospital. I want my children around me. I need their touch, their love. [a seventy-six-year-old woman]

Mum needed to be hostess and be in charge in her home even while dying. She continued to direct and guide her children about her care. While we held a cup to her mouth, she would urge, 'Eat with me.' When she needed more care, we got help from hospice nurses. When I introduced my mum to the new nurse, Mum was already in her 'withdrawal from the world stage'. But she drew herself together from her foetal position under the blankets to peek at this new person, and, in her weak, raspy voice, said, 'Welcome to my home.' These were her final words to the world. What a magnificent, independent woman this mother of mine was. She showed us how to live and how to die. Mum passed on as peacefully as possible considering her pain and weakness. [a fifty-seven-year-old woman, the daughter of the woman quoted above]

A woman who is a midwife wrote the following account of her mother's death:

This past year brought serious illness to my mother, Marion Cunningham. We sought conventional medical attention, plus an array of alternative healing practitioners. After months of misdiagnosis, Marion diagnosed herself as dying. We admitted her to the hospital and, alas, the diagnosis of lung cancer was finally acknowledged. My brother, my sister, and I stood in disbelief at her side. A pioneer in natural childbirth and in single parenting, she had always been our source of strength and inspiration. We all cried together that day. Then Marion spoke to me, words which would affect our caring of one another in the months to follow: 'Why don't they have midwives for what I've got?' We decided to care for her at home.

One night at midnight, I received a call from my brother . . . 'Mom says she will die today and that you all should come.'

And thus it was that we gathered round. My brother requested that I sing 'The Goodbye Song,' which I had written just a month before.

> *I'll see you in the babies' faces*
> *I'll feel you in the wind*
> *I'll hear you in the quietest places*
> *I'll hold you in my friend.*

I played on my guitar and sang to Marion, and in the midst of the song I could hear her breathing relax and I knew she would die. We watched one tear roll down her face and then she took her last breath.[10]

Hospices

A relatively new institution called the hospice has developed in response to the growing interest in dying at home. The hospice is modelled after medieval way stations that accommodated both travellers and those who were dying (death being, metaphorically, another form of travel).

Following the pioneering work of Dr Cicely Saunders at the St Christopher's

Hospice in South London, many hospices are now operating in different parts of the country. They are usually founded and supported by individuals and community groups, and staffed by experienced doctors, nurses and voluntary workers. The Marie Curie Memorial Foundation (see Organizations) runs hospices especially for cancer patients and they also have a service providing nurses for the terminal care of patients in their own homes. They liaise with Macmillan Nurses (see Organizations) who also provide regular care for patients in the last stages of illness, either because they want to die at home or before they go into hospital.

Help the Hospices (see Organizations) gives direct financial support to help hospices and hospice teams, funds relevant research, and provides training.

One of the major goals of a hospice programme is to maintain the quality of life through spiritual and emotional support, medication, and methods such as meditation and visualization for pain control. They will also provide temporary relief for carers.

Our son died of Hodgkin's disease two years ago. Toward the end he said he didn't want to go back into the hospital, no matter what. We called the hospice and they sent a volunteer who came to visit John two days a week at first and then, at the end, every day. He was almost like a member of the family, and the help he gave made a big difference to all of us – especially to John. [a seventy-six-year-old woman]

Some of these services have always been available from visiting-nurse and home-care agencies, clergy, church-visitation committees, and other local sources. But a hospice programme co-ordinates all these services.

Hospices do not charge fixed fees – in fact in some circumstances there is no charge. But those who can afford to pay are asked to make financial contributions, and of course donations and legacies in memory of those they have helped are always welcomed.

Choosing the Time of Our Death

Two years ago my mother, who was then eighty-three, told me that she planned to end her life by taking an overdose of pills. Her health was failing rapidly and she was going blind. She didn't want to become weak and dependent. She had always been a fierce and active woman. She wrote her intentions in a letter to me – I was her only close family member – and she told two friends and her doctor. We all told her that we would not help her accumulate enough pills to do the job. And I think we all worked very hard to help her find new reasons to be happy to be alive. But finally I understood that she really wanted to do what she had planned, and in the end, after she gathered together enough pills and took them, I sat with her for the last thirty-six hours as she slipped away. I can't tell you how many of her friends and acquaintances told me how graceful my mother was in her life to the very end. For my mother, given her personality, staying in control of her own life made her graceful. [a forty-one-year-old woman]

There is a great difference between someone, terminally ill and in pain, who says, 'I've lived a full, long life and I think this is my time to die,' and someone who is viewing life through the fog of depression and says, 'I don't want to go on living.' For a depressed person, a suicide attempt may be a call for help in finding resources to regain pleasure in living. You can get help for such a person through a suicide-prevention organization like the Samaritans (see Organizations).

It is very difficult to know what to do when a loved one wants to end her or his life. Talking with this person can help us distinguish temporary feelings of discouragement from the conviction that a life of pain and deterioration would be unbearable.

However, it has to be recognized that in the United Kingdom it is still illegal to assist, in any way, a person to end her own life and there have been a few cases in which relatives or friends who were alleged to have helped in a voluntary death have been prosecuted. To protect their loved ones, some dying persons have chosen to go off by themselves and take a fatal substance. They have had to do without the loving support and the talking and planning that would have eased the transition for everybody.

Claiming the right to control the end of our lives in no way minimizes the seriousness or the finality of the decision, nor the pain and grief of those we leave behind. The Voluntary Euthanasia Society (see Organizations) continues to publicize the issue, despite fierce opposition from some religious bodies, and can help us to deal with the problem personally.

Practical Matters

Before we die, some of us may want to donate vitally needed organs, such as kidneys and corneas, for transplant purposes. A donor's card can be supplied by a doctor's surgery or Health Centre, and should be carried at all times. If an organ is to be donated for transplant, it must be removed almost immediately after death – a kidney within half an hour and an eye within six hours. It is obvious, therefore, that some written instructions will speed things up, and, of course, save relatives some indecision and anxiety.

A growing number of people today want to keep matters relating to death under the control of their immediate circle of friends and family. Preparing the body for burial, the burial or cremation itself, and last rites and memorial services can all, within broad limits, be designed to suit the wishes of the person who has died and her or his survivors.

The person I talked to about renting a place for the memorial service told me sharply that I had no business planning a memorial while my mother was still alive. But I am very thankful that we did plan it when we did. First of all, I was amazed to find that I was in absolutely no condition to make sensible plans after she died. . . . Planning the forms of the memorial beforehand helped me face the reality of my mother's death. Thinking about and writing what I would say brought the love we had shared back to me once more. Participating in the memorial gave me a kind of peace and acceptance I hardly dared hope for.[11]

If you have preferences about your burial or cremation, it will be much easier for your family and friends to carry out your wishes if you make them known in writing. This will also protect your loved ones from having feelings of guilt, because they will be assured they are following your wishes.

This is especially important if you want a particular kind of religious ceremony or none at all. A growing number of people who have professed no religion in their lifetime find it hypocritical to 'make use' of religion when they die. The arrangements for the funeral of someone who has not been a regular worshipper are often unsatisfactory and impersonal. Some families and friends of non-believers make satisfactory and satisfying arrangements for the funeral themselves. Others can get help in arranging the funeral, or have it actually conducted by, an experienced member of the British Humanist Association (see Organizations).

Remember that the funeral business is just that – a profitable business. When arranging a funeral, make sure that the undertaker is a member of the Funeral Directors' Association, who have a code of practice, which should ensure reasonable standards and charges.

What to Do When Someone Dies is a Consumers Association book which should be in your public library. *On Your Own* (see below) and the leaflets you will be given when registering a death are useful in the immediate aftermath.

Those of us who are struggling to come to a better understanding of the great, universal transition at the end of life have many opportunities to ponder the matter. Experiences such as watching persons we are close to approach death, becoming aware of symptoms that might signal the beginning of life-threatening illness, putting our affairs in order in a written will, working as a volunteer in a hospice or hospital, or being part of a supportive network for a dying friend or relative, all can help us come to a peaceful, personal understanding of death.

NOTES

[1]Tish Sommers, *Death – A Feminist View*. Paper presented at Drake University Law School, Des Moines, Iowa, 27 March 1976.

[2]Elisabeth Kübler-Ross, *On Death and Dying*. New York: Macmillan, 1969.

[3]Carolyn Ruth Swift, unpublished manuscript.

[4]Mickey Spencer, 'Plan Ahead'. *Broomstick*, Vol. 7, No. 6, November–December 1985, pp. 40–2.

[5]J. W. Worden and William Proctor, *Personal Death Awareness*. Englewood Cliffs, NJ: Prentice-Hall, 1976.

[6]Swift, op. cit.

[7]See Stephen Jay Gould, 'The Median Isn't the Message'. *Discover*, Vol. 6, No. 6, June 1985, pp. 40–2.

[8]George Annas and Joan Densberger, 'Competence to Refuse Medical Treatment: Autonomy vs. Paternalism'. *University of Toledo Law Review*, Vol. 15, 1984, pp. 561–96.

[9]Joseph F. Sullivan, 'Wishes of Patient in Refusing Care Backed in New Jersey: Right to Die is Extended. Rulings in Three Cases Give Interests of Individuals Priority Over State's'. *The New York Times*, 25 June 1987, pp. 1, B12.

[10]Roxanne Cummings Potter, 'To Life – To Death'. *California Association of Midwives Newsletter*, Spring 1984, p. 7.

[11]Spencer, op. cit.

BOOKS AND PUBLICATIONS

Colin Murray Parkes, *Bereavement: Studies of Grief in Adult Life*. London: Penguin, 1986.

Elisabeth Kübler-Ross, *On Death and Dying*. London: Tavistock Publications, 1973.

Cicely Saunders and Mary Baines, *Living With Dying: Management of Terminal Disease*. Oxford: Oxford University Press, 1983.

Consumers Association, *What to Do When Someone Dies*. (See Organizations.)

Anthony Wright, Jennifer Cousins and Janet Upward, *Matters of Death and Life: a Study of Bereavement Support in NHS Hospitals in Eng-*land. King's Fund Centre, 1988. (See Organizations.)

Dr Trish Reynolds, *Your Cancer: Your Life*. London: Macdonald Optima, 1988. Discusses causes, treatments, options (including right to refuse life-prolonging treatment) from a radical viewpoint.

Dr R. G. Owens and F. Naylor, *Living While Dying*. Wellingborough: Thorsons, 1988.

Margaret Torrie, *Helping the Widowed*. Cruse. (See Organizations.)

30
Changing Society and Ourselves

How far have women – and particularly older women – achieved equality, respect and dignity in our lifetime? The autumn 1988 BBC programmes, *Out of the Dolls' House*, the book accompanying the series, and the exhibition staged in conjunction with it, gave many of us some cause for pride. We were there! The changes in our lives so graphically shown in words and images were achieved not only through technological progress, but through the initiatives and campaigns of women themselves – from the suffragettes of the early 1900s to the feminist movement of the 1970s and 1980s, women's voices have been heard as never before. Women are now a force to be reckoned with.

Yet in the face of the attacks on living standards and the quality of life of most older women – what has been called the 'feminization of poverty' – we can hardly be complacent. Reduction in social services and benefits, the Poll Tax, the running down of the health service – all affect the lives of most except the very rich. It's of little comfort to the elderly woman waiting in daily pain for two years for a hip replacement operation to know that a few women can now be members of the Stock Exchange or sit on the Board of Directors of an advertising agency. Poorer women and those from 'ethnic minorities' have never occupied a 'dolls' house'. Exploited at work and at home, their lives have been one long struggle. Instead of a comfortable old age, all they can look forward to is increasing deprivation as the cuts bite deeper.

But this need not be a permanent state of affairs. We can take our lives into our own hands. We can decide what kind of an older woman we want to be. Is she the powerless, discriminated-against victim of an increasingly uncaring society, or someone who knows her rights, stands up for them, and works as an individual and with others to halt the erosion of the welfare state that was a central target of government throughout the 1980s? If we look around us we will see strong, active, energetic, caring older women who are not defeated by the myths of ageing; whose involvement in the politics of health, education, freedom and peace is as strong as that of any of the past pioneers of women's rights. Such women can be our role models.

No woman is an island. All our lives we depend on others for emotional as well as physical sustenance. The only way we can combat the loneliness and isolation that are the saddest aspect of so many women's older years is to look to our fellow-women for friendship, support and understanding. To offer each other the precious gifts of tolerance and love.

Armed with a strong sense of personal worth, knowledge and experience, we can withstand the onslaughts of the establishment, the media and the official and unofficial put-downs most of us meet every day. Only by getting together, though, can we create an impact that will force recognition that we older women are part – and a part to be reckoned with – of the fabric of Britain in the 1990s.

In the United States older women have got together on a state-wide or national scale in ways that we in Britain have not yet achieved. Of course there are long-standing organizations like the Women's Institutes, the Townswomen's Guilds and the Co-operative Women's Guilds, many of whose members are older women; but their form of organization, their aims and campaigns have so far not focused specifically on the needs of older women.

The women's movement that was revived in the 1970s was composed mainly of young women, whose campaigns on issues affecting them, such as abortion and child care provision, put them on the map. Local and national groups raised consciousness and provided a forum for discussion of current issues, sparking off a variety of political activities. But older women often felt excluded, and even looked down upon, by young feminists. It was in response to these feelings that two members of the *Spare Rib* magazine collective initiated a meeting of older readers, which resulted in the formation of the Older Feminists' Network.

The Network meets in London at roughly five-week intervals throughout the year, and although most of its members live in the South East, some women travel long distances to attend. The meetings are partly social occasions – through which new friendships are formed – but they also provide workshops and discussions on topics that concern older women. As a result of contacts made at the London meetings, some local groups have been formed, and the Older Lesbian Network, too, has grown out of OFN. At last some older feminists feel that their particular needs are being met, and isolation and loneliness broken down. It is this sense of being odd and out of step with today's society that was the strongest motivation in many women for joining the Networks.

Another very positive result of this getting together of older women has been the support it has engendered for peace and anti-nuclear activities – some Older Feminists have joined the Greenham Common women and worked for conservation and 'green' issues, as well as becoming closely involved in local government.

Although action by and for older women on a national scale is still largely unco-ordinated, there are signs that this situation may be rectified. The National Council for Voluntary Service has set up a national interest group; there's a loose consortium of further education bodies working in the field of over-sixties health and general education; the Pre-Retirement Association is active in promoting the interests of older people (though until recently the emphasis has been on *men* on the verge of retirement).

In those areas where local authority Women's Committees have not been axed, they have backed local initiatives, especially on issues affecting minorities. In London the Older Women's Project, part of Pensioners' Link, is providing a model for the rest of the country. Initiated in 1985, the Project, sometimes in conjunction with other bodies such as the London University Centre for Extra-Mural Studies, Age Concern, and the Standing Conference of Ethnic Minority Senior Citizens, has organized or participated in study days, conferences, women's festivals, health and housing meetings. It has supported a number of local older women's projects in the Greater London area.

These projects campaign on local issues, getting local groups and individuals together to lobby councils and councillors. They have participated in national lobbies of MPs on matters that affect all of us as older women. Campaigns can take many forms: one success, for instance, resulted from a campaign against the closure of women's public lavatories in a London borough. When the women managed to meet their councillors, and to point out that men's needs were being met far more generously than theirs – and that older women were just as prone as men to be 'caught short' in the High Street, it was a revelation to the male councillors. They weren't only surprised to learn these physical facts of life, but by the strength of feeling and the organized and articulate ways in which it had been expressed. It is from such small victories that our experience and, above all, our confidence in our own power grows. Some of us who have never before organized action, spoken in public, or tackled authority, ever after cease to be passive recipients of whatever local and national government decides to hand out.

In the hostile political climate of the 1980s we have to learn to work together with all other organizations whose aims broadly coincide with ours. We have to try to do this without losing our own particular identity. And we have to remember that other groups and individuals have their own identities, too. Their experiences and backgrounds may be different from ours, but are just as valid. Middle-aged and older women have much to learn from the experiences of the black movement, the mainstream feminist movement and the campaigns of women in the past. We must join together to ensure that our distinctive voices are heard, and in fighting for a better world for everyone we can demonstrate not only what we need from society, but what we can give.

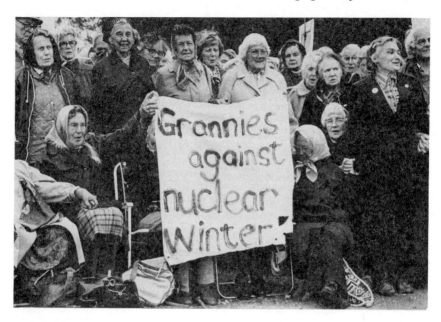

BOOKS AND PUBLICATIONS

Angela Holdsworth, *Out of the Dolls' House: The Story of Women in the Twentieth Century.* London: BBC Publications, 1988.

Pensioners' Link, Information Pack on Older Women's Project. For individuals or groups planning similar projects. Free leaflet: send s.a.e. (See Organizations.)

Organizations

Accept Services UK (ACCEPT), Accept Clinic, 200 Seagrave Road, London SW6 1RQ 01-381 3155

Action Against Allergy (AAA), 43 The Downs, London SW20 8HG 01-947 5082

Action for Benefits, 124–130 Southwark Street, London SE1 0TU 01-928 9671

Action for Victims of Medical Accidents, 24 Southwark Street, London SE1 1TY 01-403 4744

Action on Smoking and Health, 5–11 Mortimer Street, London W1N 7RH 01-637 9843/6

Afro-Caribbean Education Resource Centre (ACER), Wyvil School, Wyvil Road, London SW28 2TJ 01-627 2662

Afro-Caribbean Resource Centre Ltd (ACRC), 339 Dudley Road, Winson Green, Birmingham B18 4HB 021-455 6382

Age Concern England, 60 Pitcairn Road, Mitcham, Surrey CR4 3LL 01-640 5431

Age Concern Scotland, 33 Castle Street, Edinburgh EH2 3DN

Age Exchange, 11 Blackheath Village, London SE3 9LA 01-318 3504

Al-Anon Family Groups UK and Eire, 61 Great Dover Street, London SE1 4YF 01-403 0888

Albany Trust, 24 Chester Square, London SW1N 9HS 01-730 5871

Alcohol Concern, 305 Gray's Inn Road, London WC1X 8QF 01-833 3471

Alcoholics Anonymous, PO Box 1, Stonebow House, Stonebow, York YO1 2NJ 0904-644026

Alzheimer's Disease Society, 158/160 Balham High Road, London SW12 9BN 01-675 6557/8/9

Amarant Trust, 14 Lord North Street, London SW1P 3LW

Anatomia Ltd, 21 Hampstead Road, London NW1 01-437 0310

Anchor Housing Association, Anchor House, 269a Banbury Road, Oxford OX2 7HU 0865-311511

Anorexia and Bulimia Nervosa Association (ABNA), Tottenham Women's Health Centre, Annexe C, Tottenham Town Hall, London N5 4RX 01-885 3936

Anorexic Aid, The Priory Centre, 11 Priory Road, High Wycombe, Bucks. HP13 6SL

Arthritis and Rheumatism Council (ARC), 41 Eagle Street, London WC1R 4AR 01-405 8572

Arthritis Care, 6 Grosvenor Crescent, London SW1X 7ER 01-235 0902

Asian Women's Resource Centre, 124 Minet Avenue, London NW10 01-961 6549

Association for Improvements in the Maternity Services, 163 Liverpool Road, London N1 0RF 01-278 5628

Association for Self Help and Community Groups, 14 Hillfield Park, London N10 01-444 8664

Association of Carers, 21–23 New Road, Chatham, Kent ME4 4JQ 0634-813981

Association of Community Health Councils for England and Wales (ACHEW), 30 Drayton Park, London N5 1PB 01-609 8405

Association of Crossroads Care Attendant Schemes Ltd, 10 Regent Place, Rugby, Warwickshire CV21 2PN 0788-73653

Association of Disabled Professionals, The Stables, 73 Pound Road, Banstead, Surrey SM7 2HU 0737-352366

Association of Radical Midwives (ARM), 62 Greetby Hill, Ormskirk, Lancs. L32 2DT 0695-72776

Asthma Society and Friends of Asthma Research Council, 300 Upper Street, London N1 2XX 01-226 2260

Back Pain Association, 31–33 Park Road, Teddington, Middlesex TW11 0AB 01-977 5754

Bangladesh Women's Association, 91 Highbury Hills, London N5 1SX 01-359 5836

Black Women's Centre (Brixton), 41a Stockwell Green, London SW9 01-274 9220

Breastcare and Mastectomy Association of GB, 26a Harrison St, London WC1 01-837 0908

Breast Cancer Research Trust, 7 Soho Street, London W1V 5FA 01-437 9727

Bristol Cancer Help Centre, Grove House, Cornwallis Grove, Clifton, Bristol BS8 4PG 0272-743216

British Acupuncture Association and Register, 34 Alderney Street, London SW1 4EU 01-834 1012

British Agencies for Adoption and Fostering, 11 Southwark Street, London SE1 1RQ 01-407 8800

British Association for Counselling, 37a Sheep Street, Rugby, Warwickshire CV21 3BX 0788-78328/9

British Association of Cancer United Patients (BACUP), 121/123 Charterhouse Street, London EC1M 6AA 01-608 1785

British Association of the Hard of Hearing, 7–11 Armstrong Road, London W3 7JL 01-743 1110/1353

British Association of Plastic Surgeons, Royal College of Surgeons, 35–43 Lincoln's Inn Fields, London WC2A 3PN 01-405 6507

British Cancer and Mastectomy Association of Great Britain, 26 Harrison Street, London WC1H 8JG 01-837 0908/01-278 3529

British Council of Organizations of Disabled People (BCODP), St Mary's Church, Greenlaw Street, London SE18 5AR 01-316 4184

British Deaf Association, 38 Victoria Place, Carlisle, Cumbria CA1 1HU 0228-48844

British Dental Health Foundation (BDHF), 88 Gurnard's Avenue, Fishermead, Milton Keynes MK6 2BL 0908-667063

British Diabetic Association, 10 Queen Anne Street, London W1M 0BD 01-323 1531

British Epilepsy Association, Anstey House, 40 Hanover Square, Leeds LS3 1BE 0532-439393

British Foundation for Age Research, 48 Queen Victoria Street, London EC4N 4SA 01-236 4365

British Geriatrics Society (BGS), 1 St Andrew's Place, Regent's Park, London NW1 4LB 01-935 4004

British Heart Foundation, 102 Gloucester Place, London W1H 4DH 01-935 0185

British Herbal Medical Association (BHMA), PO Box 304, Bournemouth, Dorset BH7 6JZ 0202-433691

British Holistic Medical Association, 179 Gloucester Place, London NW1 6DX 01-262 5299

British Homoeopathic Association (BHA), 27a Devonshire Street, London W1N 1RJ 01-935 2163

British Humanist Association, 13 Prince of Wales Terrace, London W8 5PG 01-937 2341/938 4791

British Insurance Brokers Association, 10 Bevis Marks, London EC3 01-623 9043

British Kidney Patient Association (BKPA), Bordon, Hampshire GU35 9JP 04203-2021/2

British Library of Tape Recordings for Hospital Patients, 12 Lant Street, London SE1 1QH 01-407 9417

British Migraine Association, 178a High Road, Weybridge, Surrey KT14 7ED 09323-52468

British Pensioners and Trade Union Action Association, Norman Dodd's House, 315 Bexley Road, Erith, Kent 0747-61802

British Pregnancy Advisory Service, Austy Manor, Wootton Wawen, Solihull, West Midlands B95 6BX 05642-3225

British Red Cross Society, 9 Grosvenor Crescent, London SW1X 7EJ 01-235 5454

British Sport Association for the Disabled, Haward House, Barnard Crescent, Aylesbury, Bucks. HP21 9PP 0296-27889

British Tinnitus Association, 105 Gower Street, London WC1E 6AH 01-387 4803

British Touch for Health Association (BTFHA), c/o Adrian Voce, 8 Railey Mews, London NW5

British United Provident Association (BUPA), Provident House, Essex Street, London WC2 01-353 5212

British Wheel of Yoga, Grafton Grange, Grafton, York YO5 9QQ 09012-3386

Camden Chinese Community Centre (CCCC), 173 Arlington Road, London NW1 7EY 01-267 3019

Campaign for Freedom of Information, 3 Endsleigh Street, London WC1H 0DD 01-278 9686

Campaign for Homosexual Equality (CHE), 274 Upper Street, London N1 2UA 01-359 3973

Campaign for Lead-Free Air, see *CLEAR*

Cancer Help Centre, Bristol, see *Bristol Cancer Health Centre*

CancerLink, 17 Britannia Street, London WC1X 9JN 01-833 2451

Cancer Prevention Society, Volunteer Centre, 25/27 Elmbank Street, Glasgow G2 4PB 041-226 3431

Cancer Relief Macmillan Fund, Anchor House, 15 Britten Street, London SW3 3TY 01-351 7811

Caribbean House Group and West Indian Concern Ltd, Caribbean House, Bridport Place, London N1 5DS 01-729 0986

Caring for the Carers, St James the Less Centre, Moreton Street, London SW1V 2PT 01-931 7440

Centre for Policy on Ageing, 25–31 Ironmonger Row, London EC1V 3QP 01-253 1787

Chemical Cancer Hazard Information Service, Department of Cancer Studies, University Medical School, Birmingham B15 2TJ 021-472 1010

Chest, Heart and Stroke Association, Tavistock House North, Tavistock Square, London WC1H 9JE 01-387 3012

Child Poverty Action Group, 4th Floor, 1–5 Bath Street, London EC1B 9PY 01-253 3406

Chile Solidarity Campaign Women's Section, 129 Seven Sisters Road, London N7 7OG 01-272 4298

Chinese Information and Advice Centre (CIAC), 152–156 Shaftesbury Avenue, London WC2 01-836 8291

CLEANAIR – Campaign for a Smoke-Free Environment, 33 Stillness Road, London SE23 1NG 01-690 4649

CLEAR – Campaign for Lead-Free Air, 3 Endsleigh Street, London WC1H 0DD 01-278 9686

College of Health, 18 Victoria Park Square, London E2 9PF

Colostomy Welfare Group, 38–39 Eccleston Square, London SW1V 1PB 01-828 5175

Community Resources Centre, Mary Burnie House, Westhill College, Birmingham B29 6LL

Company Pensions Information Centre, 7 Old Park Lane, London W1 01-493 4757

Consumers Association, 14 Buckingham Street, London WC2 01-839 1222

Co-operative Women's Guild, 342 Hoe Street, Walthamstow, London E17 9PX 01-520 4902

Coronary Artery Disease Research Association (CORDA), Tavistock House North, Tavistock Square, London WC1H 9TH 01-387 9779

Coronary Prevention Group (CPG), 60 Great Ormond Street, London WC1N 3HR 01-833 3687

Council for Involuntary Tranquillizer Addiction, Cavendish House, Brighton Road, Liverpool L22 5NQ 051-949 0102

Council for Voluntary Service, National Association, 26 Bedford Square, London WC1B 3HU 01-636 4066

Counsel and Care for the Elderly, Twyman House, 16 Bonny Street, London NW1 9LR 01-485 1566

Cruse – Bereavement Care, Cruse House, 126 Sheen Road, Richmond, Surrey TW9 1UR 01-940 4818

DAWN (Drugs, Alcohol and Women Nationally), Omnibus Workplace, 39–41 North Road, London N7 01-700 4653

Depressives Associated, 19 Merley Ways, Wimborne Minster, Dorset BH21 1QN 0202 883957

Disability Alliance, 25 Denmark Street, London WC2H 8NJ 01-240 0806

Disabled Living Foundation (DLF), 380–384 Harrow Road, London W9 2HU 01-289 6111

Disablement Income Group, Millmead Business Centre, Millmead Road, London N17 9QU 01-801 8013

Drugline, 9a Brockley Cross, London SE4 2AB 01-692 4975

Elderly Accommodation Council (EAC), 1 Durward House, 31 Kensington Court, London W8 5BH 01-937 8709

Endometriosis Society, 65 Holmdene Avenue, Herne Hill, London SE24 9LD 01-737 4764

Family Planning Association, Margaret Pyke House, 27–35 Mortimer Street, London W1N 7RJ 01-636 7866

Family Welfare Association, 501–505 Kingsland Road, London E8 4AU 01-254 6251

Farm and Food Society (FAFS), 4 Willifield Way, London NW11 7XF 01-455 0634

Fat Women's Support Group, c/o Beverley Duguid, 53 Sandbourne, Essex Gardens' Centre, London W11 1DS 01-382 7513

Fawcett Library, City of London Polytechnic, Old Castle Street, London E1 7NT 01-283 1030, ext. 570

Fawcett Society, 46 Harleyford Road, London SE11 5AY 01-587 1287

Federation of Black Housing Organizations (FBHO), 374 Gray's Inn Road, London WC1X 8BB

Federation of Housing Co-operatives, see *Shelter*

Feminist Audio Books (FAB), 52–54 Featherstone Street, London EC1Y 8RT 01-251 2908/0713

Feminist Library and Information Centre, Hungerford House, Victoria Embankment, London WC2N 6PA 01-930 0715

Food and Chemical Allergy Association (FCAA), 27 Ferringham Lane, Ferring-By-Sea, West Sussex BN12 5NB 0903-41178

Friends of the Earth, 26–28 Underwood Street, London N1 7JQ 01-490 1555

Gay Bereavement Project, Unitarian Rooms, Hoop Lane, London NW11 8BS 01-455 6844 (admin.) – 01-455 8894 (clients)

GEMMA (Lesbians with/without Disabilities), BM Box 5700, London WC1N 3XX

GRACE, PO Box 71, Cobham, Surrey KT11 2JR 01-0932 62928

Greenpeace, 30–31 Islington Green, London N1 8XE 01-251 3022/3020

Guide Dogs for the Blind Association, Alexander House, 9 Park Street, Windsor, Berks. SL4 1JR 0753-855711

Haemophilia Society, 123 Westminster Bridge Road, London SE1 7HR 01-928 2020

Health Information Trust, 18 Victoria Park Square, London E2 9PF 01-980 6263

Help the Aged, 16–18 St James's Walk, London EC1R 0BE 01-253 0253
Help the Hospices, BMA House, Tavistock Square, London WC1H 9JP 01-388 7807
Herpes Association (The HA), 41 North Road, London N7 9DP 01-609 9061
Holiday Care Service, 2 Old Bank Chambers, Station Road, Horley, Surrey RH6
9HW 0293-774535
Housing Association Charitable Trust, 175 Gray's Inn Road, London WC1X 8UX 01-
278 6571
Hysterectomy Support Group (HSG) (London), 11 Henryson Road, London SE4
1HL 01-690 5987
Hysterectomy Support Group (Merseyside), Riverdell, Warren Way, Lower Heswall,
Wirral, Merseyside

Ileostomy Association of Great Britain and Ireland (IA), Amblehurst House, Black Scotch
Lane, Mansfield, Notts. NG18 4DF
India Welfare Society (IWS), 11 Middle Row, London W10 5AT 01-969 9493
Institute for Complementary Medicine (ICM), 21 Portland Place, London W1N 3AF 01-
636 9543
Invalids at Home, 17 Lapstone Gardens, Kenton, Harrow HA3 0EB 01-907 1706

Jewish Welfare Board, Stuart Young House, 221 Golders Green Road, London NW11
9DW

Keep Fit Association, 16 Upper Woburn Place, London WC1H 0QG
King's Fund Centre for Health Services Development, 126 Albert Street, London NW1
7NF 01-267 6111

Latin American Women's Rights Service, Priory House, Kingsgate Place, London NW6
4AT 01-372 6408
Law Centres Federation, Duchess House, 18–19 Warren Street, London W1P 5DB 01-
387 8570
League of British Muslims, 41 Cecil Road, Ilford, Essex 01-594 9080 and Webber
House, 37 North Street, Barking, Essex IG11 8JG 01-592 3050
Lesbian and Gay Employment Rights (LAGER), Room 23, South Bank House, Black
Prince Road, London SE1 7SJ 01-587 1636 (lesbians) – 01-587 1643 (gay men)
Let's Face It Support Network for the Facially Disfigured, 10 Wood End, Crowthorne,
Berks. RG11 6DQ 0344-774405
London Food Commission, 88 Old Street, London EC1V 9AR 01-253 9513
London Irish Women's Centre, 59 Church Street, London N16 01-249 7818
London Lesbian Line, Box BM 1514, London WC1N 3XX 01-251 6911

Macmillan Nurses, Anchor House, 15 Britten Street, London SW3 3TY 01-351 7811
Marie Curie Memorial Foundation, 28 Belgrave Square, London SW1X 8QG 01-235
3325
Mastectomy Association, 26 Harrison Street, London WC1H 8JG 01-837 0908/01-278
3529

Menopause Collective, see Women's Health & Reproductive Rights Information Centre

Menopause Self-Help Groups in London. Contact Jayne Nelson, 50 Mercer's Road, London N1G 01-272 3919

Midlifestyle, Birmingham Settlement, 318 Summer Lane, Birmingham B19 3RL

Migraine Trust, 45 Great Ormond Street, London WC1N 3HD 01-278 2676

MIND (National Association for Mental Health), 22 Harley Street, London W1N 2ED 01-637 0741

Multiple Sclerosis Society of Great Britain and Northern Ireland, 25 Effie Road, Fulham SW6 1EE 01-736 6267

Myalgic Encephalomyelitis Association (ME Association), PO Box 8, Stanford-le-Hope, Essex SS17 8EX 0375-642466

National Advisory Centre on Careers for Women, 8th Floor, Artillery House, Artillery Row, London SW1P 1RT

National Association for Premenstrual Syndrome (NAPS), 25 Market Street, Guildford, Surrey GU1 4LB 0483-572715

National Association of Grandparents, 8 Kirkley Drive, Ashington, Northumbria NE63 9RD

National Association of Widows/Widows' Advisory Trust, 1st Floor, 14 Waterloo Street, Birmingham B2 5TX 021-643 8348

National Council for Carers, 29 Chilworth Mews, London W2 3RG 01-724 7776

National Council for Carers and their Elderly Dependants, 29 Chilworth Mews, London W2 3RG 01-262 1451

National Council for the Divorced and Separated, 13 High Street, Little Shelford, Cambs. CB2 5ES 021-5885757

National Council for Voluntary Organizations, 26 Bedford Square, London WC1B 3HU 01-636 4066

National Council of Women of Great Britain, 36 Danbury Street, Islington, London N1 8JU 01-354 2395

National Ethnic Minority Advisory Council (NEMAC), 2nd and 3rd Floors, 13 Macclesfield Street, London W1V 7HL 01-349 8765

National Federation of Housing Associations, 175 Gray's Inn Road, London WC1 01-278 6571

National Federation of Housing Co-operatives, 88 Old St, London EC1V 9AX 01-608 2494

National Federation of Retirement Pensions Association, 14 St Peter St, Blackburn BB2 2HD 0254 52606

National Federation of Self-Help Organizations (NFSHO), Central Information Office, 150 Townmead Road, London SW6 2RA 01-731 4438/9/40

National Federation of Women's Institutes, 39 Eccleston Street, London SW1 9NT 01-730 7212

National Friend (FRIEND), BM Friend, London WC1N 3XX

National Institute of Adult Continuing Education, 19b de Montfort Street, Leicester LE1 7GE 0533-551451

National Osteoporosis Society (NOS), PO Box 10, Barton Meade House, Radstock, Bath, Avon BA3 3YB 0761-32472

National Schizophrenia Fellowship, 79 Victoria Road, Surbiton, Surrey KT6 4NS 01-390 3651/3

National Tranquillizer Advice Centre, 25a Masons Avenue, Wealdstone, Harrow, Middlesex HA3 5AH 01-427 2065 (answer phone 01-427 2065)

National Union of Townswomen's Guilds, Chamber of Commerce House, 75 Harbourne Road, Birmingham B15 3DA 021-456 3435

National Women's Register, 245 Warwick Road, Solihull, West Midlands B92 7AH 021-706 1101

New Approaches to Cancer, Addington Park, Maidstone, Kent ME19 5BL 0732-848336

New Ways to Work, 309 Upper Street, London N1 01-226 4026

Occupational Pensions Advisory Service (OPAS), 8a Bloomsbury Square, London WC1

Older Feminists' Network, c/o London Women's Centre, Wesley House, 4 Wild Court, London WC2B 5AU 01-831 7863

Older Lesbian Network, c/o London Friend, 274 Upper Street, London N1

Organic Living Association (OLA), St Mary's Villa, Hanley Swan, Worcs. WR8 0EA

Over Forty Association for Women Workers, Mary George House, 120–122 Cromwell Road, London SW7 01-370 2556/2507

Pain Relief Foundation (PRF), Rice Lane, Walton, Liverpool, Merseyside L9 1AE 051-523 1486

Pakistan Welfare Association (PWA), 181 Haydons Road, London SW19 8TS 01-542 6176

Parents Enquiry, 16 Honley Road, London SE6 2HZ 01-698 1815

Parkinson's Disease Society, 36 Portland Place, London W1N 3DG 01-255 2432

Patients Association, Room 33, 18 Charing Cross Road, London WC2H 0HR 01-240 0671

Pellin Centre, 43 Killyon Road, London SW8 2XS 01-720 4499

Pensioners' Link, 17 Balfe Street, London N1 9EB 01-278 5501/4

Pensioners' Voice, Melling House, 14 St Peter Street, Blackburn, Lancs. BB2 2HW 0254-52606

Phobic Action, Greater London House, 547/551 High Road, Leytonstone, London E11 4PR 01-558 3463/6012

Pregnancy Advisory Service, 13 Charlotte Street, London W1P 1HD 01-637 8962/8999

Pre-Retirement Association of Great Britain and Northern Ireland (PRA), 19 Undine Street, London SW17 8PP 01-767 3225

Private Patients Plan, Tavistock House, South Tavistock Square, London WC1 01-388 2468

Ramblers Association, 1/5 Wandsworth Road, London SW8 2XX 01-582 6878/6826

REACH, Retired Executives Action Clearing-House, 89 Southwark Street, London SE1 0HD 01-928 0452

Relate (National Marriage Guidance Council), Herbert Gray College, Little Church Street, Rugby, Warwickshire CV21 3AP 0788-73241

Release, c/o 347a Upper Street, London N1 0PD 01-289 1123 (24-hr emergency 01-603 8654)

Rights of Women, 52–54 Featherstone Street, London EC1Y 8RT 01-251 6577

Royal Association for Disability and Rehabilitation (RADAR), 25 Mortimer Street, London W1N 8AB 01-637 5400

Royal National Institute for the Blind (RNIB), 224 Great Portland Street, London W1N 6AA 01-388 1266

Royal National Institute for the Deaf (RNID), 105 Gower Street, London WC1E 6AH 01-387 8033

Royal Society for Mentally Handicapped Children and Adults (MENCAP), Mencap National Centre, 123 Golden Lane, London EC1Y 0RT 01-253 9433

St John Ambulance, 1 Grosvenor Crescent, London SW1X 7EF 01-235 5231

Samaritans, 17 Uxbridge Road, Slough, Berks. SL1 1SN 0753-32713 (see telephone directory for local numbers)

SHAC (The London Housing Aid Centre), 189a Old Brompton Road, London SW5 0AR 01-373 7276/7841

Shelter National Campaign for the Homeless, 88 Old Street, London EC1V 9HU 01-253 0202

Socialist Health Association, 195 Walworth Road, London SE17 1RP 01-703 6838

Society for Environmental Therapy (SET), 521 Foxhall Road, Ipswich, Suffolk IP3 8LW 0473-723552

Society of Pension Consultants, Ludgate House, Ludgate Circus, London EC4 01-353 1688

Soil Association, 86 Colston Street, Bristol BS1 5BB 0272-290661

Spitalfields Housing Co-operative, 170 Brick Lane, London E4 01-247 1040

SPOD (Association to Aid the Sexual and Personal Relationships of People with a Disability), 286 Camden Road, London N7 0BJ 01-607 8851/2

Standing Conference of Ethnic Minority Senior Citizens, Ethnic Minority Resource Centre, 5–5a Westminster Bridge Road, London SE1 7XW 01-928 0095/8108, ext. 34

Standing Conference of Women's Organizations, 20 Moorgate Avenue, Bamford, Rochdale, Lancs. OL11 5JY 0706-57192

Standing Conference on Drug Abuse (SCODA), 1–4 Hatton Place, Hatton Garden, London EC1N 8ND 01-430 2341/2

Terrence Higgins Trust, BM Aids, London WC1N 3XX 01-831 0330 (admin.) – 01-242 1010 (helpline)

300 Group, 9 Poland Street, London W1V 3DG 01-734 3457

TRANX (UK) Ltd, National Tranquillizer Advice Centre, 25a Masons Avenue,

Wealdstone, Harrow, Middlesex HA3 5AH 01-427 2065 (answer phone 01-427 2065)

U and I Club, 18 Southcote Way, Tylers Green, Bucks.
Union of Turkish Women in Britain (UTWB), 110 Clarence Road, London E5 01-986 1358
University of the Third Age (National Office), 13 Stockwell Road, London SW9 9AU 01-737 2541

VDU Workers' Rights Campaign, City Centre, 32/35 Featherstone Street, London EC1Y 8QX 01-608 1338
Vegan Society, 33–35 George Street, Oxford OX1 2AY 0865-722166
Vegetarian Society of the United Kingdom Ltd, Parkdale, Dunham, Altrincham, Cheshire WA14 4QG 061-928 0793
Voluntary Euthanasia Society, 13 Prince of Wales Terrace, London W8 5PG 01-937 7770
Volunteer Centre, 29 Lower King's Road, Berkhamsted, Herts. HP4 2AB 04427-73311

Western Provident Association, 160 Piccadilly, London W1 01-409 0414
West Indian Women's Association (WIWA), 71 Pound Lane, Willesden, London NW10 2HU 01-451 4827
Winged Fellowship Trust (Holidays for Disabled People), Angel House, Pentonville Road, London N1 9XD 01-833 2594
Wireless for the Bedridden, 81b Corbets Tey Road, Upminster, Essex RM14 2AJ 04022-50051
Woman's Place, Hungerford House, Victoria Embankment, London WCN 6PA 01-836 6081
Women for Life on Earth (WFLOE), 2 Bramshill Gardens, London NW5 1JH 01-281 4018
Women's Aid Federation (England) Ltd, PO Box 391, Bristol BS99 7WS 0272-420611 (helpline 0272-428368)
Women's Alcohol Centre (WAC), 254 St Paul's Road, Islington, London N1 2LJ 01-226 4581
Women's Environment Network, 287 City Road, London EC1 01-490 2511
Women's Health and Reproductive Rights Information Centre (WHRRIC), 52–54 Featherstone Street, London EC1Y 8RT 01-251 6332/6580
Women's Information Referral and Enquiry Service (WIRES), PO Box 20, Oxford, Oxon 0865-240991
Women's National Cancer Control Campaign, 1 South Audley Street, London W1Y 5DQ 01-499 7532
Women's Natural Health Centre, 1 Hillside, Highgate Road, London NW5 1QT 01-482 3293
Women's Nutritional Advisory Service (WNAS), PO Box 268, Brighton, East Sussex BN3 1RW 0273-771366

Women's Research and Resources Centre, Hungerford House, Victoria Embankment, London WC2N 6PA 01-930 0715

Women's Sports Foundation (WSF), c/o London Women's Centre, Wesley House, 4 Wild Court, London WC2B 5AU 01-831 7863

Women's Therapy Centre (WTC), 6 Manor Gardens, London N7 6LA 01-263 6200

Yoga for Health Foundation, Ickwell Bury, Northill, Biggleswade, Beds. SG18 9EF

Public and Professional Advisory Organizations

Voluntary Sector

Northern Ireland Council of Voluntary Action, 127 Ormeau Road, Belfast BT1 5H 0232-321224

Scottish Council for Voluntary Organizations, 18–19 Claremont Crescent, Edinburgh EH7 4HX 031-556 3882

Wales Council for Voluntary Action, Llys Ifor, Heol Crescent, Caerffili, Canol Morgannwg CF8 1XL 0222-869224/5/6 and 869111

Consumer Affairs

National Consumer Council, 20 Grosvenor Gardens, London SW1W 0DN 01-730 3469

Education

Adult Literacy and Basic Skills Unit, 229–331 High Holborn, London WC1V 7DA 01-405 4017

Advisory Centre for Education, 18 Victoria Park Square, London E2 9PB 01-980 4596

British Council, 10 Spring Gardens, London SW1A 2BN 01-930 8466

Central Bureau for Educational Visits and Exchanges, Seymour Mews House, Seymour Mews, London W1H 9PE 01-486 5101 or Edinburgh 031-477 8024, Belfast 0232-664418

Open University, Walton Hall, Milton Keynes MK7 6AA

Employment and Industry

British Institute of Management, Management House, Parker Street, London WC2B 5PT 01-405 3456

Trades Union Congress, Congress House, Great Russell Street, London WC1 3LS 01-636 4030

Equal Opportunities

Commission for Racial Equality, Elliot House, 10–12 Allington Street, London SW1E 5EH 01-828 7022

Equal Opportunities Commission, Overseas House, Quay Street, Manchester M3 3HN 061-833 9244

Medicine and Health

British Dental Association, 63 Wimpole Street, London W1 01-935 0875

British Medical Association, BMA House, Tavistock Square, London WC1H 9JP 01-387 4499

General Medical Council, 44 Hallam Street, London W1 01-580 7642

Health Education Authority, Hamilton House, Mabledon Place, London WC1H 9JX 01-631 0930

Health Visitors Association, 50 Southwark Street, London SE1 1WN 01-378 7255

Medical Women's Federation, Tavistock House North, Tavistock Square, London WC1H 9HX 01-387 7765

National Association of Women Pharmacists, c/o Pharmaceutical Society of Great Britain, 1 Lambeth High Street, London SE1 7JN 01-735 9141

Royal College of Midwives, 15 Manfield Street, London W1M 0BE 01-580 6523/4/5

Royal College of Nursing of the United Kingdom, 20 Cavendish Square, London W1M 0AB 01-409 3333

Scottish Health Education Group, Woodburn House, Canaan Lane, Edinburgh EH10 4SG 031-447 8044

Recreation

Arts Council of Great Britain, 105 Piccadilly, London W1V 0AE 01-629 9495

Sports Council, 16 Upper Woburn Place, London WC1H 0QP 01-388 1277

Scottish Sports Council, Caledonia House, South Gyle, Edinburgh EH12 9DQ 031-317 7200

Index

NB f before a number denotes reference in footnote
  numbers in bold indicates a major discussion of the topic